INTRODUCTION TO HEALTH SERVICES

ISBN 0-8273-4387-6

90000

9 780827 343870

INTRODUCTION TO HEALTH SERVICES

THIRD EDITION

Edited by

Stephen J. Williams, Sc.D.

Professor of Public Health
Head, Division of Health Services Administration
Graduate School of Public Health
San Diego State University
San Diego, California

Paul R. Torrens, M.D., M.P.H.

Professor of Health Services Administration
School of Public Health
University of California, Los Angeles
Los Angeles, California

DELMAR PUBLISHERS INC.®

NOTICE TO THE READER

Publisher and author do not warrant or guarantee any of the products described herein or perform any independent analysis in connection with any of the product information contained herein. Publisher and author do not assume, and expressly disclaim, any obligation to obtain and include information other than that provided to them by the manufacturer.

The reader is expressly warned to consider and adopt all safety precautions that might be indicated by the activities described herein and to avoid all potential hazards. By following the instructions contained herein, the reader willingly assumes all risks in connection with such instructions.

The publisher and author make no representations or warranties of any kind, including but not limited to, the warranties of fitness for particular purpose or merchantability, nor are any such representations implied with respect to the material set forth herein, and the publisher and author take no responsibility with respect to such material. The publisher and author shall not be liable for any special, consequential or exemplary damages resulting, in whole or in part, from the readers' use of, or reliance upon, this material.

For information, address Delmar Publishers Inc.
2 Computer Drive West, Box 15-015
Albany, New York 12212

Printed in the United States of America
Published simultaneously in Canada
By Nelson Canada
A Division of The Thomson Corporation

10 9 8 7 6 5 4 3 2 1

ISBN 0-8273-4387-6

For D. and N. Williams
and J., C., J. C., and N. Torrens

Contributors

Lu Ann Aday, Ph.D.
Associate Professor of Behavioral Sciences
School of Public Health
The University of Texas Health Science Center
Houston, Texas

A. E. Benjamin, Jr., Ph.D.
Assistant Adjunct Professor and Associate Director
Aging Health Policy Center
Department of Social and Behavioral Sciences
University of California, San Francisco
San Francisco, California

Thomas W. Bice, Ph.D.
Professor
Graduate Program in Health Services Administration and Planning
School of Public Health and Community Medicine
University of Washington
Seattle, Washington

Robert H. Brook, M.D., Sc.D., F.A.C.P.
Chief of the Division of Geriatrics
Professor of Medicine and Public Health
U.C.L.A. Center for the Health Sciences
Los Angeles, California
Deputy Health Program Director
The RAND Corporation
Santa Monica, California

William L. Dowling, Ph.D.
Clinical Professor of Health Services
School of Public Health and Community Medicine
University of Washington
Vice-President, Planning and Policy Development
Sisters of Providence Corporation
Seattle, Washington

Connie J. Evashwick, Sc.D.
President
CEA—Consulting & Evaluation Associates
Los Angeles, California

Claudia L. Haglund, M.H.A.
Director, Corporate Planning
Sisters of Providence Corporation
Seattle, Washington

Arnold D. Kaluzny, Ph.D.
Professor
Department of Health Policy and Administration
School of Public Health
University of North Carolina
Chapel Hill, North Carolina

Alma L. Koch, Ph.D.
Associate Professor of Public Health
Graduate Program in Health Services Administration
Graduate School of Public Health
San Diego State University
San Diego, California

Philip R. Lee, M.D.
Professor of Social Medicine
Director, Institute for Health Policy Studies
University of California, San Francisco
San Francisco, California

James P. LoGerfo, M.D.
Professor of Medicine and Health Services
Schools of Medicine and Public Health and Community Medicine
University of Washington
Seattle, Washington

Bryan R. Luce, Ph.D.
Senior Research Scientist
Director, Medical Technology Assessment Program
Batelle Human Affairs Research Centers
Washington, D.C.

Lawrence A. May, M.D., F.A.C.P.
Assistant Clinical Professor
University of California, Los Angeles
Los Angeles, California

Ira Moscovice, Ph.D.
Associate Professor and Associate Director
Division of Health Services Research and Policy
University of Minnesota
Minneapolis, Minnesota

Mary Richardson, Ph.D.
Instructor, Department of Health Services
Director, National Institute on Children with Handicaps
Child Development and Mental Retardation Center
University of Washington
Seattle, Washington

William Shonick, Ph.D.
Professor
Division of Health Services
School of Public Health
University of California, Los Angeles
Los Angeles, California

Stephen M. Shortell, Ph.D.
A.C. Buehler Distinguished Professor of Hospital and Health Services Management
Professor of Organization Behavior
J.L. Kellogg Graduate School of Management
Professor of Sociology
Department of Sociology
Northwestern University
Evanston, Illinois

Paul R. Torrens, M.D., M.P.H.
Professor of Health Services Administration
School of Public Health
University of California, Los Angeles
Los Angeles, California

James E. Veney, Ph.D.
Professor
Department of Health Policy and Administration
School of Public Health
University of North Carolina
Chapel Hill, North Carolina

Stephen J. Williams, Sc.D.
Professor of Public Health
Head, Division of Health Services Administration
Graduate Program in Health Services Administration
Graduate School of Public Health
San Diego State University
San Diego, California

Foreword

We Americans have prided ourselves on, and indeed believe we have, the wealth, the intellectual and technological capacities, the organizational skills, and the determination to provide health care to every citizen in need. This fine text, *Introduction to Health Services*, with its expert authors and editors, affords a clear and illuminating trek across the broad sweep of critical issues confronting health policy makers and care givers. The third edition has been updated to reflect the extraordinary dynamism of health services in our contemporary society. It is hard to conceive of any set of organized human endeavors that has been more heavily impacted by the inexorable forces of change than the seemingly uncomplicated task of delivering health care to each citizen whose personal well-being and acceptable health status is the quintessential foundation for daily living. As we prepare for the 1990s, it is not quite so clear that this basic human service—namely, the delivery of health information and health care to each and every American—is a sure bet.

This text provides both beginning students and health care professionals with a valuable set of data and insights into the major features and idiosyncrasies of American health services. We are gently reminded throughout the chapters that health services as we know them are really a post-World War II phenomenon. In less than 50 years we have created a host of physician specialists, an amply distributed hospital system, new health care delivery organizations, a patchwork of government and private funding systems, hospices and intensive care units, and high-tech home health care that allows patients to self-manage some of their most severe chronic health problems. Health services have also benefited from very substantial investments in bioscientific research by government and private industry and, in recent years, by a cadre of well-trained social scientists who have the tools to perform health services research and policy analysis for the health professions, the consumers and the buyers of health care. The results of their work form part of the base for the concise, and indeed precise, text that follows.

Informed observers and critics of health care in America will all agree that the 1980s have been the most turbulent and wrenching period for those who serve as the direct deliverers of health care. Pressures to reduce health expenditures have emanated from every quarter—federal and state governments, employers and their insurers, retirees, health and welfare trusts, and an increasing number of uninsured. Simultaneously, the supply of health personnel, with the notable exception of registered nurses, has more than met the demand for services that are now being financed. Without doubt, there are some serious deficiencies in access to personal medical and dental services and wide ranging variability in the quality and amenities that are available. Yet the big story of the 1980s is the paradox of increased spending; large numbers of providers of care searching for larger market shares of paying consumers and insurers; overcapacity of physicians and hospitals in many metropolitan communities; decline of our public health system at a time when the greatest public health problem of the century, AIDS, is upon us; and a more price sensitive system that is challenging the historical values of a somewhat benevolent and charitable set of organizations, agencies, and physicians who seem less able or maybe less willing to fill the gaps in a still quite imperfect health services system.

Never has the need for ingenuity and creative talent in health care been higher. At a time when many, including myself, expect shrinkage and reformation in health care services, there will be ample opportunities to influence the changes that will be required. We are going to have to refit the health system in better balance with societal, not provider, needs and offer care in quantity and quality that is affordable and necessary. That is the challenge for students and practitioners in the years ahead. That is the challenge that will be raised by a careful reading and understanding of the Williams and Torrens *Introduction to Health Services.*

Robert A. Derzon
Vice President
Lewin and Associates, Inc.
San Francisco, California

Preface

A constantly changing environment for health care in the United States has continued to be experienced by our nation since the publication of the second edition of this book. We continue to witness change in such areas as the technological armament of medicine, financing mechanisms, the politics of health care, and the structure of the delivery system itself. This third edition of the book reflects those changes and their implications for the health care system.

Few would argue against the importance of the health care system to our national well-being. On the other hand, there is much trepidation in the land as we observe and monitor these dramatic changes. Few people, including those in positions of power, have a complete understanding of the full extent of the changes and, more importantly, of their potential impact on the nation's health. As a result, it is probably more important than ever for students and practitioners in health-related fields to have a complete understanding of the structure, operation, and outcomes of the nation's health care system. That remains the principal goal of this book.

The fundamental structure of the book has been retained from previous editions. The book begins with an overview (in Part One) of the nation's health care system, as presented in Chapter 1. The overview provides an opportunity to set the stage for the chapters that follow as well as to present a coherent and relatively comprehensive perspective on the nation's health care system; each of the system's components is dissected and discussed individually in subsequent chapters. While the bulk of the book presents detailed analyses of each component of the system, it is always important to remember the larger contexts and interrelationships within which each of these components functions.

Part two discusses the causes and characteristics of health services utilization in the United States. The nature of disease and illness is discussed in Chapter 2, particularly in the context of the principal categories of illness that lead to the use of health care services. Chapter 3 presents a comprehensive and integrated examination of the characteristics of utilization of services in the United States with particular emphasis on the variables that are associated with utilization. The chapter is a completely new version for this edition, although the principal themes of the earlier version are retained. An understanding of the variables associated with the utilization of health services is critical to program planning, institutional strategic planning, and community needs assessment.

Part Three presents detailed discussions of individual provider settings within which health care is offered to patients. The first chapter in this section, Chapter 4, discusses the history and current functions of public health services. Public health services remain our principal line of defense against disease and illness in society. Although public health services account for a relatively small fraction of health care expenditures, their importance far outweighs our spending in this area. In addition, the history and role of public health services in the United States is of immense importance in helping us address such societal issues as the priorities that we should assign to health care versus other activities in our economy, the obligations of government to protect the population collectively, and the responsibilities for assuring access to care for individuals who lack services.

Chapter 5 focuses on the provision of ambulatory health care services. The increasing importance of ambulatory care in facilitating the integration of care is a key theme of this chapter and parallels the increasing focus of the book on the competitive market place, systems of care, and the financing of health care services.

Chapter 6 discusses the role of the hospital as well as the internal structure and operation of these important institutions. The hospital, too, has changed dramatically over the past few years as reflected by the changing content of this chapter. Hospitals have increasingly sought a more competitive posture for themselves individually and collectively, have aligned themselves with other organizations, and have battled for market share to ensure their long-term viability. The hospital is also changing in response to technological developments, changes in the role and power of the physician, and other recent developments. And, of course, as discussed throughout the book, dramatic changes in the way hospitals are paid, by both the private and public sectors, are forcing equally dramatic responses by all institutional providers of care.

Both long-term care and mental health services are undergoing change; the rate of change in these two areas is probably accelerating at a somewhat slower pace than is the case for the hospital or ambulatory care. Nevertheless, very significant changes have occurred since the last edition of the book in both long-term care and mental health services. To reflect these changes in the long-term care area, an entirely new chapter has been commissioned that takes a much broader perspective on the provision of long-term care. The focus in Chapter 7 on the continuum of care is particularly germane to the increasing integration of providers in organized systems of care.

Chapter 8 is an up-to-date and comprehensive discussion of the history and current status of mental health services in the United States. Change in this area has been more evolutionary than revolutionary, but the challenges for our society continue to grow.

Part Four deals with the resources needed to provide health care services. One of the most important of these resources is the technology utilized by physicians and other providers in identifying and combating illness. Technology is integral to the health care system since the nature of the technology often determines how care is provided, affects the structure of the institutions that provide care, and influences financing mechanisms. Advancements in technology and their critical evaluation can lead to lower morbidity and mortality and increased rationalization of resources. These key issues are discussed in detail in Chapter 9.

The second major area of resources utilized in the provision of health care is people. The health care system is one of the largest employers in the United States and as such is key to the economic well-being of the nation. In addition, of course, the increasingly specialized personnel required today make possible the provision of sophisticated, high-quality care. Trends and issues regarding health care personnel are discussed in detail in Chapter 10.

Chapter 11 discusses the all-important issue of health care financing. This chapter probably represents the area of greatest change since the last edition. An entirely new chapter has been commissioned. This new chapter takes a somewhat different approach to the issues of health care financing, consistent with the dramatic change that has occurred in the nation.

Part Five deals with the regulation and evaluation of health care services. Financing health care services, as discussed in Chapter 11, could readily fall either in Part Four or Part Five as a regulatory mechanism since payment modalities are increasingly being used to alter the function of the system. Chapter 12 discusses the history and current status of both regulation and planning in the health care field. These areas have undergone tortuous changes over the past few years, and the history of planning and regulation represents a fascinating study of attempts by government to modify the operation of the health care system. The current emphasis on a competitive system raises additional important societal issues that are discussed in this chapter as well.

Chapter 13 discusses the evaluation of the quality of care in health services. Both quality assessment and quality assurance are discussed as are various studies that reflect the current status of the quality of services provided in the United States. Chapter 14 discusses the important role of evaluating health care programs and services. The chapter has been modified from previous editions to decrease the emphasis on specific evaluation techniques, which are available from other sources, and to focus instead on the importance of evaluation and examples of evaluation studies.

Part Six, the final section of the book, consisting of Chapter 15, is a cogent and thought-provoking discussion of health care policy and politics in the United States. The nation has undergone many years of significant and wide-ranging changes in health care. Most Americans would probably like a health care system that is somewhat apolitical and more focused on meeting the health care needs of the American population. The reality, of course, is that politics are integral to all decision making. As a result, understanding the political process, and its implications, is critical to any realistic appraisal of where our health care system has been and where it is headed in the future. Thus Chapter 15 serves a very important function in helping the reader to evaluate the shifting political winds and the implications for the nation's health care system.

Finally, the Epilogue presents some thoughts on the nation's health care system and pulls together a number of key integrating concepts discussed throughout the book. The Epilogue only sets the stage for the reader's further integration of knowledge and personal assessments of the health care system and thoughts about his or her role in that system.

It is important for readers to think through their value systems and personal ethical perspectives in reading this book. Health care cannot be divorced from individual and societal opinions and biases. Understanding one's personal perspectives is the key to forming assessments about where the health care system has been and the directions that are appropriate for the future. As a nation, we have made dramatic changes in how we provide health care services. The rate of change may itself change in the future; but the fact remains that we will likely continue to modify the delivery system, attempt new approaches, discontinue old approaches, and make other judgments that will significantly affect how health care is provided, who services are provided to, and how the bill is paid. Everyone—providers, payers, and consumers alike—has a key active role in the health care system. The better everyone understands his or her role and the system itself, the better prepared all Americans will be to develop the best possible system.

As in the previous edition, a multidisciplinary approach is used. Empirical research is presented and summarized. The comments of colleagues, readers, and students have been integrated into the book.

Many people assisted in the preparation of the manuscript, reviewing drafts prepared for this edition, and in putting together the final manuscript itself. We are grateful to all who helped, especially to Ellen Katz Brown, who was assistant to the editors in California and so ably pulled together all the pieces. We also continue to be appreciative of the support and enthusiasm of our editors at John Wiley & Sons: Andrea Stingelin, who first recognized that we might have had something worthwhile to contribute, and Janet Walsh Foltin who has guided us through the last couple of editions.

The goal of this book, to reiterate, is to provide a basis of information and understanding for a useful perspective from which readers can analyze what they do as a part of providing or consuming services. It is hoped that whatever this book can contribute to each individual's understanding of the system and its complex interactions will lead to a more rational, fair, and equitable system for all Americans.

Stephen J. Williams
Paul R. Torrens

Contents

PART THREE
PROVIDERS OF HEALTH SERVICES   83

PART ONE

Overview of the Health Services System

CHAPTER 1

Historical Evolution and Overview of Health Services in the United States

Paul R. Torrens

This chapter introduces the development, background, concepts, and issues of health care in the United States. The first section presents the historical evolution and development of health services in this country; the second section describes the current organization of services. Combined, these sections set the stage for the detailed analyses of the latter chapters in the book.

HISTORICAL EVOLUTION OF HEALTH SERVICES IN THE UNITED STATES

In *The Tempest*, a Shakespearean character is portrayed as saying, "What's past is prologue," suggesting that the events of the past merely set the stage for the future. In a more pertinent sense, George Santayana has written, "Those who cannot remember the past are condemned to repeat it." This is particularly true of the American health care system, since many of the issues and forces that have shaped and formed it in the past continue to influence us today. If we are to understand the future better, it seems appropriate to look at the past first.

The modern American health care system has had three important periods of development and now seems to be entering a fourth. The first period began in the mid-nineteenth century (1850) when the first large hospitals, such as Bellevue Hospital in New York City and Massachusetts General Hospital in Boston, began to flourish. The development of hospitals symbolized the *institutionalization of health care* for the first time in this country. Before this time, health care in the United States was a loose collection of individual services functioning independently and without much relation

3

to each other or to anything else. By today's standards, the first hospitals were not very remarkable, but they did provide the first visible institution around which health care services could be organized.

The second important historical period began around the turn of the century (1900) with the *introduction of the scientific method into medicine* in this country. Before this time, medicine was not an exact science, but was instead a rather informal collection of unproved generalities and good intentions. After 1900, stimulated by the opening of the new medical school at the Johns Hopkins University in Baltimore, medicine acquired a solid scientific base that eventually transformed it from a conscientious but poorly equipped art into a detailed and clearly defined science.

With the coming of World War II, the United States underwent a major social, political, and technological upheaval whose effect was so marked that it ended the second and signaled the beginning of the third period of health care development. The scientific advances continued unabated, but now they were paralleled by a *growing interest in the social and organizational structure of health care*. During this time, attention was first directed toward the financing of health care, with the resultant formation of health insurance plans such as Blue Cross and Blue Shield. This was also the time of increasing concentration of power in the federal government, as witnessed by the Hill-Burton Act (Hospital Survey and Construction Act), by the huge research budgets of the National Institutes of Health (NIH), and, more recently, by the passage of Medicare. Finally, during this period the principle of health care as a right, not a privilege, was widely discussed and generally accepted.

Since the early 1980s, the health care system of this country has appeared to be moving into the fourth phase of its development, an era of *limited resources, restriction of growth, and reorganization of the methods of financing and delivering care*. Before this period, it had been presumed that the health care system would always be encouraged to grow and expand, both in size and in complexity, and that there would always be sufficient resources to support that expansion. Now it seems that the limits of our resources are being approached and that the health care system is being forced to consider options or alternatives to unrestricted growth and expansion.

Indeed, recent reimbursement policies introduced by Medicare and by employer-controlled insurance systems have caused a decrease in the numbers of inpatient days provided by hospitals each year and a reduction in the operating size of many hospitals. In the same vein, expert observers have suggested that the United States is rapidly approaching a major surplus of physicians and that the numbers of new physicians being produced each year be greatly reduced. On all sides, there are pressures for smaller size, pressures to use less, and pressures to reduce expenditures in health care.

At the same time, the 1980s have seen the appearance of many new organizational models in health care. The idea of the multihospital system has spread rapidly, and more than two-thirds of the country's hospitals are affiliated with some kind of system. The Health Maintenance Organization (HMO) model, previously limited mostly to the West Coast, has spread all over the country and in many instances is now sponsored by commercial companies whose stock is actively traded on various stock exchanges. The term "joint venture" has become an accepted part of our health care language, now used to describe new forms of partnership activities between hospitals and physicians, hospitals and insurance companies, and hospitals with other hospitals. Virtually no health care organizational model has been left untouched by recent trends and changes.

Since the dawn of recorded history, human beings have repeatedly suffered the sudden and devastating appearance of epidemics of infectious disease. Plague, cholera, typhoid, smallpox, influenza, yellow fever, and a host of other diseases raged almost at will, creating havoc wherever they struck.

During the period 1850–1900 in this country, these epidemics of acute infectious diseases were the most critical health problem for the majority of Americans. Of particular importance were those diseases related to impure food, contaminated water supply, inadequate sewage disposal, and the generally poor condition of urban housing. During this time, for example, a cholera epidemic occurred throughout the country, resulting in an official death toll of 5071 in New York City alone and an unofficial toll several times higher. During this same period, yellow fever killed 9000 in New Orleans in 1853, 2500 in 1854 and 1855, and another 5000 in 1858. Abraham Lincoln regularly sent his family away from the White House during the summer months to escape the "fevers," probably malaria, that swept through Washington.

By 1900, the epidemics of acute infectious disease had been brought under control due to improving environmental conditions. In the latter years of the nineteenth century, cities had begun to develop systems for water purification, for sanitary disposal of sewage, for safeguarding the quality of milk and food, and for monitoring the quality of urban housing. Health departments had begun to grow in numbers and in strength, and had begun to apply the methods of case finding and quarantine with satisfying results. Indeed, by 1900, as Table 1-1 shows, those epidemics that had plagued humanity for centuries were now eliminated as major causes of death in the United States.

After 1900 the predominant health problems that attracted the attention of the health services system were those acute events, either infectious or traumatic, that affected individuals one by one. The pendulum had swung away from epidemics of acute infections that affected large numbers of people toward conditions of a personal nature that require individualized treatment. As Table 1-1 shows, pneumonia and tuberculosis were the primary causes of death in 1900, with heart disease, nephritis, and accidents close behind.

Relieved from the burden of epidemic illnesses, the newly developed medical sciences turned their attention to better surgical techniques, the discovery of new sera for the treatment of pneumonia, and the development of new tests for more accurate and rapid diagnoses. Hospitals began to grow rapidly, medical schools flourished, and there was a general air of excitement that suggested the world was on the brink of significant advances in the treatment of individual illnesses.

Significant advances *were* being made. In Baltimore and Boston, the students of William Halsted, the pioneer surgeon at Johns Hopkins Hospital, began to operate on patients whose disease had previously been beyond the ability of surgeons. Advances in obstetrics now made it safer for women to have babies, and for the first time women did not approach childbirth with the fear of dying in delivery. Research work by two physicians, Banting and Best, in the laboratories of the University of Toronto led to the discovery of insulin in 1922, and for the first time diabetes could be effectively treated. Other research by Whipple, Minot, and Murphy on the causes of pernicious anemia led to successful medical treatment for that condition and further spurred the rush to find new treatments for other age-old conditions.

There were new discoveries on all fronts, each of which contributed some new advances in medical treatment. In 1928, however, in a cluttered laboratory at St. Mary's

TABLE 1-1. Death Rates for Leading Causes of Death, 1900 and 1985; United States

1900		1985	
Causes of Death	*Crude Death Rate per 100,000 Population per Year*	*Causes of Death*	*Crude Death Rate per 100,000 Population per Year*
All causes	1719.0	All causes	874.8
Pneumonia and influenza	202.2	Diseases of heart	325.0
Tuberculosis	194.4	Malignant neoplasms	191.7
Diarrhea, enteritis, and ulceration of the intestine	142.7	Cerebrovascular accidents	64.0
Diseases of the heart	137.4	Accidents	38.6
Senility, ill defined or unknown	117.5	Chronic obstructive pulmonary diseases	31.2
Intracranial lesions of vascular origin	106.9	Pneumonia and influenza	27.9
Nephritis	88.6	Diabetes mellitus	16.2
All accidents	72.3	Suicide	12.0
Cancer and other malignant tumors	64.0	Chronic liver disease and cirrhosis	11.2
Diphtheria	40.3	Atherosclerosis	9.9

SOURCES: *Vital Statistics of the United States.* Washington, DC, U.S. National Center for Health Statistics, August 1972; National Center for Health Statistics, Monthly Vital Statistics Report, Vol. 34, No. 13, September 10, 1986.

Hospital in London, a Scottish researcher, Alexander Fleming, produced the first of several discoveries that were to lead to the treatment of patients with penicillin for the first time in 1941. This discovery absolutely revolutionized medical care and totally changed the patterns of disease that threatened humanity. Within a few years after the treatment of the first patients with penicillin, antibiotics became readily available, and acute illnesses that had previously caused serious illness and possible death now meant nothing more than the discomfort of an injection and a few days of disability. Many older people experienced the incredible effects of the antibiotic era. When they had contracted pneumonia as children, their families had admitted them to hospitals and despaired for their lives; now, as older adults, they were told they had "a little pneumonia," given an injection of penicillin, and treated at home.

With the arrival of the antibiotic era in the 1940s and the subsequent conquest of acute infectious disease, the predominant problems of Americans became chronic illnesses. Since acute infections were no longer snuffing out the lives of children, people were living longer and beginning to manifest long-term chronic diseases such as heart disease, cancer, and stroke. As shown in Table 1-1, these three conditions alone now account for two-thirds of all deaths. A similar review of the causes of disability would show arthritis, blindness, arteriosclerosis, and other chronic diseases to be the predominant causes of morbidity and limitation of function.

The rather sudden appearance of acquired immune deficiency syndrome (AIDS) in almost epidemic proportion in the early 1980s has further highlighted the changing pattern of disease. AIDS is apparently initiated by a viral infection that triggers extensive damage to an individual's immune system, leading to susceptibility to other infections and various forms of cancer. This combination of viral disease, immune system defects, and cancer as manifest in AIDS is probably only the first of many such new combinations of disease causation we must face. Chronic illness will certainly continue to be the predominant health problem of the American people in the future. Increasingly important will be chronic illness related to genetic makeup, personal lifestyles, and environmental hazards. Evidence is accumulating that suggests that many of the important chronic illnesses are related to how we live our personal lives, what hazards we subject ourselves to, and what dangers we allow our environment to impose on us.

The predominance of chronic illness as the major threat to health in the future raises a number of issues relevant to health professionals. First, as May points out in Chapter 2, the entire method of defining a chronic illness and determining its prevalence must be reexamined to obtain a more accurate picture of the situation. At the present time, a chronic disease is identified or documented on the basis of the first appearance of symptoms or on positive laboratory test results. In most cases, however, it is known that the disease process started long before the appearance of symptoms. In a practical sense, this forces one to ask: when should a chronic disease be considered to be present? The implications of the answer to this question for the planning and financing of health services could be enormous.

Chronic illnesses also have two important characteristics that directly affect both prevention and treatment. First, as was just pointed out earlier, they often begin early in life, long before overt symptoms appear; the exact starting date for a chronic disease is never known. For example, many studies of apparently healthy young people who were victims of automobile accidents or other sudden death show that large percentages have already begun to develop early signs of chronic illness, detectable by pathological examination but not yet by clinical tests. Second, once a chronic illness is present, it remains with the patient forever. The *disease* is not cured by medical treatment; rather, its more prominent *symptoms* or external manifestations are treated.

Unfortunately, although the pattern of predominant illnesses has changed from epidemics of acute infections in the 1850s, to individual acute conditions in the 1900s, to chronic illnesses generally in the 1950s, and to special chronic illnesses in the 1980s, thinking about prevention and treatment has only recently begun to change. Acute infections very conveniently have a clear-cut beginning, middle, and end; as a result, they are amenable to one-shot solutions. If there is an epidemic caused by contamination of the water supply, the construction of a sewage treatment facility will eliminate it completely. If there is a threat of poliomyelitis infection, the ingestion of polio vaccine once or twice will permanently protect a population.

With chronic illnesses, however, prevention and treatment cannot be a one-shot affair, even though this is still how our health care system approaches them. Arteriosclerotic heart disease, for example, begins early in life and is probably affected by diet, cigarette smoking, stress, obesity, and several other factors that are directly related to personal habits and life style. Prevention of these conditions cannot be accomplished by giving a person a single lecture on the evils of high-cholesterol food or the dangers of heavy cigarette consumption. Rather, prevention must be long-term, continuous, and aimed at bringing about major changes in an individual's knowledge of disease, personal values, and behavior patterns. Unfortunately, that understanding has been a long time in coming, but now seems to be taking hold quite strongly. The death rates from heart disease have been dropping each year for the last ten years or so, a result that is generally attributed to more aggressive early treatment and to major improvements in the prevention of some of the important causative factors.

Optimal treatment for long-term, continuous illness requires a system of health care that is, in itself, long-term and continuous. Unfortunately, the organization of our health services is still modeled on the disease patterns that were predominant in the 1900–1945 period and concentrates on individual episodes of illness as if they were separate and distinct entities. As a result, the health care system is primarily short-term and discontinuous in nature, and it treats chronic illness as if it were merely a series of separate acute episodes. This trend is further reinforced by the current method of financing of health services, with its great emphasis on paying for individual services rendered rather than on the long-term, continuous nature of the underlying disease process.

It should be noted that efforts are beginning to be made to develop longer-term and more continuous systems of financing and organizing patient care. For the first time, there have been serious discussions of developing a system of health insurance for long-term care. Persons eligible for Medicare, the federally sponsored health insurance for those over 65 years of age, are being encouraged to join HMOs. State and local governments are encouraging the creation of new case-management programs to improve the coordination of health and welfare services for the elderly.

It is entirely possible (and, indeed, probable) that the predominant disease patterns will be changing again in the future, creating an entirely different set of conditions that may require an entirely different array of services and interventions. It will be important for future generations of health professionals to watch for changes in predominant disease patterns to ensure a health care system that is genuinely pertinent and responsive to the problems of the day.

TECHNOLOGY AVAILABLE TO THE AMERICAN PEOPLE

During the various developmental periods of the American health care system, what technology was available to handle the diseases that affected the American people? What tools were available to heal workers to conquer these conditions?

In the period 1850–1900, only a very rudimentary technology was available for the treatment of disease. The scientific base of medicine was still very narrow, and the number of effective medical treatments was very limited. Indeed, a great deal of energy and effort was expended on treatment, but whether a patient recovered from an illness usually depended more on the patient and the disease rather than the treatment.

Physicians during this period of time were poorly trained. They usually obtained their skills by serving apprenticeships with physicians already in practice and then taking short courses at unsophisticated medical colleges. What physicians had to offer was usually contained in their black bags, which they took with them wherever they went. They spent a good deal of time in patients' homes and almost no time at all in hospitals. In general, their practice was little different from that of their predecessors for centuries before them.

Nurses during the period 1850–1900 were not much better trained. Generally they were members of religious groups who volunteered to work in the few hospitals that existed, or they were poor, desperate, discarded women who frequented these institutions anyway and were pressed into service. Their work was nonscientific in the extreme and consisted simply of assisting patients with their usual bodily functions in any way possible. Not until the first training program for nurses was organized at Bellevue Hospital in the 1860s was there any formal preparation for this important role anywhere in the country.

As for the hospitals themselves, they were merely places of shelter and repose for the sick poor who could not be cared for at home. Anyone who could stay at home usually did so, since hospitals had little to offer that would not be obtained at home if one had the money. Indeed, the hospitals of those days were often a direct threat to the lives of patients, since they were dirty, crowded, and disease-ridden. Infectious diseases frequently spread rapidly among hospitalized patients, and during the typhus epidemics of 1852 in New York City, for example, the highest mortality for the disease was among the patients and staff of the hospitals themselves.

After 1900 conditions began to change, spurred on by the new discoveries that were emerging from the research laboratories in this country and in Europe. In 1912, for example, a Polish chemist, Casimir Funk, published a paper, "The Etiology of Deficiency Diseases," in which he described "vitamines" and opened a whole new field of disease conditions to treatment. In 1980, James MacKenzie, in London, published his famous book *Diseases of the Heart*, and patients throughout the world were the beneficiaries. In countless medical schools and hospitals throughout this country and Europe, major scientific advances were achieved, each of which contributed to easier and safer diagnosis and treatment of acutely ill patients.

The medical schools led the way in many of these advances as a result of some basic reforms that took place in the early 1900s. Before this time, a large number of small, poorly staffed, free-standing medical colleges existed throughout the country, 14 in Chicago alone in 1910 and 10 each in Missouri and Tennessee. In 1910, Alexander Flexner undertook a study of medical education for the Carnegie Foundation for the Advancement of Teaching and in his report, *Medical Education in the United States and Canada*, recommended that medical education in this country undergo radical reform. In particular, he strongly urged that the training of physicians be made a university function and that it be based on a firm scientific foundation. On the basis of Flexner's recommendations and the support of the Rockefeller Foundation, many of the small unaffiliated schools began to close and many of the remaining ones became part of universities, with the important result that physicians began to be trained as scientists as well as practitioners.

Gradually, physicians began to have more effective tools with which to work, and the range of their capabilities expanded rapidly. They still continued to spend the majority of their time in their offices or in patients' homes, but they now also began to look toward the hospital for the care of their more severely ill patients. A small but gradually increasing number of physicians began to specialize in a particular area of medicine; however, by 1940, more than 80 percent were still in general practice.

Hospitals in the 1900s began to play an increasingly important role in health care. As more technology developed, it tended to be concentrated in hospitals, with the result that patients and physicians began going to hospitals for the technology to be found there. St. Luke's Hospital in New York City, for example, was 50 years old in 1906 when it opened its first private patient pavilion. Before that time, there had been no reason for private patients to go to a hospital, because they could usually get the same type of care in their homes. Now, however, hospitals began to offer services and skills that were not available anywhere else.

Although the period 1900–1940 was one of rapid growth in scientific technology, it was nothing compared to what happened with the advent of World War II. With the start of the war, this country mounted a massive effort to organize the best talents available for the care of the wounded and for the solution of the health care problems generated by the war. For the first time, relatively large efforts in research were begun under the direction of the federal government, and the results were impressive. The development of antibiotics accelerated rapidly, new surgical techniques for the treatment of trauma and burns were discovered, and new approaches to the transportation of the sick and wounded were developed. The range and breadth of problems that were subjected to organized investigation were remarkable, opening the way for an even more greatly expanded research effort after the war ended. In 1950, the size of the research commitment begun during World War II had risen to $73 million per year, $35 million of which was distributed through the NIH. By 1974, this expenditure had risen to an annual research budget of $2.5 billion, with $1.6 billion coming from a now greatly expanded NIH.

After World War II, hospitals were no longer the same. Previously, they had been places for the care of patients, with great emphasis being placed on the caring function. Now they became extensions of research laboratories, places where medical science was practiced and where curing was the order of the day. New procedures, new equipment, and new techniques all flourished to such a degree that the hospitals were now captured by their technology. The technology itself was the motivating force for hospitals, and most major decisions were based on that technology.

The operation of these newly complex institutions called for waves of new workers, each more specialized and more highly skilled than the last. Before the war there had been approximately 20 major categories of health workers; by the 1970s there were hundreds. With the increasing specialization of services and skills, there was also an increasing interdependence of health workers on each other and an increasing reliance on the health care systems to integrate the work of so many separate groups.

Physicians were severely affected by these trends. With the explosive growth of scientific knowledge after World War II, it was impossible for one physician to know everything, and so the trend toward specialization in a particular subarea of medicine had a strong impetus. Before the war, approximately 80 percent of physicians had been general practitioners and 20 percent specialists. In the years after the war, these percentages were reversed. In their training and practice, physicians focused increasingly on the scientific aspects of diagnosis and treatment, and as a result spent more time in hospitals and less time in patients' homes. The hospital became the emotional center of the physician's life, since it was here that the most important, most challenging, and most interesting aspects of training or treatment occurred.

These trends affected nursing and the other health professionals to only a slightly lesser degree. The training of nurses and other health professionals became increasingly more scientific, more specialized, and more lengthy during the years after World War II. The desire to be recognized as competent in a particular area led to the proliferation of professional groups and to formal accreditation on the basis of scientific training and ability. It also led to university-based training programs in all of the health professions.

Today the technology available to the American health care system has advanced to an incredible degree. Intrauterine diagnosis of fetal malformation, laser beam surgery of the eyes, and use of sound waves in lithotripters to crush kidney stones without surgery . . . are all accepted as merely the expected developments of the technological age. The merging of technologies from fields other than medicine, such as the development of computerized axial tomographic systems and magnetic resonance imaging systems, has further added to the immense range of technology available to the health care system. However, this explosion of technology in recent years has not been without its problems. Indeed, the technology itself has *caused* a rather serious set of problems with which future generations of health care professionals must grapple.

One interesting problem introduced by technology is evaluation of the various new discoveries and techniques. Much new (and even some old) technology is adopted without appropriate evaluation of how effective it really is, and even more important, how much more effective it might be than already existing technology. Only limited examination of the cost implications of new technology is usually done before that technology is widely distributed throughout the health care system. Although it has not been customary to evaluate the effectiveness and the cost of technology in the past, economic pressures on the health care system in the future will certainly demand more careful evaluation and scrutiny of technology before it is put into place for regular use.

Possibly a more important problem of medical technology is its impact on the form and configuration of the health care system and on the values and patterns of practice of the professionals in that system. In many ways, the American health services system has been captured by its technology and has been subtly and seductively shaped by its demands. Decisions regarding the design of programs and institutions, the training of personnel, and the distribution of services have been governed by technological considerations that loom larger every year.

A still more profound effect of technology is its ability to insinuate itself into the values of not just the system but also of the people who work in the system. The student entering a health profession rapidly learns that academic success and, later, professional success, comes from mastery of the scientific technology. Increasingly, the student views excellence as being reached through technical achievements and gives decreasing importance to the more personal, nontechnical aspects of disease. By the time the student becomes a fully accepted member of the profession, a value system has been established that views illness as a series of technical problems to be solved by the application of specific technical solutions. This value system is then reinforced in practice by the expectations of the public and by the requirements of the regulators, both of whom have come to view quality in terms of technical excellence. The result frequently is a professional performance that is excellent in technical terms and rather poor in human terms.

A quite different problem of technology arises not from its excessiveness but rather from its inefficient distribution to society. If there is indeed more technology available than can be provided equitably to all people due to limits on funding, then large portions of society do not benefit as much as they should from technologic knowledge. Marked differences exist, for example, in mortality and morbidity measures for white and nonwhite segments of society, possibly indicating an unequal access to modern health care technology. The answer obviously is to improve the health services system to ensure adequate distribution of available resources.

In summary, virtually no technology was available to treat disease before the 1900s. Technology began to appear and grow rapidly after the turn of the century. World War II fostered an incredible surge of research endeavors, with the result that the health care system began to be overwhelmed by the range and diversity of available technology. By the 1980s, the American health care system had been captured by its technology, and the challenge was to regain mastery over the giant that had been created.

SOCIAL ORGANIZATION FOR THE USE OF TECHNOLOGY

How has our society organized to use the technology available to it? What has been the predominant view of the role of society in health care? During the period 1850–1900, no organized program was available for the use of whatever technology existed. Public services were rudimentary and were concentrated on a very narrow range of problems. There were hospitals in a few areas, but they were generally started by religious or charitable groups for the care of those who were obviously and publicly impoverished. The predominant ethic of the time was that people should care for themselves and be self-sufficient. If they become dependent, they should take advantage of and be grateful for the various charities established for these purposes.

This philosophy of rugged individualism and relative lack of large-scale social organization for health care predominated in this country until the 1930s, when the Great Depression struck with full force. At that time, economic forces beyond the comprehension of most Americans struck down many people, destroying their lives and leaving them destitute. The traditional belief in being totally and personally responsible for all aspects of one's life was badly shaken by the events of the Depression.

With the arrival of Franklin Roosevelt in the White House, the New Deal was launched and a wide array of social programs appeared, all aimed at repairing the damage of the Depression. The importance of the New Deal in terms of American social thought cannot be underestimated since, for the first time, American society created large scale national programs to assist those who could not assist themselves.

In health care, governmental activity was still minimal, limited to a few specific areas of grant-in-aid programs to states to improve certain public health services such as infectious disease control and maternal and child health. Although the services were limited and aimed primarily at the poor, this small start did signify an assumption of responsibility by the national government for health care, at least for those who could not care for themselves.

The next major change in social organization and social thinking came with the arrival of World War II. As part of the mobilization effort, millions of men and women entered military service and in return received a wide array of health services simply by virtue of that service. The significance was twofold: (1) the services themselves were provided without charge by salaried physicians working for the government; and (2) they were provided as a right of those in the service and were clearly not charity for people who could no longer take care of themselves, as previous governmental efforts had been.

Not only did World War II accustom the country to large-scale health care programs provided by the society to its members, it also encouraged the growth of the health insurance industry. During the war, a freeze was imposed on wages and salaries so that very little collective bargaining for increases in salary could occur. However, considerable activity did occur in the development of pensions, disability programs, and health insurance plans, with the result that the health insurance industry began to flourish. This industry provided the American public with a new form of social organization—the "third party," or fiscal intermediary. Before the development of health insurance, the public had no form of social organization to protect it from a sudden onslaught of medical bills. With the arrival of this new phenomenon, health insurance, the American public began to gain experience in the cooperative effort of pooling many individual contributions for a common group objective—protection from financial disaster.

The period immediately after World War II witnessed the slow, tentative growth of the "Blue" plans, Blue Cross and Blue Shield, nonprofit community-based health care plans that insured against hospital and medical costs. With the success and growth of Blue Cross and Blue Shield, commercial insurance companies also entered the field, offering health insurance plans to employers and industry as part of their life/health/retirement/disability packages. With the rapid advances made by Blue Cross/Blue Shield and the commercial insurance carriers, the percentage of Americans covered by some form of health insurance rose from less than 20 percent before World War II to more than 70 percent by the early 1960s.

In the early 1960s, a major battle was fought and won by those advocating a greater societal role in the organization of health services. The battle involved the creation of government-sponsored health insurance plans for people over the age of 65 and resulted in the passage of legislation that created Medicare. Although Medicare itself was directed primarily to the needs of the country's elderly, its impact was soon felt throughout the entire health care system. The creation of the Medicare program had two immediate major social implications. First, Medicare provided financing for health care for all persons over the age of 65 simply on the basis of age; need was not a factor. The American society, in effect, determined that there were certain things the society should do for all of its members, regardless of individual need, since society could ensure equity. The second major effect of Medicare was the assumption by the federal government of the responsibility for planning, financing, and monitoring a significant portion of the health care services in this country. The society not only wanted social insurance programs for health care, but also wanted the federal government to assume a central role in operating these programs.

A further significant change in the social organization of health care in this country occurred in the mid-1960s with the development of the Neighborhood Health Centers program of the U.S. Office of Economic Opportunity. In the War on Poverty, a number of health programs were funded for underserved areas of the country, each of which was required to have significant participation of consumers, often through governing boards and committees. This involvement of consumers was a substantial change from the past and soon became standard policy in new governmental programs. This philosophy was vigorously put forward in the National Health Planning and Resources Development Act of 1974, which required a majority of consumers on all local health planning boards. Although the health planning effort in this country has recently been dismantled to a large degree, the involvement of consumer advocates in health policy matters continues and will clearly be an increasingly important aspect of the U.S. health care system in the future.

It is interesting to note that, although consumer participation in local, state, and national health policy has decreased as a result of the demise of the health planning network, its decrease has been more than compensated for by the growth of employer and industrial involvement in health affairs. The growth of employer health care coalitions, and the more active involvement of various large employer purchasers of health insurance in matters of health policy, have created a new consumer advocacy force that promises to become an important part of the U.S. health care system in the future.

In the late 1970s and early 1980s, the health care system of this country, as noted previously, entered the fourth phase of its development, an era of *resource limitation, restriction of growth, and reorganization of systems of financing and of providing health care*. With the federal Medicare program experiencing increases in expenditures of 20 percent or more per year, interest has shifted toward a reduction of benefits, greater cost sharing by the elderly themselves, and a limitation on reimbursements to providers of service. Energies have now become focused less on the development of new services or the expansion of coverage and more on the control of costs through limitations and reductions. Indeed, recent changes in the manner in which Medicare reimburses hospitals have been designed to encourage hospitals and doctors to provide less in the way of services and to sharply curtail or limit the number of services provided. In turn, this has led to a gradual shrinkage in the actual supply of staffed and operating hospital beds in the United States within the last few years.

These developments, to be discussed in detail in later chapters that deal with health care financing, planning, policy, and regulation, have also served to reinforce the increasingly powerful central role played by the federal government in the direction of health services. The federal government now not only controls a significant amount of the financial support for health care (approximately one-third of the total health care expenditures from all sources) but also, by using these massive resources in a unified and centralized manner, is able to set many of the rules by which health care, governmentally funded or not, is provided. The health care system of this country, although by no means federally operated, certainly is federally dominated.

This country entered the twentieth century with the social philosophy that people should care for themselves or be satisfied with charity. In midcentury, it adopted the philosophy that society should care for those who, through no fault of their own, could no longer take care of themselves. Finally, toward the end of the century, it had moved to a philosophy that society, operating through the national government, should assume responsibility for solving certain large-scale problems of life for all of its members, even if some individual members can solve these problems for themselves. In very recent years, the country has begun to realize that some of the programs that it proposed earlier to solve one set of problems (for example, the development of a Medicare health insurance plan to protect the elderly from the economic effects of illness) have, in turn, created new problems (such as the rising cost of health care for everybody).

SUMMARY OF HISTORICAL TRENDS

The past 125 years of history have witnessed major changes in the American health care scene (Table 1-2). The predominant health problems of our people have changed from epidemics of acute infections to a different kind of "epidemic," chronic illness. The range of technology available has mushroomed from almost none in 1850 to a condition of such abundance now that the health care system has been virtually overwhelmed and captured by the technology it has created. Society's social values have changed from a *laissez-faire* approach in the 1850s that depended on individual initiative or organized private charity to one now that assumes the central role of the federal government in the organizing and financing of health care in the United States by means of various health insurance and regulatory mechanisms.

TABLE 1-2. Major Trends in the Development of Health Care in the United States, 1850 to Present

Trends	1850–1900	1900 to World War II	World War II to Present	Future
Predominant health problems of the American people	Epidemics of acute infections	Acute events, trauma, or infections affecting individuals, not groups	Chronic diseases such as heart disease, cancer, stroke	Chronic diseases, particularly emotional and behaviorally related conditions
Technology available to handle predominant health problems	Virtually none	Beginning and rapid growth of basic medical sciences and technology	Explosive growth of medical science; technology captures the health care system	Continued growth and expansion of technology, with attempts to repersonalize the technology
Social organization for the use of technology	None; individuals left to their own resources or charity	Beginning societal and governmental efforts to care for those who could not care for themselves	Health care as a right; governmental responsibility to organize and monitor health care for everyone	Greater centralization of responsibility and control in federal government; greater use of organized systems of health insurance and financing to shape and control developments within the health care system

SOURCE: Torrens PR: *The American Health Care System: Issues and Problems.* St Louis, Mosby, 1978.

15

OVERVIEW OF HEALTH SERVICES
IN THE UNITED STATES

When visitors from abroad, particularly those engaged in health services in their own country, come to the United States, they frequently want to know about the American health care system and how it works. They are usually puzzled by the answer they get:

> There isn't any *single* "American health care system." There are many separate subsystems serving different populations in different ways. Sometimes they overlap; sometimes they are entirely separate from one another. Sometimes they are supported with public funds, and at other times they depend solely on private funds. Sometimes several different subsystems use the same facilities and personnel; at other times, they use facilities and personnel that are entirely separate and distinct.

It should not be surprising that there is a multiplicity of health care systems (or subsystems) in the United States, given the historical development of health services in this country. In the earliest days, health care was entirely a private matter, and people were expected to take care of themselves by obtaining services of private physicians and nurses when needed, purchasing medications from drugstores and chemist shops, and paying for all these services personally. For those persons who could not take care of themselves, charitable institutions were established as voluntary, nonprofit corporations to provide charity health care. These groups usually centered their efforts on hospitals and were usually located in the larger towns and cities of this country.

In the early twentieth century, a new element was added with the development of the city/county hospitals. These hospitals were established by local governments to care for the poor in their area who could not get care either by their own efforts or from the voluntary nonprofit charity hospitals. These public facilities were generally large, acute care, general hospitals, with busy clinics and emergency rooms and with close connections to local government ambulance services, police departments, and other community services. At the same time, state governments were developing mental hospitals. The cities had previously been responsible for the care of lunatics and the insane, but after the turn of the century, state governments began to assume this burden. Every state soon had at least one mental hospital where the emotionally disturbed were offered what little care was available.

With the explosive growth in the size of the federal government and in the numbers of persons in the armed forces during World War II, a separate system of care developed for active-duty military personnel and their dependents, retired military personnel, and veterans. These were almost entirely self-contained systems, employing salaried physicians and nurses, working entirely in military or veterans hospitals directly operated by the federal government.

As the cost of health care began to increase rapidly after World War II, the United States experienced a rather sudden and somewhat bewildering development of a wide variety of health insurance plans. The first to be operated were community-based nonprofit Blue Cross and Blue Shield plans, developed by hospital and physician associations to spread the cost of health care more widely among the population. These were followed by labor union health and welfare trust funds, established as a consequence of benefit negotiations for union members. At the same time, the private, for-profit commercial insurance companies expanded their efforts on behalf of both individuals and large groups of employees. Finally, several large government-sponsored and publicly supervised health insurance plans evolved, such as Medicare and Medicaid, the latter to aid the medically indigent.

Private medical practitioners, voluntary nonprofit hospitals, city and state government hospitals, military and veterans hospitals, and health insurance plans with a variety of forms and origins all developed in the United States at the same time, separately, and for specific purposes. The resulting picture has been described as having a rich diversity of opportunities and approaches for meeting the health care needs of a population that has in itself a rich diversity of people and situations. It has also been described as chaotic, uncoordinated, overlapping, unplanned, and wasteful of precious personal and financial resources. The reality probably lies somewhere in between.

If there is no single, easily described American health care system, at least some of the subsystems that compose the larger entity can be identified. Although an endless set of variations is possible, it seems appropriate to examine four models or subsystems of health care in the United States, each of which serves a different group. By looking at the components, the system as a whole may be better understood. These systems serve (1) regularly employed, middle-income families with continuous programs of health insurance coverage; (2) poor, unemployed (or underemployed) families without continuous health insurance coverage; (3) active-duty military personnel and their dependents; and (4) veterans of U.S. military service. For each of these systems, the manner in which basic elements of health care are provided is reviewed.

EMPLOYED, INSURED, MIDDLE-INCOME AMERICA (PRIVATE PRACTICE, FEE-FOR-SERVICE)

It is appropriate for two reasons to consider the system of health care used by the typical employed, insured, middle-income individual or family. First, this system is frequently described as *the* American health care system (all others, therefore, immediately becoming somehow secondary to it); second, this system is frequently said to include the best medical care available in the United States and perhaps anywhere in the world.

The most striking feature of the employed, insured, middle-income system of care is the absence of any *formal* system. Each family puts together an *informal* set of services and facilities to meet its own needs. The system, therefore, has no formal structure or organization and is different for each individual or family. Indeed, each family's system may vary widely according to the particular situation in which it is used. The only constant feature of this system is the family itself, all other aspects are transient, changeable, and widely varied.

Two other characteristics are also immediately noteworthy. First, the service aspects of the system focus on and are coordinated by physicians in private practice. Second, the system is financed by personal, nongovernmental funds, whether paid directly by consumers or through private health insurance plans. As the system is described, it will become readily apparent that these two features are not only important descriptively; they have been important in shaping the system into its present form.

Public health and preventive medicine services for the middle-class, middle-income system are provided by two different sources. Those services designed to protect large numbers of people, such as water purification, sewage disposal, and air pollution control, are provided by local or state governmental agencies. Frequently, these agencies are called *public health departments*. They usually provide their services to the entire population of a region, with no distinction between rich and poor, simple or sophisticated, interested or disinterested. Indeed, these mass public health services are common to all the systems of health care to be discussed. Those public health and preventive medicine services that are aimed at individuals, such as well-baby examinations, cervical cancer smears, vaccinations, and family planning, are provided by individual physicians in private practice. If a middle-income family desires a vaccination in preparation for a foreign trip or wants the blood cholesterol level of its members checked, the family physician is consulted and provides the service. If it is time for the new baby to have its first series of vaccinations, the family pediatrician is usually the one who provides them.

Ambulatory patient services, both simple and complex, are also obtained from private physicians. Many families use a physician who specializes in family practice, while others use an array of specialist physicians such as pediatricians, internists, obstetrician/gynecologists, and psychiatrists who provide both primary care and specialty services. When special laboratory tests are ordered, x-ray films required, or drugs and medications prescribed, private commercial for-profit laboratories or community pharmacies are used. Many of these services, from individual preventive medicine services to complex specialist treatments, are financed by individuals through out-of-pocket payment, since most health insurance plans do not provide complete coverage for these needs. When the middle-income family begins to use institutional services, such as hospital care, the source of payment shifts almost completely from the individual to third-party health insurance plans.

Inpatient hospital services are usually provided to the employed, insured, middle-income family by a local community hospital that is usually voluntary and nonprofit. The specific hospital to be used is determined by the institution in which the family physician has medical staff privileges. Generally, the smaller, less specialized, more local hospitals will be used for simpler problems, whereas the larger, more specialized, perhaps more distant hospitals will be used for more complicated problems. Many of these larger hospitals have active physician training programs, conduct research, and may have significant charity or teaching wards. The employed, insured, middle-income family obtains its long-term care from a variety of sources, depending on the service required. Some long-term care is provided in hospitals and, as such, is merely an extension of the complex inpatient care the patient has already received. This practice was more common in the past, but utilization review procedures have increased the pressure on hospitals to reduce the length of time people are hospitalized. More commonly, long-term care is obtained at home through the assistance of a visiting nurse or voluntary nonprofit community-based nursing service. If institutional long-term care is needed, it is probably obtained in a nursing home or a skilled nursing facility, usually a small (50–100 patients) institution, operated privately, for profit, by a single proprietor or small group of investors. Recently, there has been a general increase in size (100 + patients per facility) and a trend toward absorption of individual facilities into larger multifacility proprietary chains. The employed, insured, middle-income family usually pays for its long-term care with its own funds, since most health insurance plans provide relatively limited coverage for long-term care.

When middle-class families require care for emotional problems, they will again use a variety of mostly private services. However, as the illness becomes more serious, families may, for the first time, rely on governmentally sponsored service. When emotional problems first begin to appear in the middle-class family, the patient will probably turn to the family physician, who may provide simple supportive services such as tranquilizers, informal counseling, and perhaps referral for psychological testing. The physician may even arrange for the patient to be hospitalized in a general hospital for a rest, for "nervous exhaustion," or for some other nonpsychiatric diagnosis. As the emotional problems become more severe, the family physician may refer the patient to a private psychiatrist, or to a community mental health center that most likely will be a voluntary nonprofit agency or under the sponsorship of one (such as a voluntary nonprofit hospital). If hospitalization is required, the psychiatrist or the community mental health center is likely to use the psychiatric section of the local voluntary nonprofit hospital if it seems that the stay in a hospital will be a short one. If the hospitalization promises to be a long one, the psychiatrist may use a psychiatric hospital, usually a private, nongovernmental community facility.

In those cases in which very extended institutional care is required for an emotional problem and the patient's financial resources are relatively limited, the middle-class family may request hospitalization in the state mental hospital. This event usually represents the first use of governmental health programs by the middle-income family, and as such it frequently comes as a considerable shock to patient and family alike.

In summary, the employed, insured, middle-income family's system of health care is an informal, unstructured collection of individual services put together by the patient and the private physician to meet the needs of the moment. The individual services themselves have little formalized interrelationship, and the only thread of continuity is provided by the family's physician or by the family itself. In general, all the services are provided by nongovernmental sources and are paid for by private funds, either directly out-of-pocket or by privately financed health insurance plans.

For all of its apparent looseness and lack of structure, the middle-class family's system of health care allows for a considerable amount of decision and control by the patient, more than that of the other systems to be discussed. The patient is free to choose the physician, the health insurance plan, and frequently even the hospital. If additional care is required, the patient can seek out and use (sometimes overuse) that care to the limit of the financial resources available. If the patient does not like the particular care being provided, dissatisfaction can be expressed in a more effective manner: the patient can seek care elsewhere from another provider. Even with the newer Preferred Provider Organization approach to health insurance, which attempts to influence people to obtain care from lower cost physicians and hospitals, the influences are indirect and economic in nature (i.e., a discount for using the lower cost providers) and certainly not coercive or directive (i.e., mandating that a person can use only certain providers in order to be insured at all).

On the other hand, the middle-class family's system of care is a poorly coordinated, unplanned collection of services that frequently have little formal integration with one another. It can be very wasteful of resources and usually has no central control or monitor to determine whether it is accomplishing what it should. Each individual service may be of very high quality, but there may be little evidence of any "linking" taking place to ensure that each service complements the others as effectively as possible.

One special subset of the middle-class, middle-income model now involves millions of patients in this country. When people reach age 65, they are automatically eligible for Medicare, the federally sponsored and supervised health insurance plan for the elderly. A patient covered by Medicare benefits can utilize the same system of care as the middle-income family, including private practice physicians and voluntary nongovernmental hospitals. The main difference now is that the bills are paid by a federal government health insurance plan, rather than the usual private plan in which the typical middle-class family is enrolled. The physicians are the same and the hospitals are the same; only the health insurance plan is different.

Many middle-class, middle-income families no longer receive their various health services in piecemeal fashion, one at a time, from various independent practitioners who have no formal relationship to one another. Now, instead, many people belong to HMOs that contract to provide an organized package of health services in an integrated and intentionally coordinated program. These HMOs usually do not provide much in the way of long-term care but do provide just about everything else to some degree. It should be noted that, whereas in the past, HMO membership was usually made up of people under the age of 65, recent changes in the Medicare program have created incentives for people over the age of 65 to join HMOs as well as incentives for HMOs to enroll them. As a result, elderly people are now joining HMOs in the same fashion as younger people have in the past.

UNEMPLOYED, UNINSURED, INNER CITY, MINORITY AMERICA (LOCAL GOVERNMENT HEALTH CARE)

A second major system of health care in the United States serves those people who are not regularly employed, don't have continuous health insurance coverage, and often are minority group members living in the inner city. While the specific details may vary from city to city, the general outline is well known in all major cities of the country. If it was important to study the system of health care for the employed, insured, middle-income population because it represented the *best* health care possible in this country, it is equally important to study the care of the poor, unemployed, and uninsured, since it frequently represents the *worst*.

The most striking feature of the health care system of the poor, inner-city resident is exactly the same as that characterizing the middle-class system: there is no *formal* system. Instead, just as in the middle-class system, each individual or family must put together an *informal* set of services, from whatever source possible, to meet the health care needs of the moment. There is one significant difference, however: The poor do not have the resources to choose where and how they will obtain their health services. Instead, they must take what is offered to them and try to put together a system from whatever they are told they can have.

There are two important characteristics of the system. First, the great majority of services are provided by local government agencies such as the city or county hospital and the local health department. Second, the patients have no real continuity of service with any single provider, such as a middle-class family might have with a family physician. The poor family is faced with an endless stream of health care professionals who treat one specific episode of an illness and then are replaced by someone else for the next episode. While the middle-class system of health care can establish at least some thread of continuity by the ongoing presence of a family physician, the poor family cannot.

The poor obtain their mass public health and preventive medicine services, including a pure water supply, sanitary sewage disposal, and protection of milk and food from the same local government health departments and health agencies that serve the middle-class system. In contrast to the middle-class system, however, the poor also get their individual public health and preventive medicine services from the local health department. When a poor family's newborn baby needs its vaccinations, that family goes to the district health center of the health department, not to a private physician. When a low-income woman needs a Papanicolaou smear for cervical cancer testing or when a teenager from a low-income family needs a blood test for syphilis, it is most likely that the local government health department will give the test.

To obtain ambulatory patient services, the poor family cannot rely on the constant presence of a family physician for advice and routine treatment. Instead, they must turn to neighbors, the local pharmacist, the health department's public health nurse, or the emergency room of the city or county hospital. It has often been said that the city or county hospital's emergency room is the family physician for the poor, and the facts generally support this contention: When the poor need ambulatory patient care, it is quite likely that the first place they will turn is the city or county hospital emergency room.

The emergency room also serves the poor as the point of entry to the rest of the health care system. The poor obtain much of their ambulatory services in the outpatient clinics of the city and county hospitals. To gain admission to these clinics, they must frequently first go to the emergency room and be referred to the appropriate clinic. Once out of the emergency room, they may be cared for in two or three specialty clinics, each of which may handle one particular set of problems but none of which will take responsibility for coordinating all the care the patient is receiving.

When the poor need inpatient hospital services, whether simple or complicated, they again usually turn to the city or county hospital to obtain them. Admission to the inpatient services of these hospitals is usually obtained through the emergency room or the outpatient clinics, thereby forcing the poor family to use these ambulatory patient services if they wish later admission to the inpatient services. The poor may also turn to the emergency room, the outpatient clinics, and the inpatient ward or teaching services of the larger voluntary nonprofit community hospitals. Since these hospitals are frequently teaching hospitals for the training of physicians, they often maintain special free or lower-priced wards. It is to these wards that the poor are usually admitted. Since the care in the teaching hospitals is generally as good as or better than any that might be obtained at the local city or county hospitals, many poor are willing to become teaching cases in the voluntary nonprofit hospitals in exchange for better care in better surroundings. By and large, however, city and county hospitals carry the largest burden of inpatient care for the poor.

If the long-term care situation of middle-income people is generally inadequate, the long-term care of the poor can only be described as terrible. In contrast to the middle class, much of the long-term care of the poor is provided on the wards of the city and county hospitals, although not by intent or plan. The poor simply remain in hospitals longer because their social and physical conditions are more complicated and because the hospital staffs are reluctant to discharge them until they have some assurance that continuing care will be available after discharge. Since this status is often uncertain, poor patients are likely to be kept longer in the hospital so that they can complete as much of their convalescence as possible before discharge.

Most of the long-term care of the poor is provided in the same types of nursing homes or skilled nursing facilities that are used by the middle class—either the smaller (50–100 patients) facilities, operated for profit by a single proprietor or the larger (100+ patients) facilities operated by a proprietary chain. One major difference between the systems used by the poor and the middle class is the quality of the facility used. The middle class generally has access to better equipped and better staffed nursing homes, while the poor are admitted to less expensive, less well-equipped facilities. Another important difference between the middle class and the poor is that middle-class, middle-income patients are more likely to pay for their own care in these institutions, while the poor have their care paid by welfare, Medicaid, or other public funds.

It is interesting to note that the system of health care for the middle class utilizes entirely private, nongovernmental facilities until long-term care for mental illness is required; at that point, a governmental facility, the state mental hospital, is used. By contrast, the system of health care for the poor is composed almost entirely of public, government-sponsored services until long-term care is required. This care is usually provided in private, profit-making facilities, the first such use of private facilities by the poor.

The convergence of poor and middle-class systems of care in the private profit making nursing homes is important, since it represents an important feature of our multiple subsystems of health care. In many cases, several systems of health care that are otherwise separate and distinct will merge in their common use of personnel, equipment, and facilities. The emergency rooms of the city or county and voluntary nonprofit teaching hospitals, for example, will serve as the source of emergency medical care for the middle-class family that cannot reach its own family physician. It will also serve as the family physician for the poor family that has none of its own. The private, for-profit nursing home will serve as the source of long-term care for the middle-class family, and may provide the same function for the poor. The radiology department of the voluntary nonprofit teaching hospital will provide x-ray tests for the middle-class patient whose care is supervised by the private family physician, as well as for the poor patient whose care is supervised by a hospital staff physician in training. This does not mean that there is any real, functional integration of the separate systems of care because of their common use of the same facility or personnel. Rather, the model is more like that of a busy harbor in which a variety of ships will berth side by side for a short period of time before going their separate ways for separate purposes.

In their use of services for emotional illnesses, the poor return once again to an almost totally public, local governmental system. Initial signs of emotional difficulties are haphazardly treated in the emergency rooms and outpatient clinics of the city or county hospital. From here, patients may be referred to the crowded inpatient psychiatric wards of these same hospitals, but are just as likely to be referred to community mental health centers operated by local governmental or voluntary nonprofit community agencies. When long-term care in an institution is required, the poor are sent to the psychiatric wards of the city or county hospital, and from there to the large state government mental hospitals, frequently many miles away.

In the past, health services for the poor were usually free, at least to the patients. Neither the local health department, the city or county hospital, nor the state mental hospital generally charged for its services, regardless of the patient's ability to pay. In the last few years, both local health departments and city and county hospitals have been forced to initiate a system of charges for services that were previously free. They have done this to recapture third-party payments to which the poor patient might be eligible, and patients who are unable to pay are still ordinarily provided the services they need. The imposition of these charges for previously free health services has probably changed the perception of these programs by the poor, but it is still too early to determine the implications of these changes.

As with the middle-class, middle-income system, there is a subset of the health care system of the poor that requires special comment. Certain persons who are poor enough by virtue of extremely low income or resources may qualify for Medicaid, the federal-state cooperative health insurance plan for the indigent, frequently termed Title 19 in reference to the section of the federal legislation by which it was created (Medicare, an entirely different program, is termed Title 18). Under Medicaid people whose income and resources are below a level established by the individual states can use a state government-sponsored health insurance program to purchase health care in the private, middle-class marketplace. The purpose of this program is to move the poor out of their usual local government health care system and into the supposedly better private practice health care system of the middle class. Unfortunately, the ability of Medicaid to move the poor into a better system of care had been limited by the reluctance of private physicians and private hospitals to assume responsibility for many Medicaid patients. This reluctance has been based on what has been seen as a low rate of reimbursement by Medicaid for services provided, an often cumbersome system of paperwork and prior authorizations in order to provide care and a frequently irrational system of retroactive denials of payment for services already provided.

Medicaid has succeeded to a degree in helping poor patients move from local government hospitals into voluntary nonprofit teaching hospitals, but its greatest effect has probably been in moving poor patients into private, profit-making nursing homes and skilled nursing facilities. In some states, for example, more than 60 percent of all patient bills in private nursing homes are now paid by the Medicaid program, providing some indication of the importance of this program to the provision of long-term care. And for all its problems, the Medicaid program has allowed certain aspects of the middle-class, middle-income system of health care to be shared with the poor, inner city minority system of health care—a blending, merging, or sharing of resources and services that is characteristic of the American health care system and that makes it so difficult to evaluate any one subsystem cleanly and separately.

Unfortunately, with the recent tendency to cut back on the Medicaid program, at both the national and state levels, this movement of poor patients into the middle-class system may abate considerably and may even be reversed. As less and less Medicaid money becomes available to purchase care in the middle-class system for poorer patients, they may increasingly have to fall back once again on the resources of the city and county public hospital, as in the past.

A second subset of the system of care for the poor and uninsured is that system that exists for poor people who turn 65. Immediately on reaching age 65, they are eligible for Medicare and ostensibly should be able to take their new insurance coverage and move into the private, middle-income system of care. Unfortunately, this movement from public to private provider systems by poor people who become 65 years of age is limited by the deductible and coinsurance features of Medicare. Under Medicare everyone (poor included) is expected to spend several hundreds of dollars for health care first, before Medicare begins to pay bills. Even when this deductible requirement is met, the elderly person is also required to pay the first $500 or so for each hospitalization, in addition to the previously mentioned deductible. The level of available cash to pay these deductibles and coinsurance limits the ability of many poor people to take full advantage of the benefits of Medicare when they become eligible at age 65.

A third subset of the system of care for the unemployed, uninsured, poor involves the use of the HMO to deliver a "package" of health care services to the poor, much as the HMO does for the middle-income group. The major difference here is the fact that the sponsor of the HMO may be a public agency or may be a private organization that is specifically providing HMO services to the poor to take advantage of public funds that have been earmarked for just that purpose. HMOs now are being organized by all sectors of the health care system, both public and private, and their services are being offered to both middle-income and poor individuals.

In summary, the system of health care for the poor is as unstructured and informal as that for the middle class, but the poor have to depend on whatever services the local government offers them. The services are usually provided free of charge or at low cost, but the patient has relatively little opportunity to express a choice and exercise options. Poor patients often cannot move to another set of services if they dislike the one first offered, since those first offered are usually the only services available.

Like the system of health care for the middle class, the system for the poor is poorly coordinated internally and almost completely unplanned and unmonitored. It is certainly as wasteful of resources as the middle-class system, but because it is a low cost, poorly financed system, the exact amount of waste is difficult to document. At the same time, the great virtue of the health care system for the poor—its openness and accessibility to all people at all times for all conditions (albeit with considerable delays) —is difficult to evaluate adequately as well.

Certainly, the most important issue for the system of care that presently serves the poor is whether or not it will be able to survive much longer without a new source of financial support. As more and more city and county governments find themselves in deep financial difficulties, as more and more states and local areas pass laws limiting the amount of tax revenue a local (or even a state) government can raise, the financial situation of local government units becomes increasingly shaky; so too does the financial situation of the public health and hospital services they provide. The key issue in the survival of the system that provides care for the poor is financial, and the prospects are increasingly bleak.

MILITARY MEDICAL CARE SYSTEM

A person joining one of the uniformed branches of the American military sacrifices many aspects of civilian life that nonmilitary personnel take for granted. At the same time, however, this person receives a variety of fringe benefits that those outside the military do not enjoy. One of the most important of these fringe benefits is a well-organized system of high quality health care provided at no direct cost to the recipient. Certain features of this military medical care system (the general term used to include the separate systems of the U.S. Army, Navy, and Air Force) deserve comment. First, the system is all inclusive and omnipresent. The military medical system has the responsibility of protecting the health of all active-duty military personnel everywhere and of providing them with all the services they may eventually need for any service-connected problem. The military medical system goes where active-duty military personnel go, and assumes a responsibility for total care that is unique among American health care systems.

The second important characteristic of the military medical care system is that it goes into effect immediately whether the active-duty soldier or sailor wants it or not. No initiative or action is required by the individual to start the system; indeed, the system frequently provides certain types of health services, such as routine vaccinations or shots, that the soldier or sailor would really wish not to have. The individual has little choice regarding who will provide the treatment or where, but at the same time, the services are always there if needed, without the need to search them out. If a physician's services are needed, they are obtained; if hospitalization is required, it is arranged; if emergency transportation is necessary, it is carried out. There is little that the individual can do to influence how medical care is provided, but at the same time, there is never any worry about its availability.

The third important characteristic of the military health care system is its great emphasis on keeping personnel well, preventing illness or injury, and finding health problems early while they are still amenable to treatment. Great stress is placed on preventive measures such as vaccination, regular physical examinations and testing, and educational efforts toward prevention of accidents and contagious diseases. In an approach that is unique among the health care systems of this country, the military medical system provides health care and not just sickness care.

In the military medical system, the same mass public health and preventive medicine services that are provided to a locality or a community by a local government health department or health agency may also be provided to the active-duty military personnel. However, whenever the personnel are actually within the boundaries of a military reservation or post, an additional set of mass public health and preventive medicine services may be provided by the military itself. Sanitary disposal of sewage, protection of food and milk, purification of the water supply, and prevention of vehicular or job-related accidents may be provided for by a local government agency, but each military installation will usually have a second separate system of its own, staffed by its own public health and safety officers. Individual public health and preventive medicine services are also provided by the military medical system according to a well-organized, regularly scheduled routine of yearly examinations, surveys of patient records, vaccinations, and other measures. The persons providing the specific preventive service (for example, a routine tetanus shot) are usually medical corpsmen or other nonphysician personnel; however, their work is carried out according to carefully developed guidelines and will be monitored by well-trained supervisory medical personnel.

Routine ambulatory care is usually provided to most active duty military personnel by the same medics who provide the individual preventive services. These services are usually provided at the dispensary, sick bay, first aid station, or similar unit that is very close to the military personnel's actual place of work. These ambulatory services may also be provided by physicians or nurses at the same locations, but this is less likely. More complicated ambulatory patient care services are usually provided by physicians, frequently specialists, working at the same dispensary or medical station as the medics or, more likely, in a clinic or outpatient department of a larger facility such as a military hospital. Patients are usually referred by medics or physicians who have first cared for the patients for more simple problems; laboratory tests, x-ray examinations, and medications are obtained at the same military facility to which the patient is referred.

The most simple hospital services are provided using short-stay beds at base dispensaries, in sick bays aboard ship, or at small base hospitals on various military installations around the world. Usually the range of services that can be offered at these installations is limited, and referral to larger institutions is routinely carried out if a more complex problem is suspected. More complicated hospital services are provided to active-duty military personnel in regional hospitals that possess a wide variety of specialized services and facilities. Frequently, these hospitals also have large teaching and training programs, where the atmosphere and the quality of care are similar to what might be expected at a university hospital or a large community teaching hospital.

The military medical system does not pretend to offer the same extensive range of long-term care services that it provides for more acute short-term problems. The military medical system does provide care for potentially long range problems in military hospitals, as long as there is some reasonable expectation that the patient will some day be able to return to full active duty. Whenever it is determined, however, that the problem is genuinely long term in nature and that complete return to active duty is not possible, the patient is given a medical discharge from the service and long-term care will be provided through the Veterans Administration (VA) facilities.

If military personnel develop emotional difficulties, care is most likely to be provided initially by the medical corpsperson and then by a physician assigned to that military unit. These personnel will provide short-term nonpsychiatric support and counseling, and possibly prescribe certain medications, such as tranquilizers. For more severe problems, the patient is referred to the psychiatric services of larger military hospitals where the severity of the problem will be determined. If the problem is short term and is not believed to affect the patient's work seriously, an attempt may be made to provide the short-term treatment at the military hospital itself, first on an inpatient and later on an outpatient basis. More likely, if there is a significant psychiatric diagnosis, the patient will be given a medical discharge, with follow-up care to be provided through the psychiatric services of the VA hospitals.

In general, the military medical system is closely organized and highly integrated. A single patient record is used, and the complete record moves from one health care service to another with the patient. Once the need for health care is identified, the system itself arranges for the patient to receive the required care and usually even provides transportation to the services. The patient does not have to search out the necessary service or determine how to use it. This service is provided at no cost to the patient, requires little effort by the patient to initiate it, and generally involves a high-quality product. The system is centrally planned, uses nonmedical and nonnursing personnel to the utmost, and is entirely self-sufficent and self-contained. The services are provided by salaried employees in facilities that are wholly owned and operated by the system itself. The system is not generally available to persons who are not active-duty military personnel or their dependents, although in cases of emergency or pressing local need, they can be. Generally, the patient has little choice regarding the manner in which services will be delivered, but this drawback is counterbalanced by the assurance that high-quality services will be available when needed.

In recent years, the military medical system has been affected by the termination of the physician draft that previously kept it well supplied with high-quality young physicians who had just completed their specialty training. With the end of the physician draft, the military medical systems have had to compete with all other health care systems for physicians, and their choice of physicians has been narrowed considerably.

Dependents and families of active-duty military personnel are served by a special subsystem of military medicine that combines the services of the middle-class middle-income system and the active-duty military system. The dependents and families of active-duty military personnel are covered by an extensive health insurance plan, the Civilian Health and Medical Program of the Uniformed Services (CHAMPUS), provided, financed, and supervised by the military. This health insurance plan allows dependents and families of active-duty military personnel to purchase medical care from private medical practitioners and from local community nonmilitary hospitals when similar services cannot be provided at a military installation within reasonable distance. The dependents and families of active-duty military personnel can also use the same military services that the active-duty personnel use, provided space and resources are available and military authorities determine that this procedure is appropriate. The resulting subsystem of care for military dependents and families generally allows them to participate to some degree in two separate systems of care: the middle-class, middle-income private practice system and the military medical system. Their participation in either is generally not as clearly focused or as active as it would be for someone firmly planted in either system exclusively, but it still provides them with two viable options for obtaining care.

VETERANS ADMINISTRATION HEALTH CARE SYSTEM

Parallel to the system of care for active duty military personnel is another system operated within the continental United States for retired, disabled, and otherwise deserving veterans of previous U.S. military service. Although the VA system is in many respects larger than the system of care for active duty military personnel, it is not nearly as complete, well integrated, or extensive. At the present time, the VA system of care is primarily hospital oriented and not really a health care system. The VA operates 171 hospitals throughout the country that provide most VA care. In recent years, the VA has increasingly provided outpatient services and now maintains more than 200 outpatient clinics; however, the majority of VA health care is still focused on the hospitals.

A second important characteristic of the VA system is the great preponderance of male patients with long-term care problems. By and large, the patients using the VA health care system are older, inactive men in whom the occurrence of multiple and chronic physical and emotional illnesses is much higher than in the general population.

A third important feature of the VA system is its existence as only one part of a much larger system of social services and benefits for veterans. Many of the people eligible to utilize the VA health care system are also receiving other kinds of financial benefits as well; indeed, access to the VA health care system is sometimes directly dependent on eligibility for financial benefits. The VA paid for health care for over 1 million veterans annually during the period 1975–1980. During this same time period, 2.5 million veterans also received educational assistance, more than 3 million veterans received VA disability compensation, and more than 3.5 million veterans had VA home loans outstanding annually. Since health care is only one of many VA programs, a great variety of social services interact with and compete for all available resources.

A further feature of the VA health care system is its unique relationship with organized consumer groups. Since the VA is organized to provide care exclusively for veterans, and since many of those veterans are members of local and national veterans' clubs and associations, the VA health care system is constantly in direct communication with groups representing the interests of veterans. In a manner that is unparalleled in any other health care system in this country, the interests of the veterans are constantly conveyed to individual VA hospitals, to the VA administration in Washington D.C., and to the U.S. Congress. In no other health care system in this country does organized consumer interest play such a constant, important, and influential role.

Since the VA system is primarily a hospital system, there are few attempts to provide general public health services or routine ambulatory care services. Veterans usually obtain these services from some other system of care, either the middle-class, middle-income system or the local government system that serves the urban poor. The VA does provide the more complicated ambulatory services, usually through its hospital outpatient clinics. This care is in preparation for possible hospital admission or as follow-up after hospitalization. Many veterans who require these services obtain them from other systems of care and come to the VA system only after a condition is apparent and hospitalization is required. Admission to VA hospitals can be gained either through the ambulatory patient care services operated by the VA itself, by direct referrals from physicians in private practice, or by referrals from hospitals in the community. The services in VA hospitals are provided by salaried, full-time medical and nursing personnel; as in the military medical system, most of the VA hospitals are self-contained, relatively self-sufficient units that require little outside support or staff.

The VA health care system provides a tremendous quantity of long-term care for both physical and emotional illnesses. Indeed, the VA is probably the largest single provider of long-term care in the country, if not the world. In addition to providing considerable long-term care in the acute, short-term care hospitals, the VA also operates a number of domicilaries and nursing homes and pays for care in local community nursing homes and skilled nursing facilities. As of early 1982, 18 VA hospitals also offered hospice or hospice-like care to their patients who were dying of cancer.

The VA system of care is difficult to describe fully for two important reasons. First, it is a system that does not attempt to provide a complete range of services, but instead concentrates on acute hospital services and on long-term care for physical and emotional problems. Second, eligibility for entry into the system is somewhat unclear and sometimes open to variable local interpretation. The system is designed to serve veterans with service-connected disabilities, but offers services to other veterans if they cannot obtain adequate care elsewhere and if adequate VA resources are available. In practice, the actual eligibility requirements and patient mix vary substantially from one VA hospital to the next.

If the system of health care for active duty military personnel focuses on preventive, ambulatory, and acute inpatient care, the VA system of care stresses long-term, chronic inpatient care for both physical and emotional problems. Whereas the military medical system offers a complete, well-integrated, well-coordinated package of health care services, the services that the VA offers are primarily hospital related. In contrast to the military medical system, which actively seeks out and offers services to patients as part of their work environment, the VA provides its services to patients only when they come forward to seek them. If they do not seek out the care, the VA system does not actively pursue them. Despite these reservations about the VA as a complete system of health care, it should be stressed that the VA serves as the primary source of inpatient hospital care for 1 million veterans a year and is a potential source of inpatient care for many millions more. As such, it is the largest single provider of health care services in this country and must be considered an integral, important component of the American health care scene, both now and in the future.

HEALTH SERVICES: A SUMMARY OF PERSPECTIVES

In reviewing each of these four major systems of health care for Americans, the middle-class, private practice system, the local government system for the urban poor, the military medical system for active duty military and their dependents, and the VA health care system, it becomes apparent that there are a number of additional systems that could have been included as well. Other systems of health care include the one used by rural farming families and the Indian Health Service operated for native Americans by the federal government. There are also many possible variations within the four systems discussed here. The purpose, however, is not to be exhaustive in describing the systems themselves but rather to point out that there are multiple systems providing services to different populations with different needs. No one system predominates in terms of persons served or benefits provided. Indeed, the purpose here is to point out that there is no one single American health care system but rather a mosaic of subsystems, each with its own characteristics and moving in its own direction.

Is it bad to have so many separate subsystems? Why is it even worth pointing out the obvious fact that many such systems exist? Several pressing reasons exist for reviewing this country's compartmentalized organization of health care. The first and most important is quite simple: To improve health services to everyone in this country, an understanding of the entire situation is essential; otherwise, piecemeal solutions will be proposed to specific problems without recognizing the possible long-range potentials for the entire system. In a system that could be compared to a jigsaw puzzle, it would be foolish and perhaps even dangerous to consider individual pieces of the puzzle without first viewing the puzzle as a whole.

The second reason for considering the various separate systems of health care in this country is the vigorous competition for scarce resources of money, people, and facilities. Although the four systems described are separate from one another, they all compete for the same resources since they are all dependent on the same economy and the same supplies of health personnel and skills.

Whenever there is vigorous competition for resources, two things frequently happen. First, the stronger, more vigorous, more aggressive, or better connected competitors obtain the larger portion of the resources, whether or not this outcome is justified by their needs. In practice, this has meant that the middle-class, private practice system, the military medical system, and the VA system have all done relatively well, while the local government health care system has not. Indeed, as has already been pointed out, the local government health care system for the poor has always been severely underfinanced and understaffed, a situation that seems to be getting progressively worse.

Second, intense competition for resources frequently results in wasteful duplication and ineffective use of resources. For example, in the same region, a city or county hospital, a private teaching hospital, a military hospital, and a VA hospital may all be operating exactly the same kind of expensive service, although only one facility might be needed and where undoubtedly one large integrated service would provide more efficient use of resources than four smaller ones. Because each institution is part of a separate system, serves a different population, and approaches the resource pool through a different channel, no really purposeful planning or controlled allocation of resources is possible. In the past, this situation might have been acceptable because the resources seemed endless, but in these days of very limited resources, this is no longer acceptable.

In addition to this economic inefficiency, there are other reasons for looking with a critical eye at multiple systems of care, reasons that are related to quality and accessibility of services. Unfortunately, not all of these subsystems of care serve people in the same way with the same results. There is great inequality among the various systems of health care, with the result that different people receive different levels of care simply by accident of birth or membership in a special group. Since all the separate systems of health care in this country ultimately depend on public funds for their continued existence, it is imperative that the inequalities among them be removed as rapidly as possible. This does not necessarily mean eliminating the various separate subsystems of care, but rather requires that all the systems rise to a common high level and equitably share responsibilities and resources.

In recent years, there have been various approaches to the problem of reorganizing these separate subsystems of care so that they function together in a more integrated and effective fashion. Although these proposals have often been limited to specific aspects, such as financing or quality of care, their overall purpose has generally been to move the various pieces of the American health care system into a better and more efficient relationship with each other. These approaches are interesting not in themselves but in how they will shape health care in the future. The specific scenarios for particular issues will undoubtedly change, but the overall effort to develop a more rationally integrated system will certainly continue unabated and will, indeed, expand as resources are stretched to the limit.

Two proposals can be mentioned briefly, not because they are unimportant but rather because the possibility of their implementation is so slight that they have relatively little practical impact. The first of these might be described as a *laissez-faire*, free-market approach that implies in effect, "Leave everyone alone, stop meddling, stop regulating, and let the workings of the marketplace with its active competition eventually force the health care system to reorganize." The second approach, at the other political and social extreme, implies, "What this country needs is a single, governmentally controlled health care system, such as the British National Health Service, which would allow for greater centralized control and planning for all aspects of the system." Although certain specific aspects of the marketplace approach have been adopted, both of these approaches as total systems have been viewed as so politically impractical for this country at this time that they have not been seriously considered.

Another approach that has been considered has been the "health planning" approach. With the passage of the original Comprehensive Health Planning legislation and, more important, with the passage of the National Health Planning and Resources Development Act of 1975, it had been thought that providers, consumers, and public officials might come together and develop plans for all states and localities that would then become blueprints for a more rationally organized system of care. This hope did not turn into reality, and with the demise of the health planning system, this approach toward more rational coordination of health care services has been virtually abandoned for the time being, as discussed further in Chapters 12 and 15.

A somewhat different approach to rationalizing the American health care system focuses on the use of financing mechanisms to encourage or force increased coordination of effort throughout the system. The proponents of this approach suggest that the power to withhold financial reimbursement to providers who do not comply with efforts to improve the system would be so strong as to be irresistible. Although the argument is used most visibly by many of the proponents of a national health insurance plan, this approach has become more apparent in the way the Health Care Financing Administration (HCFA) uses Medicare funds to encourage compliance with its long range objectives. It is also becoming increasingly obvious in the way certain employer health care coalitions are using their influence over the industrial concerns' health insurance dollars as a means of making their wishes known. Indeed, it would have to be said that the greatest forces shaping the organization and functions of the health care system today are financial, and the greatest power to affect how the system will work in the future is in the hands of the large third party payers for health care.

Another possible solution, which has yet to receive considerable attention, is the "public utility" approach. In this approach toward a more rational health care system, all the components of the health care system, or at least the large institutional ones, would be placed under the regulatory supervision of public bodies that would have total control over licensing, financing, mode of function, packages of services to be offered, personnel development, and so forth. Both public and private components could continue to exist as they do at present under their own auspices (just as individual utilities do now, for example), but what they would be able to do and how much they would be allowed to charge would be controlled by a single regulatory agency. A strong argument for this approach is that all of these regulatory efforts are now conducted in a poorly coordinated and often conflicting fashion by multiple regulatory agencies. Having one single body would remove much of the present jungle of regulatory efforts. A strong argument *against* such a body is that immense power over the system would be given to a single superagency. Practically speaking, in the present antiregulatory political climate in this country, there is little enthusiasm for this approach.

A final approach toward rationalization of the present system might be called "incremental tinkering" and it is one that tacitly assumes that no major, sweeping, overall reorganization is possible. The proponents of this approach try instead to do whatever they can to increase rationality whenever an opportunity occurs anywhere in the system. A new piece of state legislation here, a new form of federal health insurance there, a new form of local cooperative planning are all added in piecemeal fashion, with no great effort to relate them to each other or to some underlying master plan. The hope in this approach is that all the individual accretions to the system will provide for a more efficient and integrated end product.

These six approaches are obviously not mutually exclusive, so it is entirely possible that someone might support several of them because they work well together. Someone interested in reorganizing the health care system through health planning might also want to institute a national health insurance program because it would provide the centralized financial leverage for mandatory health planning. In the same fashion, someone might propose a mostly *laissez-faire* approach to any intentional reorganization and also support a national health insurance plan that would allow all people to make their own choices in an open market.

In the future, all six approaches (and possibly more) will probably continue to be fostered and most likely no single approach will predominate. What certainly will continue, however, will be efforts to bring the various pieces of the subsystems and the various subsystems themselves into a more efficient and effective new relationship with one another and with the consumers who must use them. Indeed, this issue is so important and so central to all our other interests that the future of health care in this country will be shaped by the direction our society decides to follow in this regard.

The remaining chapters of this book describe, dissect, and analyze the health services system of the United States. Trends, issues, interrelationships, and problems are revealed and assessed. Only by thoroughly understanding the evolution, structure, attributes, and deficiencies of the system, or systems, can the fundamental decisions facing the nation be addressed.

PART TWO

Causes and Characteristics of Health Services Use in the United States

CHAPTER 2

The Physiologic and Psychological Bases of Health, Disease, and Care Seeking

Lawrence A. May

In this chapter, the physiological bases of disease and the psychological characteristics of care-seeking behavior are explored. The concepts of illness and disease and the complexities surrounding the exact definitions of diseases are discussed. The orderly relationship between pathologic abnormality, physiologic alteration, and clinical manifestations of disease are presented, especially as they relate to care-seeking behavior. The influence of biologic, pharmacologic, and environmental factors on changing disease patterns is reviewed, and some of the effects of these changing disease patterns on the health services system are demonstrated as a prelude to the remaining chapters of the book.

DEFINING ILLNESS AND DISEASE

The distinction between illness and disease is essential for the understanding of care-seeking behavior. Illness is a lay experience that connotes both a physical and a social state (1). It is an individual's reaction to a biologic alteration and is defined differently by different people according to their state of mind and cultural beliefs. The term *illness*, therefore, is imprecise and represents a highly individual response to a set of physiologic and psychological stimuli.

By contrast, *disease* is a professional construct. It is perceived as being precise and reflecting the highest state of professional knowledge, particularly that of the physician. The definition of disease is used as the vehicle for informing the patient of the presence of pathology, as a means for deciding on a course of treatment, and as a basis for comparing the results of therapy. It becomes an essential element in the

35

planning and organization of the health care system and in the allocation of resources within that system.

The accurate definition of disease is so important that it is crucial to recognize that considerable imprecision exists in the process of medical diagnosis. An individual physician using the best professional judgment available may diagnose a disease in a particular patient, but this definition may not be shared by other physicians. Even when the definition of a particular disease is similar in different patients, the impact of the diagnosis on those patients may vary widely depending upon how the definition is applied and on the unique social and biologic characteristics of individual patients.

Attempts to link illness (the individual's perception of loss of functional capacity) with disease (the professional's definition of a pathologic process) is even more complicated. Illness may occur in the absence of real disease, and disease may be present in the absence of perceived illness. It is illness, the individual's perception of impaired function, and not disease that stimulates care-seeking behavior, making the relationship between these two concepts important to understand.

There can be difficulty in defining illness and disease, and significant cognitive dissonance between physician and patient may result. Mitral valve prolapse, a rather common abnormality of a heart valve with a prevalence of 5–10 percent of the population, has had an assortment of symptoms attributed to it. Fatigue, irritability, dizziness, and palpitations have all been suggested as symptoms of this condition. However, a study at Duke University failed to reveal any difference in symptoms in the patients with objectively confirmed mitral valve prolapse from a group that had been referred for echocardiographic studies in which no mitral valve prolapse was discovered (2). Although the control group in this study was not selected randomly, it illustrates that symptoms may exist and be attributable to a medical disease that are, in fact, equally prevalent in a similar population without the disease.

This problem is further illustrated in the case of hypertension, which physicians acknowledge as an asymptomatic condition, but one to which patients attribute a wide variety of symptoms. The generally acknowledged symptoms of headache, ringing in the ears, and nosebleeds failed to be confirmed as having any greater prevalence in those with hypertension than those without. The need for patients who perceive themselves as ill to have a disease explanation for their symptoms can pose a major challenge to physicians; and if a medical explanation for essentially functional symptoms is provided, notable care-seeking behavior can result.

A powerful example of this has been the possible association of chronic fatigue with persistent infection with the Epstein-Barr virus (3). This was originally reported in a group of 90 patients who were evaluated for persistent fatigue by several physicians near Lake Tahoe in California (4). The media coverage of this situation created a tremendous interest on the part of patients in determining whether they might be suffering from a disease for which there is admittedly no cu₁e, and for which such poorly defined parameters exist, that physicians cannot conclude that the disease actually exists. (A similar historical example was hypoglycemia, which produced numerous physician visits for glucose tolerance tests that are generally felt to be unnecessary; true hypoglycemia is rare and symptoms are generally absent in patients with blood sugar levels below the reported normal levels.)

The complexity of defining disease and its interaction with care-seeking behavior are well illustrated by the condition diabetes mellitus. Both the general public and the health care professional understand that diabetes results in an elevated blood sugar level, but the physiologic bases of this metabolic alteration can vary widely (5). In one person, the disease may result from impaired secretion of insulin by the pancreas, or it may be caused by a resistance to sufficient amounts of insulin in a patient who is obese.

Diabetes mellitus may result from the imposition of a normal physiologic condition such as pregnancy, or it may be due to the use of exogenous drugs such as diuretics or steroids.

Aside from the varying causes of an elevated blood sugar level (referred to as *hyperglycemia*), an important issue is the amount of hyperglycemia that defines a patient as diabetic. Various criteria have been suggested to define who is diabetic, using different numerical measures of elevated blood sugar level, but these criteria do not necessarily separate those who feel healthy, nor do they define a level at which treatment is indicated (6). The myriad criteria that have been applied to diabetes at one time or another would define anywhere between 4 percent and 40 percent of the population over age 60 as having diabetes. In recognition of the fact that even objective measures of disease or health such as a blood sugar determination are variable, great effort was expended to reach a consensus on what level of blood sugar elevation defines diabetes. The criteria state that the level must be consistently elevated in the fasting and postprandial states and that this level must be found on two occasions. The current criteria for diagnosing diabetes are a fasting blood sugar level of 140 and a blood sugar level of more than 200 measured two hours after eating on two separate occasions. The previously widely used glucose tolerance test is expensive, unnecessary, and results in an excessive number of false-positive readings sacrificing specificity in a way that is unacceptable (7).

The problem illustrated by diabetes extends to many other disease conditions that are defined by an abnormal laboratory measurement or blood test result. Hypertension is a common medical problem resulting from a variety of physiologic bases, including abnormalities in hormone production and use, improper resetting of neurologic control centers, or acquired loss of blood vessel elasticity secondary to atherosclerosis.

In view of the variety of causes of hypertension, the selection of an arbitrary number to define individuals or members of a population as having an abnormal condition is a difficult and possibly futile effort. The blood pressure reading of 140/90 has been offered as the boundary of normality, but the meaning of this reading in different persons may vary markedly. A blood pressure of 150/100 in a 72-year-old woman has quite different implications from the same reading in a 26-year-old man. An elevated blood pressure after half hour of bed rest means something quite different from an elevated blood pressure in a person waiting anxiously for half an hour in a physician's office.

To complicate matters further, as with diabetes, there is no direct relationship between the presence of elevated blood pressure and the development of either perceived symptoms or actual pathologic damage to body organs, at least at the lower ranges of hypertension. Some people with only slight hypertension will attribute a variety of functional complaints to their "blood pressure," whereas others with dangerously elevated levels may not have any symptoms and perceive themselves as being well (8).

The definition of diabetes or of hypertension is relatively straightforward when compared to diseases that cannot be numerically defined, such as rheumatoid arthritis. The definition of this disease is clinical rather than numerical and is based on the presence of four or more diagnostic characteristics determined by the American Rheumatism Association to be valid criteria for the disease. Even with the use of this symptom aggregation approach, there are still many professionals who confuse rheumatoid arthritis with degenerative joint disease and with other forms of arthritis. Further, even with this more orderly approach to the definition of this disease, the ability to measure its impact on a population is comparatively limited.

In summary, the definition of disease is a more imprecise and inexact process than is usually thought. Although it is frequently associated with apparently solid, objective measurements such as blood sugar levels or blood pressure, the implications of these values may vary widely. Finally, the relationship between illness, which is a personal observation by patients, and disease, which is a scientific judgment by professionals, needs to be understood and constantly remembered.

DISEASE PROCESSES: THE PHYSIOLOGIC BASES OF DISEASE

The major pathophysiologic processes involved in disease production are vascular, inflammatory, neoplastic, toxic, metabolic, and degenerative. These processes give rise to disease conditions, but their expression is modified by factors in the host such as age, immunologic status, medication ingestion, concurrent disease, or psychological perceptions. The combination of the pathophysiologic processes and the different host factors creates the various disease patterns.

Vascular abnormalities may produce disease in a variety of ways in multiple-organ systems. The gradual narrowing and eventual blockage of blood vessels by the deposit of fatty materials in the walls and lumina of the vessels is a characteristic of arteriosclerotic cardiovascular disease. Vascular disease may also be produced by the more rapid occlusion of a blood vessel by an embolus, material from a distant site floating in the bloodstream. Other disease pictures may be produced by bleeding from a ruptured blood vessel in the brain or elsewhere. In some disease conditions, such as stroke, the same clinical picture may result from any one of these three causes. Whatever the initial cause, gradual occlusion, embolus, or rupture, the result is damage to brain tissue and resultant paralysis. It is usually easy to determine that a cerebrovascular accident (stroke) has occured, but it is frequently impossible to determine whether it was caused by gradual occlusion, embolus, or rupture of a blood vessel.

Inflammation is the basis of disease in many organ systems, but the physiologic basis of that inflammation may be infectious, autoimmune, traumatic, or something else. A single inflamed joint may be due to autoimmune inflammation, the presence of uric acid crystals, or degeneration of cartilage as a consequence of age and use, or it may be due to infection with bacteria or viruses. The failure to identify the specific etiologic factor can be highly destructive to the patient or at least fail to resolve the problem in the appropriate amount of time. Therefore, having defined both the type of disorder and the mechanism of inflammation, physicians must seek to identify the underlying agent in the process of inflammation.

Neoplastic disease is caused by an abnormal new growth of tissue. Benign neoplasms are abnormal growths that remain localized and do not spread to distant locations in the body. Malignant neoplasms, generally called *cancer*, by contrast, not only grow locally and invade surrounding tissues but also spread to distant sites in the body, producing metastases. Benign neoplasms may cause considerable damage by continued local growth and pressure on surrounding tissues, such as pressure on the brain from a benign growth on its surface. Malignant neoplasms, by contrast, invade the organs directly and disrupt their normal functioning by replacing normal tissue with diseased tissue. Neoplasms may occur spontaneously or may be caused by environmental, toxic, or host factors (9–14).

Toxic bases for disease involve the presentation to individual organs of chemical materials that are inherently damaging. These materials may originate from environmental pollutants, from the use of potentially damaging materials such as alcohol or cigarettes, or from the ingestion of medications. Alcohol, for example, is toxic to the liver under appropriate conditions, causing hepatitis, fibrosis, and eventual cirrhosis. Cobalt in beer can be toxic to heart muscle cells, bee stings may damage the glomerulus of the kidney, and asbestos may contribute to the development of lung cancer. Cigarette smoking may destroy, inflame, or alter the cells of the lung, producing emphysema, chronic bronchitis, or cancer. Digitalis, an ordinarily useful drug in the treatment of various heart conditions, in excess doses may produce toxicity and life-threatening arrhythmias. In a society with an increasing amount of environmental pollution, drug use, and industrial exposure, toxins are unfortunately becoming a more common cause of disease.

Metabolic diseases are caused by chemical disorders within body cells, usually secondary to some excess or deficiency of a hormone or important nutrient. The excess or deficiency of a thyroid, parathyroid, or adrenal cortical hormone causes clinical disease pictures that are easily recognized by well-trained physicians. A deficiency of insulin, secreted by glands in the pancreas, gives rise to diabetes, as mentioned earlier. Deficiency of important nutrients, caused either by a scarcity of the elements in the diet or by an inability to absorb and use them, results in a wide variety of clinical pictures ranging from anemia to pellagra.

Degeneration is the final pathophysiologic cause of disease, and may occur as a primary idiopathic disorder or secondary to another process such as aging. Physicians generally resist accepting degeneration as an explanation for disease, but there are many diseases that currently cannot be otherwise explained. For example, many people with senile dementia have a pathologic process of unexplained primary degeneration of brain cells. Degenerative joint disease is usually related to age and may be accelerated by unusual use or trauma, but it remains primarily a degenerative process with no specific vascular, metabolic, or inflammatory explanation.

It should also be clear that a particular disease may be caused or affected by a variety of pathophysiologic mechanisms. Peptic ulcer, for example, is a common disease with a multifactorial physiologic basis. The ulceration of the mucosal lining of the duodenum is caused by gastric acid, may occur in genetically predisposed people, and may be abetted by the toxic effect of drugs such as aspirin or corticosteroids that impair the protective barrier of the mucosa. There may be a secondary inflammation producing pain or obstruction, and the ulcer may erode a blood vessel, producing bleeding. To say that any single pathophysiologic process "causes" ulcers would be misleading.

Once the initial pathophysiologic process has given rise to a particular disease entity, its clinical manifestations are modified by a variety of host factors such as age, immunologic status, medication ingestion, concurrent disease, or psychological makeup. For example, in a healthy person with high tolerance for pain, a case of herpes zoster (shingles) may be perceived as a minor discomfort, whereas in a person with a low threshold for pain, it may become a disabling illness for which professional attention and potent analgesics are required. Under the influence of a concurrent disease or the ingestion of drugs such as steroids that suppress the immunologic response, a usually nonpathogenic fungal infection may produce serious illness. A minor inflammation of the connective tissue such as cellulitis, for example, may become a serious, life-threatening problem in a diabetic with an impaired vascular, sensory, or immunologic status. In a genetically susceptible host, an infectious agent may precipitate an inflammatory response and antibody production leading to systemic lupus erythematosus, whereas in a genetically nonsusceptible host it may not produce any effect.

Thus, there are a variety of pathophysiologic processes that can initiate disease, but the expression of the disease itself may be modified by a variety of factors in the host. Any review of a particular disease entity, therefore, should include consideration of both aspects, so that a complete understanding of the disease can be developed.

SYMPTOM PRODUCTION AND THE PATHOLOGIC PROCESS

A pathologic process may begin and exist silently for some time without producing any evidence of physiologic alteration. Although the disease is present and active, it may be undiscovered. In many chronic disease situations, it is now well known that the disease condition may be present for a considerable length of time before becoming detectable by current diagnostic procedures. Atherosclerosis, for example, has been detected at autopsy in healthy young 18-year-olds dying from accidental causes (15–17); many prostatic cancers are discovered at autopsy that were never recognized during life.

After a pathologic process has been present for a time, it may not only begin to produce physiologic alterations that can be discovered by appropriate diagnostic tests but may also begin to produce clinical symptoms that are, for the first time, recognized by the patient or the physician. There can be a significant time lag, however, between the onset of physiologic alteration and the production of symptoms, just as there was between the onset of the pathologic process and the physiologic alteration. A pathologic process may be present and discoverable by diagnostic tests long before it produces sufficient symptoms for a patient to feel its presence. Atherosclerosis and atherosclerotic vascular disease illustrate this continuum of pathologic process, physiologic alteration, and symptom production and are reviewed to provide further insight into the disease process.

Atherosclerosis is a pathologic process characterized by focal accumulation of lipids and complex carbohydrates, producing a secondary narrowing of the arteries. The process affects arterial vessels of the body in the cerebral, coronary, peripheral, and abdominal circulations and is now the leading cause of death in the United States.

As mentioned previously, atherosclerosis without physiologic alteration has been documented in 18-year-olds. At this stage, it is a subclinical or presymptomatic process and can be identified only by direct examination of the blood vessels.

Coronary artery disease is a specific manifestation of atherosclerosis in the arteries that provide blood to the heart muscle. As it becomes progressively more serious, it interferes with arterial capability for providing sufficient oxygen to meet the heart muscle's metabolic demands. As the reduction in oxygen supply worsens, ischemia of the heart muscle may occur. With still further progression, any increased demand on the cardiac muscle, as in any kind of exertion, may produce angina pectoris, or chest pain, the cardinal symptom of coronary artery disease.

Long before the angina is present, coronary artery disease may be identified by an abnormal electrocardiogram (EKG). If an EKG with the patient at rest does not produce evidence of disease, frequently an EKG during controlled exercise will yield the necessary evidence. In these cases, the coronary artery disease may not be sufficiently serious to produce EKG changes during normal demands on the heart, but the increased cardiac demands associated with exercise will provide the necessary diagnostic evidence.

These clinical changes may not evoke any symptoms, but eventually the patient may experience intermittent chest pain on exertion and seek medical care. At this time, the chances of obtaining an abnormal EKG and confirming the presence of coronary artery disease become much greater, but even at this stage a patient may have typical angina pain with an apparently normal EKG. The difficulty of defining the specific relationship between pathology and symptoms may be even greater. Both resting and exercise EKGs produce a number of false-positive and false-negative results. The absolute criterion for the definition of coronary artery disease becomes arteriography, the injection of dye to outline the coronary artery and the areas of narrowing. However, it should be understood that many people with no symptoms have demonstrable coronary artery disease, and that many others with classic anginal symptoms and characteristic EKG abnormalities have coronary arteries free of atherosclerosis. It has been well established in the literature that the same objective alterations in the EKG and classic symptoms may be produced by spasm rather than occlusion of the coronary arteries (18).

In patients with occlusive coronary artery disease, atherosclerosis may eventually occlude a coronary artery completely, causing the heart muscles supplied by the artery to die. This clinical event is known as *myocardial infarction*, commonly called a "heart attack," and is accompanied by prolonged chest pain, nausea, sweating, shortness of breath, and weakness. However, the arterial occlusion and subsequent tissue death may occur silently and without symptoms, to be discovered by EKG at some later date.

Following the pathologic process a step further, loss of heart muscle function secondary to coronary artery disease may affect the heart's ability to maintain adequate circulation to the rest of the body and may produce a range of secondary signs and symptoms in other organs. As the heart becomes weaker, there may be progessive difficulty in breathing, swelling of the legs and feet, inability to maintain blood supply to the brain and subsequent faintness, and impairment of kidney function with reduction of urinary output. These events are sometimes labeled by the single clinical description of *heart failure*.

Atherosclerosis is a generalized disease and is usually not limited to the coronary arteries; similar events occur in the blood vessels of other organs. This process may produce primary effects in organs that are not related to the secondary effects of heart failure described above. Abdominal pain, bowel necrosis, neurologic deficits, strokes, renal failure, calf pain, and aortic aneurysms may all be produced by atherosclerotic damage to the arteries of various organs. The combination of this primary damage to the organs themselves and the secondary effects of heart failure is complicated and serious, dramatically illustrating why atherosclerosis is such a major cause of morbidity and mortality.

THE PHYSIOLOGIC BASES OF DISEASE

Over the years, the pattern of diseases affecting the U.S. population has changed profoundly, generally as a result of changes in the environment, in the population's demographic composition, and in medical practice. Infectious diseases as the major cause of mortality have been replaced by chronic diseases associated with aging. At the turn of the century, infectious diseases struck the young and healthy and spread rapidly, often resulting in death. The confluence of improved sanitation, a higher standard of living, antibiotics, and vaccines reduced death and disability from infectious diseases so markedly that they are now a comparatively minor cause of death (see Chapter 1).

The treatability of syphilis, for example, has reduced its incidence and impact markedly, and cases with the secondary or tertiary manifestations of this potentially devastating disorder are now increasingly rare. Smallpox, polio, mumps, diphtheria, measles, pertussis, rubella, tetanus, typhoid, and cholera, all once highly prevalent, have now all but disappeared. Bacterial infections of childhood and infantile diarrheas of all kinds are now effectively treated with antibiotics and intravenous feedings; as a result, they do not present the threat they did at the turn of the century.

While these disease entities have been diminishing or disappearing, new disease patterns have been emerging to take their place as the most important threat to life and health. Some of these patterns have resulted from the removal of diseases in early life (e.g., childhood infections), which has allowed time for diseases in later life (e.g., atherosclerosis) to appear. Other disease patterns, however, are comparatively new, are far more prevalent than they once were, and are the result of new forces in modern life and environment.

Changes in the incidence and prevalence of some cancers, for example, provide dramatic evidence of these patterns (19). In the early part of the century, cancer of the lung was not a major cause of death, but it began to increase in men as the rate of cigarette smoking in men increased. The incidence of lung cancer in women lagged behind that of men until recently, when it began to rise to a comparable level, probably secondary to the increase in cigarette smoking among women.

In the same vein, there has been a rise in endometrial carcinoma in women, attributed at least in part to the increased use of estrogens by postmenopausal women (20). Pancreatic cancer has increased in recent years and is occurring at a younger age than previously, but no clear explanation of this changed disease pattern has been proposed. The etiologic factors contributing to the increased risk of pancreatic cancer have been subject to vigorous epidemiologic debate. Coffee in its caffeinated and decaffeinated forms has been implicated, with considerable refutation of these arguments (21). Again, recent years have seen a marked rise in mesothelioma, a previously rare type of lung cancer, probably secondary to the markedly increased use of asbestos in manufacturing and construction.

In the same fashion, improvement in our medical technology has changed the patterns of disease, not just by wiping out previously existing scourges but also by creating new ones (see Chapter 9). The morbidity and mortality of common diseases such as pneumonia and wound infections have been replaced by serious infections with once nonpathogenic bacteria that are now resistant to antibiotics. Patients whose own defense mechanisms have been compromised by corticosteroids, immunosuppressive agents, and cancer chemotherapy are now susceptible to serious infections with fungi, yeast, protozoa, or bacteria that are not normally harmful (22).

A dramatic expression of a new disease pattern is illustrated by acquired immune deficiency syndrome (AIDS), a state of serious impairment in an individual's immune mechanisms, giving rise to greatly increased susceptibility to a variety of infectious and neoplastic diseases (23–26). The initial descriptions of a series of previously rare infections in young and otherwise healthy homosexual men gave rise to a discovery of a condition with a myriad of pathologic manifestations as well as profound social and economic implications (27,28).

The human immunodeficiency virus (HIV) infects individuals and in selected cases produces a profound alteration and suppression of the host's natural immunity. The entity might therefore be considered an infectious disease because there is a specific infectious agent responsible for initiating the disease process. It must, however, also be acknowledged as an immunologic entity because the virus seems to produce no signs or symptoms but rather alters the immune system. The prevalence of infection seems to be far greater than the development of clinical expression, since there is a large population who have antibodies from the infection but who have no medically defined disease and another large population who have much milder manifestations of infection in a condition termed AIDS-related complex (ARC). Among actual AIDS patients, the manifestations of the illness cover a wide clinical spectrum, including *Pneumocystis carinii* infections of the lung, *Cryptosporidium* infections of the bowel, *Cytomegalovirus* infections of the eye, and Kaposi's sarcoma of a generalized nature.

While AIDS illustrates a fascinating new disease, its impact on care-seeking behavior may be greater than anticipated and, indeed, greater than any previous disease condition. Its existence and rapid spread have markedly changed social and sexual behavior among both the homosexual and heterosexual communities. Many people are voluntarily seeking blood tests for confirmation of possible AIDS, and serious consideration is being given to the imposition of mandatory testing for AIDS in certain special situations of travel or employment. The onset of an unexplained febrile illness in a sexually active person increasingly raises the fear of AIDS and stimulates a request for medical care for diseases that may be self-limited and for which no care would have previously been sought or needed. Recognition of the importance of the immune system as a critical link in the body's response to disease has increased society's awareness of possible immunity-related illnesses and has generated greater interest and greater use of health services in this regard.

A substantial percentage of hospitalizations are now attributable to drug toxicity and the secondary effects of new surgical procedures such as ileojejunal bypass for morbid obesity or the complications of kidney dialysis for chronic renal disease. Cardiac pacemakers prolong life but also produce a new spectrum of morbidity, as do other new prosthetic devices such as cardiac valves, artificial joints, or silicone implants. Organ transplantation has created an entirely new spectrum of biologic diseases based on intentional destruction of the body's immunologic system, its own basic protection from disease. Patients with bone marrow or renal transplants require considerable care and present diseases that are rare if they occur at all in normal, nonimmunosuppressed populations. The potential for transplanting other organs creates considerable flux in the biologic nature of disease and has frightening implications for the ability of persons to provide and pay for these services. The most dramatic example is the artificial heart, developed and implanted in a patient in December 1982 by a team at the University of Utah.

The increased effectiveness of medical intervention is also having a considerable effect on the patterns of disease by changing the gene pool controlling the incidence of certain diseases. Improvements in prenatal and high-risk obstetric care allow completion of pregnancies in diabetic women who otherwise may not have reproduced. This development may increase the prevalence of an already common disease such as diabetes. The successful introduction of vigorous physical therapy and prophylactic antibiotic use have increased the survival of patients with cystic fibrosis, and a few have successfully reproduced. The impact of the longer-term survival on the gene pool for this disease remains to be seen, but it is a good example of some of the potential hazards caused by new technology.

An additional powerful influence affecting our patterns of disease is environmental change. Motor vehicle accidents are an increasingly important cause of morbidity and mortality, and directly reflect our increasing use of the automobile for transportation. Pollution of air and water has already been suggested as at least partially causative in a number of conditions, and toxic aspects of industrial work environments have been suggested as the cause of many more. Indeed, it has been argued that as many as three-fourths of all cancers may be in part environmentally determined.

Dietary habits have also been suggested as contributing to changes in disease patterns in recent years. The most obvious result of dietary change is obesity, which is associated with hypertension, heart disease, and diabetes. Burkitt and associates have suggested that diverticulosis, hemorrhoids, appendicitis, and even cancer of the colon may be a consequence of changes in the amount of fiber in the Western diet. Epidemiologists have implicated certain foods as possible causes of atherosclerosis (29). Increased salt intake has already been indicted in certain aspects of hypertension, and increased ingestion of refined sugars has definitely been associated with increased incidence of dental caries and possibly with several other conditions.

In summary, in addition to a wide variety of causes of disease and a wide variety of responses in individual hosts, the overall pattern of disease in a society can change markedly over time. In this country, the pattern of disease has moved from one of acute infectious disease several generations ago to one of chronic disease today. Further, the pattern of disease has been influenced by our ability to wipe out certain diseases, thereby allowing others to be expressed. Finally, many aspects of modern life, such as improved medical technology and environmental pollution, have caused disease patterns that have never existed before.

SOCIAL AND CULTURAL INFLUENCES ON DISEASE AND BEHAVIOR

It has been estimated that 70 percent to 90 percent of all self-recognized illness is not generally treated in the conventional medical care delivery system (30). Conversely, it is reported that more than half of the visits to physicians are related to patient-identified problems for which no ascertainable biologic basis can be determined. It is clear, from this finding, that seeking medical care may or may not be associated with actual pathologic processes, and that social and cultural values greatly influence the individual's decision to visit a physician (31,32).

A large number of physician visits are for complaints in which the physiologic function is well within normal limits, but for which the patient feels that some abnormality exists. Many people seek medical attention for example, when bowel function is basically normal and no serious pathology can be documented. For some reason, either internally generated or imposed by the prevailing culture, these patients believe that the situation is not quite right and seek medical attention. They have somehow been led to expect bowel function that is different from what they are experiencing, and a medical remedy is sought.

Symptoms of fatigue may be attributed by the patient to a nondisease such as hypoglycemia (33). Conversely, a disease with a well-defined physiologic basis may not produce care seeking, since it may not be interpreted as a disease. The teenager with acne, for example, has a problem with a well-understood physiologic basis and an obvious clinical manifestation. The potential patient, however, may interpret it as a normal consequence of adolescence that will eventually resolve and for which treatment is either ineffective or unavailable (34). Seeking care for serious conditions is often delayed because of fear or uncertainty (35).

Disease and the perception of illness are not the only reasons people seek medical care. Normal physiologic processes frequently are the occasion for seeking care. Pregnancy or contraception are certainly not pathologic or disease processes, but they usually require professional attention. Heavy menstrual flow, missed or irregular periods, and menopause are usually the result of basically normal physiologic processes, and yet medical attention is frequently sought concerning them.

An event of modern times illustrates how medicalized normal physiologic processes can become and the interaction of social factors in creating the need for medical care. The increasing rates of infertility and the frighteningly high incidence of cesarean sections are modern medical problems. Many have attributed the current rates of infertility to the frequent delay in childbearing (36). This decrease in fertility has been well documented and has created substantial medical and psychologic problems and a tremendous base for care seeking. The rate of cesarean section is sometimes linked to this phenomenon and to the complex interaction of physician fear of litigation, the presence of monitoring equipment that allows detection of abnormalities that might not have affected the outcome, and the technologic advances that allow cesarean section to be performed with less morbidity than formerly existed. It is not only the perception of illness or the presence of disease, but also the alterations in normal physiologic functions and changes in medical practice influenced by social and technologic interventions, that create some of the reasons for care-seeking behavior.

Indeed, in many cases, medical care is sought because the patient is healthy and wants to remain that way. Parents bring infants and small children to the pediatrician for routine evaluations in order to ensure that the child is developing normally. Adults visit their physician periodically for an examination, a chest x-ray film, a Papanicolaou smear, and possibly other tests because they have been told it is important to do so. Indeed, all care seeking behavior is carried out in a framework that is intensely affected by current social, cultural, and political values, regardless of the type or severity of the pathologic process. Cultural influences frequently determine what society considers to be a medical problem, whereas economic or political realities determine whether or not medical care is sought. The complex interactions of people and doctors, the personal and cultural influence on disease, and the perception of symptoms have been well reviewed in the literature (32).

Zborowski (37) studied the differences in attribution between Italian and Jewish patients. Italians were generally satisfied and ceased demanding medical care once pain relief was obtained. Jews were reluctant to take medication and continued to be concerned with the underlying cause of their discomfort rather than simply relief of pain. It can be anticipated that they would continue to seek care until they were reassured that there was no serious underlying pathology.

The deep psychologic meaning of disease was explored by Cassel (38) in an article on suffering. He argued that suffering was experienced by people. It was not a physical construct, and it was often underappreciated by practicing physicians. He illustrated his point by suggesting that pain in circumstances such as childbirth, in which it is expected, rarely produces suffering and does not call for much care seeking because of discomfort. In contrast, situations in which pain is unexplained may give rise to considerable suffering and continued care seeking. He again argues that the physician's failure to appreciate and deal with the bases of suffering may lead to a failure to reassure the patient.

The complex psychologic underpinnings of care seeking are indicated by the remarkable ability of patients to respond to placebos. Placebos, which have been effective in reducing not only subjective symptoms but also objective test results, are a testament to the importance of symbolic intervention. They argue for a complex interaction between physician and patient on both verbal and nonverbal levels and demonstrate that the encounter itself and the therapeutic relationship have meaning to the individual who seeks medical services (39). Many authors have recently argued that physicians do not fully recognize the social and cultural determinants of care seeking. An illuminating article on the couvade syndrome demonstrated failure by physicians in a prepaid practice to recognize the influence of a woman's pregnancy on the husband's medical complaints (40). In the couvade syndrome, husbands of pregnant women have symptoms such as nausea, vomiting, anorexia, pain, and bloating—feelings often experienced by their wives—while having no objective organic abnormalities. In this study, husbands of pregnant women had two times the number of physician visits, four times the number of symptoms, and two times the number of prescriptions without any increase in actual pathology during the period of their wives' pregnancy as compared to other periods. The study illustrates the myriad influences on the production of symptoms and the need to seek medical care. It has increasingly been argued that consumerism and a critical analysis of health care needs and physician limitations can give rise to a more productive physician-patient relationship (41). Health care administrators must understand the complex influences on care seeking and design systems that identify both the physical abnormalities and the cultural determinants that provide the impetus for seeking medical services.

As social and cultural values change, the understanding of what constitutes disease and the subsequent care-seeking patterns may change as well (42,43). The transference of marital adjustment and childrearing problems from the category of family problems best handled by a member of the clergy to psychologic problems best handled by a physician or psychologist is one example of this trend. The recent shift toward the description of alcoholism as a disease requiring medical treatment is another. A further example is the court decision changing abortion from a criminal act to a recognized medical service. The numerous manifestations of psychological problems, discussed further in Chapter 8, represent many examples of difficult to define illness with a substantial political and value-laden component.

In all of these examples, it should be noted that the underlying pathologic process has not changed; rather, it is the perception of these processes as disease or not that has been altered. In other circumstances, even our perception of certain conditions as illnesses does not change; instead, external social values change the way we react to them.

For example, the increased mobility and weakened family structure of modern American life have made it more difficult to care for elderly and infirm family members at home. Smaller housing units, increased numbers of families in which both adults are employed, and a variety of other social pressures have altered the ability to handle the health problems of the elderly in the fashion of the past. Instead, society has created a new network of health institutions—nursing homes—to provide professional care for pathologic processes that previously were handled at home. The underlying pathologic processes have remained the same. It is the societal response to them that has changed (44).

THE INFLUENCE OF SUPPLY

Within the total spectrum of pathologic processes that affect the health of people in this country, it is important to note that some processes receive much more interest and attention from the health care system than others. It is also important to speculate about why this occurs.

The structure and availability of health services contribute significantly to the amount and nature of the care that will be sought. Once the patient makes the initial decision to seek professional attention, much of the additional medical care results directly from the decisions of the physician (43). The physician usually decides what laboratory tests, x-ray films, treatment procedures, and hospitalizations are necessary, and in so doing shapes a particular pattern of care for each patient. In some ways, these decisions by the physician also shape the health care system itself by creating a demand for certain services. As long as the demand exists, the institutions, programs, and services will expand to fill the need.

But does the process work this way, or is the reverse true? Do pathologic processes stimulate patients to visit physicians, who, in turn, demand certain services as a result of their decisions? Or do the specialized services become available to physicians, thereby influencing the manner in which they approach disease, and do physicians then shape patients' perceptions and demands on the basis of what they know is available (45)? There is some evidence to suggest that the latter is true, at least in part, and is becoming progressively more important.

Physicians generally do most of their training in hospitals and are introduced early to the use and benefits of sophisticated procedures and tests. The availability of these tests and treatments then influences the physicians' view of disease, since they now make possible the treatment of conditions that were previously beyond consideration. The surgical treatment of degenerative processes such as hip replacement for osteoarthritis, laser treatment for diabetic retinopathy, and replacement of diseased heart valves with prosthetic devices have all created many new options for the physician. They have also created new reasons for patients to seek care.

Unfortunately, the development of these new approaches is not always in keeping with the real need for care among patients, as determined by the pathologic processes that threaten them. The mere fact that a particular process, such as arthritis or alcoholism, has a major impact on public health does not necessarily mean that sophisticated technology will be developed to deal with it. Instead, the more sophisticated technologies are frequently developed in areas of lesser importance, leaving more serious problems relatively less well attended. Patients' perceptions of illness and its importance are then shaped more by areas where major technology is available than by areas of perhaps greater need.

The influence of suppliers on the demand for medical care has increased in the past several years. There has been a significant increase in the offering of specialized "boutique" medical services, which may not be appreciated initially by the public but which are actively marketed and eventually widely used. The proliferation of weight control programs, substance abuse programs, and eating disorder programs are but a few examples of providers generating a perception of need and stimulating care-seeking behavior.

Eating disorder—with its hallmark disease, bulimia—illustrates the complex interface between physiology and psychology. How does a normal behavior that results in episodic weight gain and weight loss differ from the behavior of those individuals who binge-eat and use diuretics, laxatives, and enemas as a means of accelerating weight loss. At what point does a natural interest in weight and appearance become a pathologic process in need of costly professional intervention? While physicians and psychologists may debate the definition of disease, the frequent bombardment of radio and television advertising creates the perception of illness in a certain number of individuals who would not previously label themselves as ill. While advertising may make a segment of the population aware of an advance, such as intraocular lens implants for the elderly who might have otherwise considered it unaffordable, the consistent interest in generating new sources of income by health care institutions and providers may be creating an unnatural emphasis on illness for which biologic and behavioral variation are more likely explanations.

It is unclear whether the development of pathologic processes or the availability of services to treat them creates the demand for health care. It is clear, however, that the use of medical services is the result of a unique interaction involving the pathologic processes themselves, the patient's and the physicians's perceptions of them, and the availability of services to deal with them (46). Each of these elements must be considered if the use of health services is to be better understood by all concerned.

REFERENCES

1. Apple D: How laymen define illness. *J Health Hum Behav* 1960; 1:219–225.
2. Retchin SM, Fletcher RH, Earp JA, et al: Mitral valve prolapse: Disease or illness? *Arch Intern Med* 1986; 146:1081.
3. Tobi M, Straus SE: Chronic Epstein-Barr virus disease. A workshop held by the National Institute of Pathology and Infectious Disease. *Ann Intern Med* 1985; 103:251–254.
4. Centers for Disease Control: Chronic fatigue possibly related to Epstein-Barr virus in Nevada. *Mort Morb Weekly Rep* 1986; 35:350–352.
5. Siperstein MD: The glucose tolerance test: A pitfall in the diagnosis of diabetes mellitus. *Adv Intern Med* 1975; 20:297–323.
6. O'Sullivan JB, Mahan CM: Prospective study of 352 young patients with chemical diabetes. *New Engl J Med* 1968; 278:1038–1041.
7. National Diabetes Data Group: Classification and diagnosis of diabetes mellitus and other categories of glucose intolerance. *Diabetes* 1979; 28:1039–1057.
8. Mabry J: Lay concepts of etiology. *J Chronic Dis* 1964; 17:371–386.
9. Lowenfels AB: Alcoholism and the risk of cancer. *Ann NY Acad Sci* 1975; 252:366–373.
10. Merliss RR: Talc-treated rice and Japanese stomach cancer. *Science* 1971; 173:1141–1142.

11. Selikoff IJ, Churg J, Hammond EC: Asbestos exposure and neoplasia. *JAMA* 1964; 188:22–26.

12. Poskanzer DC, Herbst AL: Epidemiology of vaginal adenosis and adenocarcinoma associated with exposure to stilbestrol in utero. *Cancer* 1977; 39(suppl):1892–1895.

13. Dungal N: The special probelm of stomach cancer in Iceland with particular reference to dietary factors. *JAMA* 1961; 178:789–798.

14. Lowenfels AB, Anderson ME: Diet and cancer. *Cancer* 1977; 39(suppl): 1809–1814.

15. Enos WF, Beyer JC, Holmes RH: Pathogenesis of coronary disease in American soldiers killed in Korea. *JAMA* 1958; 158:912–914.

16. Enos WF, Holmes RH, Beyer JC: Coronary disease among United States soldiers killed in action in Korea. *JAMA* 1953; 152:1090–1093.

17. McNamara JJ, Molot MA, Stremple JF, et al: Coronary artery disease in combat casualties in Vietnam. *JAMA* 1971; 216:1185–1187.

18. Meller J, Pichard A, Dack S: Coronary arterial spasm in Prinzmetal's angina: A proven hypothesis. *Am J Cardiol* 1976; 37:938.

19. Kritchevsky D: Metabolic effects of dietary fiber. *West J Med* 1979; 130:123–127.

20. Schwarz BE: Does estrogen cause adenocarcinoma of the endometrium? *Clin Obstet Gynecol* 1981; 24:243–251.

21. McMahon B, Yen S, Trichopoulos D, et al: Coffee and cancer of the pancreas. *New Engl J Med* 1981; 304:630–633.

22. Stamm WE: Nonsocomial infections: Etiologic changes, therapeutic challenges. *Hosp Pract* 1981; 16:75–88.

23. Centers for Disease Control: Update: acquired immunodeficiency syndrome—United States. *JAMA* 1987; 257:433–441.

24. Bowen DL, Lane HD, Fauci AS: Immunopathogenesis of the acquired immuno-deficiency syndrome. *Ann Intern Med* 1985; 103:704–708.

25. Laurence J: The immune system in AIDS. *Sci Am* 1985; 253:84–90.

26. Montagnier L: Lymphadenopathy-associated virus: From molecular biology to pathogenicity. *Ann Intern Med* 1985; 103:689–704.

27. Centers for Disease Control: *Pneumocystis* pneumonia—Los Angeles. *Mort Morb Weekly Rep* 1981; 30:250–252.

28. Centers for Disease Control: Kaposi's sarcoma and pneumocystis pneumonia among homosexual men—New York City and California. *Mort Morb Weekly Rep* 1981; 30:305–308.

29. Turpeinen O: Effect of cholesterol-lowering diet on mortality from coronary heart disease and other causes. *Circulation* 1979; 59:1–7.

30. Dingle JH, Badger GF, Jordan WS: Illness in the home: A study of 25,000 illnesses in a group of Cleveland families. Western Reserve University, 1964.

31. Zola IK: Culture and symptoms: An analysis of patients' presenting complaints. *Am Sociol Rev* 1966; 31:615–630.

32. Stocker JD, Barsky AJ: Attributions: Uses of social science knowledge in the "doctoring" of primary care, in Eisenberg L, Kleinman A (eds): *The Relevance of Social Science for Medicine*. Hingham, Mass: D Reidel Publishing Co, 1980, pp 223–240.

33. Meador CK: Art and science of nondisease. *New Engl J Med* 1965; 272:92–95.

34. Ludwig EG, Gibson G: Self perception of sickness and the seeking of medical care. *J Health Soc Behav* 1969; 10:125–133.

35. Battistella RM: Factors associated with delay in the initiation of physicians' care among late adulthood persons. *Am J Public Health* 1971; 61:1348–1361.

36. DeCherney AH, Berkowitz GS: Female fecundity and age. *New Engl J Med* 1982; 306:424–426.

37. Zborowsky M: Cultural components in responses in pain. *J Social Issues* 1952; 8:16–30.

38. Cassell EJ: The nature of suffering and the goals of medicine, *New Engl J Med* 1982; 306:639–644.

39. Brody H: The lie that heals: The ethics of giving placebos. *Ann Intern Med* 1982; 97:112–118.

40. Lyokinji M, Lamb GS: The Couvade syndrome: An epidemiologic study. *Ann Intern Med* 1982; 96:509–511.

41. Jensen PS: The doctor-patient relationship: Headed for impasse or improvement? *Ann Intern Med* 1981; 95:769–771.

42. Parsons T: Definitions of health and illness in the light of American values and social structure, in Jaco EG (ed): *Patients, Physicians and Illness.* Glencoe, Ill, Free Press of Glencoe, 1958, pp 165–187.

43. Fuch V: *Who Shall Live? Health, Economics and Social Choice.* New York, Basic Books, 1974.

44. Somers AR: Long term care for the elderly and disabled: A new health priority. *New Engl J Med* 1982; 307:221–226.

45. Stoeckle JD, Zola IK, Davidson GE: On going to see the doctor, the contributions of the patient to the decision to seek medical aid: A selective review. *J Chronic Dis* 1963; 16:975–989.

46. Rosenstock IM: Why people use health services. *Milbank Mem Fund Q* 1966; 44 (Part 2):94–127.

CHAPTER 3

Indicators and Predictors of Health Services Utilization

Lu Ann Aday
Stephen M. Shortell

The utilization of health services is concerned with who does and does not receive medical care and why; and, for those who do, how much and what types of care they consume. Utilization data may be obtained from surveys asking people about their health care; from files of practicing physicians; or from hospital or other institutional record sources.

From the point of view of health policy, planning, program administration and evaluation, and knowing who did not receive care and why are equally as or more important than describing the actual utilization patterns for those who do.

Health policy analysts and program evaluators, for example, want to know the impact of health policies or programs or changes in these over time (e.g., Medicaid, Medicare) on whether the people most directly targeted by the programs are actually served and/or use services at higher or lower rates as a result. Health planners are concerned with identifying areas of greatest need or highest potential demand in the target communities for new health care delivery organizations. Health care program administrators want to know the share of the health care market captured by their facility and whether special programs they may have developed are having the desired impact in changing patterns of care (e.g., seeing women earlier in their pregnancy, reducing inpatient utilization). Physicians and nurses are concerned with patients who delay obtaining care in response to serious symptoms and with those who fail to comply with prescribed medical regimens. Social workers, discharge planners, and case managers need to take into account the social and psychological, as well as physiological, factors in formulating appropriate patient care plans. All of these issues are informed by understanding approaches to conceptualizing, measuring, and predicting health services utilization behavior.

The discussion that follows reviews (1) ways in which the utilization of health services have been conceptualized and measured, (2) major analytic models that have been developed to explain health care-seeking behavior, (3) selected empirical findings on utilization, and (4) current policy issues that can benefit from studies of health care utilization.

CONCEPTUALIZATION AND MEASUREMENT OF HEALTH SERVICES UTILIZATION

Utilization may be characterized in a number of different ways. Four principal dimensions of the concept are, however, reflected in most empirical indicators of utilization: the type, purpose, site, and time interval of use.

The *type* of utilization refers principally to the category of service rendered—physician, dental or other practitioners' services, hospital or long-term care admissions, prescriptions, medical equipment, and so on. The *purpose* refers to the reason care was sought: for health maintenance in the absence of symptoms (primary prevention), for the diagnosis or treatment of illness in the interest of returning to a previous state of well-being (secondary prevention), or rehabilitation or maintenance in the case of a long-term health problem (tertiary prevention). Another reason for rendering care is the maintenance or custodial care of medically fragile or dependent adults or children, in which the personal, as well as medical care, needs of the patient are met. The *site* or organizational unit refers to the place services were received. It might be in an inpatient setting (e.g., short-term-stay hospital, mental institution, nursing home) or ambulatory setting (e.g., hospital outpatient department or emergency room, physician's office, Health Maintenance Organization (HMO), public health clinic, community health center, free-standing emergency center), or the patient's home. The *time interval* refers to measures of (1) contact, based on whether the service was received during a particular time period (e.g., proportion seeing a physician within the last year); (2) volume, the total units of service received during that period (e.g., mean number of visits in a year for those seeing a physician); or (3) episodic patterns, based on the patterns of providers, referrals, and continuity of care for a given occurrence or episode of illness.

These dimensions are not mutually exclusive. A single utilization indicator may, in fact, be descriptive of a number of different dimensions. The "proportion seeing a physician in the year for a particular symptom" reflects, for example, the type, purpose, and time interval of utilization. It is important to understand, however, that different indicators may well reflect different stages of or reasons for seeking care. In choosing a relevant utilization indicator, it is important to consider the precise dimension(s) one is interested in examining and what measures best operationalize it. Further, the process of selecting the appropriate models and variables for predicting or explaining utilization should be guided by their relevance to the particular dimension(s) of utilization being considered.

ANALYTIC MODELS OF
HEALTH SERVICES UTILIZATION

Over the past 20 years there has been considerable interest in integrating the multiplicity of factors found to be associated with health services utilization into conceptual models to guide the conduct of research for understanding who uses health care services and who does not and why. The development of these models is of interest from both more theoretical and applied points of view. They contribute to an understanding of health care behavior in a broad sense by clarifying how it might be influenced by social, psychological, economic, institutional, and other factors. They also provide guidance for practical health policy decisions about what might be changed to facilitate individuals' or groups' receiving care when they need it.

There has been a considerable interest expressed in recent years with developing a systems approach to understanding utilization behavior that would integrate the range of institutional and individual factors associated with decisions to seek care. This systems perspective is represented to a considerable extent by the Behavioral Model of Health Services Utilization introduced by Ronald Andersen in 1968 and expanded by Andersen, Aday, and their colleagues to have broad applicability for measuring access to medical care (1–7). The discussion that follows describes the Andersen and Aday framework and the contributions and limitations of this and other major conceptual models in understanding health care utilization behavior.

BEHAVIORAL MODEL OF HEALTH SERVICES UTILIZATION

The expanded Behavioral Model of Health Services Utilization is portrayed in Figure 3-1 and the principal indicators used to operationalize various aspects of the model appear in Table 3-1.

Utilization, particularly as it might indicate the population's or a subgroup's access to medical care, is often evaluated in a political context. For example, major health care financing (e.g., Medicare and Medicaid) and organizational programs (e.g., community health center, preferred provider arrangements) have been concerned with improving target groups' ability to obtain care when it is needed. It is the effect of health policy on altering the utilization of and access to medical care that health policymakers and administrators often wish to evaluate. Thus it may well be appropriate to view health policy as the starting point for consideration of utilization behavior.

The delivery system component of the model refers to those arrangements for the potential rendering of care to consumers. It includes both their availability (volume and distribution of services) and organization (mechanisms for entry and movement through the system). These characteristics are aggregate, structural properties. The community, or a particular delivery organization, is the unit of analysis rather than the individual.

The characteristics of the population-at-risk are the predisposing, enabling, and need components in Andersen's original Behavioral Model of Health Services Utilization (5).

Predisposing variables include those that describe the propensity of individuals to use services—including basic demographic characteristics (e.g., age, sex, family size),

TABLE 3-1. Operational Indicators of the Expanded Behavioral Model

I. Characteristics of health delivery system
  A. Availability
    1. Volume
      a. Personnel
        i. Number of primary care physicians
        ii. Number of specialists
      b. Facilities
        i. Number of hospitals
        ii. Number of hospital beds
    2. Distribution
      a. Number of personnel per 1000 population
      b. Number of facilities per 1000 population
  B. Organization
    1. Entry
      a. Convenience of regular source of care
        i. Availability of services at night, on weekends, and in emergencies, house calls
        ii. Mode of transportation
        iii. Travel time
        iv. Appointment system and waiting time
        v. Office waiting time
        vi. Time physician spends with the patient (on average)
      b. Sources of medical care used by those with no regular source
        i. Reasons for not having a regular source
        ii. Places that people without a regular source did or will go to for care
    2. Structure
    a. Type of regular source of care
        i. Location of provider
        ii. Type of provider
        iii. Types of paramedical provider
        iv. Specialty of attending physician
      b. Type and extent of third-party coverage
        i. Type of health plans
        ii. Extent of coverage
        iii. Out-of-pocket cost of care

II. Characteristics of population at risk
  A. Predisposing
    1. Mutable
      a. General health care beliefs and attitudes
      b. Knowledge of health care information
    2. Immutable
      a. Age
      b. Sex
      c. Family size
      d. Race and ethnicity
      e. Education
      f. Employment status
  B. Enabling
    1. Mutable
      a. Family income
      b. Type and convenience of regular source of care[a]
      c. Type and extent of third-party coverage[a]
    2. Immutable
      a. Residence
      b. Region
      c. Length of time in community
  C. Need
    1. Perceived
      a. Health status
      b. Episode of illness
      c. Symptoms of illness
      d. Disability days
    2. Evaluated
      a. Physician severity ratings of condition
      b. Physician severity ratings for symptoms

III. Utilization of health services
  A. Type
    1. Physician
    2. Dentist
    3. Hospital
    4. Long-term care
  B. Site
    1. Location of nonhospital visits with physician in the year
    2. Location of visits to a physician in connection with illness episode

[a] A fuller description of these indicators is provided under the entry and structure heading for the characteristics of the health delivery system.

54

TABLE 3-1. (Continued)

C. Purpose
 1. Prevention
  a. General preventive exam
  b. Diagnostic procedures
 2. Illness-related
  a. Response to symptoms experienced in the year
  b. Use in response to disability
 3. Custodial
  a. Nursing home stays reported in connection with illness episode
  b. Other long-term stays
D. Time interval
 1. Contact
  a. Percent seeing provider in the year
  b. Percent hospitalized in the year
 2. Volume
  a. Mean visits in the year
  b. Mean admissions and hospital days in the year
 3. Continuity
  a. Profile of care in response to illness episodes
  b. Summary indexes of continuity of care
IV. Consumer satisfaction
 A. On most recent visit to usual source of care
 B. With medical care in general

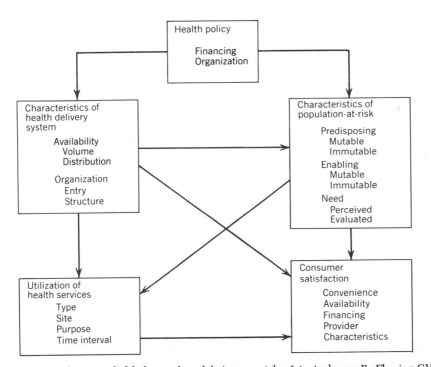

Figure 3-1. The expanded behavioral model. (SOURCE: Aday LA, Andersen R, Fleming GV: *Health Care in the U.S.: Equitable for Whom?* Copyright © 1980 by Sage Publications, Inc. Reprinted by permission of Sage Publications, Inc.)

social structural variables (e.g., race and ethnicity, education, employment status and occupation), and beliefs (e.g., general beliefs and attitudes about the value of health services', and/or of physicians' knowledge of disease). For example, age is highly correlated with the need for care. Variables such as ethnicity, education, and occupation suggest the importance of life style and environmental influences on individuals' decisions to seek care. People who believe strongly in the value of health care or physicians might be more likely to seek care than those who do not have these beliefs.

The enabling component describes the means individuals have available to them for the use of services. Both resources specific to individuals and their families (income, insurance coverage) and attributes of the community or region in which an individual lives are included here. Place of residence—for example, whether one lives in a rural or urban area—may indicate geographic proximity to a source of care as well as local attitudes about health care.

Need refers to health status or illness, which is the most immediate and important cause of health service use. The need for care may be perceived by the individual and reflected in reported symptoms or disability days, for example, or evaluated by the provider in terms of the actual diagnoses or severity of presenting complaints.

Those characteristics that are biological or social givens, such as one's age, sex, race, or place of residence are termed *immutable*. Health policy cannot directly alter these attributes, but they are defining of target groups of interest. The more manipulable beliefs and enabling variables, such as insurance coverage, are characteristics which health policy seeks to change in order to affect these groups' access to care. They are "mutable" to or alterable by health policy.

This model has been applied to evaluate whether services are fairly or equitably distributed. To the extent that differences in utilization are explained primarily by medical need variables and demographic correlates of need (e.g., age, sex), the distribution of services is said to be equitable. If other factors (e.g., insurance coverage, income) are the most important predictors of who gets care, then an inequitable system is said to exist (8,9).

In the expanded Behavioral Model, applied to measuring the concept of access, the principal outcomes of interest were objective measures of health services utilization, as well as subjective assessments by consumers of their recent utilization experiences.

A number of criticisms have been offered of this framework. Wolinsky (10) and Becker and Maiman (11) have, for example, argued that because of the range of variables and differing levels of analysis included, it is difficult to gather data to test the complete model. Mechanic (12) notes that major multivariate studies of health services utilization applying this and other comprehensive models of utilization behavior have failed to confirm the importance of certain psychosocial and organizational factors borne out in other studies. He offers a number of explanations for these results: (1) the measures of perceived *need* used actually incorporate concepts of psychological distress as well but are not interpreted as such, (2) the use of aggregate system-level resource availability indicators for large areas does not adequately capture the experience of individuals in their local communities, and (3) the large-scale multivariate studies fail to adequately model patient decision making about the care-seeking process. He argues that in bringing the literature on larger-scale quantitative studies and smaller-scale qualitative approaches together, it is important "to recognize that what are characterized as 'illness' variables in the multivariate studies are more appropriately seen as illness-behavior measures incorporating various learned inclinations, and life events as well as physical illness" (12:395).

In the discussion that follows other efforts to develop comprehensive, systems models of health services utilization, as well as those that focus more directly on modeling the processes for decision-making surrounding illness that Mechanic describes, are reviewed.

OTHER COMPREHENSIVE MODELS OF HEALTH SERVICES UTILIZATION

In a comprehensive review of the literature on health services utilization in the early 1970s, McKinlay (13) identified six major approaches to characterizing the predictors of health services utilization: (1) demographic, (2) social structural, (3) social psychological, (4) economic, (5) organizational, and (6) systems (see Table 3-2). They may be identified principally by the types of predictors they emphasize.

Many of these indicators are ones that appear in the Behavioral Model described earlier. Of particular interest is how the systems approach facilitates the specification of the causal linkages between variables and their direct and indirect impact on the ultimate utilization outcomes of interest. Anderson (14:197), for example, concludes, "What is sorely needed is careful, theoretically based attempts to explicate causal structures that incorporate major features of all [the] approaches. The social systems approach appears to provide a valuable framework in which such research can be undertaken."

A number of studies have been carried out in recent years attempting to specify and test the causal relationships implied in the Behavioral Model directly (15–23). Others attempt to model a somewhat different set of relationships in specifying the operation of the health care system (24–26). The relative impact of selected indicators considered separately and in the context of analyses controlling for other factors is summarized in the discussion of empirical findings on utilization later in the chapter.

What is important to underline here is that various factors may account for who ultimately obtains care; considerable progress has been made in measuring and specifying the relationships among these different factors, and the systems perspective provides an integrative framework for considering many of these factors and their interrelationships; however, more focused studies are required to adequately model the causal relationships and internal processes associated with individual patients' decisions to seek care. The discussion that follows reviews a number of these efforts. [It

TABLE 3-2. Six Approaches to Characterizing the Predictors of Health Services Utilization

Model	Predictors
Demographic	Age, sex, marital status, family size, residence
Social structural	Social class, ethnicity, education, occupation
Social psychological	Health beliefs, values, attitudes, norms, culture
Economic	Family income, insurance coverage, price of services, provider/population ratios
Organizational	Organization of physicians' practices, referral patterns, use of ancillaries, regular source of care
Systems	All or most of the above considered in the context of set of interrelationships

draws heavily from review articles by Becker and Maiman (11), Becker et al. (27), and Janz and Becker (28).]

MODELS OF PATIENT DECISION-MAKING

Suchman

The dimension of utilization that is the focus of Suchman's framework for stages of decision making about seeking medical care is an episode of illness. In Suchman's paradigm, the sequence of seeking medical care for illness is divided into five stages: (1) the experience of the symptom, (2) assumption of the sick role, (3) medical care contact, (4) dependent-patient role, and (5) recovery or rehabilitation. At each stage, the patient makes certain decisions and engages in particular types of health care behavior (29,30).

At the first stage, one perceives that something is wrong, based on the physical sensation of pain or discomfort; this is followed by a cognitive interpretation of the symptom's importance given its impact on one's functioning and finally by an emotional reaction of fear or anxiety. During this stage the patient may use nonprescribed home remedies to deal with the symptoms. Theoretically one would then move to the next stage of response and assume the sick role, although one could also deny having the illness or delay, beginning to act like someone who is ill.

At the point of assuming the sick role, however, one would begin to relinquish one's usual roles and obligations, such as stay in bed or not go to work and request provisional validation for the sick role from family members or friends that constitute one's lay referral system. One may continue to use home remedies, based on their advice as well.

In the next stage, help is sought from a professional medical provider to provide legitimation for the sick role and negotiate the proper treatment for the condition. As in the previous two stages, the individual may not accept the recommended therapies and might shop around for another professional opinion.

In the dependent-patient role stage, the individual accepts professional judgment and undergoes the recommended treatment. This stage is seen as necessary to restore the patient to good health. A variety of factors, including the quality of the physician–patient relationship itself might, however, interfere with patient compliance with the recommended regimens.

In the final stage of recovery and rehabilitation, the patient is called on to relinquish the sick role and resume normal activities. Some people may refuse to give up the sick role at this point, however, and become chronic malingerers.

Suchman then proceeds to pose a theoretical explanation for the impact that social structure and associated medical orientations might have on the patient's progression through these stages. A group with more parochial or traditional, in contrast to more cosmopolitan, affiliations and a popular, rather than more scientific, orientation toward medical care would, he suggests, be more likely to delay in recognizing the seriousness of the symptoms initially, linger longer in the stage in which one uses home remedies and seeks support from family and friends, be suspicious of medical providers and maybe shop around more, fail to adhere to prescribed regimens, and relinquish the sick role as soon as possible (31).

Suchman's model is an interesting conceptual framework for the various stages many patients might go through in responding to illness. There has not, however, been strong empirical support for Suchman's formulation of the impact of the social structure and medical orientation on these stages of care seeking (33–34).

Kosa and Robertson

Kosa and Robertson (35) have formulated another model for explaining decisions to seek medical care in the context of an episode of illness. Whereas Suchman's model tended to offer more sociological or social structural explanations for why individuals might respond differently at different stages of the illness episode, Kosa and Robertson's explanation is more psychological in focus. Behavior is motivated by the individual's psychological need to reduce the anxiety aroused by the threat of illness. Anxiety might be of two kinds: "floating anxiety" (generalized anxiety that is not directly connected with the illness episode) and "specific anxiety" (the psychological response to physical discomfort proportionate to the seriousness of the symptoms experienced).

The Kosa–Robertson formulation is a process model as well with stages organized around the episode of illness. The principal components include (1) an assessment of a disturbance in usual functioning, (2) anxiety arousal based on a perception of the symptoms, (3) the application of one's medical knowledge to address the problem, and (4) the performance of activities to alleviate the anxiety. Activities may be of one of two kinds: "therapeutic interventions" that are directed at the removal of a particular health problem and its concomitant anxiety or "gratificatory interventions" aimed at relieving the anxiety or satisfying other needs without addressing the underlying health problem directly. The model does not deny the importance of external social factors, however. Each stage of the process is influenced by these psychological dynamics as well as the culture and social groups of which one is a part (e.g., family) or with which they come in contact (e.g., professional medical providers). There has, however, not been substantial empirical verification of the Kosa–Robertson framework.

Mechanic

Mechanic is concerned more generally with the variety of factors that influence individuals' experiences of symptoms in seeking care for illness-related reasons. It is not a process model in the context of an illness episode as are the Suchman and Kosa–Robertson formulations. It addresses, however, a variety of social and psychological factors that influence patients' perceptions of the need to seek medical care. These include the following:

> (1) visibility, recognizability, or perceptual salience of deviant signs and symptoms; (2) the extent to which symptoms are perceived as serious (that is, the person's estimate of the present and future probabilities of danger); (3) the extent to which symptoms disrupt family, work, and other social activities; (4) the frequency of the appearance of deviant signs or symptoms, their persistence, or their frequency or recurrence; (5) the tolerance thresholds of those who are exposed to and evaluate the deviant signs and symptoms; (6) available information, knowledge, and cultural assumptions and understandings of the evaluator; (7) basic needs that lead to denial; (8) needs competing with illness responses; (9) competing possible interpretations that can be assigned to the symptoms once they are recognized; and (10) availability of treatment resources, physical proximity, and psycho-

logical and monetary costs of taking action (included are not only physical distance and costs of time, money, and effort, but also such costs as stigma, social distance, and feelings of humiliation) (36:268–269).

These variables are identified as influencing "help seeking" from the point of view of the patient. They may or may not be associated with the need for care as defined by the provider, however. Further, Mechanic distinguishes "other-defined" from "self-defined" illnesses. The former differs from the latter in that the definition of illness originates with others in the environment, and the sick individual may resist this labeling and have to be brought into treatment involuntarily. It is, therefore, applicable to mental illness as well as situations when dependent children or adults may resist required medical treatment (37).

HEALTH BELIEF MODEL

One of the more social psychological oriented models for explaining decisions to seek medical care that has been subject to considerable empirical testing as well is the Health Belief Model (HBM). As originally conceived, it was applied to understanding preventive care (health behavior) but has subsequently been applied to explaining care seeking in response to illness (illness behavior) and those activities required for recovery from illness (sick role behavior) (11,27,28,38–42). In the HBM (see Fig. 3-2), a variety of diverse demographic, sociopsychological, and structural factors may influence behavior. They are, however, believed to work through their effects on the individual's subjective perceptions and motivations (beliefs), rather than functioning as direct causes of the behavior themselves.

The basic perceptual components of the model are as follows:

1. The individual's subjective state of readiness to take action, which is determined by both the individual's perceived likelihood of "susceptibility" to the particular illness and perceptions of the probable "severity" of the consequences (organic and/or social) of contracting the disease.
2. The individual's evaluation of the advocated health behavior in terms of its feasibility and efficaciousness (i.e., subjective estimate of the action's potential "benefits" in reducing susceptibility and/or severity), weighed against perceptions of physical, financial, and other costs ("barriers") involved in the proposed action.
3. A "cue to action" must occur to trigger the appropriate health behavior, coming from either internal (e.g., symptoms) or external (e.g., interpersonal interactions, mass media media communications) sources (11).

There is a large body of empirical evidence testing the applicability of the HBM to explaining preventive, illness-related, and sick role (especially compliance) behavior. "Perceived barriers" appeared to be an important predictor across all of the types of behavior examined. In most of the studies perceived susceptibility to illness was associated with engaging in a variety of preventive behaviors, such as having a Papanicolaou (Pap) test, influenza vaccination, preventive dental visit, and screening for Tay-Sachs disease. The other components of the model were less strongly or consistently associated.

In prediction of illness behavior (in response to perceived symptoms), the perceived benefits of seeking care appear to be associated, while the results for the

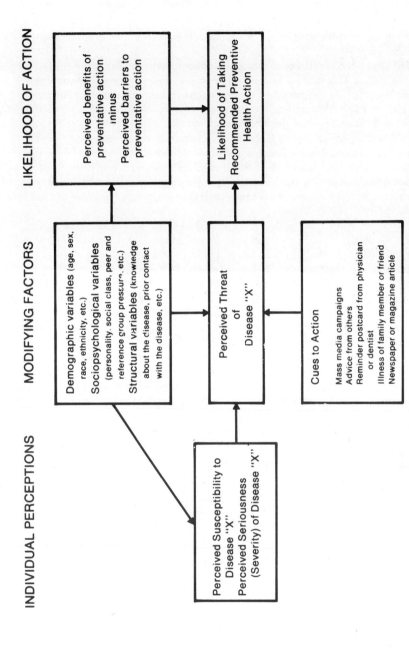

INDIVIDUAL PERCEPTIONS | MODIFYING FACTORS | LIKELIHOOD OF ACTION

Demographic variables (age, sex, race, ethnicity, etc.)
Sociopsychological variables (personality, social class, peer and reference group pressure, etc.)
Structural variables (knowledge about the disease, prior contact with the disease, etc.)

Perceived Susceptibility to Disease "X"
Perceived Seriousness (Severity) of Disease "X"

Perceived Threat of Disease "X"

Cues to Action
Mass media campaigns
Advice from others
Reminder postcard from physician or dentist
Illness of family member or friend
Newspaper or magazine article

Perceived benefits of preventative action minus Perceived barriers to preventative action

Likelihood of Taking Recommended Preventive Health Action

Figure 3-2. The health belief model. (SOURCE: Rosenstock IM: Historical origins of the health belief model, *Health Educ Monogr* 1974; 2:344. Adapted from Becker MH, Drachman RH, Kirscht JP, et al: A new approach to explaining sick role behavior in low income populations. *Am J Public Health* 1974: 64:205–216. Reprinted by permission.)

impact of perceived susceptibility are less clear and consistent across studies of this type of behavior.

The HBM has been applied to studying compliance, in particular in the context of sick role behavior. The studies in general bear out that perceived susceptibility, severity, and benefits are associated with compliance in taking prescribed medications. Findings are more mixed regarding the impact of aspects of the model in predicting compliance with other types of prescribed regimens (27,28,29).

Many of the studies testing the HBM do not include all of the components of the framework, nor do they adequately empirically model the implied causal relationships among the variables. Less than half of the studies are prospective in design in that attitudes are measured prior to the behaviors they are supposed to predict. The issue of whether the attitudes are a cause or a consequence of behavior has, therefore, not been adequately resolved (11,27,28,39).

These and the other models discussed that deal with patient decision making concerning medical care differ in the type (lay or professional contact), purpose (preventive or illness-related), or time interval unit (contact or episode) of use being considered and the components of the decision-making process itself. They do, however, in contrast to the systems models described earlier, attempt to clarify the social psychological processes in which the individual patient engages in when deciding to seek medical care. The systems framework, which begins with issues in the organization and financing of care, represents a macro perspective; and the patient decision-oriented frameworks concerned with the psychosocial dynamics that underly decisions to seek medical care present a more micro perspective in understanding health care utilization behavior. Depending on one's perspective, both approaches are useful. From a macro public policy perspective, identifying the likely effects of changes in financing and major organizational forms for delivering care are necessary. At the same time, it is important to recognize that the way in which consumers in local communities will react to such changes will also depend on a number of micro-level social psychological factors. As David Mechanic points out, perhaps these efforts should be viewed as different but complementary ways of illuminating and understanding utilization behavior:

> The traditional medical sociology literature on physician utilization would be enriched by examining psychosocial processes within an economic context that takes into account enabling variables such as access to care, the availability of providers, and scope of insurance coverage. Examining the role of cultural and social-psychological processes within the constraining influences of economic and organizational factors will result in better theory and, it is to be hoped, more adequate prediction (12:395).

In the section that follows, major empirical findings on the array of predictors of health services utilization are summarized separately and, when available, their effects controlling for other factors reported are discussed as well.

SELECTED EMPIRICAL FINDINGS ON HEALTH SERVICES UTILIZATION

This summary of selected empirical findings on health services utilization will (1) review national data on the principal types of health care services—physician, dentist, hospital, and long-term care—and, when available, report data on the other major dimensions of health services utilization (purpose, site, and time interval) as they relate to these indicators; and (2) summarize the importance of a variety of predictors of health services utilization for each of these indicators, based on a review of empirical studies of their relationships to the respective use measures. These summaries draw upon a number of excellent bibliographies and reviews of health services utilization in recent years (2,14,43–51) as well as major national surveys of health care utilization and access (3,4,52–57). It should be noted that comparisons over time or between studies may well be affected by methodologic differences or changes in question wording across studies.

FINDINGS: SELECTED INDICATORS OF HEALTH SERVICES UTILIZATION

Physician Utilization

The proportion of the population that had seen a physician at least once during the year remained relatively stable from 1958 to 1963, prior to the introduction of Medicaid and Medicare. It did, however, increase slightly from 1963 (65 percent) to 1970 (68 percent), and then substantially to around three-fourths of the population in 1976 (76 percent) (3). This proportion has remained relatively stable over the last decade—at around 75 percent (56,57).

The average number of visits to a physician has also remained relatively stable—at around five (e.g., 4.9 in 1971 and 5.3 in 1985)—over the past 15 years (56–58). There have, however, been substantial changes in the sites or organizational settings in which patients see physicians. In the early part of the century (1928–1931), it is estimated that 40 percent of all physician visits occurred in the home. By 1971, this proportion had dropped to less than 2 percent. During this same period, office visits increased from 50 to 70 percent of all visits (59). By 1985, the proportion seeing a physician in the office had declined to around 58 percent, but the percent of visits to hospital outpatient clinics or emergency rooms had increased to approximately fifteen percent, similar to the proportion of patient contacts with providers handled over the phone (around 13 percent (57).

Around half of the U.S. population reported having a general physical exam in 1963, 1970, and 1976. However, during this period, the most frequently cited reason for having the physical tended to shift from concern about symptoms of illness to preventive care in the absence of illness per se (3,53). The percent of women seeing a physician during the first trimester of their pregnancy has also increased substantially— from 68 percent in 1970 to 76 percent in 1983, as has the proportion of children 1 to 4 years of age immunized for measles (57.2 percent in 1970 to 62.8 percent in 1984), rubella (37.2 to 60.9 percent) and mumps (48.3 percent in 1976 to 58.7 percent in 1984). There have, however, been declines over the past fifteen years in the proportion of children having diphtheria-tetanus-pertussis (DTP) and polio vaccinations (76.1 to 65.7 percent and from 77.5 to 54.8 percent, respectively) (56). The proportion of adults having selected preventive procedures (e.g., blood pressure test or Pap smears and breast examinations for women) has also increased since the early 1970s. The proportion of adults reporting that they had a blood pressure check in the year, for example, increased from approximately 62 percent in 1974 to 74 percent in 1985. Corresponding changes for Pap smears and breast examinations were from 54 to 63 percent, and from 56 to 68 percent, in 1973 and 1985, respectively (60,61). Questions have been raised, however, about the appropriate intervals and efficacy in detecting or preventing illness of these various screening procedures relative to their cost (4).

Dentist Utilization

The percent of the U.S. population having seen a dentist in the year increased from 42 percent in 1964 to 49.9 percent in 1978 and 51.8 percent in 1983. The proportion of the U.S. population that had *never* seen a dentist also declined during this period (from 15.6 percent in 1964 to around eleven percent in 1978 and 1983). The average number of visits for those seeing a dentist has remained close to two over this same period, however—from 1.6 in 1964 and 1978 to 1.8 in 1983 (56).

The proportion of dental visits for preventive reasons (e.g., cleaning and fluoride treatment) did increase substantially from 1964 (25 percent) to 1974 (36 percent). The rate of seeing a dentist to obtain fillings or inlays remained around 25 percent during this period, while the proportion receiving other restorative procedures, such as extractions and dentures, declined from 18 percent to 12 percent from 1964 to 1974 (62). Unpublished data from the 1983 National Health Interview Survey showed the percent of dental visits on which selected procedures were performed for people 2 years of age or older to be as follows: examination (35.6 percent), cleaning (32.1 percent), x-ray (27.9 percent), fluoride treatment (7.6 percent), filling (21.2 percent), extraction (7.3 percent), straightening (10.0 percent), and crown/cap (8.2 percent).

Over the last 20 years, there have been major changes in how both physician and dental services are organized and delivered. Dentists have, for example, increasingly employed dental assistants to handle preventive (e.g., examination and prophylaxis) procedures especially. In addition, an increasing number of dentists are practicing in partnerships or corporately funded settings (63,64).

Hospital Utilization

In general, the proportion of the population hospitalized has declined since the early 1970s. In 1971–1972 13 percent of the U.S. population had been hospitalized in that year (65). In 1976 the rate was 11 percent (3). It dropped to ten percent in 1978 and has remained around that proportion since then (4,66).

The total number of hospital discharges per 1000 population similarly tended to increase steadily until the mid-1970s, at which point it began to level off, and then has declined from the early 1980s on. The total days of care has declined as well since the mid-1970s, as has the average length of stay in the hospital (57,67,68). [Data in Table 3-3 on hospital discharges and lengths of stay are based on the National Health Interview Survey (NHIS) of the civilian noninstitutionalized population of the United States. Estimates from this source will differ from those obtained directly from hospitals in the National Hospital Discharge Survey. They do, however, confirm the trends reflected in the NHIS data.]

According to the National Hospital Discharge Survey, rates of discharge per 1000 population for diseases of the heart tended to increase from 1979 to 1983 (12.8 to 14.2), as did discharges for malignant neoplasms (7.5 to 8.3). The numbers of operations per 1000 males for cardiac catheterizations and the insertion of prosthetic lenses for cataracts also increased substantially over this same period (from 1.9 to 3.0 and from 0.5 to 1.7, respectively). There were increases in the rates of cesarean sections for females (from 4.7 to 5.9), but declines in inpatient operations for diagnostic dilation and curettage of the uterus (from 7.6 to 4.8) from 1979 to 1983. In 1983 both men and women were increasingly likely to have certain diagnostic and nonsurgical procedures while hospitalized [e.g., computerized axial tomographic (CAT) scan, diagnostic ultrasound] than had been the case 4 years earlier—when these diagnostic procedures were relatively new technologies (56).

There has been an increasing interest in outpatient surgery for certain conditions in recent years. Also, as mentioned previously, hospital outpatient departments and emergency rooms have come to be important sources of ambulatory physician care. The growth of freestanding emergency centers represent one effort to serve those individuals who tend to use hospital emergency rooms especially on an intermittent basis for nonurgent primary care (70).

Long-Term Care

Long-term care encompasses principally the utilization of nursing and personal care homes and mental health facilities.

The number of residents in nursing and related care homes increased from approximately 759,000 in 1969 to 1.4 million in 1982. (The estimate of 865,930 in Table 3-3 excludes those for whom age and sex information were not available; therefore, rates are not computed by population subgroup.) The demand for nursing home care is expected to increase as the proportion of the population 65 and over increases and lives longer (71).

The rates of inpatient utilization of mental health facilities has declined substantially in recent years, reflecting efforts to deinstitutionalize this population. The rates of use of outpatient and day treatment mental health facilities, on the other hand, increased substantially from the late 1960s (1969) to the late 1970s (1979): from 575.9 per 100,000 civilian population to 1188.4 and from 27.8 to 77.6, respectively. There have been particularly substantial declines in the rates of inpatient utilization of state and county mental hospitals over the past 15 years (56).

FINDINGS: SELECTED PREDICTORS OF HEALTH SERVICES UTILIZATION

In the discussion that follows, the importance of a number of variables that are considered most often in describing or explaining how utilization differs for different groups are summarized. The major types of utilization emphasized in this summary will be those just reviewed (physician, dentist, hospital, and long-term care utilization). The predictors are, in general, grouped according to the categories of the Behavioral Model of Health Services Utilization. To the extent possible, data available on the importance of the respective variables, controlling for other associated factors, are presented.

Characteristics of the Population: Predisposing Variables

Age. Age is significantly associated with all the different types of health services utilization, primarily because it is an important indicator of age-associated morbidity.

In general, the relationship between age and physician contacts and visits is curvilinear (see Table 3-3). Young children and older people are more apt to contact a

TABLE 3-3. Utilization Indicators for Selected Subgroups: United States

Selected Subgroups	Physician[a]		Dentist[b]		Hospital[c]		Nursing Home[d]
	Percent Visiting in Year	Mean Visits	Percent Visiting in Year	Mean Visits	Discharges per 100 Population	Average Length of Stay	Number of Residents 65+
Total	75.4%	5.3	51.8%	1.8	12.4	6.7	865,930
Age (years)							
<5	92.3	6.7	23.1	0.5	8.1	5.1	—
5–17	73.6	3.3	66.1	2.6	3.8	5.2	—
18–44	—	—	56.6	1.8	—	—	—
18–24	71.2	4.2	—	—	11.2	4.3	—
25–44	71.1	4.9	—	—	10.9	5.3	—
45–64	74.4	7.1	51.9	2.0	16.2	8.0	—
≥65	—	—	37.8	1.5	—	—	—
65–74	83.0	7.7	—	—	24.7	8.4	164,155
≥75	86.9	9.3	—	—	33.6	9.1	—
75–84	—	—	—	—	—	—	345,706
≥85	—	—	—	—	—	—	356,069
Sex							
Male	69.9	4.4	49.9	1.7	10.5	7.4	226,257
Female	80.5	6.1	53.7	2.0	14.1	6.3	639,673

Race							
White	75.7	5.4	54.0	1.9	12.5	6.6	—
Black	73.9	4.7	37.7	1.2	12.4	7.6	—
Family income							
>$10,000	75.9	6.2	37.4	1.2	17.5	8.4	—
$10,000–$19,999	73.8	5.3	—	—	14.2	6.8	—
$10,000–$14,999	—	—	41.9	1.4	—	—	—
$15,000–$19,999	—	—	46.6	1.6	—	—	—
$20,000–$34,999	75.3	5.2	57.5	2.2	11.4	5.8	—
≥$35,000	78.1	5.2	70.4	2.7	8.9	5.6	—
Geographic region							
Northeast	77.4	5.2	57.0	2.3	11.8	7.8	178,605
North Central	75.7	5.4	54.7	1.8	12.6	6.9	278,803
South	73.9	5.0	46.0	1.5	13.6	6.7	257,626
West	75.5	5.6	52.7	2.08	10.6	5.2	150,896
Location of residence							
Within SMSA	76.0	5.4	53.7	2.0	11.9	6.8	—
Outside SMSA	73.3	4.9	48.0	1.6	13.9	6.5	—

[a] 1985 data in Tables 71 and 72 in Ref. 57.
[b] 1983 data in Table 47 in Ref. 56. Age categories differ as follows: <6, 6–16, 17–44, 45–64, ≥65.
[c] 1985 data in Table 77 in Ref. 57.
[d] 1982 data in Table 4 in Ref. 69.

physician and average more visits, reflecting their age-related need for medical services. Very young children (under 6) and older adults (55 and over) are also more likely to report having a general physical simply because it was "time to get a checkup" (3). A larger proportion of older adult visits are to the physician's office, compared to younger adults or especially very young children, for whom rates of telephone contacts with physicians for medical advice are much higher (56,57).

The relationship between age and dentist office visits is the opposite of that observed for physician office visits. The youngest and oldest are least likely to see a dentist and average fewer visits overall (see Table 3-3). Children, however, are more likely to visit a dentist for preventive reasons (examinations and cleaning) than are adults. Restorative visits for fillings and dentures tend to increase up to age 40 and then decline in the older years (62,72, unpublished NCHS data).

Excluding hospitalizations for delivery, the rates of admissions, discharge, and length of stay for adults tend to increase with age (see Table 3-3). The rates for specific types of operations, and diagnostic and other nonsurgical procedures also vary considerably by age (56,57).

The vast majority of nursing home residents are elderly. The rate for those 65 and over is, in fact, highest for the oldest old (85 or older) (see Table 3-3). Rates of institutionalization in inpatient psychiatric facilities tend to be highest for middle-aged adults (25–44 years of age) and lowest for children (under 18) (56).

Sex. Women use more health services than do men in general, which is to some extent (but not totally) a function of their obstetrics-related care.

Women are more likely to see physicians than are men and have at least one more visit on average (see Table 3-3). Findings on the relationship of sex to the use of preventive services are not consistent. In some instances, women appear to be more likely to have certain preventive procedures than do men, but in other cases, there are no sex differentials. There is substantial evidence, however, that men are less likely to see a physician in response to symptoms of illness than are women (49,50). Further, a larger proportion of men's visits are to hospital outpatient departments or emergency rooms. Women, on the other hand, are more likely to contact the physician by phone for medical advice (56,57). Overall, women are more likely to have seen a dentist and average more visits than men (see Table 3-3).

Women are also much more apt to be hospitalized (see Table 3-3). When admissions for obstetrical reasons are excluded, the difference diminishes, however. In 1985, the National Center for Health Statistics Hospital Discharge Survey reported discharge rates of 123.5 per 1000 for men and 170.7 per 1000 for women, including deliveries. Excluding deliveries, the rate for women was around 139 per 1000, or only 12 percent higher than that for men. Men, on the other hand, average longer lengths of stay in the hospital. The rates in 1985 were 6.9 days for men and 6.2 for women, including deliveries. The average length of stay for women for deliveries was 6.8. In general, rates of inpatient surgery are higher for women than men (67).

The number of women in nursing and personal care homes is almost three times that of men (see Table 3-3) (69). There are, in particular, many more of the oldest old (85 and older) among female residents of nursing homes. The admission rates to state and county mental hospitals for males (219.8 in 1980) is almost twice that of females (111.1). Women, on the other hand, are likely to have slightly higher rates of admission than men to private psychiatric (63.3 vs. 61.9) or nonfederal general hospitals (265.1 vs. 233.8) for inpatient psychiatric treatment (56).

Race. Whites are more likely to use certain services than are nonwhites, although the differences have narrowed considerably in recent years.

In 1985 75.7 percent of whites had seen a physician in the year, compared to 73.9 percent of blacks (see Table 3-3). This represents a substantial narrowing of the differences between whites and blacks over the last 20 years, however. For example, in 1964, the rates for whites and blacks were 67.3 and 57.0 percent, respectively. On the other hand, the gap in the average number of visits has widened since the early 1980s. In 1983 the rates for whites and blacks were 5.1 and 4.8, respectively (56). In 1985 the average number of visits for whites who saw a physician was 5.4, compared to 4.7 for blacks (57)—a differential more comparable to that almost 15 years earlier in 1971— 5.0 and 4.4, respectively (58). Recent national survey data show that blacks may be as likely to have certain preventive procedures (blood pressure checks) or more likely to have others (Pap smears or, to some extent, breast examinations for women) than are whites (4,7). Although the gap has narrowed considerably, smaller proportions of black women (61.5 percent in 1983), compared to white women (79.4 percent), see a physician during the first trimester of pregnancy (56). There is also evidence that blacks have lower rates of use relative to their experienced need for care (measured by disability days and reported symptoms) than do whites (3,7). Blacks are much more likely to receive care in hospital outpatient departments and emergency rooms than are whites, whereas whites more often visit or telephone physicians (56,57).

Whites are much more likely to have contacted a dentist than blacks and to average more visits once they go (see Table 3-3). Whites also have higher rates of preventive dental visits than do blacks, while blacks usually see a dentist for more serious conditions and have higher rates of visits for restorative procedures (62, unpublished NCHS data).

There is evidence that hospital discharge rates for blacks, which had been higher than the rate for whites since the late 1970s, have begun to decline to be more comparable to those for whites (56,57). The average length of stay, on hospital admission, remains higher for blacks compared to whites (see Table 3-3). However, the number of elderly blacks in nursing homes (30.4 per 1,000 population in 1977) is lower than the number of whites (49.7) [56].

Ethnicity. Despite improvements in the levels of access to medical care among Hispanics, there is evidence that they continue to experience barriers to obtaining care.

National Health Interview Survey data from 1978 to 1980 showed that Mexican-Americans were least likely, compared to other all major Hispanic groups, blacks, or whites to have seen a physician in the year—33.1 percent had not seen a physician. They also averaged the smallest number of visits overall (4.3). Corresponding proportions and mean visits for other groups were as follows: Puerto Ricans (20.4 percent; 6.1), Cuban-Americans (23.3 percent; 5.8) other Hispanics (23.9 percent; 5.1), blacks (23.8 percent; 4.8) and whites (23.3 percent; 4.8) (73).

In 1978–1980, among people four years of age and older, Mexican-Americans were least likely to have seen a dentist in the year (34.5 percent), compared with whites (55.8 percent), blacks (36.9 percent), or any other Hispanic groups—Puerto Ricans (45.6 percent), Cuban-Americans (45.5 percent), or other Hispanics (49.8 percent). The rates of never having seen a dentist were also highest for Mexican-Americans (17.4 percent), compared with only 2.5 percent for whites, for example (73).

NCHS data confirm that Mexican-Americans were least likely to be hospitalized and also tended to spend fewer days in the hospital than most other Hispanic or non-Hispanic groups (73).

The literature on Hispanic health care suggests that language barriers, the middle-class values and attitudes of providers, longer waiting times to see a physician, and the assignment of different doctors to patients on different visits tend to characterize many Hispanics' contact with the health care system. Further, a disproportionate number of Hispanics do not have medical insurance, which is also frequently a significant barrier to their use of traditional medical services (74).

Education. The relationship of education to utilization in general varies by the type of indicator examined. It does, however, seem to be an important predictor of preventive health care utilization.

Better educated people are, for example, more likely to have had general physicals, immunizations, tests, and procedures for preventive purposes and (for women) to have seen a physician early in pregnancy. They are also more likely to have been to a dentist and to have more visits, once they go. The relationship between education and hospital utilization tends to mirror that for income (described below). People with less education are likely to have more hospitalizations (43,49).

Characteristics of Population: Enabling Variables

Income. In the past, people with higher incomes used more health services than those with lower incomes. Since the enactment of Medicaid and Medicare in the mid-1960s, lower-income people have come to use certain services at even higher rates than those with high incomes.

In 1964, 57.5 percent of people with family incomes of less than $10,000 (in 1983 dollars) had seen a physician in the year, compared to 73.0 percent of those with family incomes of $35,000 or more (56). The corresponding percentages some twenty years later (1983) were 73.6 and 78.1 percent, respectively. Further, whereas in the past the poor tended to report fewer visits to a physician on average than did the nonpoor, they now report more (see Table 3-3). The proportion of low-income adults undergoing certain preventive procedures (e.g., blood pressure check, or Pap smear and breast examination for women) continues to be lower than that for higher-income persons (4,7). The rates of physician contact in general, the mean number of visits, and use both of illness-related and preventive services tend to be lower for low-income, compared to high-income, children. Although the proportion of low-income women seeking prenatal care in the first trimester of pregnancy has increased substantially over the past 30 years, the rates remain lower for low-income, compared to high-income, women. There is evidence as well that low-income people continue to see physicians at lower rates, relative to the disability days or symptoms they experience, than do high-income people (43,49). Low-income people report having fewer of their visits at physicians' offices (49.8 percent for those with less than $10,000 income in 1983) than do high-income individuals (59.6 percent for those with incomes of $35,000 or more). They are, however, much more likely to use hospital outpatient departments or emergency rooms (18.4 and 11.5 percent, respectively) and less likely to use the phone to consult with the physician (12.3 vs. 18.8 percent) (56).

The proportion of low-income persons reporting having seen a dentist in the year remains much lower than the proportion for high-income people (see Table 3-3). The proportion reporting they had *never* seen a dentist in 1983 was also much higher for those with incomes under $10,000 (14.4 percent), compared to those with incomes of $35,000 or more (6.2 percent) (56). The number of visits to a dentist also varied directly with income, with higher-income people having more and low-income people fewer visits (see Table 3-3). People with higher incomes are also more likely to see dentists for preventive reasons, while lower-income people are more likely to present more serious problems and require restorative procedures once they visit dentists. These differences by income appear to be particularly pronounced for low-income, compared to high-income children (62, unpublished NCHS data).

The numbers of hospital admissions, total days of care, and average lengths of stay are higher for low-income people, reflecting their poorer health status and more severe medical problems (Table 3-3).

Residence. Rates of utilization for most types of services tend to be lower for people who live outside major metropolitan areas, especially those who live on farms or in rural communities.

The proportion of people seeing physicians and the average number of visits reported did tend to be higher for residents of Standard Metropolitan Statistical Areas (SMSAs) compared to those who live outside these areas (see Table 3-3). There is evidence as well that non-SMSA residents, especially those who live on farms, are less likely to have had certain preventive procedures (e.g., blood pressure check or Pap smear and breast examination for women) (3,4). Rates of contacting a physician in response to disability days or symptoms have also tended to be lower for people who live in rural areas, relative to those who live in cities (3,4). People who live outside major metropolitan areas are also more likely to see physicians at their offices and less likely to go to hospital emergency rooms or outpatient departments than are those who live in cities (56).

The proportion of people seeing dentists and the average number of visits for those who do, tend to be higher for people who live in SMSAs, compared to the rates for people who live outside SMSAs (see Table 3-3).

Hospital discharge rates are higher for people who live outside SMSAs, although their average lengths of stay are shorter (see Table 3-3). This probably reflects the propensity of physicians in less densely populated areas to hospitalize their patients so they can see more patients on a single visit to the hospital.

Characteristics of the Population: Need Variables

Need is consistently borne out to be the most important predictor of the use of health services. Need indicators may be based on patient self-perceptions of their health, as well as clinical diagnoses and evaluations by medical professionals.

Perceived Need. Patient self-reports of health status include indicators of whether they perceive their health to be excellent, good, fair, or poor; the extent to which they worry about their health; whether they had to go to bed or otherwise limit their usual activities because of illness or injury; and the particular symptoms or conditions they say they have experienced.

These measures tend to be highly correlated. People with poorer health, measured in these ways, are consistently more likely to have contacted a physician in the year, average more visits when they go, have been hospitalized, and tend to stay in the hospital longer once admitted (7,43,48,49).

Evaluated Need. Providers' and patients' evaluations of medical need may not always agree. Indicators of providers' evaluations of the patients' condition include their assessment of the actual severity of presenting symptoms or complaints and diagnoses, based on laboratory tests and clinical judgments (7,43,48,49).

The type of diagnosis or disease category affects the number of physician visits and the types of provider seen. The National Center for Health Statistics reports that chronic illness, especially hypertensive disease, arthritis and rheumatism, and other diseases of the musculoskeletal system, as well as acute conditions, such as influenza, the common cold, and infectious and parasitic diseases, tend to be the most frequently mentioned reasons for seeing a physician for illness-related diagnosis or treatment (75).

Normal delivery constituted (for women) the major reason for hospitalization. Other major diagnoses for which people were hospitalized related to malignant neoplasms, fractures, pneumonia, and cerebrovascular diseases. Most of the inpatient surgery performed is gynecologic, abdominal, and orthopedic (68).

In general, as the physician-evaluated severity of a condition increases, the use of physician services also increases, although many conditions for which physicians see patients are not deemed as particularly serious by the providers (49,76).

CHARACTERISTICS OF THE HEALTH CARE DELIVERY SYSTEM: SPECIAL UTILIZATION ISSUES

The beginning point for the consideration of the correlates of health services utilization in the Behavioral Model (Fig. 3-1) is health policy as it relates to the organization and financing of medical care. There have been a number of major changes under way in how medical care is organized and financed in this country in recent years, which are apt to have a profound impact on the types and volume of services consumed as well.

The numbers and kinds of Health Maintenance Organizations (HMOs) and other primary care alternatives are increasing. Outpatient surgery and other alternatives to traditional inpatient care are being encouraged. A variety of new preferred provider alternatives are being offered to the poor. Diagnosis-related groups (DRGs) under Medicare have radically altered the systems of the public financing of care for the elderly. Private insurers are becomingly increasingly concerned about cost shifting and are themselves beginning to forge selective contracts with providers to contain costs. Hospitals are becoming increasingly concerned about the level of uncompensated care they provide and consumers about the increasing share of health care costs they are paying out of their own pockets. The Gramm-Rudman budget bill promises to even more drastically reduce the level of support for many health and human services programs over the next few years.

These changes portend profound changes for the access and utilization of medical care for those groups most apt to be affected by these developments—the poor, the uninsured, those with some form of public third-party coverage, and people who have tended to use hospital outpatient services for their regular source of care.

The most immediate operational indicators for the individual patient of how care is organized and financed, and which are used quite often in social surveys of individual's health care utilization, are whether one has or does not have a regular source of medical care and insurance coverage, respectively, and if so, what type of care and coverage. These are the most immediate expressions for the individual of the health care policy-oriented organizational and financial resources potentially available to that individual to enhance access (7).

In the discussion that follows some of the major issues relating to the organization and financing of care and their probable relationship to the utilization of health care services are reviewed. We discuss the findings, in general, for the relationship of regular source of care and insurance coverage to utilization and then other special issues relevant to the changing organization and financing of services in the United States that may have significant impacts on the volume and mix of health care services consumed in this country.

ORGANIZATION OF MEDICAL CARE

Regular Source of Medical Care

Having a regular source of medical care is a strong and consistent predictor of health services utilization. Recently extensive secondary analyses of data collected in a 1982 national survey of health care utilization and access were conducted by researchers at the Center for Health Administration Studies, The University of Chicago, using the Behavioral Model of Health Services Utilization as the conceptual basis for the analysis. A variety of predisposing, enabling, and need factors were entered in multiple-regression equations for physician, hospital, and selected preventive services utilization indicators. The results demonstrated that for the range of contact measures considered (seeing a physician, being hospitalized, having a blood pressure check, or for women having a Pap smear or breast examination in the year), people who did not have a regular medical provider were much less likely to have had the service. Further, people who regularly used hospital emergency rooms for primary medical care were much less apt than those with private physicians to have seen a physician or had selected preventive procedures (e.g., blood pressure reading or breast examination) performed in the previous year. These multivariate analyses confirm descriptive findings from a variety of sources as well that document the importance of having a regular source of care in predicting health services utilization. Once entry is gained, having a regular source of care appears to be less significant in predicting the subsequent number of visits to a physician or the length of time in the hospital (7).

There have been questions raised in the literature about the causal ordering of the regular source and utilization measures—is having a regular source of care a determinant or a result of using services? Empirically based models to examine the directionality of these relationships have confirmed that having a regular source of care does indeed have a direct and causally prior impact on the decision to seek medical care (15,77).

Prepaid Systems of Care

In recent years, there has been considerable interest in encouraging the development of prepaid capitated systems of care. These generally provide for services to be rendered by a particular set of providers to an enrolled population for a set fee per person paid in advance of delivering care. These may take a variety of forms, including having salaried physicians working for a particular delivery organization, groups of physicians contracting with the plan to provide care to enrollees, fee-for-service physicians who contract to deliver services for a negotiated fee, or arrangements in which contracting providers serve as managers or gatekeepers for the type and amount of care that plan enrollees can receive. These alternatives are being touted as promising avenues for containing the costs of medical care through encouraging more cost effective medical practice. [See entire issue of *Health Affairs*, Vol. 5, No. 1 (Spring 1986).]

Studies conducted on HMO enrollees indicate that they receive at least as many ambulatory visits as do enrollees in conventional fee-for-service plans. There also appears to be a tendency for HMOs to encourage patient-intiated and preventive service-related visits and fewer follow-up and illness-related visits.

Utilization studies provide strong and consistent evidence that HMOs are associated with lower rates of hospitalization, compared to fee-for-service arrangements. In the vast majority of studies, HMOs had lower admission rates in particular, but there was not a clear difference in average length of stay (78,79).

Questions have been raised about whether differences observed for HMO users are a function principally of the fact that HMO enrollees are often younger and in better health and have higher incomes and more education than do fee-for-service users. In the Rand Health Insurance Study (Rand Corp., Santa Monica, CA), eligible persons were randomly assigned to various levels of coverage in either a fee-for-service or an experimental group and then compared with those who had enrolled in the HMO (Group Health Cooperative in Seattle) by choice. Admission rates and hospital days per 100 persons were equivalent for the two groups of HMO patients but about 40 percent less than in the fee-for-service group. The Rand investigators concluded that population characteristics can be ruled out as an explanation for the lower hospitalization rate at Group Health Cooperative. They also concluded that the HMO did, in fact, stimulate a less hospital intensive style of medical practice (80).

The proliferation of these modes of practice, as well as efforts in general to encourage the use of outpatient alternatives to traditional inpatient services, are apt to have major impacts on the volume and mix of services consumed in this country.

FINANCING OF MEDICAL CARE

Insurance Coverage

There is increasing concern that the number of people who do not have insurance coverage of any kind has increased in recent years, resulting principally from cutbacks and more restrictive eligibility criteria in the Medicaid program, as well as the loss of coverage by working people during periods of high unemployment in the early 1980s. Estimates of the uninsured vary considerably—from 10 to 34.4 million, depending on the source and definitions used. In general, however, approximately 1 in 10 Americans (some 21.5 million people), are said to have no form of third-party coverage for their medical expenses. Being uninsured is one of the principal criteria used in defining the medically indigent in this country. Increasing concern is being expressed about individuals who cannot afford to pay because of not having such coverage and the impact that their inability to pay has on their access to needed services, as well as the financial viability of institutions or providers that continue to serve them. [See Bazzoli (81) for a review of these issues.]

In the multivariate analyses of the 1982 national survey data on access and utilization described earlier, insurance coverage was another important predictor that was considered. These analyses, holding other factors constant, demonstrated that people who did not have insurance were much less likely to have seen a physician or be admitted to the hospital, to have shorter stays once admitted, and to have had routine preventive screening procedures (e.g., blood pressure checks or, for women, a Pap smear and breast examination). These findings confirm the results of many national and local studies demonstrating a positive relationship between being insured and using health care services (7,43,48,49). There is evidence in recent years as well that people with public insurance coverage, especially Medicaid, tend to average more ambulatory physician visits than do people with private insurance coverage. This may be due to the more discontinuous patterns of care used by the publicly insured or to the fact that ambulatory physician visits are more likely to be covered by Medicaid than is the case for most private insurance policies (7). Various alternatives have been considered in many states to attempt to extend coverage to the uninsured. These include providing some type of catastrophic coverage at a minimum, requiring insurers to participate in insurance pools to make coverage available to high-risk individuals, setting minimum standards for insurance plans offered in the state, and requiring insurers to extend group coverage to workers leaving the firm (81:377). These and other alternatives may serve to considerably increase the ability of the uninsured to obtain care when they need it.

Methods of Payment

There has been an increasing interest in recent years in reducing the amounts that public and private third-party payers have to pay for medical care. This has taken the form of fixed, predetermined (prospective) rates of reimbursement by service or diagnosis (e.g., DRGs) or by encouraging greater cost sharing on the part of consumers.

Empirical findings on the impact of the major prospective pricing initiative in recent years (reimbursement for hospital services under Medicare on the basis of DRGs) on hospital utilization and expenditures appear mixed. Hospital admission rates, total days of care, and average length of stay have declined since the advent of DRGs. These changes may reflect a function of secular trends under way prior to the introduction of this medical program or other changes in the organization and delivery of medical care in this country in recent years (e.g., increased emphasis on nonpatient alternatives). On the other hand, there have been concerns expressed as well that providers might attempt to "game" the system by modifying the diagnoses assigned to particular cases or encouraging early discharges and frequent readmissions as necessary to obtain desired levels of reimbursement (82–89).

The evidence regarding the impact of consumer cost sharing on the patterns and amount of health services utilization are much more consistent and convincing, however. A number of studies in both the United States and Canada document as inverse the relationship between the amount of physician and hospital services consumed and the amount of consumer copayment—the more consumers had to pay out of their own pockets, the less medical care they had (90–92). The Rand Health Insurance Study provided the most comprehensive test of the impact of consumer cost sharing on utilization. Some 2756 families in six sites across the country, representing 7706 individuals, were randomly assigned to five different groups representing different levels of cost sharing: those with (1) free care; (2) 25 percent coinsurance; (3) 50 percent coinsurance; (4) 95 percent coinsurance; and (5) 95 percent coinsurance with a maximum out-of-pocket expense of $150 for an individual and $450 for a family. The results of the study demonstrated that those with no or minimal coinsurance had much higher rates of physician and hospital use, and expenditures as a whole, compared to those with higher coinsurance rates (93).

The National Medical Care Expenditures Survey has similarly documented that the financial burden of out-of-pocket outlays for medical care tend to fall hardest on the low income. Medical care expenses tend to comprise a larger proportion of their total income than is the case for higher-income individuals (94). Policies that encourage greater cost-sharing by consumers will then undoubtedly lower their overall use of relevant services. Questions about how equitable this impact might be relate to (1) considerations of whether the utilization of necessary or more discretionary services result and (2) what the disproportionate economic consequences for low-income families and individuals might be.

This chapter has reviewed the major conceptual and empirical approaches to determining who uses medical care and why. Health services utilization measures are important indicators for evaluating the need for and impact of both national and local health policy and programmatic activities. Major changes are underway in this country in the organization and financing of medical care. These changes are apt to have a substantial impact on the types and amount of health care consumed in general and for certain subgroups in particular. The concepts and correlates reviewed here can be used by health care policymakers, evaluators, and program designers to assess the impact of these changes for the U.S. population as a whole and the groups particularly vulnerable to these developments both now and in the future.

REFERENCES

1. Aday LA, Andersen R: A framework for the study of access to medical care. *Health Serv Res* 1974; 9:208–220.

2. Aday LA, Andersen R: *Development of Indices of Access to Medical Care.* Ann Arbor, MI, Health Administration Press, 1975.

3. Aday LA, Andersen R, Fleming GV: *Health Care in the U.S.: Equitable for Whom?.* Beverly Hills, CA, Sage Publications, 1980.

4. Aday LA, Fleming GV, Andersen R: *Access to Medical Care in the U.S.: Who Has It, Who Doesn't.* Chicago, IL, Pluribus Press, 1984.

5. Andersen R: *A Behavioral Model of Families' Use of Health Services.* Research Series No. 25. Chicago, IL, Center for Health Administration Studies, The University of Chicago, 1968.

6. Andersen R, Newman J: Societal and individual determinants of medical care utilization in the United States. *Milbank Memo Fund Quart—Health Society* 1973; 51:95–124.

7. Andersen R, Aday LA, Lyttle CS, et al: *Ambulatory Care and Insurance Coverage in an Era of Constraint.* Chicago, IL, Pluribus Press, 1987.

8. Aday LA, Andersen R: Equity of access to medical care: A conceptual and empirical overview. *Med Care* 1981; 19 (suppl):4–27.

9. Andersen R, Kravits J, Anderson OW (eds): *Equity in Health Services: Empirical Analysis in Social Policy.* Cambridge, MA, Ballinger, 1975.

10. Wolinsky FD: *The Sociology of Health: Principles, Professions, and Issues.* Boston, MA, Little, Brown, 1980.

11. Becker MH, Maiman LA: Models of health-related behavior, in Mechanic D (ed): *Handbook of Health, Health Care, and the Health Professions.* New York, The Free Press, 1983, pp. 539–568.

12. Mechanic D: Correlates of physician utilization: Why do major multivariate studies of physician utilization find trivial psychosocial and organizational effects? *J Health Soc Behav* 1979; 20:387–396.

13. McKinlay JB: Some approaches and problems in the study and use of services—an overview. *J Health Soc Behav* 1972; 13:115–152.

14. Anderson JG: Health services utilization: Framework and review. *Health Serv Res* 1973; 8:184–199.

15. Andersen R, Aday LA: Access to medical care in the U.S.: Realized and potential, *Med Care* 1978; 16:533–546.

16. Evashwick C, Conrad D, Lee F: Factors related to utilization of dental services by the elderly. *Am J Publ Health* 1982; 72:1129–1135.

17. Markides KS, Levin JS, Ray LA: Determinants of physician utilization among Mexican-Americans: A three generation study. *Med Care* 1985; 23:236–246.

18. Stoller EP: Patterns of physician utilization by the elderly: A multivariate analysis. *Med Care* 1982; 20:1080–1089.

19. Wolinsky FD: Health Service utilization and attitudes toward health maintenance organizations: A theoretical and methodological discussion. *J Health Soc Behav* 1976; 17:221–236.

20. Wolinsky FD: Effects of predisposing, enabling, and illness-morbidity characteristics on health service utilization. *J Health Soc Behav* 1978; 19:384–396.

21. Wolinsky FD: Racial differences in illness behavior. *J Commun Health* 1982; 8:87–101.

22. Wolinsky FD, Coe RM, Miller DK, et al: Health services utilization among the non-institutionalized elderly. *J Health Soc Behav* 1983; 24:325–336.

23. Wolinsky FD, Coe RM, Mosely RR, et al: Veterans' and nonveterans' use of health services: A comparative analysis. *Med Care* 1985; 23:1358–1371.

24. Anderson JG: Causal models and social indicators: Toward the development of social systems models. *Am Sociol Rev* 1973; 38:285–301.

25. Shortell SM, Richardson WC, LoGerfo JP, et al: The relationships among dimensions of health services in two provider systems: A causal model approach. *J Health Soc Behav* 1977; 18:139–159.

26. Williams S, Shortell SM, LoGerfo JP, et al: A causal model of health services for diabetic patients. *Med Care* 1978; 16:313–326.

27. Becker MH, Haefner DP, Kasl SV, et al: Selected psychosocial models and correlates of individual health-related behaviors. *Med Care* 1977; 5(Suppl):27–46.

28. Janz NK, Becker MH: The Health Belief Model: A decade later. *Health Educ Quart* 1984; 11:1–47.

29. Suchman EA: Social patterns of illness and medical care. *J Health Soc Behav* 1965; 6:2–16.

30. Suchman EA: Stages of illness and medical care. *J Health Soc Behav* 1965; 6:114–128.

31. Suchman EA: Health orientation and medical care. *Am J Publ Health* 1966; 56:97–105.

32. Farge EJ: Medical orientation among a Mexican-American population: An old and a new model reviewed. *Soc Sci Med* 1978; 12:277–282.

33. Geersten R, Klauber MR, Rindflesh M, et al: A reexamination of Suchman's views on social factors in health care utilization. *J Health Soc Behav* 1975; 16:226–237.

34. Reeder LG, Berkanovic E: Sociological concomitants of health orientations: A partial replication of Suchman. *J Health Soc Behav* 1973; 14:134–143.

35. Kosa J, Robertson LS: The social aspects of health and illness, in Kosa J, Zola IK (eds): *Poverty and Health: A Sociological Analysis.* Cambridge, MA, Harvard University Press, 1975, pp. 40–79.

36. Mechanic D: *Medical Sociology: A Comprehensive Text.* New York, The Free Press, 1978.

37. Mechanic D: *Medical Sociology: A Selective View.* New York, The Free Press, 1968.

38. Becker MH (ed): *The Health Belief Model and Personal Health Behavior.* Thorofare, NJ, Charles B Slack, 1974.

39. Becker MH, Kirscht JP, Haefner DP, et al: Patient perceptions and compliance: Recent studies of the health belief model, in Haynes RB, Taylor DW, Sackett DL (eds): *Compliance in Health Care.* Baltimore, MD, Johns Hopkins Press, 1979, pp. 78–109.

40. Kasl SV, Cobb S: Health behavior, illness behavior, and sick role behavior. I. Health and illness behavior. *Arch Environ Health* 1966; 12:246–266.

41. Kasl SV, Cobb S: Health behavior, illness behavior, and sick role behavior. II. Sick role behavior. *Arch Environ Health* 1966; 112:531–541.

42. Rosenstock I: Why people use health services. *Milbank Mem Fund Quart* 1966; 44:94–127.

43. Aday LA, Eichhorn R: *The Utilization of Health Services: Indices and Correlates— A Research Bibliography.* DHEW Publ. No. (HSM) 73-3003. Washington, DC, U.S. Government Printing Office, 1972.

44. Andersen R, Anderson OW: Trends in the use of health services, in Freeman HE, Levine S, Reeder L (eds): *Handbook of Medical Sociology,* 3rd ed. Englewood Cliffs, NJ, Prentice-Hall, 1979.

45. Anderson OW, Andersen R: Patterns of use of health services, in Freeman HE, Levine S, Reeder L (eds): *Handbook of Medical Sociology,* 2nd ed. Englewood Cliffs, NJ, Prentice-Hall, 1972.

46. Freeburg LC, Lave JR, Lave LB, et al: *Health Status, Medical Care Utilization, and Outcome: An Annotated Bibliography of Empirical Studies,* Vols. I–IV. DHEW

Publ. No. (PHS) 80-3263. Washington, DC, U.S. Government Printing Office, 1979.

47. Hankin J, Oktay JS: *Mental Disorder and Primary Medical Care: An Analytical Review of the Literature.* DHEW Publ. No. (ADM) 78-661. Washington, DC, U.S. Government Printing Office, 1979.

48. Hulka BS, JR Wheat: Patterns of utilization: The patient perspective. *Med Care* 1985; 23:438–460.

49. Maurana CA, Eichhorn RL, Lonnquist LE: *The Use of Health Services: Indices and Correlates—A Research Bibliography, 1981.* Rockville, MD: National Center for Health Services Research, 1981.

50. Muller C: Review of twenty years of research on medical care utilization. *Health Serv Res* 1986; 21(Part I):129–144.

51. Zuvekas A, Arnold J, Bracken BW, et al: *Second Generation Project for Identifying Medically Underserved Populations.* Washington, DC, Lewin & Associates, 1986.

52. Andersen R, Anderson OW: *A Decade of Health Services.* Chicago, IL, The University of Chicago Press, 1967.

53. Andersen R, Lion J, Anderson OW: *Two Decades of Health Services: Social Survey Trends in Use and Expenditure.* Cambridge, MA, Ballinger, 1976.

54. Anderson OW, Feldman J: *Family Medical Costs and Voluntary Health Insurance: A Nationwide Survey.* New York, McGraw-Hill, 1956.

55. Anderson OW, Collette P, Feldman J: *Changes in Family Medical Care Expenditures and Voluntary Health Insurance.* Cambridge, MA, Harvard University Press, 1963.

56. National Center for Health Statistics: *Health, United States, 1985.* DHHS Publ. No. (PHS) 86-1232. Washington, DC, U.S. Government Printing Office, 1985.

57. National Center for Health Statistics: *Current Estimates from the National Health Interview Survey, United States, 1985.* DHHS Publ. No. (PHS) 86-1588. Washington, DC, U.S. Government Printing Office, 1986.

58. National Center for Health Statistics: *Physician Visits: Volume and Interval Since Last Visit.* Series 10, No. 97. DHEW Publ. No. (HRA) 75-1524. Washington, DC, U.S. Government Printing Office, 1975.

59. Donabedian A, Axelrod SJ, Wyszewianski L, et al: *Medical Care Chartbook,* 8th ed. Ann Arbor, MI, Health Administration Press, 1986.

60. National Center for Health Statistics: *Health, United States, 1981.* DHHS Publ. No. (PHS) 82-1232. Washington, DC, U.S., Government Printing Office, 1981.

61. National Center for Health Statistics; Thornberry OT, Wilson RW, Golden P: Health promotion data for the 1990 objectives: estimates from the National Health Interview Survey of Health Promotion and Disease Prevention: United States, 1985. *Advance Data from Vital and Health Statistics.* No. 126. DHHS Publ. No. (PHS) 86-1250, Hyattsville, MD, Public Health Service, September 19, 1986.

62. U.S. Department of Health and Human Services: *A Decade of Dental Service Utilization: 1964–1974.* DHHS Publ. No. (HRA) 80-56, Washington, DC, U.S. Government Printing Office, 1980.

63. Balit HL: Traditional and emerging forms of dental practice: Another view. *Am J Publ. Health* 1982; 72:662–664.

64. Rovin S, Nash J: Traditional and emerging forms of dental practice: Cost, accessibility, and quality factors. *Am J Publ Health* 1982; 72:656–662.

65. National Center for Health Statistics: *Differentials in Health Characteristics by Marital Status, United States, 1971–72.* Series 10, No. 104. DHEW Publ. No. (HRA) 76-1531. Washington, DC, U.S. Government Printing Office, 1976.

66. National Center for Health Statistics: *Current Estimates from the Health Interview Survey, United States, 1978.* Series 10, No. 130. DHEW Publ. No. (PHS) 80-1551. Washington, DC, U.S. Government Printing Office, 1979.

67. National Center for Health Statistics: *Utilization of Short-Stay Hospitals, United States, 1983.* Series 13, No. 83. DHHS Publ. No. (PHS) 85-1744. Washington, DC, U.S. Government Printing Office, 1985.

68. National Center for Health Statistics: 1985 Summary: National Hospital Discharge Survey. *Advance Data from Vital and Health Statistics.* No. 127. DHHS Publ. No. (PHS) 86-1250. Hyattsville, MD, Public Health Service, September 25, 1986.

69. National Center for Health Statistics: An overview of the 1982 National Master Facility Inventory Survey of nursing and related care homes. *Advance Data from Vital and Health Statistics.* No. 111. DHHS Publ. No. (PHS) 85-1250. Hyattsville, MD, Public Health Service, September 20, 1985.

70. Ermann D, Gabel J: The changing face of American health care: Multihospital systems, emergency centers, and surgery centers. *Med Care* 1985; 23:401–420.

71. Andersen R, Aday LA, Chen MS: Health status and health care utilization. *Health Affairs* 1986; 5:154–172.

72. Rosen HM, Sussman RA, Sussman EJ: Capitation in dentistry: A quasi-experimental evaluation. *Med Care* 1977; 15:228–240.

73. National Center for Health Services: *Health Indicators for Hispanic, Black and White Americans.* Series 10, No. 148. DHHS Publ. No. (PHS) 84-1576. Washington, DC, U.S. Government Printing Office, 1984.

74. Andersen R, Giachello A, Aday LA: Access of Hispanics to health care and cuts in services: A state-of-the-art overview. *Public Health Rep* 1986; 101:238–252.

75. National Center for Health Statistics: *Physician Visits: Volume and Interval Since Last Visit, United States, 1980.* Series 10, No. 144. DHHS Publication No. (PHS) 83-1572. Washington, DC, U.S. Government Printing Office, 1983.

76. Wartman SA, Morlock LL, Malitz FE, et al: Impact of divergent evaluations by physicians and patients of patients' complaints. *Publ Health Rep* 1983; 98:141–145.

77. Kuder JM, Levitz GS: Visits to the physician: An evaluation of the usual source effect. *Health Serv Res* 1985; 20:579–596.

78. Luft HS: How do health maintenance organizations achieve their savings: Rhetoric and evidence. *New Engl J Med* 1978; 298:1336–1343.

79. Luft HS: *Health Maintenance Organizations: Dimensions of Performance.* New York, Wiley, 1981.

80. Manning WG, Leibowtiz A, Goldberg GA, et al: *A Controlled Trial of the Effect of a Prepaid Group Practice on the Utilization of Medical Services.* R-3029-HHS. Santa Monica, CA, Rand Corporation, 1985.

81. Bazzoli GJ: Health care for the indigent: Overview of critical issues. *Health Serv Res* 1986; 21:353–393.

82. Anderson HJ: Majority of hospitals are better off under prospective pricing—surveys. *Mod Healthcare* 1985; 15:72–74.

83. Davis K, Anderson GF, Renn SC, et al: Is cost containment working? *Health Affairs* 1985; 4:81–94.

84. Dolenc DA, Dougherty CJ: DRGs: The counterrevolution in financing health care. *Hastings Center Rep* 1985; 15:19–29.

85. Iglehart JK: Early experience with prospective payment of hospitals. *New Engl J Med* 1985; 314:1460–1464.

86. Newcomer R, Wood J, Sankar A: Medicare prospective payment: Anticipated effect on hospitals, other community agencies, and families. *J Health Politics, Policy and Law* 1985; 10:275–282.

87. Simborg DW: DRG creep: A new hospital-acquired disease. *New Engl J Med* 1981; 304:1602–1604.

88. Spiegel AD, Kavaler F: The debate over diagnosis-related groups. J Commun Health 1985; 10:81–92.

89. Wennberg JE, McPherson K, Caper P, et al: Will payment based on diagnosis-related groups control hospital costs? *New Engl J Med* 1984; 311:295–300.

90. Beck RG, Horne JM: Utilization of publicly insured health services in Saskatchewan before, during, and after copayment. *Med Care* 1980; 18:787–806.

91. Lairson D, Swint JM: A multivariate analysis of the likelihood of volume of preventive visit demand in a prepaid group practice. *Med Care* 1978; 16:730–739.

92. Scheffler RM: The United Mine Workers' Health Plan: An analysis of the cost-sharing program. *Med Care* 1984; 22:247–254.

93. Newhouse JP, Manning WC, Morris CN, et al: Some interim results from a controlled trial of cost-sharing in health insurance. *New Engl J Med* 1981; 305:1501–1507.

94. Rossiter LF, Wilensky GR: Out-of-pocket expenses for personal health services. *NCHSR National Health Care Expenditures Study Data Preview 13.* DHHS Publ. No. (PHS) 82-3332. Washington, DC, U.S. Government Printing Office, 1982.

PART THREE

Providers of Health Services

CHAPTER 4

Public Health Services: Background and Present Status

William Shonick

Public health services have traditionally focused on the prevention of disease. A new capitalist society—one seeking a more comfortable life for more people with its dynamism and mobility—evolved out of the decline of the relatively stable and immobile feudalism in Europe, bringing with it new ways of living and traveling and, subsequently, the side effects of new threats to health. Disease threatened whole communities and regions with severe illness and death. Early efforts in Europe, and later in America, were directed at preventing or mitigating epidemics of acute infectious diseases such as smallpox, bubonic plague, cholera, typhoid fever, malaria, yellow fever, venereal disease, tuberculosis, and the childhood diseases of measles, mumps, scarlet fever, diphtheria, and whooping cough. [The current status of the battles against infectious disease is described in Last (1).]

The change in living conditions created by capitalism—rapid growth of city life, worldwide exploration and trade, and formidable technology— was accompanied by an ever-changing set of diseases as people struggled to adapt to their new environment (2,3). These threats to health changed over time. During the earlier stages of capitalism, the greatest scourges were epidemics of acute, infectious, and highly lethal disease. With the advent of better public health measures and other factors, such as the development of genetic immunity in large portions of the population, these threats were replaced by chronic and debilitative diseases such as emphysema, asbestosis, and other pulmonary diseases; cancer; stroke; heart disease; arthritis; and mental and emotional dysfunction associated with modern life. Throughout these changes, public health practitioners, policymakers, and researchers have attempted to learn the nature of the new threats and to organize public measures to combat them. To be fully effective, these measures had to be based on a correct assessment of what caused the disease and how it spread, and methods to control its spread had to be developed. In most cases, some form of organization was necessary to combat the spread of disease. Since this organization usually involved governmental authority, the term public health arose. Thus the development of public health services had four aspects: (1) identifying the diseases that were the leading causes of death and debility, (2) learning their cause and method of transmission, (3) finding methods to prevent or control them, and (4) learning how to organize society to apply the controls effectively.

As each new threat to public health arose, it drew a response from lay people and professionals who tried to organize preventive services for mitigating or eliminating it with varying degrees of success. In describing the organization and development of public health services in the United States, this chapter follows the pattern suggested by the actual evolution of public health programs described above. First, we identify the major threats to health existing during a particular period, the social conditions that led to prevailing patterns of disease, and the scientific discoveries that revealed what caused the disease, how it was transmitted, and how it could be combatted. Subsequently, we show how the understanding of the disease patterns, the state of scientific knowledge, and the current status of the society shaped the organization of public health services in response to the prevailing threats to health.

The organization of American public health agencies has involved an interplay of federal, state, and local governments and authorities. Although the form and functions of public health organizations were determined largely by the nature of the diseases and the knowledge of their causes, as well as the relationships among medical professionals, the structure of the public health system was also strongly affected by the roles played by these three levels of government. Great changes in these roles have occurred over time, but the most significant one for the development of U.S. public health services was the passage of the Social Security Act of 1935. For the first time, the federal government began to play a major role in the development of state and local public health services. The following discussion of the development of public health services is therefore arranged in two major sections: the period before 1935 and the period after 1935.

THE PERIOD BEFORE 1935

LOCAL PUBLIC HEALTH SERVICES

During the colonial period (1620–1781), small agricultural communities generally existed. In addition to farming, they engaged in some trade, and a few port towns, such as Boston, New York, Philadelphia, and Charleston, were beginning to develop into cities. The principal health threats were epidemics of infectious diseases, probably resulting from a combination of unsanitary and unhealthy local conditions—unsafe water supplies, swamps, and poor sanitation in housing—and diseases brought in by ships anchored in the harbors. The port towns were the sites of some of the more serious epidemics.

Local organization to counter these epidemics consisted of voluntary boards of health set up, for the most part, on a temporary basis to meet particular threats. These ad hoc boards applied what were considered to be the appropriate sanctions, namely, sanitation measures and quarantine. Quarantine was the practice of confining persons who were suspected of harboring a communicable disease to restricted quarters—a house or a ship—until there was no further evidence there of such disease. All persons who had had contact with the infected person would also be confined. Only special persons such as physicians, nurses, and ministers were permitted to enter the house or board the ship as it lay in the harbor.

After the American Revolution, local public health services were carried on much as before. Community boards, meeting as the occasion required, used their powers of quarantine and summons to force compliance with a sanitary code. In time, a practicing local physician occasionally came to be designated as the local public health officer. For his public duties he was recompensed, always modestly and often not at all. However, the continued development of sea trade increased the frequency and severity of epidemics in the port cities. This threat was abetted by the initially slow but accelerating industrial development that further increased the size and congestion of the cities—both ports and others—in which manufacturing was developing. However, the epidemics in the port cities continued to be especially severe, indicating that the most serious epidemics were imported at this time. Yellow fever attacked these port cities in a series of epidemics, of which the Philadelphia epidemic of 1793 "was in many ways the worst calamity of its kind ever suffered by an American city" (4:216). It was particularly serious because Philadelphia was then the capital and cultural center of the infant United States, and virtually the entire government deserted the city. One-tenth of the population died. The usual measures of quarantine and sanitation were followed, with emphasis on sanitation.

Before about 1850, local public health activities were largely reactive to the onset of epidemics. Local elected officials, aldermen, or council members generally passed ordinances establishing house quarantine, ship quarantine, and sanitation measures during epidemics. On an outgoing basis, they passed ordinances providing for street drainage, cleanliness of public markets, and waste disposal. With the development of biologic science in Europe, methods of preventing and controlling outbreaks of contagious disease became more effective. As a consequence, professional health departments arose during the years 1850–1900, and full-time officials who came to be known as *health officers* were appointed to head them. The use of quarantine and sanitation was guided by the rapidly developing bacteriologic and pathologic sciences and the new knowledge of animal and human disease carriers. The development of vaccines and antitoxins made the giving and promotion of immunizing innoculations a standard public health function. Increased knowledge about the causes and method of transmission of venereal diseases and tuberculosis led local health departments to engage in case finding and some treatment of these diseases. These practices were later included under the category of "communicable disease control."

In addition to sanitation, quarantine, and communicable disease control, the collection and analysis of vital statistics was becoming a standard local public health activity. Like many other measures, this was an American adaptation of European and especially British public health practice. Records were kept of deaths by cause and demographic classification, and, in later years, physicians were required to report the incidence of communicable diseases to the local public health authority. These data were used to monitor disease rates and to alert governmental authorities to the developments of epidemics. They were also used to establish causes of disease by association with environmental factors. The increasing sophistication of bacteriologic and pathologic science created a growing appreciation of the importance of appropriate laboratory facilities to determine the communicable disease agents that were prevalent in the environment or in the population. This method, in turn, led to the addition of a fifth function for local public health departments—maintenance of a public health laboratory. Since most private physicians had no laboratories, a public health department laboratory that could test human tissue or fluid samples—sent by private practitioners—and water or food samples—submitted by health authorities or other citizens—became an important local public health facility.

By 1925, most of the leading communicable diseases that had afflicted humanity for thousands of years, producing devastating epidemics in Europe and America since about 1300, had been identified in terms of their causes and methods of transmission. Preventive measures had been developed for most of these: water and food sanitation; identification, treatment, and perhaps isolation; immunization; and control of disease carriers (principally the mosquito, louse, and rat). The requirements for applying these controls helped to shape the structures and operations of health departments. By the 1920s, worldwide epidemic and widespread endemic occurrence of acute communicable diseases were due to the failure to organize public health services for an entire population. Thus the very presence of these diseases was considered to be a social rather than a scientific or medical problem because methods for preventing them were known.

As mentioned previously, given these developments, localities increasingly found it necessary—or at least desirable—to employ full-time, professionally trained staff. The size of this staff grew, especially in the large cities. Toward the end of the 1800s, a medium-sized to large community with a fairly adequate public health organization had a voluntary board of health, policymaking members appointed by the executive of the local government, and a department of public health with full-time professional staff headed by a medically trained health officer. Large departments often had more than one health officer heading bureaus or divisions that specialized in various aspects of public health work such as communicable disease control. The head of the agency might then be designated the commissioner of health or chief health officer. Helping the health officer were the public health nurses, who in large departments might be organized in a bureau or division of public health nursing. They aided in administering immunization, managing clinics, and making home visits to determine the need for quarantine or to encourage immunization and perform other health education functions. Together with the local coroner, they were frequently the main collectors of vital statistics.

In a large city, sanitation functions were typically headed by civil engineers who specialized in sanitation. Working under these sanitary engineers were specially trained technicians known as *sanitarians*. Sanitary engineers framed the ordinances and planned the water works and waste disposal systems to ensure freedom from contamination. If they did not actually plan sanitary construction, they were consulted on proposals. The sanitarians inspected places of business (especially food establishments), houses, streets, and other areas for violation of the sanitary code. They often had the power to collect food and water samples and send them to the local or state public health department laboratory for analysis. They also reported violations to the health department, where the reports were routed to the appropriate health officer or sanitary engineer. The vital statistics were assembled by trained personnel known as *registrars*.

The typical bureau or division of communicable disease control operated diagnostic clinics for identifying venereal disease and tuberculosis, provided or arranged for treatment, and enforced isolation or hospitalization for identified cases. In many places, attempts were made to identify and locate the persons from whom the disease had been acquired. It also offered immunization against those diseases for which vaccines and antitoxins were available and supervised vector (disease carrier) control measures such as drainage of stagnant water to control mosquitoes and rat and louse eradication.

The division of public health laboratories provided diagnostic services for physicians, public health clinics, and sanitarians. Samples sent to such laboratories were tested for contagious disease organisms. Many laboratories also distributed vaccines to private physicians, although in some places this was done by the division of communicable disease control.

Smaller health departments rarely had a full complement of bureaus or divisions, each performing a major specialized function and headed by a highly trained specialist. They usually operated with only sanitarians and had no sanitary engineers on staff. General clerks, instead of specially trained registrars, handled whatever vital statistics were collected; communicable disease control was most likely handled by the health officer who also headed the agency; and tissue, food, and water samples were sent to the state public health laboratory for analysis. In very small health departments, a single health officer—often a local private practitioner serving part time—handled all these functions or shared them with a single public health nurse and perhaps a clerk.

In addition to changes in local public health practice resulting largely from scientific advances, the approach of the turn of the century brought with it a marked change in local health department practice due to social developments in the U.S. population. Important demographic changes were taking place in the large cities of the East Coast and the Midwest. Immigration had been an important factor in the population growth of the United States throughout the 1800s (5), but particularly large waves of immigrants began arriving in New York City and other cities by 1892. Immigration peaked during 1901–1910 and then subsided slowly, reaching its low point during 1931–1940. Working in the factories and mills, these immigrants were predominantly poor and settled into many urban ghettos, especially in New York City. The resulting slum conditions produced illnesses similar to those that had arisen in Great Britain during the Industrial Revolution of 1750–1850, when the cities became very unhealthy and unsafe because of massive immigration from the countryside. Reformers and volunteer organizers worked and propagandized to alleviate the living conditions of the tightly packed slums. The health condition of the immigrants—a principal concern—focused on communicable disease and infant mortality; housing, especially sanitation; and nutrition. Volunteer agencies opened milk stations in slum areas to provide uncontaminated milk and established clinics for child care. The outpatient departments of public and some private hospitals were inundated with patients seeking primary care.

This period saw the first sign of schism in public health professional circles concerning a basic issue: the appropriateness of including personal health care in a public health department. As noted previously, until about 1900 the functions of local public health departments had generally focused on communitywide control measures—sanitation, quarantine, and immunization. Sanitation was an engineering and inspection activity; quarantine called for examination at times, but it was basically an administrative and police activity (the government's right to quarantine superseded even property rights); and much immunization was done by private physicians with vaccines obtained from the health department. Thus, most health departments were operating out of one or perhaps a few centers.

Given the overwhelming problems of slums in the big cities after 1890, many in public health were saying that the most significant new need for the immigrants was that of preventive health centers in their neighborhoods, and that public health departments in large cities should develop chains of neighborhood public health centers. Furthermore it was suggested that additional preventive services of a personal nature—maternal and child health (well care only) and health education, including nutrition—should be offered at these centers. The subject remained controversial until about 1910, when the New York City Health Department implemented a system of neighborhood health centers in poor areas that offered maternal and child health care, examinations (and even some treatment) for venereal disease, and tuberculosis detection. These latter programs, involving the part-time use of private clinicians, rapidly gained almost unanimous acceptance in professional public health circles as the sixth function considered to be basic to public health services.

Although the issue of public health departments providing general personal health (i.e., medical) services became a more serious policy issue in public health circles after 1935, the expansion of local public health departments into any aspect of curative or therapeutic general medicine, as opposed to preventive services, was watched closely and nervously by local medical societies even before 1935. The local and national medical societies jealously guarded their exclusive right to give medical care, and their resistance to perceived challenges often took on a truculent tone. Their insistence on the sole right to dispense personal medical treatment was largely responsible for the restriction of public health departments to communitywide activities such as communicable disease and sanitation control. If a patient was completely indigent and could not afford to pay for treatment, the organized medical profession had no objection to local or other government agencies providing treatment in clinics or via government-reimbursed physicians. But the preference was for fee-for-service reimbursement to private physicians rather than the use of salaried physicians, and for welfare department rather than health department sponsorship. During the relatively prosperous 1920–1929 period, the operation of general medical care clinics by local health departments was occasionally tolerated by the medical profession. However, during the Depression years many of these programs were effectively discontinued, and the public health profession was sharply reminded that its scope of function did not extend to curative care.

STATE PUBLIC HEALTH AGENCIES BEFORE 1935

Permanent state health departments developed later than did their local counterparts, as states were being pressed to exercise their police powers under the Constitution with respect to health. The power of the state to carry out functions such as protecting the health of its citizens "is generally referred to as the state's police power . . . i.e., the power 'to enact and enforce laws to protect and promote the health, safety, morals, order, peace, comfort, and general welfare of the people'. . . and local agencies, including state and local public health departments and agencies, derive their power by delegation from the state legislature" (6:5–6). The permanently organized state health department became a familiar part of state government during the years 1870–1910 when it was becoming increasingly apparent that many health problems were wider in geographic scope than the local community. As commercial and industrial development became statewide and regional rather than local, statewide public health action came to be needed. One of the principal immediate factors leading to the formation of a state public health organization often was a request "from a comparatively large number of localities which shared a common problem, or when some powerful local jurisdiction such as a large city, demanded state action" (7:91).

The first permanent state board of health was organized in 1869 in Massachusetts. It is not surprising that this should have happened since the functions and structure of such a department were first formulated in that state. Lemuel Shattuck, a bookseller and a student of the work of the English public health reformer Edwin Chadwick, had been campaigning for the improvement of public health measures in Massachusetts when, in 1849, he was appointed chairman of the Massachusetts Sanitary Commission, which had been appointed by the governor to make a "sanitary survey" of the state. The report of this commission, issued in 1850, "has become a classic in public health literature and documents" (7:93), with many of its recommendations serving as guides for the organization of subsequent state and local health departments. The recommendations were remarkably comprehensive. In fact, many of them formed the basis for the later organization of public health departments, and others are still regarded as desirable even though they remain largely unrealized to the present day.

By 1900, 40 states had state health departments, and by 1909, all states had organized some form of health department. The previously cited study of public health departments by Ferrell et al. (8) found that in 1925 a total of 17 states had separate bureaus of county health work with a full-time director in charge. This finding was highlighted because of the importance attached by the authors to the promotion of local health work as a function of the state health department. The interrelationship of the state and local public health agencies remains an important aspect of the public health system to the present day. The Ferrell Study found the proportion of the funds for local full-time health departments provided by the states to vary greatly—another condition that still prevails. One state met 48 percent of the total expenses for full-time county health service, and in 10 states, the state's share of county budgets ranged from 20 to 30 percent of the total. The study revealed that "the trend toward increasing the aid from the state is growing." Functions found to be performed or promoted most often by the state health departments in 1925 were rural or district health work: development of local health units; communicable disease control, particularly tuberculosis and venereal disease; vital statistics; public health laboratories; sanitary engineering; child hygiene; public health nursing; public health education; and food and drug regulation and control. In many states, full-time divisions were organized in the state health department to direct some of these functions.

Because this report described the situation existing before the Social Security Act of 1935 began pumping federal monies into the states—thus expanding state and local health department facilities and functions—it was used as a benchmark to measure later progress ascribed to the availability of such funds.

FEDERAL ROLE IN LOCAL AND STATE
PUBLIC HEALTH SERVICES BEFORE 1935

Although the primary focus of this chapter is on public health services supervised or delivered by state and local health departments, some discussion of the federal role is required, as the pattern and nature of these services have, over the years, been formed largely by federal government policy. The discussion of federal health policy is therefore focused on those aspects that affected state and local health departments directly. This section describes the pre-1935 period, during which the foundations for a greater federal role were established, so that that after 1935, federal grants-in-aid and the regulations accompanying them increasingly determined the direction of state and local policy; federal policy was rapidly becoming dominant.

An intricate and unique federal system was created in which states were to supervise public health, set standards, and do only a small amount of direct service delivery; localities were to deliver most of the direct services; and the federal government was to pay for these services and, in the process, set national policy. The intergovernmental relations involved were sometimes baffling. Under the U.S. Constitution the protection of public health is, as a general proposition, implicitly reserved to the individual state under its police powers, since a health function is not explicitly assigned to Congress. Whenever constitutional authorization was invoked to justify early federal action in public health matters, one or both of two sections of the Constitution were cited. Under the first of these sections, Congress is specifically given the power "to regulate commerce with foreign nations, and among the several states." This proviso was used to justify the earliest federal activites centering on control of communicable diseases at ports of entry and, somewhat later, included attempts to control communicable disease in interstate commerce. Under the second proviso, that of Article I, Section VIII, Congress is empowered "to . . . provide for the general welfare of the United States." This clause was the justification advanced by those who sought federal intervention in health problems in the interests of countrywide uniformity, equity, and efficiency (6).

Early federal legislation, beginning in 1796, concentrated on attempting to control the introduction into the United States of communicable diseases such as malaria, yellow fever, and cholera. To this end, various laws were passed establishing aid for quarantine procedures at the major ports of entry. The 1796 law merely provided for cooperation of the federal government with states and localities in enforcing state and local laws of ship quarantine. Quarantine authority itself was still regarded by Congress as resting with the states, but opposition to this view also existed. In 1878 the Marine Hospital Service—which had been established in 1798 to provide medical care for merchant seamen—was designated as the agency that would assist any state or community that requested its services in helping to prevent the introduction of contagious or infectious diseases into this country. In 1879, a National Board of Health with a 4-year term of office was voted by Congress. Its duties included having "charge of interstate and foreign quarantine" (7:54). Because of serious dissent among its participants and various public health bodies, it became effectively defunct at the end of the mandated 4 years and officially ceased to exist in 1893. At the end of its effective life in 1883, quarantine duties were restored to the Marine Hospital Service (7:54). Under an act of 1893, ship quarantine became a federal function, and by 1921, all quarantine stations had been acquired and were being operated by the federal government.

Congress also passed laws regulating interstate quarantine measures, with enforcement powers delegated to the National Board of Health in 1879. These powers were strengthened and specifically given to the Marine Hospital Service in 1893. Thereafter the public health aspects of the work of the Marine Hospital Service were concerned primarily with control of communicable diseases with respect to both introduction of disease from abroad and its spread among the states. The agency used this internal power very cautiously, and for the most part, assisted states with advice and personnel only when asked, despite the 1893 law entitling it to use enforcement.

Another aspect of the Marine Hospital Service's work in communicable disease control consisted of administering federal grant-in-aid to localities and lending personnel for demonstration projects in the various states, thereby hoping to encourage better practice. This was a relatively minor facet of its operations, however.

Despite the change of name of the marine Hospital Service, first to the U.S. Public Health and Marine Hospital Service in 1902 and finally to the U.S. Public Health Service in 1912, it continued to concentrate mainly on medical care for seamen and other stipulated eligible persons and on foreign quarantine. Beginning in 1913, however, a gradual broadening of perspective occurred when Congress began to appropriate funds for local research in public health. During the years 1914–1916, the Service conducted a series of field studies in typhoid fever control with the cooperation of about 16 states. These field investigations contained a large demonstration component, and by 1917, funds were appropriated annually by Congress for rural sanitation work by the U.S. Public Health Service. The grants had to be matched in equal amount by the states receiving them. This arrangement lasted through 1934.

Between the years 1915 and 1935, two other sources of federal stimulation for state and local public health activity were in place: grants for both venereal disease control and maternal and child hygiene. Grants for venereal disease control began with the Chamberlain-Kahn Act of 1918, which allocated funds to the states according to population. Although the appropriations for this program eventually dwindled away and ultimately disappeared by 1926, venereal disease control laws were strengthened, and programs remained in effect in many states. Grants for maternal and child health began in 1921 with passage of the Sheppard-Towner Act. Administration of the act was assigned to the Children's Bureau which was established in 1912 as part of the Department of Labor. The Children's Bureau had been doing research and educational work on matters pertaining to the welfare of children, and had been a leading proponent of the 1921 legislation. The act provided for allocation of the appropriated money among the states by a formula. Mustard writes that "between 1922 and 1927 the Division of Maternal and Infant Hygiene carried on an aggressive and productive program" (7:76). In 1929, the program ended after the discontinuation of federal funds.

Thus the period up to 1935 was one of development of public health both as a profession to combat epidemics of acute communicable disease and as an organ of government. The organization was principally local, with many the large cities having impressive departments and boards. The states were managing organizations that concentrated on setting standards and monitoring local service, encouraging the formation of local health departments in areas where none existed. Direct local public health services were also provided via state "districts" in areas that needed the services and did not have a local department. By 1900, the federal government was working with states in performing quarantine services at major ports, providing modest amounts of aid to localities, and improving sanitation services in rural areas. This agency also supervised interstate quarantine when asked to do so.

THE GROWING DISPARITY BETWEEN THE TAX BASE AND SERVICE RESPONSIBILITIES AMONG LEVELS OF GOVERNMENT

It is important to identify two aspects of the fiscal relationship among the various levels of American government: (1) the service responsibilities of the respective levels and (2) the tax revenue resources available to them. The disparity between the responsibility for providing health services and the proportion of total tax revenue collected by the respective levels of government grew wider after the establishment of the United States. It is common sense to suppose that if a particular level of government is assigned responsibility for a specified function, a part of the total tax revenues sufficient to finance it would be allotted. Indeed, at the inception of our government, allocation of revenue roughly matched the responsibilities of each level of government. In time, however, although local governmental responsibility for providing services grew enormously, its share of total taxes collected by all governmental levels declined. Most of the taxes collected eventually went to the federal government whose service responsibilities were minimal. Moreover, the basis of much of the nation's wealth and income shifted from family-operated agriculture to commerce and industry operated by national corporations; rapid growth in the service sector of the economy was apparent. With these changes, most of the tax base shifted from land and building capital to money income and money capital. Taxes on money capital, including investment securities, were not collected at all in the United States; taxes on money income were collected primarily by the federal government and secondarily, at a far lesser rate, by the state governments. Furthermore, money income and capital were concentrated in a few states to a greater degree than were land and property values. Despite this unequal distribution, large money income was always generated by federal taxes, excluding those states whose citizens had relatively low incomes. Taxes on land and the property on it (real property) were the principal sources of taxes for local governments. Thus, whereas the proportion of the available tax base had shifted in favor of the federal government, responsibility for health services (and other social services) remained with state and local governments. The problems attendant upon this "cultural lag" will be considered in further detail.

In its early years, the federal government was assigned functions that involved mainly conducting foreign affairs, providing for national armed forces, and regulating commerce both with foreign governments and among the states. The Founding Fathers clearly seemed to believe that the basic regulatory and administrative unit of government, as far as the individual citizen was concerned, was the state, with the federal government handling only those problems that involved all or at least several of the states. It was thus entirely appropriate that the federal government's revenues came mostly from various excise taxes and tariffs. The principal function of these tariffs was to protect the development of the infant American industry; the fact that they also produced revenue was an added benefit.

As late as 1910, 54 percent of the population was still listed as rural and only 46 percent as urban. By 1970, 73 percent of the population was urban. Between 1910 and 1920, the majority of the population shifted from rural to urban and remained so thereafter. During this same period, there was a basic shift from a primarily agricultural population to one engaged in commerce, industry, and services.

With increasing regulatory functions after the Civil War to serve the burgeoning and increasingly centralizing American capitalism, and with rising military expenditures, the federal government's need for additional revenue was growing and becoming a permanent feature of national operations. As the major source of personal income shifted markedly from real property and agricultural production to money capital and nonagricultural sources, the federal government sought to tap these new sources of wealth. After an attempt in 1894 to legislate a federal income tax was struck down as unconstitutional by a 5:4 decision of the Supreme Court (*Pollock v. Farmer's Loan and Trust Co.*), the Sixteenth Amendment to the Constitution was ratified in 1913, explicitly permitting the federal government to levy income taxes. Thereafter, the federal income tax rapidly became the most important single source of tax revenue for the federal government, accounting for $26 billion out of the total $35 billion, or 75 percent of federal receipts by 1950, and $173 billion out of $201 billion, or 86 percent in 1976. Customs revenues, which accounted for 84 percent of total revenue in 1800, 91 percent in 1850, and as much as 41 percent even as late as 1900, had shrunk to less than an insignificant 1 percent by 1950.

Equally illuminating is the change over time in the percentage of total government tax revenues collected by state and local units compared with that collected by the federal government. In 1902 64 percent of total taxes were collected by the states and localities and 36 percent by the federal government. These percentages remained relatively the same until after World War II. By 1950, the picture was almost exactly the reverse of the 1900–1940 pattern, with 69 percent of all taxes being collected by the federal government. Thus, during the immediate post-World War II years, some 65 to 70 percent of all taxes were being collected by the federal government.

The shift of the major tax base from real property to money income has resulted not only in a movement in taxable resources from the states and localities to the federal level but also in a heavily unbalanced geographic distribution of these taxable money resources (tax base) among the states. States with industrial—including large-scale, industrially organized agriculture (agribusiness)—commercial, and financial centers had high per capita incomes; those that were predominantly rural and had few or only secondary centers of industry, commerce, and finance suffered from low per capita incomes. The available base for local taxes became more and more unevenly distributed, not only among states but also among localities. Furthermore, the need for health services from state and local governments was often inversely related to the available tax base. Study after study of expenditures for health services of the various states in the 1920s, 1930s, and 1940s revealed two important facts: (1) the amount spent per capita varied greatly from state to state and (2) states with a lower per capita income spent less per capita for public health than did states with higher per capita incomes and were often spending more relative to their total tax revenues and income than were the more affluent states.

Clearly, increasing local and state taxes could not equitably provide a uniform level of public health services to match local needs because local taxable income was generally inversely related to such needs. Further, although the tax base now favored the federal government, the responsibility of the states for providing public health and other services remained. A solution to the problem boiled down to a choice between two alternatives or some combination of the two: either (1) the responsibility for many health and other services could be directly transferred to the federal government by legislative, constitutional, or judicial action or (2) the states could keep their responsibilities but receive money back from the federal treasury to discharge them. Federal revenues would thus be shared with the states and localities, but program control could continue to remain largely in state and local hands. Revenue sharing did eventually occur, but with it came a shift in responsibility and program control in the public health (and other) fields to the federal government. This change corroborated the well-established maxim that "control follows the dollar."

After 1935, the principal mechanism used to correct the disparity between tax base and service responsibilities was the grant-in-aid, under which the federal government shared its revenue with the states and localities. Different schemes for distributing these grants have been used. Some formulas are better for achieving one set of goals and other formulas for other goals. Let us now consider various mechanisms and the objectives of each in supplying grants-in-aid to various levels of government.

Subsequent sections discuss how the federal health grants actually operated with respect to state and local public health work after 1935.

REDISTRIBUTION OF TAX REVENUES AMONG THE DIFFERENT LEVELS OF GOVERNMENT

Two basic methods have been used to allocate federal money among states and the two localities, the formula grant and the project grant. Formula grants are distributed among the states according to a formula established by law. The basis for distribution may be equal allocation, variable allocation, or a combination of the two. Under the infrequently used equal allocation, an equal fixed amount is allocated to each state. Under variable allocation, certain characteristics of each state determine the percentage of the total national appropriation it receives. This type of grant allocation was the more common one for health purposes until about 1965, and it is still widely used. Its main attribute is that it permits the appropriation to be distributed in a manner that helps to equalize services and tax burdens throughout the nation.

The preceding discussion deals with formulas for *distributing* money among the states. In addition, grants to states often carry stipulations about how the money may be *spent*. Formula grants have been further identified as either general purpose (block grants) or earmarked (categorical grants), depending on the restrictions imposed. Block grants may be used without detailed specific restrictions for broadly defined purposes such as improving and expanding local health department services. Categorical grants, on the other hand, if given to a local health department, may be spent only for a specific type of activity, such as cancer control. It is important to note that what may seem to be a block grant at one level of administration is viewed as a categorical grant at a higher level. For example, a general-purpose health grant to a local health department is a block grant for that department, but it is categorically restricted from the point of view of the local government, which may prefer to use part of it for law enforcement.

Project grants are principally designed to carry out a particular federal program rather than to help a local health agency accomplish its own objectives. This grant transfers money directly from the federal government to a state or local government, or to any other type of governmental or nongovernmental organization, for carrying out a specific project previously approved by the federal granting agency. Often the grant award is made to one of several competing applicants. This type of grant requires an application from a would-be recipient and is not given automatically to any governmental unit according to a present formula.

THE PERIOD AFTER 1935

LOCAL HEALTH DEPARTMENT GROWTH, 1936–1945

The Social Security Act of 1935 established annual grants-in-aid from the federal government to the states, part of whose purpose was to further the development of full-time local health departments. This landmark in the development of intergovernmental relations in the health field marked the first major entrance of the federal government into local and state public health operations. Although all of the provisions of the act were interrelated and a number of them affected health services, two sections directly mandated federal support for state and local public health departments. Title V, Part 1, provided grants to the states for aiding state and local health departments to provide maternal and child health services and was administered by the U.S. Children's Bureau, which at that time was part of the U.S. Department of Labor. These were categorical grants earmarked for maternal and child health. Title VI provided grants to the states for aiding the work of state and local public health departments. Title VI funds were administered by the U.S. Public Health Service (PHS). They were formula block or general health grants that could be spent as each public health department saw fit, within very broad limits. For both Title V and Title VI grants, the states had to match the federal money by spending a dollar of their own funds for each dollar of federal grant money.

The Mountin Report

The development of these departments through 1946 has been described by Joseph W. Mountin, an Assistant Surgeon General of the PHS well known for his public health writing, and his associates. In a PHS monograph (9), they described a substantial expansion of local and state services.

The Mountin report indicated that the number of counties covered by full-time local health services grew from 762 in 1935 to 1577 in 1940 and then to 1851 in 1946, and that the proportion of the population covered (outside the cities that had their own municipal health departments) grew from 37 percent in 1935 to 72 percent in 1946. The influence of these funds on the growth of local health department staffs, again exclusive of independent metropolitan centers, was equally marked with total full-time personnel increasing from 3435 to 10,320—more rapidly in nonmedical than in medical personnel. This improvement was accomplished in spite of the fact that "a considerable proportion of established positions for medical—and others—were vacant for war-related reasons" (9:38). The data also indicated that at least 60 cities with populations of 10,000 or greater were added to the list of cities with "some type of full-time official public health organization." Mountin et al. define municipal health departments as "those city health units which operate under full-time technical direction and are independent of county or district organization" (9:16).

Despite this progress, by 1946 approximately 30 percent of the nonmetropolitan population and almost 20 percent of the total population still remained without full-time local health coverage. Furthermore, some of the expanded coverage was of questionable depth; often it represented a reporting artifact resulting from a simple blanketing-in of additional areas via consolidation of counties into multicounty health districts without a proportionate increase in staff and other needed resources. Public health professionals and analysts were insistently and increasingly stressing that extending full-time local health services coverage of at least minimally acceptable quality to the entire population was an important and perhaps overriding goal of public health. Clearly, the extent of such coverage could not be accurately measured if standards defining minimally acceptable services were not available.

The Emerson Report

Because of this expressed professional desire to define minimally acceptable local health services more clearly, the growth of local health departments due to federal grants was accompanied by a heightened interest in defining adequate quality or depth of service. A special committee of the APHA chaired by a well-known public health officer, Haven Emerson, worked on this question. In 1945, it prepared and issued a definitive set of standards for measuring minimally adequate public health services. The committee also estimated what resources would be needed to cover the entire population with public health services that met these standards. Standards were set for staffing, types of services to be offered, organization of both the board and the department, and other matters. Staffing standards were based on ratios of personnel (by occupational categories) to population. All needed improvements were projected as increases over the 1942 data, which were used as a baseline from which such improvement might be measured. This informatin was embodied in what has come to be known as the Emerson Report (10).

The section of the report dealing with the scope of function probably had the most lasting influence. The committee defined the six basic functions (which came to be known as the "basic six" functions) of a local public health department as follows:

1. Vital statistics—recording, tabulation, interpretation, and publication of the essential facts of births, deaths, and reportable diseases
2. Communicable disease control—tuberculosis, venereal disease, malaria, and hookworm
3. Sanitation—supervision of milk, water, and eating places
4. Laboratory services
5. Maternal and child hygiene—including supervision of the health of the school-age child
6. Health education

Public health goals for the future were described in these terms: "The Committee is of the opinion that a present goal should be the creation of such number and boundaries of areas of local health jurisdiction in every state in the union as will bring within the reach of every person and family the benefits of modern sanitation, personal hygiene, and the guidance and protection of trained professional and accessory personnel employed on a full-time basis at public expense, selected and retained on a merit or civil service basis, and free from disturbance by the influence of partisan politics" (10:26). The emphasis on the merit civil service system of personnel practice as a necessary reform to curb the abuses of an earlier day is worthy of note.

DEVELOPMENTS AFTER THE EMERSON REPORT: THE PERIOD 1946–1965

The period 1936–1945 had been one of consolidating the position of local health departments. With the federal Title V and Title VI monies and the matching state contributions, local public health departments became well established in performing the standard basic six functions. The Emerson Report provided visible evidence of the progressive nature and professional vitality characterizing many of the leaders of public health departments. In general, the leaders of the federal government's health activities accepted the role of the local public health department as delineated by leading public health executives through the American Public Health Administration (APHA) and worked with local and state leaders to develop public health departments with more personnel and wider geographic coverage. Here and there, dissent was raised about the inadequate scope of function of these departments. It was noted that times were changing and that the basic six functions would no longer suffice. In particular, more attention was needed to preventing and controlling chronic and degenerative diseases and to providing general medical care in public health clinics. These criticisms began to multiply rapidly after World War II.

The mounting problems in the large cities, the growth of private health insurance that covered only the nonpoor, and the social reformism of some administrations and Congresses all combined to put pressure on local public health departments to deliver services that were essentially alien to the spirit of the Emerson Report. The recommendations of this report had stressed preventive services based on suppressing acute infectious disease. The nature of the new demands on these departments and how they were met is the subject of this section. Of course, the story must include the role of the federal government, which grew rapidly. This account is given later and includes the changing role of the states as well.

By 1960, a U.S. government study (11) indicated that some 94 percent of the population was judged to have access to the services of full-time health departments (11). Such departments numbered 1557 and included 2425 of the 3072 counties in the United States. Clearly, widespread coverage had been achieved, but the depth or quality of coverage recommended by the Emerson Report was lacking. Other data of this 1960 study indicated that the per capita personnel implied in the Emerson Report recommendations was not achieved by 1960. In the all-important categories of public health nurses and dental personnel, the staffing was far short of the recommendations; the number of dental hygienists and public health nurses per population had actually declined from 1942 levels. Indeed, the overall staff to population ratio was somewhat lower in 1960 than the Emerson Report baseline 1942 figures showed, and yet the development of the standard local public health department had gone about as far as it was to go.

Thus there is every indication that by 1960 most of nonmetropolitan America had access to full-time local public health department services, and the small part that did not appeared to have little need for it. "Full-time" continued to mean having only a separate public health department address (i.e., not a physician's private office) and at least one full-time employee, even if only a clerk. But further public sentiment for enriching standard public health department staffs in rural and semirural areas was not strong. The political pressures for improvement in public health services were coming from another quarter—the metropolitan areas. In metropolitan areas, defined here similarly to the Census Bureau's Standard Metropolitan Statistical Area (SMSA) as consisting of a large city and its surrounding trading area, two civilizations were developing: that of the central or innercity and that of the more affluent suburbs. These two cultures, although distinct, interacted with each other, usually to the detriment of the former. The members of each culture had different public health needs. The inner-city populations and their advocates were pressing for more and better public medical services, especially primary care. The social structure of what had been working-class and middle-class areas in the large cities before World War II had changed, leaving them—among other things—almost bereft of private physicians. In many places, they were also demanding better protection against unsafe and unclean dwellings and streets, but the demand for medical care was more prominent politically.

Many urban areas long had health departments that met or exceeded the minimum standards of the Emerson Report, but the standard health department was not set up to cope with the newer inner-city needs. By long-standing tradition, providing general medical care was alien to it. Fighting for improved sanitation in housing was part of the tradition and function of local public health departments, but the widespread deterioration of the inner cities overwhelmed their resources. Coping with the widespread physical devastation of slum areas and the fiscal plight of the cities was simply too much for these departments. Even standard public health activities such as public health nurse home visits often could not be properly carried out given the increasingly unsafe neighborhoods and hostile clients. The two major requirements of the inner city for public health services—medical care and aggressive enforcement of sanitation (including safety)—found the local public health department unable to respond adequately.

The demands of the suburban populations were different. Their intellectual and artistic leaders demanded environmental control (air pollution, radiation emissions, solid waste), consumer product protection, automotive safety, and similar matters. The local public health departments existing in the newly built-up suburban areas were holdovers from the previous rural environments and were operating on a relatively modest scale. They were ill-equipped and insufficiently empowered to handle these new demands and the rapid surge of development. Further, even the most efficient and forward-looking local public health leaders faced the fact that most of the problems were being caused by large, powerful industries—automotive, petrochemical, nuclear power, and extractive. They could scarcely be controlled by a local health department, even a very well managed one. Only the regional, state, and in many cases, federal (and even international for many important problems) agencies could realistically be expected to deal with them.

The confluence of these two sets of problems in the metropolitan areas, neither of which proved very amenable to the work of the standard local public health department as it had developed, greatly diminished the public standing of and federal support for these departments in performing their standard roles.

Congress and the federal executive were being pressed to consider means of using governmental powers more effectively to make better medical care available to all the people, especially those in the lower income brackets, and to improve the quality of the environment. The leadership of the local public health department, finding itself faced with a changed and seemingly intractable set of problems and rapid alterations in the composition of its clientele, became disoriented as it was pushed from all sides to do different things. Various experts and commentators were counseling different courses. Some writers and practicing professionals advised local public health departments to stick to prevention, basically as defined in the Emerson Report. Others called for a bold expansion into delivering primary medical care. Still others sought to define the fundamental role of the local public health department as one of areawide health planning, standard setting, and monitoring. Examples abound of the probing, questioning, and exhortation that was appearing everywhere, reflecting confusion about the "true" role of local public health departments. (Similar questions were being raised about the role of state health departments.)

Perhaps the most vivid indication of attempts within the ranks to redefine the function of public health departments is provided by the annual efforts of the APHA leadership to spell them out in official policy statements. Over the years, the official APHA positions on the scope of functions and proper organization of a local public health department continued to change in conformance with changing conditions.

There was a sharp decline in the amount of federal funds given to local health department operations, which dropped from $15 million (19 percent of the total spent by local health departments) in 1947 to $9 million (5 percent of the total) in 1956, so that the brunt of expenditures fell increasingly on states and especially localities. This decline in federal contributions came in spite of increased local contributions, from $54 million to $127 million, and increased state contributions, from $10 million to $40 million, during the same period. The relative decine in federal money, therefore, was even greater than the absolute reduction (12).

Public Policy Implications

The criticism of the adaptive abilities of local public health departments that were being made by the federal government was reflected in changes in its mechanisms for giving grants to local governments. This issue is discussed in greater detail later, but it is appropriately mentioned here. The federal grants-in-aid to states that had been used since 1936 largely to help local health departments develop their traditional functions—the so-called formula grants for general health purposes—declined while the formula increased (13). The latter were aimed at promoting carefully focused demonstration projects to encourage an innovative approach to expanding public health functions in directions desired by the federal government. Many articles and speeches by public health figures and federal analysts, and the changing positions of the APHA, showed that changing social conditions were placing demands on local health departments in large metropolitan areas that were perceived in Washington as not being met. These demands centered on medical care for the poor, enforcement of local environmental health conditions in the ghettos, particularly housing conditions, and regional environmental control, demanded primarily by sections of the middle classes. None of these demands were met to any great degree despite the infusion of federal and state funds, policy statements by public health organizations, and the writings of professional public health administrators, academics, journalists, and a wide assortment of general pundits. Why were changes not being made?

Solving these problems involved tackling adversaries for which the local health department was no match politically. Eliminating the unhealthy conditions of ghetto life meant fighting slum landlords, urban redevelopers, and urban political machines to obtain adequate and meaningful inspection and enforce compliance. This meant taking on the entire problem of the deterioration of the inner city. Providing adequate medical care for the poor in the cities involved tackling the entire system of medical care distribution, including the traditional treatment of the public medical care sector as a charity, second-class "track." The problem of environmental decay that was troubling the middle class was not amenable to local solution. The large corporations and their polluting activities, as well as the attendant problems of automobile transportation and housing sprawl, could scarcely be tackled by the states, let alone the local governments. Thus, despite suggestions for policy changes appearing in APHA resolutions and goading by speeches and writings of commentators—and that of officers of the federal government and grant mechanism manipulation—the local health department, as an institution, departed little from its well-beaten paths.

The fundamental problems of the health delivery system and the inner cities could not be solved by local public health departments, although vigorously and skillfully led ones could do more than others. The problem of medical care for low-income groups was also shifting to a national focus, and the battle to preserve the environment was shifting to the state and federal arenas. Local health departments continued to perform the basic six functions and reacted to developments in medical care and environmental control in a variety of ways, depending on local conditions. In some areas, they became the local agents of new federal programs for operating neighborhood and migrant health centers and became actively involved in fostering federally and state-financed systems of medical care for low-income people. In most areas they did not.

STATE PUBLIC HEALTH AGENCIES: 1946–1965—TRENDS IN ORGANIZATION AND FUNCTIONS

The previously discussed Mountin study of 1946 (9) also analyzed the effects of 10 years of the Social Security Act on the expansion of state health department activities. Mountin found that expenditures of the 48 states for health departments increased from $12.9 million in 1930 to $18.7 million in 1940 to $37.0 million in 1946. The breakdown of these expenditures by category showed that "such activities as communicable disease control (including tuberculosis and venereal disease control), sanitation, laboratory services, and maternal or child hygiene—which accounted for a majority of State expenditures in 1930—still received more than half of the funds available in 1946." According to the study, "At the same time, the growth of newer programs is illustrated by such figures as these for dental hygiene: 37,000 in 1930, 227,000 in 1941, and 708,000 in 1946.

These data represented real expansion of services and were not all due to price increases, as is shown by the corresponding increase in full-time personnel from 4672 in 1930 to 10,128 in 1940 to 12,414 in 1946. An additional indication given by Mountin that the expansion in the years 1935–1946 was real, and not merely an artifact of price increases, is the number of activities reported as "identified projects" by state health departments. Although this sort of measure taken alone does not necessarily imply an increase in total service volume, it was used by Mountin as an indicator of expanding scope of function. Of the 46 states reporting, 39 listed communicable disease control projects for 1935, 43 in 1940, and 45 in 1946. The number of states reporting tuberculosis control programs rose from 19 in 1935 to 32 in 1940 and 45 in 1946. Virtually all the traditional public health functions showed similar increases. Mental hygiene and cancer control, however, were listed by only 7 and 27 states, respectively, in 1946. (At the time of Mountin's report, the states were heavily involved in psychiatric care, maintaining large censuses in state mental hospitals. However, these functions were generally lodged in state hospital departments or special departments of mental hospitals. The organizational separation of what is today called *mental health* from *public health* is still true.)

Planning, chronic disease work, and other more modern functions did not appear as identified projects at all. If they were in effect in any state, they are subsumed in the statistics under the catchall category "other central services." Thus the increased scope of function was not mainly in areas new to public health but represented expansion in standard areas by departments that had not yet been engaging in them.

A noteworthy exception was the striking increase in the number of states operating industrial hygiene programs. In 1935 this activity was listed as an identified project by only 4 states, compared with 26 states listing it in 1940 and 38 in 1946. The two states that did not respond to the question regarding identified projects did, in fact, have industrial hygiene units in both 1940 and 1946. In addition, New York and Massachusetts provided industrial hygiene units through their departments of labor.

Thus, by 1946, 42 states had such units covering 96 percent of the country's labor force. The services most commonly supplied by such units were "general surveys or inspection of plants for occupational health hazards with recommendations for improvement" (8:25). As early as 1946, state health departments had begun to look for occupational health hazards; this was one of the relatively few new areas they had entered. (It was not until 1970 that the federal government established the Occupational Safety and Health Administration.)

The state health department of these later years may be characterized as a supervising, coordinating, equalizing, and mediating agency, whereas the local health department was the principal agency carrying the responsibility for the day-to-day operations of public health programs. There were exceptions. In some states the state health department conducted all the functions of local public health work, with no local government health departments; these cases are discussed later. (Generally the state agency provides a complete set of personal public health services directly only when local organization is lacking or inadequate, and then only as an interim measure pending local organization.) More often, it provided only isolated special services, if any. Many of the substantive areas covered by local health departments were among those also most frequently assigned by state law to the state health department, again with the exception that the state involved health department's functions have been supervisory rather than involved with direct delivery. Examples of such areas are sanitation and maternal and child health. In addition, because of the breadth of the state's police powers, many state health departments engaged in health-related functions that were never or rarely practiced by local public health departments, such as licensing and accreditation of health professionals and health facilities, standard setting for automobile safety devices, and supervision of the quality of public medical payment programs such as Medicaid.

A 1961 study Shubick and Wright (14) summarized in Hanlon (15) listed the principal activities of state health agencies in terms of how many of the 50 states were actually practicing them. Table 4-1 lists a few of the most frequently encountered activities and the number of states in which they were carried on. It should be noted that these activities are, for the most part, either the traditional programs or "the programs which are categorically funded by the federal government. On the other hand, newer programs such as "program planning, development, and evaluation" appeared in activities in only 7 state health departments, "radiologic health" in 11, and heart disease control in 25. Other programs that are infrequently encountered, such as "professional registration and licensure," appearing in only three states, represent the type of program generally administered by a special licensing body of the state.

The functions considered appropriate for state health departments were outlined in a policy statement of the governing council of the APHA adopted at its 96th annual meeting on November 13, 1968 (16). These may be summarized as (1) health surveillance, planning, and program development; (2) promotion of local health coverage; (3) setting and enforcement of standards; and (4) providing health services. The complexity of the monitoring and supervision that results from local programs operating with both state and federal support and supervision is treated in greater detail in a later discussion of the federal role. The quality of local public health work throughout a state has been strongly influenced by the quality of the state health department leadership, as constrained by its budget and the responsibilities assigned to it by the state government. This is particularly true outside of the big cities and highly urbanized counties. In urban areas, the local health department has often depended

TABLE 4-1. Sixteen Most Frequently Conducted Activities of State Health Departments, 1961

Rank	Activity	Number of States
1	Environmental health	50
2	Health education	50
3	Maternal and child health	50
4	Nursing	50
5	Vital statistics	49
6	Laboratories	47
7	Dental health	46
8	Communicable diseases	45
9	Engineering	43
10	Tuberculosis control	43
11	Hospital survey, planning, and construction licensure	42
12	Local health services	42
13	Industrial health	36
14	Personnel	34
15	Cancer control	31
16	Chronic disease control	30

SOURCE: Shubick HJ, Wright EO: Composite study of fifty health department organizational charts representing forty-nine states and the District of Columbia. Unpublished report, 1961, cited in (22:224).

less on the state health department, has had more direct ties with Washington, and has often been lax in reporting to the state health agency.

A study of the composition of state boards of health by Gossert and Miller (17), completed in 1972, revealed that the standards of Shattuck or the APHA were far from having been met. Alaska and Rhode Island had no statutory boards. In Illinois and Delaware there was statutory provision, but no board was currently appointed in Illinois, and the Delaware board consisted solely of two state officials. In 16 states, the health function was combined with at least one other agency, and four states had a conglomerate human resources agency. Of the 46 states with functioning boards, 32 had at least one-third medical doctors on them, and in 12 they constituted a majority of the board. In two states, Alabama and South Carolina, the state medical society was the board of health. Shattuck had warned in 1850 against domination of the board of health by any one profession. Only 12.5 percent of the 433 seats in 46 states were occupied by persons identified as consumers in 1972. Appointments to the board were almost always made by governors, with some form of legislative approval being required in half of the states. The trend was to merge state health departments with other departments. In 1969 there were 8 such states, and 1972 there were 16.

The previously described trends in changing attitudes regarding the functions of local health departments also occurred at the state level. Over time, there has been a shift away from a conception of function restricted to a few communitywide preventive measures toward one of responsibility for making the total system of health care available to all citizens of the state. However, a comparison of the 1968 APHA statement of policy with the actual activities of state health departments in recent years reveals that the traditional functions are still paramount—with the newer ones of community coordination for total health care, particularly medical care—becoming less evident.

THE MOST RECENT PICTURE: THE ASTHO DATA

Since 1970, annual statistics on the operation of state health departments have been assembled via questionnaire under the auspices of the Association of State and Territorial Health Officials (ASTHO). The organizational entity established by ASTHO to carry out this task in 1970 was called the National Public Health Program Reporting System (NPHPRS). In 1981 the ASTHO foundation, a nonprofit organization, was established to monitor developments in public health and facilitate the exchange of information. It continued collection and publication of the public health data that the NPHPRS system had been assembling, but it was now called the ASTHO Reporting System (ASTHO/RS). In November of 1985 the name of the ASTHO Foundation was changed to the Public Health Foundation. Because promotion of local public health department activities is so important a part of the state health agency's functions, these data also include much information about these local health departments (or LHDs, as they are referred to in these reports.) With the publication of the most recent report for fiscal year 1984, 12 consecutive years of comprehensive data are available. Most of the following remarks about the 1984 status of these departments, State Health Agencies (SHAs), as they are called in these reports, are based on November 1986 report (18).

In Fiscal year 1984, there were 55 SHAs in 50 states and five territories. Only the Northern Mariana Islands and the Trust Territory had no SHAs, although in prior years they did. Seven states (Maine, Massachusetts, Montana, New Mexico, Ohio, South Dakota, and Wisconsin) and two territories (American Samoa and Guam) did not provide expenditure data to the ASTHO/RS for fiscal 1984, and the expenditure data cover only 46 states and territories. In 1984 the 46 reporting SHAs and the local health departments (LHDs) in their states spent a total of $5.8 billion for public health, of which $4.3 billion, or 74 percent, was allocated to personal health services and the remainder to other categories such as environmental health, health resources, laboratory, and general administration. The data indicate a substantial transfer of source of funding from state and local to federal. In 1974 25.5 percent of the funds were of federal origin: by 1978 this proportion had risen to 34.8 percent; and in 1984, it was 37.1 percent. It is worth noting that in 1984, the total public health expenditures by state and local public health agencies in the 46 reporting states was $6.9 billion, so that the SHAs spent 84 percent of this amount. In 1978, by contrast, this ratio was only 65 percent. Despite the widespread discussion of the need to pay greater attention to public health, only 2.8 percent of the total $388 billion spent for health services in calendar year 1984 was spent for public health (19), and only a bit over 1.5 percent of this total was spent by SHAs.

The principal functions being performed generally continue to emphasize those areas that Mountin found predominant in 1946, in terms of both the relative distribution of the dollar and the number of SHAs involved. Comparison of the state health department functions cited by Mountin for 1930, 1940, and 1946—on one hand, with the number of states presently reporting programs and with the 1961 tabulations shown in Table 4-1, on the other hand—indicates that the scope of activities has not been significantly enlarged. In 1984 "nearly all" SHAs were concerned with maternal and child health, communicable disease control, chronic disease, dental health, public health nursing (including home visits), nutrition, consumer protection and sanitation, water quality, health statistics, and diagnostic laboratory tests. However, the amounts spent for these functions varied widely, with maternal and child health comprising 34 percent, chronic disease 3.7 percent, and dental health 0.7 percent. Local consumer protection and sanitation are still the leading environmental functions, and maternal and child health still represents the mainstay noninstitutional activities of most state health departments in the area of personal services. After maternal and child health services (excluding institutional operations), the order of SHAs expenditures for personal health are as follows: handicapped children's services, supporting personal health services (e.g., health education, home health care, public health nursing), chronic disease, alcohol and drug abuse, communicable disease control, mental health, and dental health. The "newer" functions of chronic disease that Mountin stressed is now shown as a function by 44 of the 46 reporting SHAs, but only 5 percent of the total personal health expenditures (6.4 percent of the noninstitutional expenditures) went for this function.

The dominance of a single functional area, maternal and child health, is striking. Expenditures for these programs comprise one-third of the total expenses and 46 percent of personal health care expenditures. The percentages are even higher if one includes crippled children programs. The dominating position of Maternal and Child Health program expenditures is, is turn, also largely due to a single item, Women and Infant Care (WIC) nutrition, a diet supplement program supported by the Department of Agriculture. In 1984 $1158 million of the $1978 million in MCH expenditures, or 59 percent, went for this single program. The predominance of the MCH and Handicapped Children's programs, even without the WIC component, raises provocative questions about the future. If a national medical care program, with universal eligibility and comprehensive benefits, were ever implemented, it presumably would include prenatal care, mother and infant care, and care of handicapped children. It would, parenthetically, also include much of the care now provided under categorical programs for venereal disease, dental health, chronic disease, and other personal health programs. The personal health care functions of the SHAs might then be reduced, in which event the environmental, planning, and monitoring functions would be likely candidates to become the most important functions. It is interesting, therefore, to look at the status of these programs categories in SHAs in 1984.

Environmental protection is an area that exemplifies an important trend in recent years, that is, the widespread use of agencies other than SHAs for health protection functions. In the District of Columbia all environmental services are provided by agencies other than the SHA. In 45 reporting SHAs, these services were provided in varying degrees, with at least 26 percent of the $381 million in expenditures going for consumer protection and sanitation programs. At least another 23 percent was spent on water quality programs. However, most of the environmental health activities were of the standard type. As recently as 1978, the ASTHO report stated:

> All of the SHAs reporting environmental health programs provided *consumer protection and sanitation* [emphasis in original] services, including food, or milk control, substance control and product safety, sanitation of health care facilities and other institutions, housing and recreational sanitation, or vector and zoonotic disease control. *Water quality* services, provided by 51 SHAs, were usually related to public drinking water, individual water supply, and individual sewage disposal. Public water pollution control services were more often provided by an agency other than the SHA. *Radiation control* services were

offered by 45 SHAs. Fewer SHAs provided other environmental health services: *occupational health and safety and related services* (38 SHAs), *waste management* (34), and *air quality* [emphasis added].

The question is not discussed in the report of the 1984 data, but it is unlikely that the picture has changed materially. Environmental health expenditures of state health agencies were funded predominantly (61 percent) by the state, almost 25 percent came from federal sources, and the rest originated from local government and other sources. The Environmental Protection Act of 1970 called for the governor and/or the legislature of each state to designate a "lead environmental agency" to have overall responsibility for environmental activities. There are three generally recognized models for such agency selection: an SHA, a state environmental protection agency, and a state natural resources agency (20). In 14 of the 55 SHAs that had environmental programs were designated as lead environmental agencies.

Turning to the role of SHAs in statewide health planning, the picture is similar to, but not quite the same as, that in environmental health. In many states, other agencies are mainly responsible for health planning, but more SHAs have been given this function than in environmental health. Under the Health planning and Resource Development Act of 1974 (PL 93-641), each state was to appoint a single agency as the State Health Planning and Development Agency (SHPDA). of the 55 "states," 32 designated their SHA as the SHPDA in 1984 (similar to the number that did so under the Comprehensive Health Planning Act of 1966).

One of the most important activities of state health departments is the development of local public health departments and the supervision and monitoring of their work. It is interesting to see, therefore, how these matters stood in 1984 according to the ASTHO data. The ASTHO definition of a local public health department (and therefore that which constitutes public health coverage) has been somewhat relaxed as compared to some previous definitions in that it no longer requires medical leadership. The ASTHO definition asserts a local health department to be:

> An official public health agency, responsible to a governmentality such as a city, county, city-county, federation of countries, borough, or township. To meet this definition, a local health department must have a staff of one or more full-time professional public health employees (e.g., public health nurse, sanitarian); deliver public health services; serve a definable geographic area; and have identifiable expenditures or budget in the political subdivision which it serves (18).

ASTHO is now defining a local health department even more liberally than the full-time public health department in the older literature of Ferrell, Mountin, and Emerson. The relaxation of the previous requirement for a medically trained health officer to head the agency is not merely a compromise with reality. Some of the literature in the intervening period (21,22) has reported the belief—and often strong advocacy—that it is desirable, not merely expedient, to discontinue this requirement. The health officer position has been seen by some as one largely involving administration and policy analysis, requiring a grasp of overall public health knowledge and principles of administration, rather than one of medicine.

Three types of local public health department (LHD) were identified in the 1975 report: an LHD operated by the SHA as part of a centrally directed state system of local public health agencies; a largely autonomous LHD receiving some technical assistance and consultation from the SHA; and a partly autonomous LHD that shares control with the SHA, with the latter having direct operating authority in some areas. In 1984 there were 2200 LHDs meeting the definition of NPHPRs. Forty of the 55 states had LHDs, and 6 Arkansas, Delaware, District of Columbia, Rhode Island, Vermont, and the Virgin Islands had none. Fifteen "states" reported portions of there population served by their SHAs, but only seven reported more than 13 percent of their population so served; Puerto Rico with 84 percent, New Hampshire with 72 percent, Pennsylvania with 64 percent, and Alaska with 55 percent were the largest.

About 23 percent of SHA money spent on public health went to to LHDs in the 46 states reporting for 1984. Most of this money was allocated for personal health progams (such as public health nursing, health education, maternal and child health, chronic disease, etc.) A little more than one-half of the money originated within the state itself, and 29 percent was federal money which was transmitted to the local government via the SHA. The total of $389 million in federal funds included $142.1 million from the MCH and Preventive Health block grant funds (or 37 percent of the total). These included the original Title V and Title VI funds that had been folded into the block grants (see below).

Although 55 percent of the funding of the LHDs originated from the SHAs, some of this SHA money granted to the LHDs came, in turn, from the federal government. In terms of the *ultimate* source of LHD expenditures, 30 percent came from state money, 18 percent from federal, 34 percent from local funds, and the rest from fees collected and other sources. The percentage coming from local sources varied greatly from state to state, as it always has. In New Jersey, New York, South Dakota, and 27 other states, none of the LHD expenditures originated from local sources. In Texas, 80 percent was estimated to originate locally. In other states, the percentage varied from 0 to 80 percent. (Tables 4-2 and 4-3 summarize the patterns of LHD sources of funds, and Tables 4-4 and 4-5 show the pattern of the combined SHA and LHD expenditures by source of funds.)

Public Policy Implications

At the beginning of this section, it was noted that the state's responsibilities for health protection are much broader than those of the local government. Consequently, there is a wider range of possible functions that could appear in the list of programs engaged in by any particular state health department. Despite this greater breadth of choice, the number of functions that SHAs actually perform is generally only a small proportion of the health functions carried on by different state governments, and the ones assigned to the health department vary markedly from state to state. Responsibility and control are shared with other agencies. The reasons for the wide distribution of health functions among the different SHAs are complex. They reflect a growing tendency to assign health problems to agencies other than health departments since 1960. Although much rhetoric ascribes the "need" to choose another agency to the alleged fact that the SHA is technically inadequate and/or managerially inefficient, some have argued that various special interest groups seek such a choice because they believe it to be advantageous to them. Whatever factors are actually most influential, the trend away from assigning major health-related programs to SHAs is undeniable. This issue will be further addressed in the discussion of the federal role. but it is so important in terms of the development of SHAs that it is worth pausing to review the evidence that establishes this trend as a fact.

TABLE 4-2. Expenditures[a] of Local Health Departments by Program Area, Fiscal Year 1984

Program Area	Total LHD Expenditures		SHA Intergovernmental Grants to LHDs		Additional LHD Expenditures	
	Amount	Percentage of Total	Amount	Percentage of Total	Amount	Percentage of Total
Personal health	1416.3	57.8	871.1	65.1	545.2	48.9
Environmental health	292.5	11.9	131.4	9.8	161.1	14.5
Health resources	220.1	9.0	185.8	13.9	34.2	3.0
Laboratory	42.3	1.7	26.9	2.0	15.4	1.4
General administration	132.1	5.4	35.8	2.7	96.3	8.6
Unallocated to program areas	349.0	14.2	86.9	6.5	262.1	23.5
Total	2452.2	100.0	1338.0	100.0	1114.2	100.0

SOURCE: *Public Health Foundation: Public Health Agencies 1984*, Washington, DC, Public Health Foundation, 1986.
[a]Amounts in millions of dollars.

TABLE 4-3. Expenditures[a] of Local Health Departments by Source of Funds, Fiscal Year 1984

Source of Funds	Total LHD Expenditures		SHA Intergovernmental Grants to LHDs		Additional LHD Expenditures	
	Amount	Percentage of Total	Amount	Percentage of Total	Amount	Percentage of Total
State funds	727.6	29.7	709.3	53.0	18.3	1.6
Federal grant and contract funds	430.8	17.6	388.8	29.1	42.0	3.8
Local funds	826.7	33.7	134.8	10.1	691.9	62.1
Fees and reimbursements	265.6	10.8	82.7	6.2	182.9	16.4
Other sources	50.2	2.0	22.3	1.7	27.8	2.5
Source unknown	151.3	6.2	—	—	151.3	16.4
Other sources	50.2	2.0	22.3	1.7	27.8	2.5
Source unknown	151.3	6.2	—	—	151.3	13.6
Total	2452.2	100.0	1338.0	100.0	1114.2	100.0

SOURCE: *Public Health Foundation: Public Health Agencies 1984,* Washington, DC, Public Health Foundation, 1986.

[a]Amounts in millions of dollars.

TABLE 4-4. Expenditures[a] of the Nation's Public Health Agencies, by Program Area, Fiscal Year 1984

Program Area	Total SHA and LHD Expenditures	Direct SHA Expenditures	SHA Inter- Governmental Grants to LHDs	Additional Expenditures of LHDs
Personal health	4841.8	3425.5	871.1	545.2
Environmental health	542.9	250.4	131.4	161.1
Health resources	552.0	332.0	185.8	34.2
Laboratory	212.5	170.2	26.9	15.4
General administration	399.1	267.0	35.8	96.3
Not allocated to program areas	349.0		86.9	262.1
Total public health	6897.3	4445.1	1338.0	1114.2

SOURCE: *Public Health Foundation: Public Health Agencies 1984*, Washington, DC, Public Health Foundation, 1986.

[a]Amounts in millions of dollars.

TABLE 4-5. Expenditures[a] of the Nation's Public Health Agencies, by Source of Funds, Fiscal Year 1984

Source of Funds	Total SHA and LHD Expenditures	Direct SHA Expenditures	SHA Inter- Governmental Grants to LHDs	Additional Expenditures of LHDs
State funds	3153.1	2425.5	709.3	18.3
Federal grant and contract funds	2188.5	1757.7	388.8	42.0
Local funds	830.8	4.1	134.8	691.9
Fees and reimbursements	448.4	182.8	82.7	182.9
Other sources	125.2	75.1	22.3	27.8
Source unknown	151.3	—	—	151.3
Total public health	6897.3	4445.1	1338.0	1114.2

SOURCE: *Public Health Foundation: Public Health Agencies 1984*, Washington, DC, Public Health Foundation, 1986.

[a]Amounts in millions of dollars.

One of the principal functions of the SHA, especially after the passage of the Social Security Act, has been that of liaison and administrative agent for the distribution and supervision of federal grants among local health agencies within the state. Use of the SHA health agency was generally mandated by the early post-1935 legislation. Later, beginning in the 1950s, the SHA began to be bypassed with increasing frequency as the state agency distributing federal monies to localities for health activities; project grants for local services given directly by the federal agency to the local grantee became increasingly prevalent. In addition, many subsequent health program grants distributed via the states did not specify the SHA as the mandatory administering agency. For example, the Comprehensive Health Planning Act of 1966 specified only that a single state agency in each state was to administer federal grants to that state under this act; 23 states placed this function not in their SHAs but in other agencies. Under the provision of the 1975 Planning Act, in 1978, 36 states designated the SHA as their State Health Planning and Development Agencies (SHPDAs), the remaining 21 naming other agencies.

Under the Medicaid Act, only relevant SHAs are the designated state agency for administering Medicaid, despite the fact that nearly all SHAs have their own programs of general ambulatory care, and in 1984 SHAs spent $901 million for SHA-operated institutions, including general, mental, and chronic disease hospitals; institutions for the mentally retarded; and skilled nursing facilities. Other examples could be cited, but these are sufficient to support the assertion that SHAs have often been bypassed since 1950 as the chief administrator of new statewide health programs. This tendency has been widespread even in the area of health planning, despite the fact that public health professionals and others have long advocated that areawide and state health planning be *the* basic function of state and local health departments. As was noted in 1984, only 32 of the 55 "states" designated their SHAs as their official planning agency.

FEDERAL ROLE IN STATE AND LOCAL
PUBLIC HEALTH SERVICES
AFTER 1935: 1936–1945

It was noted previously that passage of the Social Security Act in 1935 heralded the beginning of a major program of federal grants-in-aid to the states for health purposes, and that the portions of the act that affected public health departments were Titles V (Section 1) and VI. Administration of these two titles comprised the major public health activities of the federal government in the 1930s. Selected details of the original provisions of these titles, especially Title VI, are presented here to illustrate some of the characteristics of revenue-sharing grants discussed earlier.

Under Title V, federal grants could be given to the states for "promoting the health of mothers and children" (7:77). The funds were distributed by the Children's Bureau to the SHDs to be used for supporting these services in state and local health departments. These programs were subsequently expanded; amendments passed in 1965 as part of the Medicare Act later provided for project grants to state and local health agencies for comprehensive maternity care to high risk mothers and for the development of high-quality comprehensive health services to children and youths of school or preschool age. The operating agency could be a public or an appropriate nonprofit private agency. Amounts were subsequently also appropriated for research projects "relating to maternal and child health and crippled children's services." Expanded federal support of maternal and child health activities by state and local health departments continued until 1981, when these grants were consolidated with six other programs into a Maternal and Child Health Services Block Grant. This action was part of the reduction in social programs in the Reagan Administration embodied in the Omnibus Budget Reconciliation Act of 1981, which is further discussed below.

Title VI of the act directly addressed the buildup of state and local health departments, and the monies appropriated under it have been administered by the PHS. In the original act, federal funds were appropriated annually, under a block grant formula, for the years 1936–1940, "For the purpose of assisting states, counties, health districts and other political subdivisions of the states in establishing and maintaining adequate public health services" (7:63). In 1944 this title, with some changes, was transferred from the Social Security Act to Section 314 of the newly constituted Public Health Service Act. The original act required that funds be allocated among the states on the basis of a formula to be promulgated by the U.S. Surgeon General, taking into account three factors: (1) the state's population size, (2) the state's relative economic status, and (3) the prevalence of special health problems in the state. Each state health department was required to file an acceptable plan with the U.S. Surgeon General indicating how the grant was to be used and a report at the end of the year detailing how it had actually been used.

Several aspects of the allocation and administrative provisions of Title VI set important precedents for future federal governmental policy: (1) all funds were to be administered nationally by a general health agency; (2) the system of tax sharing was partially a per capita redistribution of federal tax revenues and partly an attempt to equalize relative local and state tax burdens among the states; (3) the filing of state plans and the requirement of annual reports was a modest attempt to achieve quality control and encourage statewide planning; and (4) the funds went directly to a single state agency, which was mandated to be the state health department, to be redistributed within the state.

THE PERIOD 1946–1968

The previous discussion of local public health departments noted that public health professionals, some members of Congress, and the Democratic presidents came to believe that the state and local health departments were being inordinately slow to enter the newer fields of public health work. These concerns, dealing principally with primary care in medically underserved areas, chronic disease abatement, and control of the more recent environmental threats, were being defined by students of personal health care organization and environmental control as belonging to the local health department. It has also been mentioned that attempts by the federal government to encourage local health departments to pursue these special programs led to increased use of categorical grants as opposed to general-purpose formula grants (13). The categorical grants were still formula grants and required matching—usually on a one-to-one basis—but were intended to stimulate spending for specific activities that the federal government deemed desirable nationally rather than to support the general budget of the health department. From about 1950 on, the federal grant structure increasingly encouraged state and local public health agencies to move more aggressively into areas defined by the federal government as national health priorities. The number of classes of categorical formula grants increased over the years, as did the proporiton of total formula grants so earmarked. By 1965, out of about $50 million in formula grants, only $10 million, or 20 percent, were allocated for general health; the rest were designated for specified categories (23). Considerable difficulties were experienced by some states and localities, which found these earmarked funds to be inappropriate for the programs needed in their areas. After 15 years of continued unsuccessful efforts to encourage greater activity in chronic control, pollution abatement, medical care services, and similar programs through the use of earmarked formula grants, the federal government attempted in 1966 to discontinue the use of earmarked grants funneled through state governments for accomplishing these goals.

The Comprehensive Health Planning and Public Health Service Amendments of 1966 (PL 89-749) and the Partnership for Health Amendments of 1967 (PL 90-174) abolished all categorical earmarking of formula grants (24). These amendments are discussed in the next section.

Project Grants

Development of the programs being promoted by the federal government via categorical formula grants was inhibited by the conflict between large metropolitan centers and their state governments (25). Many state legislatures were so structured that the influence of rural sections was out of proportion to the size of their populations. These states had been slow to assign comprehensive health care and wide ecologic control responsibilities to their state health departments. The population and organizations in the large municipal centers and their suburbs, on the other hand, had increasingly attempted to expand such activities. Unable to prevail in the state capital, they turned to Washington for direct aid. These factors, among others, led to the emergence of project grants as an increasingly important segment of federal grants in the 1960s.

Project grants for rural sanitation projects had been made in very modest amounts as far back as before 1935. After 1935, the first project grant to be administered by the PHS was made in 1946 for venereal disease control (9), and between 1947 and 1959, the project grant program for this purpose remained unique. "The first half of the 1960s was marked by a flood of new project grant programs." (22) Formula grants (including categorical grants) were 77 percent of the total $76 million in health grants in 1963; they were only 48 percent of the $105 million distributed in 1965. In the latter years, the proportion of total grants-in-aid for project grants exceeded that for formula grants for the first time.

The overall thrust of these amendments to Section 314 of the Public Health Service Act was not only to remove the categorical earmarking from formula grants but also to attempt to establish the project grant as a permanent form of aid and to meet the various objections to the disintegrative effects of such grants on planning. All formula grants were block grants, and no categorical formula grants were included in the 1966 act. The federal government's attempts to encourage local public health departments and other agencies to act on its high-priority targets were to be continued and intensified, but this was to be done only by the use of project grants.

It should be noted that project grants are, by their very nature, well suited to promoting categorical programs. The formula public health grants that were continued as block grants in subsequent years came to be known as "314d" monies after the section of the Public Health Act that provided for them.

The important changes in grant-in-aid structure under this act may be summarized as involving four basic elements: (1) introduction of a heavy element of planning activity, (2) abolition of categorical formula grants, (3) introduction of a state comprehensive health planning authority that need not be the same as the state health department, and (4) reinforcement of the practice of awarding health services grants directly to nongovernmental grantees through the increased emphasis on project grants.

Despite the 1966 legislation, which intended that formula grants to public health departments be of the block type, Congress was apparently unable to resist pleas of various advocates of specific programs. Categorical programs continued to proliferate, while the block 314d money continued to dwindle away.

The continued inability of the federal government structure to bring state and local public health departments more into line with federal priorities led to a number of subsequent reorgnizations that weakened the Office of the Surgeon General, the head of the US Public Health Service. The status of that office and the role of the PHS remained in a state of flux for a number of years, with the position of U.S. Surgeon General being actually abolished for a time under the reorganization of the PHS in 1973. The position was reinstated under the Carter administration, and its incumbent attempted to strengthen the role and prestige of the PHS with emphasis on prevention.

THE PERIOD 1969–1980

Following the election of Richard M. Nixon as president in 1968, the federal executive branch began to reverse certain aspects of the relationship between the federal, state, and local governments. This attempted change was directly pertinent to public health policy because of the federal grant system of supporting public health programs. The main goal of this policy, dubbed the "New Federalism" by his administration, was summarized by President Nixon early in 1969: "after over a century and a half of power flowing from the people and from the local communities and from the States to Washington, D.C., let's get it back to the people and to the cities and to the States where it belongs" (26). The legislative and organizational changes that the administration expected to use to translate the goals of the New Federalism into action had three principal elements:

1. Greater reliance on state and local governments in the operation and administration of federal grant programs. Categorical grants were to be eliminated as far as possible in favor of global block grants (revenue sharing). It should be noted that the term "block" here meant a lump sum granted to a state or local government for all purposes, health included. The amount of the grant to be used for health would be decided solely by the state or local government.
2. Streamlining federal granting programs, to make them simple to administer. Federal programs were to be decentralized to regional offices, with increased interagency standardization of requirements and procedures for federal grant applications. Local governments and regional offices were to have broad decision-making power.
3. A major realignment of federal departments "to better conform to major purposes of government and to better coordinate the managment of federal programs" (27). On October 20, 1972, general revenue sharing was enacted into law (PL 92-512) as the State and Local Fiscal Assistance Act of 1972. An amount of $30.2 billion was appropriated to states and localities to be distributed over a 5-year period beginning January 1, 1972. About one-third of the money went to the states and two-thirds to local governments. The program was extended in 1977 for 5 years through 1981. The budget program proposed by President Ronald Reagan for 1983 envisaged a continuation of the revenue-sharing program, at least through 1986, at slightly increased levels over those of 1981 and 1982 (28). It was discontinued in 1987.

The revenue-sharing programs were of great potential importance for state and local public health programs. Block grants provided to states and localities subsequently increased state and local decision-making power—a power that could be used to reduce or augment public health programs in relation to other spending areas. This potential was only modestly realized, but in some areas such as Oakland, California, it was an important source of funding for local community health centers.

Although agreeing to the president's revenue-sharing proposals, Congress opposed the elimination of appropriations for many ongoing categorical programs that had been funded in past years. President Nixon's 1974 budget had called for discontinuing many of these programs and cutting others substantially (29). It also proposed cancellations totaling about $550 millions appropriated in 1973 that the administration had not spent (recissions). An apparent truce in the administration–Congress battle over the federally funded programs was declared when the president, in June 1973, signed a law extending expiring health programs for 1 year.

Further contests between Republican President Nixon and the Democratic Congress were ended with Mr. Nixon's resignation on August 9, 1974 and the succession of Gerald R. Ford to the presidency. President Ford generally employed Nixon's health policies. The principal thrusts continued to include overall reduction of health budgets and consolidation of existing categorical programs into block formula grants. In his last State of the Union Address, President Ford called for budgetary consolidation of 16 health programs, including a number of public programs such as formula public health grants (314d), immunization, rat control, lead paint poisoning prevention, maternal and child health, state health grants, and family planning. Because the states were not required to match the federal funds under this budget proposal, they could have offset reductions in federal funds by reducing their own expenditures and curtailing programs. The proposal seemed clearly tied to a reduction of health services, and was opposed by Congress. In January 1977, President Jimmy Carter assumed office.

The Carter administration discontinued Ford's attempts to consolidate most public health categorical grants into a single block grant. However, the total sum allotted for health programs in the Carter budget for 1977–1978 was only slightly higher than it had been in the Ford budget (29). Throughout the Carter administration, three major goals were emphasized in public health: expansion of preventive and some treatment services for poor children; health promotion and prevention for the entire population; and mental health services, especially in the community.

The measures suggested to expand services for children were embodied in a proposal called Comprehensive Health Assessment and Treatment for Poor Children (CHAP). It was to have reached 1.8 million children in addition to the 12 million who were already eligible for such services through Medicaid. During 1977, CHAP bills were introduced in both the Senate and the House of Representatives and throughout President Carter's term of office, this proposal was pushed in Congress but failed to pass. A leading factor in its defeat was an antiabortion amendment that was attached by legislators opposed to abortion, a tactic that split congressional support.

The health promotion and disease prevention program consisted of stepped-up national campaigns to inform people about the importance of health matters such as smoking, eating, and exercise and a reorganization of the Communicable Disease Control section of the PHS into the Centers for Disease Control. The program was the centerpiece of the agenda of Dr. Julius Richmond, the Surgeon General of the PHS. Doctor Richmond, appointed in July 1977, set out to revitalize the PHS largely by assertively promoting the idea of prevention and health maintenance. In documents issued in 1979 and 1980 (30–32), the importance of prevention and health promotion was carefully delineated and national "achievable" goals for 1990 established. The report called for allocating a greater portion of the health dollar to prevention. The 1980 report set targets for the following priority areas: high blood pressure control, family planning, pregnancy and infant health, immunization, sexually transmitted diseases, toxic agent control, occupational safety and health, accident prevention and injury control, fluoridation and dental health, surveillance and control of infectious diseases, smoking and health, misuse of alcohol and drugs, physical fitness and exercise, and control of stress and violent behavior (32).

Using extant research writings, the reports concluded that of the 10 leading causes of death in 1976, 50 percent were due to unhealthy behavior or life style, 20 percent to environmental factors, 20 percent to human biologic factors, and 10 percent to inadequacies in the existing health care system. It seemed to follow clearly that changing unhealthy behavior was the most important way of preventing or controlling the diseases that were the leading causes of death.

The Center for Disease Control was expanded in October 1980 with a reorganization that changed the Communicable Disease Center to the Centers for Disease Control (CDC). The CDC contained six bureaus: the Center for Prevention Services, the Center for Environmental Health, the National Institute for Occupational Safety and Health, the Center for Health Promotion and Education, the Center for Professional Development and Training, and the Center for Disease Investigation and Diagnosis.

Thus was the campaign to enhance prevention as a priority of the federal health agency, organized along the lines of previous campaigns to prevent communicable disease. Included were the identification of health threats, determination of probable causes and methods for combatting them, and an organizational form with which to execute the series of operations. The early public health measures of sanitation and quarantine had often been successful even though they were based on imperfectly understood causes of acute disease and the method of their transmission. As one historian of public health once stated: "The program of the sanitary reformers was based to a large extent on a structure of erroneous theories, and while they hit upon the right solution, it was mostly for the wrong reasons" (5:225). It seemed reasonable to hope that a public health campaign to curb the ravages of degenerative disease could also result in partial success. Even though the precise mechanisms of these disease processes were only imperfectly understood, their associations with certain risk factors were applied as guides to proper preventive measures—the coming to the fore of the epidemic of the acute disease process, acquired immune deficiency syndrome (AIDS), the mysterious nature of which only adds further impetus to the approach of this "campaign."

The opponents of this view did not argue that prevention was unimportant. However, they stated that at present, and for a long time to come, persons will continue to get sick, and when they do, they need medical care. Poor people get sick more often and more seriously than do the nonpoor (33), and the only reason they often do not receive treatment is that they are socially and economically disadvantaged. The medical care problem must be solved, they argued, before real political support could be mustered behind prevention. Persons facing imminent financial ruin because of impending medical bills could not be expected to concentrate on preventing ill health in the future. The various repercussions of this rift prevented unified support for President Carter's health proposal in Congress. It may fairly be said that *financial* support for public health did not advance substantially under Carter, despite his avowed commitment to increasing public health. In fact, considering inflation, it retrogressed. Carter's own budgets for Fiscal years 1980 and 1981 mandated cuts in public health funds. The principal contribution was the *theoretical leadership* provided by the U.S. Surgeon General in beginning to define more completely what a modern program of prevention might look like.

The Reagan Administration took office in January, 1981, determined to slash all government social programs with public health as one of its main targets. The new president called for a severe cutback in federal support for public health, to be accomplished by discontinuing some programs, cutting appropriations for others, and turning as many as possible back to the states. He hoped to eventually consolidate all remaining federal money for public health given to the states into one block grant. The first major legislative result of the new administration was the Omnibus Budget Reconciliation Act (PL 97-35), passed on August 13, 1981, giving the appropriations for the fiscal year ending 1982. The Reagan Administration did not obtain its request that 26 programs be combined into two block grants for public health, but it did succeed in getting 20 programs combined into four block grants. Six programs remained categorical. The block grants were set up as a new section of the Public Health Service Act, Title XIX. The folding in of the porgrams into block grants consisted of the following:

1. Preventive Health and Health Services (PHS) Block Grant. The programs folded in were (a) rodent control, (b) fluoridation, (c) hypertension control, (d) health services and centers (rape crisis centers), (e) old 314d money, (f) home health services, and (g) emergency services. The grants were to be distributed among the states according to a formula based on population and other factors deemed appropriate by the Secretary of Health and Human Services (HHS). Each state had to apply for these grants.

2. Alcohol Abuse, Drug Abuse, and Mental Health Block Grant. The programs folded in were (a) Community Mental Health Centers Act; (b) Mental Health Systems Act; (c) Comprehensive Alcohol Abuse and Alcoholism Prevention, Treatment, and Rehabilitation Act of 1970; and (d) Drug Abuse Prevention, Treatment, and Rehabilitation Act.

3. Primary Care Block Grant. This section consisted of the Community Health Centers. States could begin to take them over beginning in Fiscal year 1983.

4. Maternal and Child Health (MCH) Block Grant (amends Title V of the social Security Act). The programs folded in were (a) maternal and child health and crippled children's services of Title V of the Social Security Act, (b) supplementary security income to provide rehabilitation services for blind and disabled children, (c) lead-based paint poisoning prevention, (d) genetic disease service, (e) sudden infant death syndrome (SIDS), (f) hemophilia treatment, and (g) adolescent pregnancy under the Health Services and Centers Amendment of 1978. The SHA was designated the administering agency, and the formula for Fiscal years 1982 and 1983 was based on the number of low-income children. Alternative bases for the formula in the future were to be submitted to Congress by the Secretary of HHS by June 1982. The states had to contribute $3 for every $4 of federal funds received.

The six programs left as categorical grants were (1) childhood immunization, (2) tuberculosis control, (3) family planning, (4) migrant health centers, (5) venereal disease control, and (6) an amount equal to 15 percent of the total Maternal and Child Health Services Grant that was to be set aside for use by HHS to fund projects of "regional or national significance" in training and research, genetic disease testing, counseling, and information development and for comprehensive hemophilia diagnostic and treatment centers. In addition, the Women, Infants, and Children (WIC) nutrition program funded by the Agriculture Department was also left categorical. As has been noted, this food supplement program is an important LHD activity. Thus six programs were left as categorical and the remaining 20 were folded into four block grants, instead of all being folded into two block grants, because of vigorous lobbying in Congress by advocates of the varying programs.

Not only were block grants being turned over to the states to administer, but their total funding for the programs in each block grant was reduced by 21 percent. Further, after accounting for inflation, the actual reduction in resources was expected to be even higher, perhaps 30 percent. When one considers the simultaneous reduction in state and local tax revenues because of the recession of the early 1980s and the tax revolt of the late 1970s and early 1980s, it is clear that local and state public health services faced a severe financial shortfall. For 1983, President Reagan's budget proposals had requested further reduction in federal grants for public health, to be accomplished by further folding remaining categorical grants into blocks and reducing the total. In his State of the Union Address, he had called for turning over 43 federal programs to the states by 1984 and giving them the choice of continuing or discontinuing them. The congressional consensus that had so quickly passed the Omnibus Budget Reconciliation Act had weakened considerably, and the request for further cuts was met with substantial opposition in Congress. After the reduction for Fiscal year 1982 contained in the Omnibus Budge Act, most of the federal money for state and local public health department work was not further substantially eroded, and in some cases, were later raised to Fiscal year 1982 or earlier levels. For example, the MCH block grant federal obligations for Fiscal year 1982 were $374 million and for 1985, were $478 million (34). Adjusting for inflation would bring the new amounts into approximate equality in terms of the resources they would command. Similar remarks apply to the PHS and Health Services and Alcohol, Drug Abuse, and Mental Health Services Block Grants.

The appropriation for fiscal 1986 and 1987 each provided $478 million for the Maternal and Child Health Block Grant and $89.5 million for the Preventive Health and Health Services Block Grant. The alcohol, Drug Abuse, and Mental Health block grant for 1987 received $720 million, a large increase of $225 million over 1986, reflecting the accent on drug abuse control prevailing in Congress and the Reagan Administration in 1986. Appropriations for disease prevention were also increased over prior years, providing $75 million for childhood immunization grants, $7 million for tuberculosis protection, and $50 million for control of sexually transmitted diseases. In addition to the last named item, $400 million was appropriated for 1987 to finance the fight on AIDS, an increase from $234 million appropriated for 1986.

Public Policy Implications

The Reagan program has represented a "basic reversal in U.S. federal policy in health," but it is important to recognize that the essentials of the Reagan administration policies, insofar as they deal with public health services, are largely continuations of policies first formulated by Presidents Nixon and Ford. What, then, are the essential features of these policies, insofar as they have important implications for public health in the United States?

First, they call for an end to federal grants to the states and localities for public health services. A transition period was to give money to the states for public health and ambulatory care services on a block grant basis, with little or no categorical restrictions on how it is to be spent by programs. Regulation of operations by the federal government would be minimal.

Second, direct federal health activities would be limited to a few programs that are clearly national in scope, such as research. Environmental protection activities would be sharply reduced. Third, federal income taxes would be substantially reduced so that persons would have more disposable income available. Thus citizens could vote for more state or local taxes if they wanted particular public health programs. Finally, federal grants would to go the states, and direct federal–local government contact would be avoided wherever feasible. The SHA would be the administering agency for the Maternal and Child Health Services Block Grant.

Persons favoring this program argue that the federal government has become too large and its influence too pervasive on the state and local health activities (and other activities, as well). Local requirements and needs are not well determined in distant Washington and should be made locally. The massive amount of federal regulation had made most programs inefficient; they were top-heavy with administrative personnel and procedures and stifled innovative initiatives for effective operation. Many of the environmental and workplace protections have been extreme and have hurt the growth of the economy, which is basic to national welfare. Furthermore, many programs did not achieve their purpose. The mechanisms of the marketplace, if unfettered by aggressive regulation, will see to it that industry's operations in a competitive world serve the American people in the best manner. In particular, the Reagan program will revitalize industry and result in an increased tax base for states and localities. They will then be able to decide for themselves what programs they want and be able to raise the taxes to pay for them.

Persons opposing the Reagan program point to the shift of the American economy from a local to a regional and a national one. These developments led to a centralization of tax revenue in the federal government, while the responsibility for public health services remained with the states and localities. This divergence led to ever-growing disparities between needs and available tax bases in states and among localities within states. All persons, especially children and youth, should have equal—or as nearly equal opportunity as possible—to develop their potential (35), regardless of the state or locality in which they were born or reared. This belief requires either that programs can be run entirely out of Washington or that federal tax money be redistributed among states and localities according to measures of need. These people also point to the fact that the American economic system is increasingly consolidating and centralizing its control. The organization needed to protect the public interest, they would argue, also needs to be increasingly centralized to correspond to this changing system. In the public health field, the emergence of chronic and degenerative diseases as the leading health threats points to nationwide causation and the need for nationwide preventive measures. Local agencies cannot act to control activities of national and international combines. Returning environmental control to the states, for example, could result in competition among the states to offer the fewest environmental controls possible in an effort to attract national industry.

This is not to say that control and administration from Washington is desirable. There should be as much local administration as possible, but with goals and aims coordinated on a national basis. That was the central idea for the federal "partnership" system, as differentiated from President Nixon's approach and President Reagan's New Federalism.

Finally, the federal partnership system grew in a typically American way: it developed as a series of responses to specific problems. The Reagan program, its opponents argue, is based on abstract ideology and consists merely of a set of assertions stemming from theoretical assumptions about the functioning of the market. The reply of Reagan policy supporters is that the federal partnership really became a federal dictatorship and that its programs have not worked. Something else must be tried.

WHERE DO WE STAND?

What does the future hold for public health? After almost 50 years of proceeding in one direction, a reversal of cooperative federalism was attempted by the Nixon and Ford Administrations and has been strongly pushed by the Reagan Administration. The question is whether this "counterrevolution" is an aberration or a harbinger. The long-term answer is unlikely to be decided by either ideology or empirical developments alone. If history is any guide, the American pattern will be to adopt solutions based on dominant ideological beliefs strongly modified by programmatic responses to changing circumstances.

With respect to the organization and content of public health services, an overriding fact is the changed nature of the major threats to health—the chronic and degenerative diseases as well as the appearance of AIDS. It may be that public health now stands with respect to those diseases where it stood with respect to acute infectious diseases in the mid-1850s. We are beginning to know something about the determinants or risk factors of these diseases and, therefore, certain preventive measures that can reasonably ba advocated. For these measures to be as effective as public health measures became against acute infectious diseases after 1915, considerably more epidemiologic and biologic research is needed. As the results of this research continue to be revealed, and as the smoke settles from the political battles being waged over the future structure of our federal system, decisions will have to be made about the structure of our public health system. The structure and roles of local, state, and federal public health agencies and of other agencies performing health-related work will need to be determined. Again, if past history is any guide, these relationships and functions will be worked out in a combination of theoretical formulation, pragmatic experiments in administrative accommodation, and political battle. After a period of change and turmoil, an attempt will be made to codify the existing arrangement into a comprehensive federal law. If this process of realignment is to be as painless as possible, the nation will need public health leaders who keep up with findings and have the political and administrative ability to incorporate the pioneering ones into public health practice, not only as experiments in individual places but also as national and state policy. The foremost leaders will need to have a good grasp of health problems and what is known about meeting them—both preventive and curative. They will also need to understand the political, social, and historical background of health services and the society as a whole. A number of developments in the federal role in public health have not been addressed here. These include the Food and Drug Administration (FDA), the Occupational Safety and Health Act (OSHA), the federal Community Mental Health Act, the Alcohol and Drug Abuse Act, and the Environmental Protection Act of 1970.

Although these are extremely important to a total understanding of government's public health roles, this chapter has addressed public health activities of the federal government only from the viewpoint of the federal system of public health agencies— the PHS, the SHAs, and the local health departments. Descriptions of many activities not covered in this brief overview may be found in other chapters of this book.

REFERENCES

1. Last JA (ed): *Maxcy-Rosenau Public Health and Preventive Medicine*, 11th ed. New York, Appleton-Century-Crofts, 1980.
2. Dubos R: *The Mirage of Health.* Garden City, NY, Doubleday, 1959; *Man Adapting.* New Haven, CT, Yale University Press, 1965.
3. Dubos R: *Man Adapting.* New Haven, CT, Yale University Press, 1965.
4. Shyrock R: *The Development of Modern Mecicine.* Madison, University of Wisconsin Press, 1979.
5. Rosen G: *A History of Public Health.* New York, MD Publications, 1958.
6. Grad FP: *Public Health Law Manual: A Handbook on the Legal Aspects of Public Health Administration and Enforcement.* Washington, American Public Health Association, 1970.
7. Mustard HS: *Government in Public Health.* New York, Commonwealth Fund, 1945.
8. Ferrell JA, Wilson GS, Covington PW, et al: *Health Departments of States and Provinces of the United States and Canada,* Public Health Bulletin 184. U.S. Public Health Service, Treasury Department, April 1, 1929.
9. Mountin JW, Hankela EK, Druzin GB: *Ten Years of Federal Grants-in-Aid for Public Health,* 1936–1946, Public Health Bulletin 300, U.S. Public Health Service, 1947.
10. Emerson H: *Local Health Units for the Nation.* New York, Commonwealth Fund, 1945.
11. Greve CH, Campbell JR: *Organization and Staffing for Local Health Services,* Public Health Service Publication 682. Washington, DC, U.S. Government Printing Office, 1961 revision.
12. Sanders BS: Local health departments: Growth or illusion? *Publ Health Rep* 1957; 74:13–20.
13. Kenadjian B: Appropriate types of federal grants for state and community health services. *Publ Health Rep* 1966; 81:9.
14. Shubick HJ, Wright EO: Composite study of fifty health department organizational charts representing forty-nine states and the District of Columbia. Unpublished report, 1961, cited in Ref. 22, p 224.
15. Hanlon JJ: *Principles of Public Health Administration.* St Louis, Mosby, 1969. (See also the 9th edition for additional information.)
16. American Public Health Association: The state health department, policy statement of the governing council of the Association, November 13, 1968. A condensed version appeared in *Am J Publ Health* 1969; 59:158–159.

17. Gossert DJ, Miller CA: State boards of health, their members and commitments. *Am J Publ Health* 1973; 63:486–493.

18. Public Health Foundation: *Public Health Agencies 1984*, Washington, DC, Public Health Foundation, November 1986.

19. Levit, KR, et al: National Health Expenditures, 1984, *Health Care Financ Rev,* 1985; 7:1–35.

20. *Book of States,* 1976–1977. Washington, DC, Council of State Governments, 1977.

21. Shonick W: Mergers of public health departments with public hospitals in urban areas: Findings of 12 field studies. *Med Care* 1980; 18(suppl):1–50.

22. Cameron CM, Kobylarz A: Nonphysician directors of local public health departments: Results of a national survey. *Publ Health Rep* 1980; 95:386–397.

23. Zwick D: Project grants for health services. *Publ Health Rep* 1977; 82:131–138.

24. Cavanaugh JH: Comprehensive Health Planning and Public Health Service Act of 1966 (PL 89-749). *Health Educ Welfare Indicators* 1967; 9–18.

25. Ingraham HS: Federal grants management: A state health officer's view. *Publ Health Rep* 1965; 80:670–676.

26. Executive Office of the President: *Restoring the Balance of Federalism*, Second annual report to the president on the federal assistance review. Office of Management and Budget, June 1971.

27. *Federal Assistance Review: A Special Report from the Department of Health, Education and Welfare*, DHEW Publication (OS) 72-38. Office of the Secretary, Department of Health, Education and Welfare, June 1972.

28. Palmer JL, Sawhill IW (eds): *The Reagan Experiment: An Examination of Economic and Social Policies under the Reagan Administration*. Washington, DC, Urban Institute Press, 1982.

29. *Washington Report on Medicine and Health*, a McGraw-Hill weekly publication. February 1973, February 1977, February 1982.

30. *Healthy People*, the U.S. Surgeon General's report on health promotion and disease prevention, DHEW (PHS) Publication 70-55071. Public Health Service, Office of the Assistant Secretary for Health and Surgeon General, 1979.

31. *Healthy People*, the U.S. Surgeon General's report on health promotion and disease prevention, DHEW (PHS) publication 79-05571A, Background Papers. Public Health Service, Office of the Assistant Secretary for Health and Surgeon General, 1979.

32. *Promoting Health/Preventing Disease: Objectives for the Nation*, U.S. Department of Health and Human Services, Fall 1980.

33. Hurley R: The health crisis of the poor, in Dreitzel HP (ed): *The Social Organization of Health*. New York, Macmillan, 1971, pp 83–122.

34. Budget of the United States, 1987. Appendix. Section I–K, Washington, DC, U.S. Government Printing Office, 1987.

35. Tobin J: Reagonomics and economics. *The New York Review of Books,* December 3, 1981, pp 11–14.

CHAPTER 5

Ambulatory Health Care Services

Stephen J. Williams

Ambulatory services are increasingly becoming the fundamental thread that ties together the delivery of health care. As discussed throughout this book, the trend toward integrated health care systems encompassing both financing and delivery mechanisms has relied on the ambulatory care component of the health care system for many key functions.

Insurers, providers, and patients themselves are increasingly seeking control over services through organized networks of care as a means of controlling costs and quality. Ambulatory care services, particularly through the controlling role of the physician, can be utilized as a gatekeeper and systems integrator. Ambulatory care services are likely to increase in importance as a result of key control and organizing functions and the increasing shift in the provision of services away from inpatient care.

Traditionally ambulatory care services have been viewed as the primary source of contact that most people have with the health care system. Although there are few concise definitions of ambulatory care, these services can be defined as care provided to noninstitutionalized patients. Sometimes ambulatory care is termed care for the "walking patient." Ambulatory care includes a wide range of services from simple routine treatment to surprisingly complex test and therapies.

This chapter presents a brief overview of the scope and history of ambulatory care services. Office-based practice is discussed, including both solo and group practice. Institutional providers of ambulatory care services are also presented, as are noninstitutional and governmentally sponsored providers. Most importantly, the role of ambulatory care services in structuring the health care system is discussed in considerable detail. The many attributes of ambulatory care which allow for the control and integration of services have received the most attention recently and are likely to become the focus of both research and management innovation in the years ahead.

HISTORICAL PERSPECTIVE AND TYPES OF CARE

Ambulatory care originated with the healing arts themselves. In primitive societies and for many years thereafter, until the advent of institutional care, all care was provided on what might be referred to as an *ambulatory care basis.* Of course, the types of care given then have little resemblance to today's health care, but the history of civilization demonstrates a consistent commitment to caring for the sick, using whatever knowledge has been available at the time. Remarkable forms of medical practice occurred in Greece, Rome, and other relatively sophisticated societies. In fact, many primitive societies had, and most, if not all, developing countries still have, their own indigenous practitioners such as religious healers and medicine men.

In more recent times, ambulatory care was provided in many new settings by a variety of more advanced practitioners. In Europe, and later in the United States, many of these services were given to wealthy patients in their homes, and poor people were cared for in dispensaries and public clinics. With the improvements in hospital care discussed in Chapter 6, more patients of all social classes received both inpatient and outpatient care in hospital settings. In the United States the poor have always been more likely than wealthier people to obtain care from the hospital versus a private physician.

In the United States, ambulatory care services were traditionally provided by individual medical practitioners working in their offices and in patients' homes and by public clinics operating primarily for poor and indigent patients. The limited technological armament that physicians required allowed them to travel easily, carrying with them their principal equipment and supplies. Thus home care was common, especially among wealthier patients. Physicians' offices were frequently located in their homes or in other small buildings, as opposed to today's medical office buildings or large medical centers (1). The general practitioner who made house calls, provided guidance, and offered available treatments was typical of the primary care provided before World War II.

Since World War II, however, an explosion of medical knowledge has led to increasing specialization, more complex technology, and rapid changes in the setting and nature of services. Fewer physicians are able or willing to travel to the patient's home, and many can no longer carry with them either the equipment and supplies or the specialized personnel available in an office. The growth of technical specialization in particular, has led to the rapid expansion of new settings for providing care, such as group practices and hospital clinics, both of which are discussed further below. Increased knowledge has led to the partial phasing out of the "traditional" general practitioner.

For the poor, in both Europe and the United States, care, when available, was often limited to public or philanthropic clinics or dispensaries. Private practitioners may have given their time to serve the poor, but their devotion to the patient was probably limited, as was the availability of care and the facilities in which services were provided.

Early efforts to link ambulatory care services and integrate them formally with inpatient care were promoted in this country and in Europe, in part, through the concept of regionalization. In Great Britain, the concept was presented in the Dawson Report (2), which eventually led to the National Health Service. In the United States, however, centralization of authority under government of the health care system has not been accepted as a politically viable alternative. In its place are many increasingly extensive networks of providers.

The increasing sophistication of insurance mechanisms and the use of ambulatory care services as a control mechanism on the use of all services has led to an increase in the degree of structure of the health care system over the past few years. This increasing structure has primarily been in the private, nongovernmental sector. The concept of social and economic regulation of the system through governmental intervention, carried to a high level of sophistication in the Dawson Report, has largely been abandoned, at least for the forseeable future. Integration of services will largely focus on multiple independently organized systems of care that are competitive with one another.

Table 5-1 demonstrates some of the diversity of services, providers, and facilities involved in ambulatory care today. Many of these services and organizations are discussed in this chapter. Particular attention is directed toward rapidly expanding and innovative settings, such as group practice, and integration of settings and services through organized systems of care.

LEVELS OF AMBULATORY CARE SERVICES

Ambulatory care services can be differentiated into a number of distinct levels or types of care. Chapter 3 discusses these levels in the context of utilization measurement. Primary prevention seeks to reduce the risks of illness or morbidity by removing disease-causing agents from our society. These activities include efforts to eliminate environmental pollutants that are suspected to cause diseases such as cancer. Other examples of primary prevention include encouraging people to use automobile seat belts, treatment of water and sewage, and sanitation inspections in restaurants. Preventive health services are more direct interventions to detect and prevent disease. Examples of these services include hypertension, diabetes, and cancer screening clinics and immunization programs. The combination of primary prevention and preventive services is our first line of defense against disease.

Medical care that is oriented toward the daily, routine needs of patients, such as initial diagnosis and continuing treatment of common illness, is termed *primary care* (3). This care is not highly complex and generally does not require sophisticated technology and personnel. The vision of the general practitioner of bygone days, traveling from house to house and ministering to the sick, represents the traditional role of primary care which is replaced in today's society by considerably better skilled practitioners in relatively complex facilities.

In addition to providing services directly, the primary care professional should serve the role of patient advisor, advocate, and system "gatekeeper." In this coordinating role, the provider refers patients to sources of specialized care, gives advice regarding various diagnoses and therapies, and provides continuing care for chronic conditions. In many organized systems of care, such as certain forms of Health Maintenance Organizations (HMOs), this role is very important in controlling costs, utilization, and the rational allocation of resources.

The evolution of technology and medicine's increasing ability to intervene in illness have led to greater specialization of health care services. These more specialized services, termed *secondary* and *tertiary care,* are provided in both ambulatory and inpatient settings. The content of secondary and tertiary care practices is usually more

TABLE 5-1. Illustrative List of Providers of Ambulatory Care Services

Settings	Principal Practitioners	Level or Type of Service
Private office-based solo and group practice	Physicians, dentists, nurses, MEDEX, therapists	Primary and secondary care
Hospital clinics	Physicians, dentists, nurses, MEDEX, therapists	Primary and secondary care
Hospital emergency rooms	Physicians, nurses	All types
Ambulatory surgery centers (hospital-based and free-standing)	Surgeons, nurses, anesthesiologists	Surgical secondary care
Communitywide emergency medical systems	Technicians, nurses, drivers	Emergency transportation, communications, and immediate care
Poison control centers, community hotlines	Physicians, technicians, nurses	Emergency advice
Neighborhood health centers, migrant health centers	Physicians, dentists, nurses	Primary care
Community mental health centers	Psychologists, social workers	Primary health services
Free clinics	Physicians, nurses	Primary care
Federal systems—Veterans Administration, Indian Health Service, Public Health Service, military	All types	All types
Home health services	Nurses	Primary care
School health services	Nurses	Primary and preventive care
Prison health services	All types	Primary care
Public health services and clinics	Physicians, nurses	Targeted programs (e.g., family planning, immunization, inspections, screening programs, health education); primary care
Family planning and other specialized clinics (nongovernmental)	Physicians, nurses, aides	Specialized services; primary care
Industrial clinics	Physicians, nurses, environmental health specialists	Preventive, primary, and emergency care
Pharmacies	Pharmacists	Drugs and health education
Vision care	Opticians Optometrists	Examinations, screening, prescriptions filled
Medical laboratories	Technicians	Specialized laboratory services
Indigenous	Chiropractors, medicine men, naturopaths	Primary and supportive care

narrowly defined than that of the primary care provider. Subspecialists, who provide the bulk of secondary and tertiary care, also often require more complex equipment and more highly trained support personnel than do primary care providers.

There are no clear dividing lines for primary versus secondary and secondary versus tertiary care. Secondary services include routine hospitalization and specialized outpatient care. These services are more complex than those of primary care and include many diagnostic procedures as well as more complex therapies. Tertiary care includes the most complex services, such as open heart surgery, burn treatment, and transplantation, and is provided in inpatient hospital facilities. Most of the care discussed in this chapter involves primary care and those secondary services that can be provided in such settings as office-based practice, hospital outpatient departments, or community clinics.

The differences between the types of services provided within the ambulatory care sector are an important concern throughout this chapter since one objective of improving or rationalizing the health services system is to match the capabilities of providers, or levels of care, with the needs of consumers. As different settings for providing ambulatory care are presented, one must consider the advantages and disadvantages of each to patient care needs and the optimal relationships that should be developed between the different levels of care. Similarly, one needs to regard the importance of these considerations as they relate to the managers of organized health care systems.

SETTINGS FOR THE PROVISION OF AMBULATORY CARE

OFFICE-BASED PRACTICE

Historically, and at the present time, most ambulatory care services are provided in solo and group practice, office-based settings. Institutional settings for care, primarily the hospital, although an important component of the health care system, remain less prominent. However, overlap between office-based practice and institutional settings is increasingly common as the dividing lines between various components of the health care system continue to blur (4).

An indication of the distribution of ambulatory care visits by type of setting is contained in Table 5-2, which presents survey results on utilization patterns, based on national data, representative of the entire U.S. population. The data in this table are taken from the National Health Interview Survey, a national survey of Americans' use of health care services, and complements the utilization data presented in Chapter 3.

Relatively little quantitative data is available on the utilization of ambulatory care services. Most utilization data is available from survey research results. However, in an attempt to obtain more detailed information on health care use in physician office settings, the federal government has conducted an ongoing survey of private, office-based physicians—the National Ambulatory Medical Care Survey (NAMCS) (5). This survey involves a random sample of the nation's office-based, nonfederal physicians. Physicians are asked to complete a data collection form for each patient treated during a 2-week interval. The most recent survey was conducted in 1985 (6).

TABLE 5-2. Physician Visits, by Source of Care and Patient Demographic Characteristics, United States, 1983

Selected Characteristic	Physician Visits (Number per Person)	Source or Place of Care		
		Physician's Office	Hospital Outpatient Department[a] (Percent of Visits)[b]	Telephone
Total[c][d]	5.0	55.9	14.9	15.5
Age				
<17 years	4.4	55.0	13.7	19.3
<6 years	6.5	54.3	12.8	20.6
6–16 years	3.2	55.8	14.7	17.9
17–44 years	4.5	54.4	16.4	14.6
45–64 years	5.8	58.7	15.2	12.5
≥65 years	7.6	58.9	12.3	11.9
Sex[c]				
Male	4.4	54.7	16.9	13.5
Female	5.7	56.5	13.6	16.7
Race[c]				
White	5.1	57.4	13.4	16.2
Black	4.8	44.1	26.5	9.7
Family income				
<$10,000	5.9	49.8	18.4	12.3
$10,000–$14,999	5.0	52.2	17.7	13.2
$15,000–$19,999	4.7	54.2	16.7	16.3
$20,000–$34,999	5.0	59.0	13.2	16.1
≥$35,000	5.4	59.6	11.5	18.8
Geographic region[c]				
Northeast	4.9	58.1	15.5	14.0
North Central	5.2	53.4	14.6	17.1
South	4.8	56.6	14.5	15.6
West	5.4	56.0	15.1	14.4
Location of residence[c]				
Within SMSA	5.2	54.7	15.6	15.9
Outside SMSA	4.6	58.8	13.2	14.5

SOURCE: Department of Health and Human Services: *Health, United States, 1985.* Washington, DC, U.S. Government Printing Office, 1986.

[a]Includes hospital outpatient clinic, emergency room, and other hospital visits.

[b]Includes source or place unknown.

[c]Age adjusted.

[d]Includes all other races not shown separately.

Tables 5-3 and 5-4 list the most common reasons and the principal diagnoses for all office visits, respectively. The relative prominence of routine care, of follow-up or ongoing care, and of relatively simple primary care is rather striking and reflects the predominance of "routine" day-to-day needs of patients seeking ambulatory care services.

Further understanding of the nature of the visits is available from additional data regarding the services provided to patients and the interactions shared between patients and physicians. Table 5-5 represents the diagnostic services provided to patients, excluding the prescription of drugs. Most visits entail relatively limited examination and some degree of testing. Table 5-6 presents certain therapeutic services, much of which is focused on counseling. This further reinforces the widely recognized importance of the primary care role of patient advising. The drugs prescribed during these visits are listed in Table 5-7. The majority of drugs prescribed comprise anti-infection agents, cardiovascular drugs, and central nervous system (CNS) agents.

TABLE 5-3. NAMCS, Most Common Reasons for Office Visits, 1985

Rank	Most Common Principal Reason for Visit	Number of Visits (in Thousands)	Percent
—	All visits	636,385	100.0
1	General medical examination	30,821	4.8
2	Prenatal examination	25,747	4.0
3	Well-baby examination	16,447	2.6
4	Symptoms referable to the throat	16,371	2.6
5	Postoperative visit	16,303	2.6
6	Cough	16,134	2.5
7	Progress visit not otherwise specified	13,638	2.1
8	Earache or ear infection	11,402	1.8
9	Back symptoms	11,311	1.8
10	Skin rash	10,350	1.6
11	Blood pressure test	9,446	1.5
12	Vision dysfunctions	9,266	1.5
13	Fever	9,050	1.4
14	Head cold, upper respiratory infection	8,902	1.4
15	Abdominal pain, cramps, spasms	8,901	1.4
16	Hypertension	8,814	1.4
17	Headache, pain in head	8,684	1.4
18	Chest pain and related symptoms	8,099	1.3
19	Knee symptoms	7,407	1.2
20	Eye examinations	7,170	1.1
—	All other reasons	382,122	60.0

SOURCE: National Center for Health Statistics; McLemore T, DeLozier J: 1985 Summary: National Ambulatory Medical Care Survey. *Advance Data from Vital and Health Statistics,* No. 128. DHHS Publ. No. (PHS) 87-1250. Public Health Service, Hyattsville, MD, January 23, 1987; and unpublished data of the 1985 National Ambulatory Medical Care Survey, National Center for Health Statistics, U.S. Public Health Service, Hyattsville, MD.

Finally, Table 5-8 suggests that the majority of office-based care requires relatively short periods of contact between patients and physicians; nearly three-fourths of all visits required 15 minutes or less. A high percentage of visits concluded with the recommendation that the patient return at a specified time interval for a follow-up visit.

The National Ambulatory Medical Care Survey thus provides some insight into the nature of office-based ambulatory care. Much more extensive documentation of the survey and results for various types of services, providers, and patient characteristics are available from the federal government. The survey data are an aid to planning health services in the ambulatory care setting and provide perspectives on national patterns of utilization. The applicability of the data to setting standards of performance in prepaid settings or under contractual agreements for service, however, is limited because of the many variables that could not be adequately measured.

The National Ambulatory Medical Care Survey aggregates physicians in private practice regardless of the specific setting in which they function. In reality, significant differences exist among physician practice settings and are discussed in the following

TABLE 5-4. NAMCS, Most Common Principal Diagnoses for Office Visits, 1985

Rank	Most Common Principal Diagnosis for Visit	Number of Visits (in Thousands)	Percent
1	Essential hypertension	26,049	4.1
2	Normal pregnancy	24,182	3.8
3	Health supervision of infant or child	17,088	2.7
4	Suppurative and unspecified otitis media	15,607	2.5
5	General medical examination	14,916	2.3
6	Acute upper respiratory tract infections of multiple or unspecified sites	14,691	2.3
7	Diabetes mellitus	12,302	1.9
8	Neurotic disorders	9,320	1.5
9	Acute pharyngitis	9,302	1.5
10	Follow-up examinations	9,277	1.5
11	Disorders of refraction and accommodation	8,268	1.3
12	Diseases of sebaceous glands	8,104	1.3
13	Allergic rhinitis	7,835	1.2
14	Bronchitis, not specified as acute or chronic	7,563	1.2
15	Other forms of chronic schemic heart disease	6,732	1.1
16	Asthma	6,503	1.0
17	Cataract	6,285	1.0
18	Certain adverse effects, not classified elsewhere	5,880	0.9
19	Special investigations and examinations	5,838	0.9
20	Contact dermatitis and other eczema	5,837	0.9
—	All other diagnoses	414,816	65.2

SOURCE: National Center for Health Statistics; McLemore T, DeLozier J: 1985 Summary: National Ambulatory Medical Care Survey. *Advance Data from Vital and Health Statistics* No. 128. DHHS Publ. No. (PHS) 87-1250. Public Health Service, Hyattsville, MD, January 23, 1987; and unpublished data of the 1985 National Ambulatory Medical Care Survey, National Center for Health Statistics, U.S. Public Health Service, Hyattsville, MD.

TABLE 5-5. NAMCS, Diagnostic Services Provided, 1985

Diagnostic Service[a]	Number of Visits (in Thousands)	Percent
None	229,926	36.1
Breast examination	43,170	6.8
Pelvic examination	54,854	8.6
Rectal examination	34,191	5.4
Visual acuity	40,945	6.4
Urinalysis	88,009	13.8
Hematology	58,983	9.3
Blood chemistry	43,913	6.9
Pap test	28,549	4.5
Other laboratory test	53,514	8.4
Blood pressure check	245,886	38.6
Electrocardiagram	20,288	3.2
Chest x-ray	17,549	2.8
Other radiology	37,806	5.9
Ultrasound	5,996	0.9
Other	67,778	10.7

SOURCE: National Center for Health Statistics; McLemore T, DeLozier J: 1985 Summary: National Ambulatory Medical Care Survey. *Advance Data from Vital and Health Statistics,* No. 128. DHHS Publ. No. (PHS) 87-1250. Public Health Service, Hyattsville, MD, January 23, 1987; and unpublished data of the 1985 National Ambulatory Medical Care Survey, National Center for Health Statistics, U.S. Public Health Service, Hyattsville, MD.

[a]May not total 100.0 percent since more than one service was possible.

TABLE 5-6. NAMCS, Therapeutic Services Provided, 1985

Nonmedication Therapy	Number of Visits (in Thousands)	Percent
None	438,406	68.9
Physiotherapy	26,485	4.2
Ambulatory surgery	41,931	6.6
Radiation therapy	656	0.1
Psychotherapy	21,343	3.4
Family planning	12,146	1.9
Diet counseling	41,294	6.5
Other counseling	59,102	9.3
Corrective lenses	10,861	1.7
Other	7,787	1.2

SOURCE: National Center for Health Statistics; McLemore T, DeLozier J: 1985 Summary: National Ambulatory Medical Care Survey. *Advance Data from Vital and Health Statistics,* No. 128. DHHS Publ. No. (PHS) 87-1250. Public Health Service, Hyattsville, MD, January 23, 1987; and unpublished data of the 1985 National Ambulatory Medical Care Survey, National Center for Health Statistics, U.S. Public Health Service, Hyattsville, MD.

[a]May not total 100.0 percent since more than one procedure was possible.

TABLE 5-7. Number and Percent Distribution of Drug Mentions by Therapeutic Categories: United States, 1985

Therapeutic Categories[a]	Number of Drugs Mentions (in Thousands)	Percent Distribution
All drugs	693,355	100.0
Anti-infective agents (systemic)	101,723	14.7
Antibiotics	85,299	12.3
Sulfonamides	10,453	1.5
All other anti-infective agents	5,971	0.8
Antineoplastic agents	5,343	0.8
Autonomic drugs	25,366	3.7
Blood formation and coagulation	8,176	1.2
Cardiovascular drugs	80,237	11.6
Analgesics and antipyretics	67,631	9.8
Psychotropic drugs	41,934	6.0
Electrolytic, caloric, and water balance	51,589	7.4
Antihistamines, antitussives, expectorants, and mucolytic agents	47,892	6.9
Eye, ear, nose, and throat preparations	30,589	4.4
Gastrointestinal drugs	26,647	3.8
Hormones and synthetic substances	52,642	7.6
Serums, toxoids, and vaccines	20,649	3.0
Smooth-muscle relaxants	11,675	1.7
Vitamins	18,873	2.7
Other or undetermined	60,858	9.1

SOURCE: National Center for Health Statistics; McLemore T, DeLozier J: 1985 Summary: National Ambulatory Medical Care Survey. *Advance Data from Vital and Health Statistics*, No. 128. DHHS Publ. No. (PHS) 87-1250. Public Health Service, Hyattsville, MD, January 23, 1987; and unpublished data of the 1985 National Ambulatory Medical Care Survey, National Center for Health Statistics, U.S. Public Health Service, Hyattsville, MD.

[a] Based on American Hospital Formulary Service Classification System.

sections of this chapter. The two primary noninstitutional settings for the provision of ambulatory care are solo and group practice. Each of these settings may be components of larger systems of care through such integrating mechanisms as referral arrangements, insurance contracts, and direct ownership of practices. An organized system of care can, in turn, be comprised of various settings or types of ambulatory care providers.

Although the solo practice of medicine has traditionally attracted the greatest number of practitioners, group practice and institutionally based services are now expanding dramatically, continuing a trend that has been building over the past 30 years. Changing life styles, the cost of establishing a practice, personal financial pressures on practitioners, contracting and affiliation opportunities, and the burdens of government regulation have enhanced the attractiveness of group practice for many physicians. With sharp increases in the number of physicians beginning practice, as discussed in detail in Chapter 10, the growth of alternate settings, and especially of

TABLE 5-8. NAMCS, Characteristics of Office Visits, 1985

Disposition and Duration	Number of Visits (in Thousands)	Percent Distribution
Disposition[a], 1985		
No follow-up planned	62,138	9.8
Return at specified time	391,142	61.5
Return if needed, prn	145,552	22.9
Telephone follow-up planned	25,229	4.0
Referred to other physician	20,075	3.2
Returned to referring physician	4,947	0.8
Admit to hospital	10,281	1.6
Other	3,416	0.5
Duration (minutes), 1985		
0[b]	14,436	2.8
1–5	65,250	10.3
6–10	181,191	28.5
11–15	190, 954	30.0
16–30	144,211	22.7
≥31	40,343	6.3

SOURCE: National Center for Health Statistics; McLemore T, DeLozier J: 1985 Summary: National Ambulatory Medical Care Survey. *Advance Data from Vital and Health Statistics,* No. 128. DHHS Publ. No. (PHS) 87-1250. Public Health Service, Hyattsville, MD, January 23, 1987; and unpublished data of the 1985 National Ambulatory Medical Care Survey, National Center for Health Statistics, U.S. Public Health Service, Hyattsville, MD.

[a]May not add to 100.0 percent since more than one disposition was possible.

[b]Represents office visits at which there was no face-to-face contact between the patient and the physician.

group practice, has been dramatic. Although solo practice remains an important avenue for providing ambulatory care services, these other settings have rapidly assumed a more prominent and visible role in the health care system, particularly as they provide a further mechanism for the integration, management, and control of health care services.

SOLO PRACTICE

Solo practitioners are difficult to characterize for a number of reasons. First, there are little data available on their practice patterns and activities. Although a few studies have been conducted, they tend to focus on specific questions, such as referral patterns or quality of care, and do not provide a comprehensive picture of what the solo practitioner does (7). The studies that do contribute to a more complete understanding of the activities of solo practitioners are based on physicians in one geographic area or a particular specialty, and the results of these studies, although interesting and useful, may not be generalizable to other practices or areas. The second problem in attempting to characterize solo practitioners is their heterogeneity; they include many types of health care professionals and provide an immense array of services.

The available evidence indicates that physicians in private solo practice generally work hard, although they often earn less, on average, than their counterparts in group practice. Many solo practitioners are subspecialists who provide secondary care primarily on referral from primary care practitioners. These practitioners include allergists, dermatologists, and surgeons. Some subspecialists provide both primary and secondary care since they have insufficient work in their own specialty to achieve desired income levels.

Many solo practitioners, including those trained in general and family practice, internal medicine, pediatrics, and obstetrics and gynecology, provide primary care services. There is some controversy and competition among practitioners concerning which specialists should be providing primary care. The specialty of family practice, in particular, represents a challenge to internal medicine in providing adult primary care and to pediatrics in child care (8).

Little detailed information exists on how the individual practitioner's time during the workday is allocated among various activities. Most solo practitioners perform a number of functions in the office, including patient care, consultations, and administration and supervision of office staff. Exactly how much time each of these activities requires is difficult to assess, but the requirements for administration and for supervision of personnel have been increasing in recent years.

Solo practice is often associated with a greater feeling that the provider cares about the welfare of the patient, possibly resulting in a stronger patient–provider relationship than occurs in other settings. There is some evidence that this situation, where it occurs, is a result of the lower level of bureaucracy or organizational complexity in solo practice (9). Since there is also some evidence that the relationship between patient and physician is related to patient compliance with medical regimens, patients who perceive that they are receiving more personalized care may respond to the care process more positively (10). Solo practitioners are also not as restricted in referrals to specialists as are providers in some other settings, such as group practice, where organizational loyalties intervene. Finally, the solo practitioner may feel a greater identification with the community served since there is a more direct relationship between patient and provider. New organizational forms that incorporate solo practitioners into larger systems of care, such as Independent Practice Plans and Preferred Provider Organizations, may be decreasing some of this physician–patient bond, especially as providers are forced to further discount fees.

From the provider's perspective, solo practice offers an opportunity to avoid organizational dependence and to be self-employed; there is also no need to share resources or income with other providers. Philosophically, solo practice is most closely aligned with the traditional economic and political orientations that have characterized medicine; younger physicians faced with discounting, contracting, and networks for care may no longer identify with the more traditional perspectives, however.

All of the increasingly complex problems of administering a practice must be dealt with in solo practice unless a professional manager is hired. Furthermore, competitive pressures in the health care industry are leading many practitioners to question the feasibility and desirability of going it alone. Thus solo practice offers distinct opportunities and has philosophical and emotional appeal but is far from devoid of problems and constraints, especially in light of the realities of medical practice today.

GROUP PRACTICE

Office-based practice includes, in addition to solo practice, group practice. This form of practice has been growing in popularity in recent years, especially as the increasing pressures of practice have led many providers to seek alternative settings in which to work.

Group practice is an affiliation of three or more providers, usually physicians, who share income, expenses, facilities, equipment, medical records, and support personnel in the provision of services through a formal, legally constituted organization (11). The formal definition of group practice, developed by the American Medical Association and the Medical Group Management Association, is three or more physicians formally organized to provide medical care, consultation, diagnosis, and/or treatment through the joint use of equipment and personnel, and with income from medical practice distributed in accordance with methods previously determined by members of the group. Although definitions of a group practice vary somewhat, the essential elements are formal sharing of resources and distribution of income (12).

Traditionally, group practice has meant participation and ownership by physicians. Increasingly, however, as new and more diversified models for the provision of services are developed, other practitioners will participate in group practices. In some communities, for example, group practices of nurse practitioners may be the only sources of health services. Dentists, optometrists, and other specialized personnel are also increasingly developing group practices. .

History of Group Practice

Some of the earliest group practices in the United States were started by companies that needed to provide care to employees in rural sites where medical care was unobtainable. For example, the Northern Pacific Railroad organized a practice in 1883 to provide care to employees building the transcontinental railroad. This industrial clinic was one of a number of such clinics founded in the nineteenth century. Even more significant, however, was the establishment of the Mayo Clinic in Rochester, Minnesota—the first successful nonindustrial group practice. The Mayo Clinic, originally organized as a single-speciality group practice in 1887 and later broadened into a multispeciality group, demonstrated that group practice was feasible in the private sector. The Mayo Clinic also represented a reputable model for group practice in a national atmosphere of fierce independence where group practice was viewed with skepticism and distrust. By the early 1930s there were about 150 medical groups throughout the country, many of which were located in the Midwest. Most included or were started by someone who had practiced or trained at the Mayo Clinic.

In 1932 a national committee—the Committee on the Costs of Medical Care—was established to assess health care needs for the nation. It issued a report that suggested a major role for group practice in the provision of medical care. The committee recommended that these groups be associated with hospitals to provide comprehensive care and that there be prepayment for all services (12). The report strongly supported the concept of regionalization that eventually gained wide recognition in the establishment of the British National Health Service, our own military health care systems, and other national models of organized health service systems.

Other constituencies, including some unions, also developed group practices. After World War II, a number of pioneering groups were established. In New York City, the

Health Insurance Plan of New York was organized to provide prepaid medical care to the employees of the city—an idea promoted by Mayor Fiorello LaGuardia. On the West Coast, the Kaiser Foundation Health Plan was established to provide health care to employees of Kaiser Industries; Kaiser is an affiliation of plans and providers that is now serving millions of Americans across the nation. In Seattle, a revolutionary development included the establishment of Group Health Cooperative of Puget Sound, a consumer-owned cooperative prepaid group practice, which now provides comprehensive care to more than 200,000 people. It was founded by progressive individuals who were dissatisfied with the private medical care available to them in the late 1940s.

Developments in medical practice also spurred the group practice movement. Perhaps most notable was the increasing specialization of medicine and the rapid expansion of technology. This increasing sophistication meant that no individual practitioner could provide all the expertise that patients would require. It also meant that more complex and expensive facilities, equipment, and personnel were needed to care for patients. Group practice provided a formal structure for sharing these costs among providers. Many people believed that resources would be used more efficiently in groups. In addition, multispeciality groups, encompassing more than one specialty, could provide patients with more of their health care under one roof and, hence, reduce problems of physical access to care and coordination of services.

Group practice was also thought to promote higher-quality care since most of the different specialists that a person required would be practicing together and would thus have the opportunity to discuss patient problems among themselves, share a common medical record, and be more able to ensure the quality and continuity of care. Therefore, group practice was viewed by many as being advantageous for the physician—offering opportunities such as easily developed referral arrangements, sharing of after-hours coverage, greater flexibility in working hours, and less financial risk—while also benefiting the patient.

Opposition to group practice has occurred mostly for political and philosophical reasons. The American Medical Association and local medical societies have, at times, opposed group practice. Many early group practices had difficulties when physicians were denied admitting privileges in local hospitals. Community-based specialists sometimes refused to treat patients referred by group practice physicians. In more recent years, however, opposition to group practice has lessened dramatically and restrictive laws have been challenged. The need to form affiliations for contracting under reimbursement programs and for achieving efficiencies in organizing health services more generally has resulted in little remaining formal opposition to group practice.

Survey of Group Practice

The American Medical Association has conducted surveys of physician oriented medical group practices in the United States on a periodic basis since 1965. These surveys represent the most comprehensive data available concerning the growth and characteristics of group practice in this country. The most recent survey was conducted in 1984. Group practices that qualified within the American Medical Association's definition were identified from a variety of data sources and were then surveyed through a mail data collection instrument. Numerous items of information were collected regarding the nature of the practice and its facilities and relationships to other entities (13).

The dramatic increase in popularity of practices is reflected in Table 5-9. The number of group practices nearly doubled during the 10-year period from 1974 to 1984. There are now over 15,000 group practices in the United States, two thirds of which are single-speciality groups.

Even more dramatic is the growth in the number of physicians practicing in a group practice setting. Approximately 140,000 physicians in the United States are now working in group practices, which represents a marked increase from 67,000 in 1975 and 88,000 in 1980. A higher percentage of all physicians in group practice work in multispecialty oriented groups as compared to the percentage of total groups that are multispecialty, largely because the average multispecialty group is substantially larger (26.6 physicians on average) than the average single-specialty (5.8 physicians on average) group. The average size of all group practices in the United States in 1984 was 9.1 physicians, demonstrating an increase from 7.9 physicians in 1975 and 8.2 physicians in 1980. These data reflect only physician "positions" and exclude other medically related professionals such as nurse practitioners.

Of all group practices in 1984, 73 percent were professional corporations, in contrast to only 15.6 percent in this category in 1969. Partnerships constituted 68.7 percent of group practices in 1969 but only 14.7 percent of practices in 1984. Sole proprietorships, associations, and foundations as well as a variety of other legal forms represent the ownership and organizational status of the remaining groups. The dramatic shift toward professional corporations is primarily a result of changes in federal and state laws pertaining to taxation, the increasing size and complexity of the practices themselves, and interrelationships among physicians participating. Changes in federal tax law may result in further shifts in patterns of legal organizational forms.

Specialty distribution of physicians in group practice has not changed dramatically over the past 10 years. The specialties that account for the largest percentage of

TABLE 5-9. Number of Medical Groups and Number of Physicians in Group Practice by Specialty Orientation of Group, United States, Selected Years

Year	Single Specialty	Multispecialty	Family or General Practice	Total
		Number of Groups		
1969	3,169	2,418	784	6,371
1975	4,601	2,976	906	8,488
1980	6,156	3,552	1,054	10,762
1984	10,635	2,781	1,770	15,186
		Number of Physician Positions in Group Practice		
1969	13,053	24,349	2,691	40,093
1975	23,572	39,311	3,959	66,842
1980	29,456	4,122	4,712	88,290
1984	59,917	69,371	9,839	139,127

SOURCE: Hwulich PL: *Medical Groups in the U.S., 1984*. Chicago, American Medical Association, 1985.

physicians participating in group practice include family and general practice, internal medicine, anesthesiology, obstetrics and gynecology, pediatrics, and radiology.

Of particular interest, in view of the changing nature of organizational relationships, is prepaid health care. A greater number of group practices indicated an involvement in prepaid health care in 1984 when compared to previous surveys, and the percentage of prepaid care provided by each group increased significantly over the past few years (14). In 1984 22.2 percent of all group practices surveyed indicated that their involvement in prepaid health care represented 1–4 percent of their total business, 48 percent indicated that prepayment represented 5–24 percent of their business, 12.6 percent indicated that prepayment represented 25–49 percent of their total business, and the remainder indicated that prepayment represented at least 50 percent of the total revenue generated. It is likely that this trend will continue with an increasing percentage of groups having some involvement in prepayment; for those groups participating, the percentage of prepaid business in relation to total business activity is likely to continue to increase.

Relatively few groups account for significant percentage of all physicians in group practice as presented in Table 5-10. There are few groups that employ more than 15 physicians. As would be expected, most of the larger groups are multispecialty while the predominance of the smaller groups are single specialty.

The geographic distribution of group practice in the United States is dominated by seven states, which account for 40 percent of all groups. These states are California, Pennsylvania, New York, Texas, Illinois, Florida, and Ohio. The origin, growth, and current distribution of group practices and group practice physicians are not homogeneous throughout the various regions, which reflects a greater acceptance of group practice in some regions as well as a varied distribution of larger urban

TABLE 5-10. Total Groups and Group Physician Positions by Size of Group

Size of Group	Groups		Group Physician Positions	
	Percent	Number	Percent	Number
3	32.6	4,795[a]	10.1	14,249[c]
4	22.2	3,266	9.3	13,064
5	12.8	1,884	6.7	9,420
6	7.2	1,054	4.5	6,324
7	4.5	666	3.3	4,662
8–15	12.6	1,854	13.6	19,112
16–25	3.6	522	7.4	10,354
26–49	2.4	354	8.6	12,037
50–99	1.0	148	7.0	9,828
≥ 100	1.1	158	29.4	41,342
Total	100.0	14,701[b]	100.0	140,392

SOURCE: Hwulich PL: *Medical Groups in the U.S., 1984*. Chicago, American Medical Association, 1985.
[a] Includes 107 groups with less than three physicians who qualified per the AMA definition of group in other important respects.
[b] Excludes 784 groups whose size was unknown.
[c] Includes 185 physician positions in groups with less than three physicians.

population centers in the country. As might be expected, physician groups and physician group practice physicians are substantially more prominent in metropolitan areas than in nonmetropolitan areas of the country. The development of prepaid group practice also varies by region (15).

Interestingly, 62.6 percent of the respondents indicated that their group practice employed a business manager or administrator, although only 26.6 percent had an identifiable medical director. Multispecialty groups were more likely to employ a group administrator, and, as might be expected, larger groups were much more likely to employ administrators and have medical directors than were smaller groups. Nearly all the larger groups did employ an administrator. With nearly 7000 group practices responding that they employed a medical director, the market for trained group practice administrators has grown substantially over the past few years, and its growth is likely to continue as the number of group practices increases.

The increasing integration of the health care system raises interesting questions regarding the affiliations of group practices with other organizations. Table 5-11 presents data from the most recent survey of group practices in terms of their relationships with hospitals. Although the data are not available over periods of time, it is interesting to note that approximately half of all groups, and more than half of all group practice physicians, are directly affiliated with a hospital. The increasing involvement of hospitals in the integration of the health care system is discussed further in other chapters in this book, but it is dramatically illustrated by these data.

An Assessment of Group Practice

A critical assessment of group practice yields distinct advantages and disadvantages for both patients and providers as compared to other modalities for providing ambulatory

TABLE 5-11. Total Groups and Group Physician Positions by Relationship of Group to a Hospital

Hospital Relationship	Groups		Group Physician Positions	
	Percent	Number	Percent	Number
Hospital operated	2.4	253	2.6	2,250
Hospital landlord	30.6	3,264	30.4	26,596
Hospital associated	5.5	584	9.0	7,889
Hospital privilege	8.6	916	7.9	6,946
Referral basis	0.9	98	0.9	753
Multiple relationships	0.6	65	0.9	754
Other	4.6	493	10.3	8,992
None	46.7	4,977	38.2	33,435
Total	100.0	10,650[a]	100.0	87,615[b]

SOURCE: Hwulich, PL: *Medical Groups in the U.S., 1984.* Chicago, American Medical Association, 1985.

[a] Excludes 4835 groups whose hospital relationship was unknown. Of these groups, 4242 responded to the short-form questionnaire and thus were not asked about hospital relationshiops.

[b] Excludes 52,777 physician positions in groups whose hospital relationship was unknown.

services (16). Some of these are summarized in Table 5-12. Specific advantages and disadvantages vary from group to group, and Table 5-12 lists major considerations generally associated with group practice. Some of the topics listed under patient or provider perspectives could readily pertain to both.

The advantages of group practice from the perspective of the provider include shared operation of the practice; joint ownership of facilities and equipment; centralized administrative functions; and, in larger groups, a professional manager.

TABLE 5-12. Some Advantages and Disadvantages of Group Practice[a]

Advantages	Disadvantages
From Perspective of Health Services Provider	
Availability of professional manager	Less individual freedom
Organizational responsibility for patient	May lead to excess use of specialists
Less physician administrative time	Fewer outside consultants
Shared capital expense	Possible reduced identity with patient and community
Shared financial risk	
Improved contracting and negotiating ability	Group rather than individual decision making
Better coverage and shared on-call shifts	Share all problems
More flexible working hours	Must work with others
More peer interaction	Less individual incentive and more security oriented
Increased access to specialists	
Broader array of ancillary services	Income limitations
Stable income for providers	Income distribution arguments
No direct financial concerns with patient	
Lower initial investment	
More time for continuing education	
More flexible vacation time	
Generally excellent benefits	
Possible efficiencies of scale	
Use of nonphysician practitioners	
From Perspective of Group Practice Patient	
Care under one roof	Possible lessening of provider patient relationship
Availability of specialists, laboratories, etc.	
Improved coverage and emergency care	Possible overuse of ancillary services
Medical and administrative records centrally located	Possible high provider turnover
Referrals simplified	Heavy patient loads and waiting times may be increased
Peer interaction among providers	Less provider incentive for care
Better administration of group	More bureaucracy
Efficiency may be promoted in patient care	
Possibly better knowledge of medical care costs	

[a]Some advantages and disadvantages could be included under both provider and patient categories.

The professional manager can provide expertise in areas often lacking among the providers such as billing; personnel management; patient scheduling; ordering of supplies; and, recently, of particular importance, negotiating, contracting, and related matters.

Financially, the group relieves the provider of the heavy initial investment often required to establish a practice. In most groups, however, co-ownership requires that new members buy into the group through purchase of a share of the group's capital over a period of time.

The burden of operating costs is also lessened for any individual member of a group. Rather than having to independently absorb the ups and downs of a practice, as do sole practitioners, those involved in a group practice share the income and expenses within the group, allowing for moderation of those fluctuations experienced in individual practices. For example, a solo practitioner who becomes ill may have no practice income aside from disability insurance, whereas a group member's income may continue during a short period of illness since other providers are simultaneously generating revenue. However, the provisions of income distribution plans vary substantially among groups.

The participation of physicians in group practice also has a significant advantage in facilitating the development of definitive arrangements for contracting and negotiating. The group can support increased levels of participation, has a knowledgeable group practice administrator to manage the contracts, and can respond to the market with a wider range of services. Even single specialty groups, with shared on-call services and subspecialization of group members, will be able to offer more to the market on a contractual basis than the individual practitioner. Having a professional manager to negotiate on behalf of the group further enhances the relative attractiveness of group practice, particularly for physicians who lack experience in interpreting and negotiating contracts.

Patient care responsibilities are also shared in group practice. This sharing results in greater flexibility of working hours for the provider, as well as more time for vacation and continuing education, without sacrificing the quality of care for the patient. For example, providers cover for each other during vacations and after normal working hours. Although most practitioners in solo practice arrange for patient care coverage, the continuity of care and the extent of coverage are probably greater in group practice since the patients' medical records and the full resources of the group are always available, even if specific providers are not working.

Sharing of patient care may have some other potential benefits. These include more peer interaction as a result of informal discussions and referral of patients among providers. The inclusion of more providers also results in the availability, by necessity, of a wider range of specialists and ancillary services, which represents a convenience for both providers and patients as well as a source of added revenue for the group.

Does the sharing of administrative and patient care activities within group practice produce better care at lower cost? Although many people believe that effective group management uses resources more efficiently than solo practice, the evidence is mixed. Some evidence tended to refute these beliefs, but more analytical research indicates some economies of scale, or efficiencies, attributable to the grouping of resources for smaller groups but possibly less so for larger and more bureaucratic groups (17). The use of personnel may be more advantageous in group rather than solo practice. Receptionists, medical records specialists, laboratory and radiology technicians, nurses, and other types of personnel may be used more efficiently and in the specialized areas of their training in many medium- and larger-sized groups. In addition, there is some question as to whether any savings that are achieved will be returned to consumers or simply represent higher income for providers. Further, the increasing supply of physicians, as discussed in Chapter 10, may reduce the desirability of employing mid-level practitioners, except in certain prepaid settings.

The effect of groups on patient care, especially on the quality of care, has been investigated more extensively in the prepaid, as opposed to fee-for-service, setting. In prepaid group practices the incentives are substantially different since providers are paid a salary and consumers pay "in advance" for all care. Sharing of medical records, peer interaction, easy referrals and consultations with specialists, more sophisticated and accessible ancillary services, and more skilled and diversified support personnel are all arguments suggested in support of higher-quality care in group practice.

Group practice also offers advantages to patients and their communities. For the patient, the group offers a wide range of services under one roof so that travel between providers is reduced and access increased. A unified medical record can contribute to continuity of care and less duplication in diagnosis and treatment. Some groups also own or operate hospitals and thus further extend the integration and scope of the services that they provide, an especially important consideration in negotiating with employers and insurers.

Group practices usually offer more accessible care after normal working hours. Some groups also offer emergency services through their own emergency rooms or clinics. Groups with a broader community perspective may even be involved in programs such as school health services and community immunization efforts.

The use of a professional manager should benefit the patient through more efficient scheduling and patient flow and improved overall management of the practice. Billing is simplified since all care received can be included on one statement.

On a communitywide basis, group practice may offer a means of attracting providers to areas with inadequate numbers of medical care personnel. By offering peer interaction, support services, and other advantages, groups may increase the appeal of practicing in rural or inadequately served urban centers.

There are also distinct disadvantages to group practice for providers, patients, and communities. From the perspective of the provider, practicing in a group implies less individual freedom, with a variety of restrictions imposed through the sharing of a practice. Ideologically, the limitations of a group in this regard may be difficult for some people to accept since medicine has traditionally been an individualistic enterprise. In addition to reduced freedom, group practice entails sharing responsibilities and problems with others. The interpersonal requirements for working out these responsibilities may not appeal to all practitioners. Older individuals who have been working in solo practice may be especially unlikely to adapt readily to group practice.

The financial advantages for group practice are a trade-off against some restrictions on income generation and the necessity of complying with the group's income distribution and practice pattern requirements. Thus there often is more security and less risk but also less incentive and reward for individual initiative and production.

The shift of some patient care responsibilities from the individual practitioner to the group also may adversely affect the patient–provider relationship by introducing a degree of impersonalization. If a group has high physician turnover, which is rare, the patient may have to change providers frequently. Groups that have too few providers for the number of patients that they serve, a common occurrence when excess capacity is being avoided, will also have waiting times for appointments in the office that the patient may believe to be excessive. The group may impose greater restrictions on referral practices, consequently limiting the practitioner's willingness to use the expertise of other specialists in the community.

From a community perspective, groups may reduce the geographic dispersion of providers and thus increase difficulties of physical access to care. In addition, groups may reduce competition in the health care marketplace by consolidating what would otherwise be competing providers. Consolidation may eventually reduce the ability of insurers, employers, and other plan sponsors to negotiate favorable terms for contracted care.

PREPAID GROUP PRACTICES AND HEALTH MAINTENANCE ORGANIZATIONS

Group practice that is reimbursed on a prepaid rather than a fee-for-service basis is an increasingly popular approach in designing health care plans. In recent years this approach has been given government encouragement through the development of HMOs (18). Although group practice requires that physicians practice together in one organization and under one roof, the concept of prepayment has also been applied to community-based solo and group practitioners through the development of Independent Practice Plans or Associations (IPPs or IPAs), a form of HMO (19). The increasing importance of prepayment has led fee-for-service group practices to participate, at least partially, in prepayment, as mentioned earlier. The rapid escalation of health care costs, increased employer interest in alternative financing methods, and encouragement of competition in health care also suggests an increasing role for prepayment, and most group practices will seek to develop responsive packages with prepayment characteristics.

Prepayment is discussed in this chapter primarily as it pertains to the organization of service providers. Other aspects of the financing of care under various forms of prepayment and of prepayment in various delivery settings are discussed elsewhere in this book, especially in Chapter 11.

Prepayment within group practice alters the incentive system for the provider organization and for the professional delivering care. Although exclusively prepaid groups, such as the Kaiser Foundation Health Plan, incorporate many of the principles of group practice, physicians and other providers are usually on salary, sometimes supplemented by an incentive reimbursement program. Since the plan itself is reimbursed prospectively through a monthly fee for all health care provided, there is an incentive to avoid unncessary use. This fact ensures that the plan's prospective budget is not exceeded and that the plan can maintain its competitiveness in the health services marketplace.

Most prepayment plans have achieved lower costs for all care through hospitalization rates that are lower than those in the fee-for-service sector (20). Ambulatory care utilization has generally been at least as high as and often higher in prepaid plans than that in fee-for-service insurance programs, especially as care has increasingly shifted from inpatient to outpatient settings. Prepaid group practices attempt to ration the availability of both ambulatory and inpatient services by using a number of mechanisms. For instance, ambulatory visits initiated by the patient can be constrained by limiting the availability of care. This result is achieved, for example, by creating longer waiting times for appointments than patients desire, although the plan must schecule in such a manner that only low-priority care is discouraged while patients with more serious or urgent problems are assured access. Other means of rationing patient services include changing practice patterns to encourage outpatient care and limiting the availability of inpatient beds. There is little or no evidence, however, that for any specific service, such as an office visit, prepaid groups can actually provide care at substantially lower costs than can fee-for-service groups or solo practitioners. Thus their primary cost advantage is in reducing hospitalizaiton rather than in achieving economies for individual services.

Prepaid group practices can assume many organizational forms. Figure 5-1 presents a simplified organizational structure of a typical health plan which incorporates a group. The fundamental components include the plan itself, which administers the health care program, recruits enrollees, and arranges all contractual relationships. The hospitals and the medical group practices are often organizationally separate from the plan administration and are the direct providers of all care. The medical groups are composed of physicians who contract with the plan to provide care and who use facilities administered by the plan. The hospitals may be owned by the plan, but in many smaller prepaid groups, community hospitals are used through contractual arrangements.

Another type of prepaid practice is the foundation or independent practice plan in which community physicians remain in private practice using their own offices but contract individually with a central plan that, in turn, contracts with prepaid enrollees (21). The physicians in this situation are reimbursed by the plan on a fee-for-service basis. This arrangement provides for prepaid services to enrolled populations without requiring that physicians either practice together or be paid on a salaried basis. Foundation-type plans were started as an alternative to prepaid group practice that

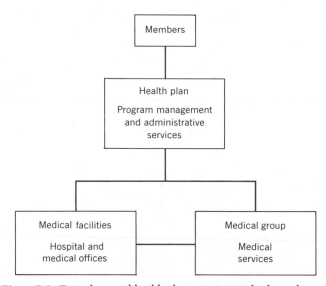

Figure 5-1. Typical prepaid health plan organizational relationships.

could preserve private fee-for-service practice within a prepayment framework. One of the first foundations was the San Joaquin Foundation in California.

The federal HMO program was instituted in 1973 to promote prepayment plans and incorporates both the group practice and foundation models. The concept was originally proposed by President Richard M. Nixon as a means of promoting private sector medicine through self-regulation, while at the same time incorporating some incentives for containment of health care costs (22,23). The HMO law provided grants and loans for the planning and establishment of HMOs and required that certain services (Table 5-13) be provided.

The HMO program and prepaid group practices had early success in providing comprehensive and acceptable quality health services at lower total costs than the fee-for-service sector (24). However, some of these plans have had difficulties attaining financial viability. This problem may be partially the result of program requirements that include offering a full range of services and having a period of open enrollment during which anyone could join. Some provisions of the program, however, helped developing HMOs. These provisions included the dual-choice requirement under which certain employers must offer an HMO as a health care option to employees in competition with other insurance plans. The most successful prepaid groups have generally been the larger plans or those serving populations with high levels of insurance coverage. Poor management and lack of commitment on the part of organizers and providers have been identified as major reasons for the failure of some early HMOs (25,26).

Under the competitive concepts of the Reagan administration, HMOs and other prepaid plans have had considerable appeal because of their internal incentives for cost containment and their ability to provide relatively comprehensive services for a predetermined monthly premium. They also have attributes with application to arranging care in governmental entitlement programs, particularly Medicare.(27–29). However, federal support for the development of HMOs has been reduced on the assumption that the appeal of HMOs will lead to their creation without external governmental financing. The original legislation has also been amended to reduce the

TABLE 5-13. Health Services Originally Required Under
the Health Maintenance Organization Act of 1973

Physician professional services

Outpatient services

Short term mental health services

Short term rehabilitative services

Certain services for substance abuse

Laboratory and radiology services

Home health services

Family planning services

Certain social services

Immunizations and preventive health services

Health education

Arrangements for emergency care

Arrangements for out-of-area coverage

restrictions on HMOs in the health care marketplace—for example, decreasing benefit requirements and allowing premiums to be computed on a more financially sound basis.

An important recent trend in prepaid programs has been a shift toward for-profit plans (30,31). Many new prepaid plans are established as for-profit entities. A large number of older, established plans have converted from not-for-profit to for-profit status or have been assimilated by for-profit entities. For-profit status allows these plans to obtain financing through equity channels and to earn and distribute profit. In some respects, public accountability may even be greater in the for-profit sector, especially when the plan offers stock ownership to the public.

Other forms of prepayment have been or are being developed. Some use prepayment to reimburse providers, while others combine fee-for-service with prepayment. Most of these innovations do not alter the structure of the provider organizations themselves, as in an HMO. Rather, they restructure, through contractual arrangements, the relationships between insurers, providers, and consumers.

The empirical evidence, although not entirely consistent throughout all studies, has accumulated over the past few years and suggests distinct advantages for prepaid plans. These advantages have been reviewed in a comprehensive and analytical manner by Luft (32,33). The results of this review are presented in brief form in Table 5-14. It is evident that although much is now known, more remains to be discovered. The accumulated evidence does support many of the proclaimed advantages of prepayment, although there are also distinct disadvantages, and many challenges remain (34). The two most important concerns for the future of prepayment in its many forms are maintenance of an acceptable level of quality of care and assuring access to care. An eclectic health care system that offers many alternatives is likely to allow both providers and consumers the opportunity to select the type of plan that is most appealing and that meets their unique needs.

INSTITUTIONALLY BASED AMBULATORY SERVICES

In addition to solo and group practice in the traditional private sector, many institutions are expanding their involvement in ambulatory care. These institutionally based settings, especially those associated with hospitals, are discussed next.

The hospital has evolved from an institution for poor people who could not be cared for at home to a provider of a full range of health services from primary to tertiary care. As technological advances have brought more services into the hospital and expanded the scope of care provided, the hospital has assumed an especially important role in the provision of highly complex health services. At the same time, an increasing number of people have sought primary care from hospitals, sometimes as a result of lack of access to other sources of care.

OUTPATIENT AND AMBULATORY CARE CLINICS

The increased demands placed on hospitals for care taxed the ability of many facilities to respond with appropriate and adequate resources. The result was overcrowded facilities, the wrong mix of services, equipment, and personnel to respond to patient

TABLE 5-14. Empirical Evidence Concerning HMOs

Area of Knowledge	Evidence
Consumer enrollment	Some people prefer HMOs due to broader coverage or types of benefits; other people prefer to maintain existing relationships with community physicians.
	Consumers selecting HMOs sometimes have used hospital services less and ambulatory care more than those selecting other plans. Adverse selection less likely in HMOs than in other plans.
Health care costs	Prepaid group practice (PGP) members have 10–40% lower costs than those in other plans. IPPs do not appear to have similar low costs.
	HMOs tend to offer broader coverage for the same premium as other plans. Consumer out-of-pocket costs are often lower and usually more predictable.
Health care use	HMOs deliver fewer units of service, due to lower hospitalization. PGPs have significantly lower rates of hospitalization. IPPs have somewhat lower rates than traditional insurance plans, but the evidence is less conclusive than for PPGs.
	Length of stay is similar to HMOs to other plans, but the case mix may differ. PGPs have lower admission rates for diagnoses and tests, suggesting more use of ambulatory care for these purposes.
	IPPs have a lower admission rate for surgical procedures than other plans, but PGPs do not. The use of discretionary surgical procedures does not seem to differ between PGPs and other plans.
	HMOs tend to have higher rates of ambulatory care use than other plans, in part due to broader coverage.
Use of resources	HMOs probably do not provide individual services, such as a hospital day or an office visit, at significantly lower cost than other types of providers.
	Fewer total resources per consumer probably exist in HMOs than in fee-for-service medicine.
	PGPs provide more laboratory tests and radiologic services than traditional plans.
	Productivity of specialists, especially surgeons, is much higher in HMOs due to more stringent staffing.
	Use of allied or mid-level health personnel probably does not differ between HMOs and other providers, although some HMOs rely on these personnel more heavily than do other providers.
Trends over time	There are few consistent patterns over time in HMO total costs, premiums, ambulatory care visits, or inpatient costs per day. Hospital admission and use rates and physician productivity have been falling, as has been the case for all health care providers.
Preventive care	HMOs probably provide more preventive care than other insurers.

TABLE 5-14. (Continued)

Area of Knowledge	Evidence
Quality of care	Limited evidence does not clearly favor HMOs. The quality of medical records, tests performed and appropriateness of care, and health status may be more favorable in HMOs. Use of drugs and outcome of care may not differ between HMOs and other providers.
Consumer satisfaction and access to care	Little conclusive evidence exists.
	PGP enrollees wait less time in the office when they have an appointment, and are less satisfied with scheduling delays in obtaining appointments.
	HMO enrollees tend to be more satisfied with their coverage and financial arrangements.
	Continuity of care may be lower in PGPs.
	PGP enrollees tend to be less satisfied with their interaction with physicians, and possibly with the quality of care.
	PGPs probably have a relatively low disenrollment rate. Out-of-plan use in PGPs is about 5 to 10%.
Physician perspectives	Physicians work fewer hours, earn less, have less autonomy, may be less happy with patient relationships, and are attracted by the prepayment concept in PGPs and HMOs in general. Turnover of physicians is not a problem, nor is recruitment.
HMOs and competitors	HMOs have generally been able to compete in the insurance marketplace. Restrictive laws have been eased, complex management has been improving, and relationships with other providers have been established. HMOs may select certain types of enrollees and providers. They may also force other providers to be more efficient.

SOURCE: Luft, HS: *Health Maintenance Organizations: Dimensions of Performance.* Copyright © 1981 by John Wiley & Sons, Inc. Reprinted by permission of John Wiley & Sons, Inc.

needs, and extremely dissatisfied consumers and providers. Most hospitals have now successfully responded to these demands by expanding outpatient services and hiring full-time providers to staff-redesigned hospital ambulatory facilities.

Traditional hospital outpatient services have been provided in clinics and emergency rooms. In many hospitals, clinics have had second-class status as compared to complex and expensive inpatient services. However, as hospitals are increasingly recognizing the important role of primary care, especially in contracting, and are seeking to expand the base of patients who are potential users of inpatient and ancillary services, more attention is being directed toward improving clinic operations and services.

Hospital clinics include both primary care and specialty clinics. Many hospitals differentiate between clinics for walk-in patients without appointments and those for scheduled visits. Specialty clinics are usually organized by department and provide services such as ophthalmology, neurology, and allergy care. In teaching hospitals, clinics serve as important settings in which house staff members provide ongoing care to patients and follow-up after hospitalization. Increasingly, clinics also provide an opportunity to expose medical students and house staff to ambulatory care services in order to complement the traditionally more extensive experience with inpatient care. In teaching hospitals, there may be more than 100 different clinics reflecting the diversity of subspecialties. In nonteaching hospitals, there are fewer specialty clinics, and there may be more emphasis on primary care.

Many hospital primary care clinics evolved from an orientation of service to the poor and were staffed by physicians who served without reimbursement in exchange for staff privileges. The level of commitment to the patient under such circumstances was, not surprisingly, less than desirable. Many hospitals now employ physicians and other practitioners as full-time clinic staff. Some hospitals have established primary care group practices to complement other outpatient services and to assume the burden of providing primary care to patients who seek most of their care from the hospital.

The development of a group practice has advantages for both consumers and the hospital by providing comprehensive and accessible care and by removing primary care patients from facilities that are not designed to serve their needs, such as emergency rooms. Development of these group practices also has the potential of increasing use of the hospital's inpatient and ancillary services, an advantage if occupancy is low (35). Hospitals with ambulatory care resources can negotiate contracts for providing a wide range of both inpatient and outpatient services. They are subsequently also able to more effectively control the use of services and thus costs. However, questions have been raised concerning the ability of hospitals to compete effectively in an arena in which they have not been overly successful in the past (36). But the increasingly competitive nature of the hospital and the health care marketplace is forcing many hospitals to enter this area of practice even if they are uncertain about doing so.

Over the past few years, especially, the competitive approach to health care has gained dramatically. Some of these new approaches are discussed in Chapter 6. In ambulatory care, these efforts have reached far beyond the traditional areas, including the construction of medical office buildings into such new areas as joint ventures, development of health plans, purchases of medical practices, and other more aggressive activities (37,38). The success or failure of these ventures will not be measurable for some time on a national scale, but they clearly place the hospital at greater financial risk, raising the stakes far above those associated with more limited initiatives. At the same time, many hospitals view these actions as logical extensions of earlier, more timid moves into ambulatory care. The long-term viability of the hospital is also felt by many to be dependent on the successful incorporation of additional components of the delivery system into the hospital, administratively and financially.

AMBULATORY SURGERY CENTERS

A further innovation in hospital-based care has been the development of ambulatory surgery centers. Originated in hospitals in Washington, D.C., Los Angeles, and elsewhere, these organized hospital units provide 1-day surgical care. Patients are usually screened for acceptability by their personal surgeon and then report at an assigned date and time for surgery. The surgeon is supported by the unit's facilities, equipment, and personnel, and the patient is discharged 1–3 hours after surgery when recovery from anesthesia is sufficiently complete.

In the early 1970s, free-standing ambulatory surgery centers were opened; one of the first was in Phoenix, Arizona. These facilities are independent of hospitals and usually provide a full range of services for the types of surgery that can be performed on an outpatient basis. Community surgeons are granted operating privileges and can perform surgery in these facilities when the patient agrees and when there are no medical contraindications.

Other facilities are also used for ambulatory or outpatient surgery. Many physicians traditionally performed surgery in their offices, although this practice has declined in some specialties as a result of malpractice concerns and the increasing availability of better equipped and staffed alternative facilities. Other specialities, such as oral surgery, plastic surgery, and ophthalmology extensively use office based facilities.

Free-standing emergency centers have also opened in many cities, paralleling the success of ambulatory surgery centers. These emergency centers sometimes provide a wide range of primary care in addition to responding to urgent problems. The future of specialized ambulatory centers, in both hospitals and as free-standing facilities, will probably include further expansion into other areas of health care, ranging from sports medicine to women's health care. The commercial success of these organizations, however, is certainly not assured, especially as the health care marketplace becomes more competitive.

EMERGENCY MEDICAL SERVICES

The emergency room, like other hospital departments, has undergone transformation in recent years. The emergency room has expanded in the range of services offered and in complexity. An especially important long-term trend has been the increasing use of the emergency room for primary care. Since the emergency room requires sophisticated facilities and highly trained personnel and must be accessible 24 hours a day, costs are high and services are not designed for nonurgent care. To reduce the burden on the emergency room and to meet patient need more effectively, many hospitals treat patients on a triage basis. In this process, often performed by a nurse, the patient's health care needs are determined and the patient is referred to a more appropriate source of care within the hospital. The misuse of the emergency room has received considerable attention over the past 20 years.

Emergency medical services have also been increasingly integrated with other community resources. Included are drug and alcohol treatment programs, mental health centers, and voluntary agencies. Most major urban centers have developed formal emergency medical systems that incorporate all hospital emergency rooms as well as transportation and communication systems. In these communities, people needing emergency care either transport themselves or call an emergency number (such as 911). An ambulance is dispatched by a central communications center that also identifies and alerts the most appropriately equipped and located hospital. In many communities, regional hospital-based trauma centers have been built with extremely sophisticated capabilities. Specialized ambulance services, including mobile coronary care units and shock-trauma vans, are also increasingly prevalent.

The Red Cross and other voluntary agencies have administered programs for many years to train people to respond to accidents, drownings, and other emergencies. In Seattle, a program was initiated—now expanding to other cities—to augment emergency capabilities by teaching as many people as possible to respond to heart attacks by administering cardiopulmonary resuscitation (CPR). Because accidents and heart attacks are major sources of mortality, these programs have the potential of contributing to reductions in deaths.

GOVERNMENTAL PROGRAMS

In addition to private sector and institutionally initiated efforts, governmental programs have been designed to increase the availability of health care resources in many communities. These programs have adapted some of the concepts of private institutional settings, especially those of group practice.

Neighborhood health centers have been funded since 1965. Originally intended to serve approximately 25 million people, this federal program never reached its initial objectives. The program was designed to provide primary medical care with a family orientation. It was targeted for population groups in need of services, as reflected by such indicators as disease prevalence and income level. At the same time, the centers were intended to employ people from the communities they serve in positions that would offer opportunities for training and advancement. Responsiveness to community needs was to be ensured by a community board or advisory panel. The centers were to recognize that the broad attributes of a community, such as housing and employment, contributed to health and illness.

Most of the neighborhood health centers are free-standing group practices, although some are affiliated with other institutions such as hospitals, medical schools, or community associations. The majority of centers are located in urban areas. There is considerable diversity in the types of service provided by the centers, but all give primary care and most offer pharmacy, laboratory, radiology, and, to a lesser extent, dental services. Some centers also provide transportation for patients and social services to address broader health needs.

Although these health centers were originally intended to serve the poor, changes in federal policy that encouraged them to collect fees from patients and from third-party insurers have broadened the socioeconomic mixture of patients obtaining care. However, the centers still predominantly serve the medically indigent. Sources of funding have been broadened to include local government as well. Pressures for achieving self-sufficiency have been very powerful in recent years.

A related category of provider, the "free clinic," evolved from a strong social commitment but has had to face similar financial realities. The combination of "former" free clinics, neighborhood health centers, public agency clinics, and some hospital clinics and groups now form an informal "safety net" of providers for individuals who lack private insurance, access to other sources of care, or simply need care from an available, sympathetic, provider. Many of these providers now contract on their own or in coalitions with other providers to provide care to various individuals under governmental entitlement programs as well.

Neighborhood health centers were subjected to considerable criticism, especially from traditional medicine. These centers were often noted as having low productivity and substandard care as compared to the private sector, unwarranted federal intervention in the provision of health services, and high administrative costs.

Although it is not possible to generalize across all the centers, some probably had high costs and low productivity. This circumstance was, at least, partially attributable to several factors, including their goals of employing and training local residents, occasionally inexperienced management, constraints imposed by the federal government, and local politics. Neighborhood health centers also had difficulties in finding adequate facilities, had problems in physician recruitment, and experienced high staff turnover. There have been practical problems in designing family-oriented comprehensive care for clients used to receiving few services and episodic care. Studies designed to measure the quality of care provided in these centers have generally concluded that the centers met acceptable standards and, in some instances, provided a higher quality of care than did local practitioners on average; succeeded in increasing access to care under difficult circumstances; and served as an interesting experimental model for the provision of ambulatory care (39).

Other community health centers that have been funded by the federal government included migrant health centers serving transient farm workers in agricultural areas and rural health centers. The National Health Service Corps supported practitioners who were placed in urban and rural areas with shortages of medical resources. Other innovations, such as mobile health vans in rural areas, have also been used to expand the scope of services. The Community Mental Health Center program was established to provide ambulatory mental health services in underserved areas. Community mental health centers were intended to provide outpatient services and emergency care and to work with other community agencies to foster action and concern for mental health (Chapter 8).

OTHER FEDERAL GOVERNMENT PROGRAMS

The federal government, in addition to supporting a variety of community-based health services organizations, directly operates many health facilities. The Veterans Administration includes the largest health services system under a unified management structure in the United States with more than 170 hospitals and clinics. This system provides needed care to millions of veterans throughout the nation. The military services also provide health care to millions of individuals in the armed forces and have developed extensive regionalized facilities throughout the world, as discussed in Chapter 1.

The government has a special responsibility for providing health care to a number of groups within the country. The Indian Health Service is charged with ensuring access to medical care on Indian reservations and in certain other locations. Although the difficulties of operating a largely rural system are immense, the Indian Health Service has succeeded in bringing modern medicine to many people.

NONINSTITUTIONAL AND PUBLIC HEALTH SERVICES

As noted in the introduction to this chapter, there are many ways in which ambulatory and community health services are provided. Although only the most prevalent types of provider and service are discussed here, each helps to meet the many health care needs of a community. The list is nearly endless, and a number of services warrant further discussion.

Home health services, discussed in more detail in Chapter 7, are provided by visiting nurse associations, proprietary companies, some hospitals, public health departments, and other agencies. These services allow people to remain in their homes and yet receive essential health services, thereby reducing costs and increasing the quality of life for many.

Rural health care has required unique and innovative solutions in many communities, especially in the absence of adequate supplies of physicians and facilities. In rural Alaska, many towns are served by physicians and other professionals who regularly fly in to treat patients. Satellites are used to facilitate communications with specialists in urban medical centers since even ordinary communications in remote areas may be difficult. Rural health care in many areas remains a challenging test of the ingenuity and resourcefulness of the health services system and of community residents.

Other community health services not discussed in detail here include—but are not limited to—school health services; prison health services; vision care; dental care provided by solo, group, and institutionally based practitioners; foot care from podiatrists; and drug dispensing from pharmacists, who often also extensively advise and educate consumers. Voluntary agencies also provide health care services such as cancer screening clinics and health education. Finally, many indigenous health practitioners offer their services in this country and abroad. These practitioners include chiropractors, "medicine men," naturopaths, and others. The supportive and sometimes curative role of these individuals is often underestimated.

Among the most important contributions to reductions in mortality and morbidity in the twentieth century have been public health measures such as the improvement of sanitation, ensurance of potable water supplies, and upgraded housing. In recent years there has also been an increased awareness of the need to control air and water pollution, to reduce exposure to carcinogens, and to improve and ensure the quality of the environment. The contribution of these efforts to health far exceeds, dollar for dollar, efforts to treat illness once it occurs (40). Their importance to ambulatory care is mentioned here, however, because public health agencies have responsibility for a remarkable range of relevant services.

ORGANIZATION OF AMBULATORY CARE SYSTEMS

The changing structure of the health services system has had tremendous implications for ambulatory care services. The increased movement toward integrated systems of care has led ambulatory care services to assume a central role in the design and operation of many insurance and delivery programs. In addition, those paying for health services, including employers and insurers, have increasingly focused attention on the role which ambulatory care services can provide in improving the coordination and control of care as well as in reducing costs through the reduction of duplication and shifting of services to lower-cost settings.

Finally, those organizations constructing large-scale, integrated systems of care are continuing to seek existing ambulatory care structures, or are building new ones, as a means to complete their systems. In particular, insurers, hospitals, and other organizational entities are developing or purchasing ambulatory care resources such as medical practices, clinics, and other existing networks. Governmental units, such as the military, have long recognized the key attributes of ambulatory care in coordinating and controlling the overall utilization of services and then, the cost and quality of care. These trends are likely to continue.

There are many key design attributes of ambulatory care that are essential for both the effective operation of ambulatory services and for the full integration of these services into larger systems of care. Table 5-15 lists many of these criteria.

Ambulatory care is important in providing access to care, particularly within larger integrated systems. Access considerations include scope of services provided and hours of operation as well as distribution of resources throughout a geographic region populated by the target group of consumers. Physical access to facilities must also be assured, including such considerations as parking, access to public transportation where appropriate, and access to physical facilities for the handicapped.

The scope of services provided must respond to population needs. These needs may differ depending on whether the population is prepaid or fee-for-service. How the population is served differs substantially in each situation. For both situations, however, decisions must be made concerning the type of care to be provided on an ambulatory versus an inpatient basis.

Marketing advantages can be achieved in the ambulatory care setting by recognizing the special needs of consumers, such as having multilingual staff available where appropriate. The friendliness of the staff and the attractiveness of the physical facilities can have dramatic effects on patient attitudes and satisfaction, with not only the ambulatory care provider but the larger system of care as well. Thus ambulatory care provides an influential marketing function in any system of care. Ambulatory care services generally also provide an opportunity for educating the consumer in terms of both health behaviors and "appropriate" utilization of the system. This educational role can contribute to cost containment by having patients help in "managing" their utilization.

Ambulatory care can provide a key role in the overall provision of coordinated and continuous care. By accepting the gatekeeper role of the primary care physician, utilizing medical records and other administrative tracking of patients, and avoiding duplication of services and unnecessary care, the ambulatory care setting can contribute handsomely to the overall effectiveness of all care provided to the patient. Centralization of responsibility for patient care thus must be clearly assigned. Mechanisms for monitoring patient and provider behaviors to assure compliance with health system operating guidelines are essential. There is also evidence that more effective continuity of care is associated with higher levels of patient compliance regarding medical regimens, which, in turn, may lead to better health outcomes and eventually lower subsequent utilization rates. Patient satisfaction is generally greater when continuity and coordination of care are achieved—both effective marketing and cost containment tools.

The quality of care should reflect not only adequate medical skills but also a caring attitude on the part of the provider. Consumers in ambulatory care are capable of detecting some aspects of the technical quality of care, but they are even more aware of provider and system attitudes and behaviors.

The challenge in ambulatory care is to effectively shift from a traditionally reactive set of providers, attitudes, and operational approaches, to the proactive leadership role needed in today's competitive environment. Ambulatory care once meant a largely unaffiliated and unstructured set of small providers responding as business walked in

TABLE 5-15. Design Criteria for Ambulatory Care Systems

Criteria Topics	Criteria Requirements
Community criteria	
Availability and distribution of resources	Adequate number of facilities and practitioners
	Geographic dispersion
	Adequate transportation
Use of resources	Integration of community resources
	Effective referral network
	Appropriate mix of services
	Constrained excess capacity (few underused services)
Consumer criteria	
Convenience and satisfaction	Physical access assured
	Availability (hours of operation, after-hours coverage) ensured
	Efficient scheduling (appointments, follow-ups, waiting times)
	Financial access (insurance coverage, reasonable prices)
	Caring providers
Quality services	Continuity and coordination of care (medical records, follow-ups, etc.)
	Comprehensive services
	Technical quality of care ensured
	Multilingual staff and other special needs ensured
	Health education and instruction provided
Provider criteria	
Work environment	Pleasant and humane
	Appropriate roles for all providers
	Adequate income
	Productivity encouraged
	Personnel duties match skills and training
Patient care services	Efficient use of resources (personnel, capital, and technology)
	Use of most appropriate personnel
	Adequate support services available
System concerns	Technological progress readily adopted
	Development of owned or contractual systems of care
	Competitive delivery of services

the door. Now ambulatory care is a key vital element in the structuring of large-scale systems. These systems require financial and contractual arrangements with providers, and these ties are critical to all parties concerned.

The system's structure itself vitally affects the role of ambulatory care services; ambulatory care can, in turn, be vital to the success of the system. Whether services are organized on a fee-for-service, prepaid, or combined fee-for-service–prepaid basis, success in the provision of services mandates building the delivery of care around the ambulatory care providers. In increasingly competitive markets, this is especially important (41). In prepayment systems such as HMOs, fee-for-service systems, and particularly in aggressively contracted and discounted arrangements such as Preferred Provider Organizations, the ability to control providers and consumers—and hence costs—is dependent on structuring the system based on the controlling role of ambulatory care and performing needed services through ambulatory delivery vehicles where feasible, hopefully while maintaining quality (42). Ideally, quality, access, and health status will attain acceptable minimum levels under any delivery system, and controls will be built in to monitor both (43,44).

From a health care delivery perspective, as opposed to the financial focus of other chapters, the demands on ambulatory care to provide a marketing, integrating, controlling, and organizing function are great. At the same time, services must retain the attributes of high quality, meeting specific patient needs and offering a stimulating and rewarding environment for the providers as well. This is no small challenge.

REFERENCES

1. Roemer M: *Ambulatory Health Services in America.* Rockville, MD, Aspen Systems Corp., 1981.
2. United Kingdom Ministry of Health: Dawson Report, interim report on the future provision of medical and allied services. London, His Majesty's Stationary Office, 1920.
3. Noble J (ed): *Primary Care and the Practice of Medicine.* Boston, Little, Brown, 1976.
4. Roemer M: From poor beginnings, the growth of primary care. *Hospitals* 1975; 49(5):38–43.
5. National Center for Health Statistics; Gagnon R, DeLozier J, McLemore T: The National Ambulatory Medical Care Survey, United States, 1979 Summary. *Vital and Health Statistics.* Series 13, No. 66. DHHS Publ. No. (PHS) 82-1727. Public Health Service. Washington, U.S. Government Printing Office, September 1982.
6. McLemore T, DeLozier J: 1985 Summary: National Ambulatory Medical Care Survey. *Advance Data From Vital and Health Statistics.* National Center for Health Statistics, No. 128. DHHS Publ. No. (PHS) 87-1250 Public Health Service, Hyattsville, MD, January 23, 1987.
7. Peterson OL, Andrews LP, Spain RS, et al: An analytical study of North Carolina general practice 1953-1954. *J Med Educ* 1956; 31(Part 2):1–165.
8. Petersdorf R: Internal medicine and family practice, controversies, conflict and compromise. *New Engl J Med* 1975; 293:326–332.
9. Mechanic D: *The Growth of Bureaucratic Medicine.* New York, Wiley, 1976.
10. Becker M, Maiman L: Sociobehavioral determinants of compliance with health and medical care recommendations. *Med Care* 1975; 13:10–24.
11. Medical Group Management Association: *The Organization and Development of a Medical Group Practice.* Cambridge, MA, Ballinger, 1976.

12. Rorem R: *Private Group Clinics.* Chicago, University of Chicago Press, 1931.

13. Hwulich, PL: *Medical Groups in the U.S., 1984.* Chicago, American Medical Association, 1985.

14. Held PJ, Reinhardt UE: Prepaid medical practice: A summary of findings from a recent survey of group practices in the United States. *Group Health J* 1980; 1:4–15.

15. Cromley EK, Shannon GW: The establishment of Health Maintenance Organizations: A geographical analysis. *Am J Publ Health* 1983; 73:184–187.

16. Graham F: Group versus solo practice, arguments and evidence. *Inquiry* 1972; 9:49–60.

17. Kimball L, Lorant J: Physician productivity and returns to scale. *Health Serv Res* 1977; 12:367–379.

18. Anderson, OW, Herold T, Butler R, et al: *HMO Development: Patterns and Prospects. A Comparative Analysis of HMOs.* Chicago, University of Chicago, Center for Health Administration Studies, 1985.

19. Mackie DL, Decker DK: *Group and IPA HMOs.* Rockville, MD, Aspen Systems Corp., 1981.

20. Cascardo D: Factors affecting cost containment in an HMO: A review of the literature. *J Ambulatory Care Management* 1982; 5:53–63.

21. Egdahl R: Foundations for medical care. *New Engl J Med* 1973; 288:491–498.

22. Bauman P: The formulation and evolution of the Health Maintenance Organization policy, 1970–1973. *Soc Sci Med* 1976; 10:129–142.

23. Mayer TR, Mayer GG: HMOs: Origins and Development. *New Engl J Med* 1985; 312:590–594.

24. Roemer M, Shonick W: HMO performance: The recent evidence. *Milbank Mem Fund Quart* 1973; 51:271–317.

25. Strumpf G, Garramone M: Why some HMOs develop slowly. *Public Health Rep* 1976; 91:496–503.

26. Meyers SM: Growth in Health Maintenance Organizations, in *Health, United States, 1981.* Washington, DC, U.S. Government Printing Office, 1981.

27. Iglehart JK: Medicare Turns to HMOs. *New Engl J Med* 1985; 312:132–136.

28. Adamache KW, Rossiter LF: The entry of HMOs into the Medicare market: Implications for TEFRA's mandate. *Inquiry* 1986; 23:349–364.

29. Luft H: Health Maintenance Organizations and the Rationing of Medical Care. *Milbank Mem Fund Quart: Health Society* 1982; 60:268–306.

30. Iglehart JK: HMOs (for-profit and not-for-profit) on the move. *New Engl J Med* 1984; 310:1203–1208.

31. Harrison DH, Kimberly JR: Private and public initiatives in Health Maintenance Organizations. *J Health Politics, Policy and Law* 1982; 7:80–95.

32. Luft HS: Assessing the evidence on HMO performance. *Milbank Mem Fund Quart* 1980; 58:501–536.

33. Luft HS: *Health Maintenance Organizations: Dimensions of Performance.* New York, Wiley, 1981.

34. Buss ML: HMOs' second decade: 1983–1993. Proposed responses to new challenges. *Group Health J* 1985; 6:17–21.

35. Williams S, Shortell S, Dowling W, et al: Hospital sponsored primary care group practice: A developing modality of care. *Health Med Care Serv Rev* 1978; 1:1–130.

36. Williams SJ: Ambulatory care: Can hospitals compete? *Hosp Health Serv Admin* 1983; 28:22–34.

37. Shortell SM, Wickizer T, Wheeler J, (eds): *Hospital Physician Joint Ventures.* Ann Arbor, MI, Health Administration Press, 1984.

38. Holl EF: Fighting off competition by a joint venture in outpatient surgery. *Topics Health Care Financ* 1985; 12:58–65.

39. Morehead M, Donaldson R, Seravalli M: Comparison between OEO neighborhood health centers and other health care providers of ratings of quality of health care. *Am J Publ Health* 1971; 61:1294–1306.

40. McKinlay J, McKinlay S: The questionable contribution of medical measures to the decline of mortality in the United States in the twentieth century. *Milbank Mem Fund Quart* 1977; 55:450–428.

41. Iglehart JK: The twin cities' medical marketplace. *New Engl J Med* 1984; 311:343–348.

42. Manning WG, Leibowitz A, Goldberg G, et al: A controlled trial of the effect of a prepaid group practice on use of services. *New Engl J Med* 1984; 310:1505–1510.

43. Ware JE Jr, Brook RH, Rogers WH, Keeler EB, and others: Comparison of health outcomes at a health maintenance organization with those of fee-for-service care. *Lancet* 1986 May 3; 1(8488):1017–1022.

44. Cunningham FC, Williamson JW: How does the quality of health care in HMOs compare to that in other settings? An analytic literature review: 1958 to 1979. *Group Health J* 1980; 1:4–25.

CHAPTER 6

The Hospital

Claudia L. Haglund
William L. Dowling

The modern hospital is the key resource and organizational hub of the American health care system, central to the delivery of patient care, the training of health personnel, and the conduct and dissemination of health-related research. The hospital represents the community's collective investment in health care resources, presumably available for the benefit of all, and it is often the first place people think of when they need medical care. Since the turn of the century, hospitals, the indispensable workshop of the physician, have become even more the economic and professional heart of medical practice as the accelerating pace of advances in medical knowledge and technology continues. In recent years, hospitals have expanded beyond their inpatient role in an effort to become comprehensive, vertically integrated community health systems. As highly advanced, scientific institutions, hospitals manifest the complexity and detached efficiency of a clinical laboratory. As human service organizations, they are charged with the emotions of life and death and of triumphs and tragedies. Hospitals are frequently the care givers of last resort for many of the nations's poor who have nowhere else to turn for health care.

Hospitals are also big business. Collectively, they are the second or third largest industry in the United States in terms of the number of people they employ. By far the largest part of the health care system, hospitals employ about three-fourths of all health care personnel and consume 39 percent of the nation's health expenditures. About 58 percent of all federal expenditures for health services and about 36 percent of all state and local government health expenditures are for hospital care (1).

Ironically, the magnitude of the hospital sector and the central role hospitals play in the delivery of health services now place hospitals at the root of many of the health care system's most pressing problems—cost increases, duplication of services, bed surpluses, overemphasis on specialized inpatient services versus primary care services, deper-sonalization of care, and so forth (2–5). Furthermore, as community or quasipublic institutions heavily dependent on public dollars, hospitals are open systems, subject to influence from outside forces and, therefore, susceptible to the efforts of community groups, external agencies, business coalitions, and insurance carriers to use them as instruments of social change and health system reform (6,7).

The hospital system is a mix of public and private for-profit and not-for-profit institutions. Hospitals range from small institutions in less populated communities and isolated rural areas providing basic medical care to large regional referral centers providing a comprehensive range of sophisticated, highly specialized services. Over one-third belong to multiunit hospital systems. Many hospitals have expanded their role to include an array of noninpatient services, including primary care clinics, home care, health promotion, and long-term care services. Other hospitals have reorganized to develop for-profit enterprises or sponsor managed care systems.

The purpose of this chapter is to characterize the hospital system in the United States, emphasizing major issues and trends. Because the character of the modern hospital reflects its past, this chapter begins with a discussion of the historical development of hospitals. The second section describes the hospital system as it exists today. The third section describes the internal organization of hospitals. The final section discusses a number of major issues confronting hospitals at the present time. It should be noted that while the discussion of hospitals in this chapter focuses primarily on their inpatient role, hospitals now play an increasingly important role in the provision of outpatient care and are evolving toward a new role as providers of a comprehensive and integrated continuum of health services (8,9). To illustrate, the number of emergency room visits and the number of outpatient referrals for diagnostic and therapeutic services in community hospitals have been increasing four times faster than the number of admissions, and the ratio of outpatient visits to inpatient admissions in community hospitals is now almost 6:1. Fully 55 percent of the nation's community hospitals have organized outpatient departments, 85 percent have emergency departments, 83 percent have ambulatory surgery units, 52 percent have health promotion programs, and 27 percent offer home health services (10).

HISTORICAL DEVELOPMENT OF HOSPITALS

The history of hospitals in this country (Figure 6-1) can be traced back to the almshouses and pesthouses that existed in some form in almost all cities of moderate size by the mid-1700s (11,12). Almshouses, also called *poorhouses* or *workhouses*, were established by city governments to provide food and shelter for the homeless poor, including many aged, chronically ill, disabled, mentally ill, and orphaned people. Medical care was a secondary function of the poorhouse; however, in some facilities, those who became ill were isolated in infirmaries where care, such as it was before the advent of modern medicine, was provided, typically by other residents. Not until the late 1800s did the infirmaries or hospital departments of city poorhouses break away to become medical care institutions on their own—the first public hospitals.

Pesthouses were operated by local governments as isolation or quarantine stations in seaports where it was necessary to isolate people who contracted contagious diseases aboard ship. During epidemics, these institutions were used to isolate victims of cholera, smallpox, typhus, and yellow fever. Their primary purpose was to control the spread of infectious diseases by removing infected individuals from the community. As in almshouses, medical care was a secondary function—in this case, secondary to protecting the community from outbreaks of contagious diseases. Pesthouses were often established during epidemics and discontinued or closed down when the threat of disease subsided. These institutions were the predecessors of the contagious disease and tuberculosis hospitals that later emerged.

SITE OF CARE
IN 1700s

TYPE OF PATIENT

SITE OF CARE
IN 1900

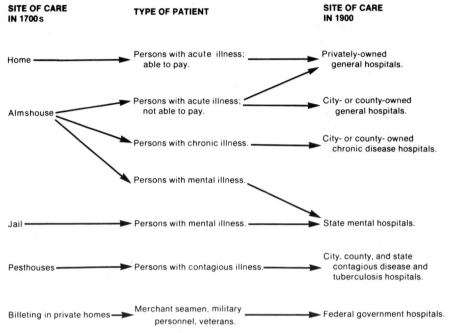

Figure 6-1. Evolution of institutional care sites.

Almshouses and pesthouses were maintained for the poor and the homeless and were avoided by everyone else. These institutions were dismal places: crowded, unsanitary, and poorly heated and ventilated. Nutrition was often inadequate, nursing care incompetent, and separation of different types of patients minimal. Contagious persons, the disabled, the dying, and the mentally ill were often crowded together. Cross-infection was rampant and mortality high. Persons who were able were cared for at home or in the homes of neighbors.

The first community-owned or voluntary hospitals in this country were established in the late 1700s and early 1800s, often at the urging of influential physicians trained in Europe who needed facilities to practice obstetrics and surgery in the manner in which they had been taught, and also to provide preceptor-type instruction for medical students. These early hospitals depended on philanthropy, and contributions were solicited from both private citizens and the local government. Voluntary hospitals generally preceded both religious and public hospitals in the United States, representing a departure from patterns in England and Europe. Voluntary hospitals admitted both indigent and paying patients. For example, in its first year of operation (1751), the Pennsylvania Hospital admitted 24 paying patients and 40 poor patients. These hospitals were supported by community contributions and philanthropy, rather than by a church or the state. Except in the largest cities, where the concentration of poor was too great, the early voluntary hospitals cared for people in their communities who were unable to pay on a charitable basis, drawing on philanthropy and donations of time by members of the medical staff (11,13).

The first hospitals of this type were the Pennsylvania Hospital, Philadelphia, 1751; New York Hospital, New York City, 1773; Massachusetts General Hospital, Boston, 1816; and New Haven Hospital, New Haven, Connecticut, 1826. Additional voluntary hospitals were established in Savannah, Georgia, in 1830; Lowell, Massachusetts, in 1836; and Raleigh, North Carolina, in 1839. Voluntary hospitals cared for patients with acute illnesses and injuries but did not admit persons with contagious diseases or mental illnesses. Isolation of these unfortunates from the rest of the community was seen as a governmental responsibility. Therefore, during the same period, a number of city, county, and state mental hospitals were established. These included hospitals in Williamsburg, Virginia, 1773; Lexington, Kentucky, 1817; Columbia, South Carolina, 1829; Worcester, Massachusetts, 1832; Augusta, Maine, 1834; Brooklyn, New York, 1838; and Boston, Massachusetts, 1839.

Although voluntary hospitals provided better accommodations and care for the sick than had the poorhouses that preceded them, the efficacy of care improved little, and it was not until the late 1800s that hospitals became accepted by persons of all economic strata as the best setting for the care of serious illness and injury. In 1873 there were only 178 hospitals with 35,604 beds in the United States. By 1909, the number of hospitals had increased to 4359, with 421,065 beds, and by 1929, to 6665 hospitals with 907,133 beds. This rapid growth was brought about by advances in medical science that rapidly transformed the hospital's role from a custodial institution in which to isolate and shelter the poor to a curative institution in which communities concentrated their health care resources in support of the practicing physician for the benefit of all (13,14). Starr (15) has characterized this redefinition of the hospital as a transformation from a social welfare facility to an institution of medical science, from a charitable organization to a business, and from an orientation toward patrons and the poor to a focus on professionals and patients.

FORCES AFFECTING THE DEVELOPMENT OF HOSPITALS

Six major developments in health care were particularly significant in transforming hospitals into the institutions of today: advances in medical science increased the efficacy and safety of hospitals; the development of technological sophistication and specialization necessitated the institutionalization of much medical care; the development of professional nursing brought about more humane treatment of patients; advances in medical education added teaching and research to the hospital's role; the health insurance industry grew; and the role of government increased (11,13,15–17).

Advances in Medical Science

Most notable in terms of their impact on hospitals were the discovery of anesthesia and the rapid advances in surgery that followed and the development of the germ theory of disease and the subsequent discovery of antiseptic and sterilization techniques. By the early 1800s, enough was known about anatomy and physiology that surgeons were able to perform a variety of fairly complex surgical procedures. However, the inability to deaden pain meant that surgery had to be carried out with extreme speed. In addition, infection from surgery was common. Ether was first used as an anesthetic in surgery by Long in 1842 and then by Morton in 1846, and its use then spread rapidly. Great advances in the efficacy of surgery followed.

Before the formulation of the germ theory of disease, a few scientists, most notably Holmes in the United States and Semmelweis in Vienna, had observed and reported that fever, infection, and mortality could be reduced through cleanliness. Both concluded that childbed fever, which was the cause of high maternal mortality, was an infection transmitted by physicians, midwives, and medical students to women in labor. In 1861 Pasteur proved that bacteria were living, reproducing microorganisms that could be carried by air or on clothing and hands. It became clear that germs were the cause rather than the result of infection and could be destroyed by chemicals and heat. Lister built on Pasteur's work and in 1867 introduced carbolic acid spray in operating rooms as an antiseptic to keep air and incisions clean. In 1886, steam sterilization was introduced, providing a means of freeing medical equipment from microorganisms. Surgical infection rates fell. Advances in surgery led to the need for skilled preoperative and postoperative care and operating room facilities, which could be provided only in hospitals. By 1900, 40 percent of all hospitalizations were for surgery.

Development of Specialized Technology

By the late 1800s, medical technology began to proliferate. The first hospital laboratory opened in 1889, and x-ray films were first used for diagnosis in 1896. These developments greatly increased the diagnostic effectiveness of hospitals. The discovery of blood types in 1901 made blood transfusions safe; the electrocardiogram (EKG) was first used in 1903 and the electroencephalogram (EEG) in 1929. In addition to increasing the efficiency of medical care, these advances in technology affected the site and the organization of care. Since the tools of the new technology could no longer be carried around in the physician's black bag, hospitals became the central resource where the equipment, facilities, and personnel required by modern medicine were housed. In addition, since one person could no longer be competent in all areas of medical practice, specialization began to occur within medicine, and new professional and technical occupations began to emerge. Again, the hospital became the place where physicians and support personnel came together to provide patient care.

Development of Professional Nursing

Humane treatment of patients awaited the development of professional nursing. Before the late 1800s, the only humane nursing care was provided by Catholic sisters and Protestant deaconesses, who were dedicated to caring for patients. Some religious orders established their own hospitals, and occasionally they were called on by city officials to provide nursing services in public institutions. Almshouses used untrained female residents to provide nursing care, and hospitals relied on poorly paid, unskilled labor.

The transformation of nursing into a profession is credited to Florence Nightingale, who completed 4 months of nurses' training in a deaconess school in Germany. In 1854, Nightingale and 38 nurses were sent by the British government to the Crimea to take charge of nursing care for wounded soldiers. The nurses found conditions deplorable and instituted cleanliness and sanitation, dietary reforms, simple but humane care, discipline, and organization. As a result, mortality dropped dramatically. On her return to England, Nightingale wrote of her experiences in the Crimea and on the contributions of sanitation to the recovery of wounded and ill patients. In 1860 she founded the Nightingale School for Nursing in England.

In the United States, President Abraham Lincoln called on Catholic religious communities to provide nursing care for the wounded during the Civil War, but more nurses were needed. Dorothea Dix was appointed Superintendent of Nursing for the Union Army. She began a recruitment program and encouraged a 1-month hospital training program for new nurses. By the end of the war, there were 2000 lay nurses in the country. The first permanent schools of nursing were established at Bellevue Hospital, New Haven Hospital, and Massachusetts General Hospital in 1873. Although there was some initial reluctance on the part of hospital administrators and trustees to establish nursing schools, the benefits of good nursing soon became apparent. In addition, student nurses provided better care and were less expensive than the untrained women previously employed to do this work. By 1883, there were 22 nursing schools and 600 graduates; by 1898, these totals had grown to 400 schools with 10,000 graduates.

Advances in nursing contributed to the growth of hospitals in two ways: (1) increased efficacy of treatment, cleanliness, nutritious diets, and formal treatment routines all contributed to patient recovery; and (2) considerate, skilled patient care made hospitals acceptable to all people, not just the poor. The public's fear of hospitals began to give way to an attitude of confidence and respect.

Advances in Medical Education

Changes in medical education brought about by the Flexner Report (18) in 1910 had a major impact on the development of hospitals. Before 1900, there was great variation in the nature and quality of medical education. There were no standards of academic training for physicians. Most medical schools were proprietary and were not connected with universities. They were dominated by influential practitioners, and most instruction was through didactic (often unscientific) lectures. Apprenticeship practices varied greatly. There was little clinical or laboratory instruction and little research.

The Flexner Report led to changes in the content and methods of instruction to emphasize the scientific basis of medicine. The standards of education established by the Flexner Report were widely accepted by both the profession and the public; as a result, schools that did not meet the standards were forced to close. State laws were established requiring graduation from a medical school accredited by the American Medical Association as the basis for a license to practice medicine. A 4-year course of study at a medical school based in a university became standard, as did clinical training in the wards of a hospital.

These changes expanded the role of the hospital to include education and research as well as patient care. The hospital's role in education became even more prominent as specialization in medicine led to a proliferation of internships and residencies in the 1920s and 1930s. The requirements of medical education necessitated the expansion of hospital facilities and services and the addition of equipment and personnel. Hospitals were called on to assume a greater responsibility for coordinating and organizing these resources. Quality of care improved through advances in medical education, especially for patients with complex and serious illnesses. On the other hand, specialization led to a fragmentation of care among different physician specialists and ancillary personnel and a lack of interest in chronic, routine, and other "uninteresting" medical conditions.

Thus the growth of hospitals in the United States was a direct result of advances in medical science that made hospitals effective and safe. These advances, particularly the discovery of sulfa drugs in the mid-1930s and antibiotics in the mid-1940s, changed the prevalent causes of death from acute, infectious diseases to the diseases of old age, particularly heart disease, cancer, and stroke. Hospitals have not been quick to respond to the chronic health care problems of an aging population. Their resources continue to be concentrated on curable, short-term illnesses that respond quickly to medical treatment, rather than on chronic, long-term illnesses that must be managed over long periods of time. Hospitals are just now beginning to expand their role to include extended or skilled nursing care units, inpatient or outpatient rehabilitation programs, day care, home care, and other nontraditional services (4,19–20).

Growth of Health Insurance

Another factor that has significantly affected the development of hospitals is the growth of the health insurance industry. Private insurance for hospital care grew rapidly, especially between 1940 and 1960, increasing both the proportion of the population with insurance and the adequacy and scope of coverage. Today, the out-of-pocket cost of hospital care at the time of use is relatively modest for most people, because most of the bill is covered by some third-party purchaser—either government or private health insurance.

A variety of factors led to the growth of hospital insurance. From the consumer's perspective, of course, a hospital stay is sufficiently expensive to warrant the purchase of insurance protection. The hospital industry's interest in insurance began with the Great Depression of the 1930s, when the number of patients who could not pay their bill increased markedly and hospital use declined. The financial solvency of many hospitals was threatened, and the number of hospitals dropped from 6852 in 1928 to 6189 in 1937. Furthermore, a study of nonprofit hospitals in 1935 revealed that total income was 3 percent less than total expenses. As a result, acting through the American Hospital Association, hospitals took the initiative in actively encouraging the development of hospital insurance plans, primarily Blue Cross (16,21,22). These developments are discussed in detail in Chapter 11.

The growth of health insurance has had a substantial impact on hospitals. First, ensuring the financial stability of hospitals, insurance subsequently provided the flow of funds that made possible the great expansion of facilities and services and the prompt implementation of new medical technology that have characterized the hospital industry since the end of World War II. Insurance also contributed to the increased demand for health services. Historically, hospital services have been better covered by insurance than services provided outside the hospital, so patients have been reluctant to substitute less expensive out-of-hospital services. This attitude resulted in a bias toward hospital use versus the use of ambulatory care services, home care programs, or nursing care facilities as sources of care and a general overuse of expensive hospital services (23,24). In the 1980s, however, concern over the rising costs of hospital care and inappropriate hospital admissions has reversed this trend. Insurance carriers are now actively promoting nonhospital alternatives for medical care and stringent utilization control over inpatient admissions. The belief that hospital admissions are unwarranted in many instances was recently underscored in a Rand Corporation study based on a sample of hospital records from 1974 to 1982. The study concluded that 23 percent of the admissions studied were inappropriate and another 17 percent could have been avoided through the use of ambulatory surgery (25).

Another problem in the hospital industry can be traced at least partially to cost-based reimbursement, the method of payment used until recently, by Medicare,

Medicaid, and most Blue Cross plans. Cost reimbursement does not provide hospitals with an incentive to contain costs. The result has been inefficiency, duplication of services, and overbuilding (26–28). To stem rising hospital costs, public and private payers have experimented in recent years with a number of regulatory and competitive approaches to cost containment (29). Regulatory approaches to cost containment, most notably certificate-of-need (CON) review for new hospital equipment, services, and beds, and hospital rate regulation, were initiated in the 1970s. As hospital costs continued to rise, however, economists, business coalitions, and policymakers began suggesting that true market competition would provide greater incentives for controlling health care spending (30). As a result, the 1980s have witnesses a weakening of regulatory approaches to hospital cost containment and a growing emphasis on competition. One hallmark of the competitive model is the centrality of the buying power of major purchasers of hospital care such as Blue Cross, Medicare, and Medicaid. These purchasers have taken swift action in the 1980s to replace payment systems based on retrospective costs with ones based on competitive prices.

A major step toward the introduction of market power occurred when the Tax Equity and Fiscal Responsibility Act of 1982 (PL 97-248) converted Medicare reimbursement to a prospective per case system based on diagnosis-related groups (DRGs). In turn, several states revised their Medicaid programs and now pay hospitals on a prospective basis. In addition, managed care programs, including Health Maintenance Organizations (HMOs) and Preferred Provider Organizations (PPOs), which emphasize strict utilization controls over hospital admissions, began to proliferate in the private health insurance sector. Hospitals now find themselves competing on the basis of price and discounts for patients covered by health insurance plans. While cost reimbursement is widely blamed as the root cause of runaway hospital costs, it nevertheless has allowed hospitals to keep up to date with advances in medical technology and demands from their communities and physicians for access to a broad range of services. A key public policy issue yet unresolved is how to balance the accessibility and costliness of hospital services, and particularly how to guarantee the poor and disadvantaged a decent standard of care in a system driven by competitive forces.

Role of Government

Government's role in the hospital industry has changed substantially in both form and level. During colonial times, government involvement was mainly at the local level through ownership of almshouses and pesthouses and grants to help construct and support voluntary hospitals. State government limited its role to running contagious disease and mental hospitals; and the federal government, to running hospitals for merchant seamen, military personnel, and veterans. Gradually, the forms of involvement have multiplied and the balance has shifted to the federal level.

The initial thrust of federal involvement began in 1935, with federal categorical grants-in-aid to state and local governments to assist in the establishment of traditional public health programs: public health departments; communicable disease programs; maternal and child health programs; and public assistance for specific groups such as crippled children, the aged, the blind, the disabled, and poor families with dependent children. These programs were part of the general social reform movement that developed during the Depression with the recognition that state and local government and voluntary efforts were not sufficient to meet social needs.

Direct federal involvement in the hospital industry began in 1946 with the Hill-Burton (Hospital Survey and Construction) Act. Few hospitals had been constructed during the Depression and World War II, and by the end of the war, it was generally felt that a severe shortage of hospitals existed. The Hill-Burton program was enacted to help states and communities plan for and construct hospitals and other health facilities by providing federal grants on a matching basis to supplement funds raised at the community level. Although the initial emphasis of the program was to provide funds for the construction of new hospitals, priorities changed over time from construction to modernization and from inpatient to outpatient facilities. Funds were available through the program for the construction of nursing homes as well.

The Hill-Burton program assisted in the construction of nearly 40 percent of the beds in the nation's short-term general hospitals and was the greatest single factor in the increase in the nation's bed supply from 3.5 short-term beds per 1000 population in 1946 to 4.5 beds per 1000 population today. Another positive impact of the program is that hospital facilities are more evenly distributed across rural and urban areas and high- and low-income states than they would have been without the program. However, the program also contributed to the overbuilding of hospitals and to the preponderance of small rural hospitals existing today.

From assisting with the financing of hospital construction, the federal government's involvement in the hospital industry has expanded to financing the provision of care and regulating the construction, operation, and use of hospitals. Of all hospital bills, 54 percent are now covered by government programs, primarily Medicare and Medicaid (1), which puts the federal government in a position to exercise a great amount of control over the operations of hospitals. The regulation of hospitals is discussed later in this chapter and in Chapter 12.

CHARACTERISTICS OF THE HOSPITAL SYSTEM

The hospital industry is complex and diverse and therefore difficult to describe simply. However, hospitals can be classified generally in one of three ways: according to length of stay, according to the predominant type of service provided, and according to ownership (31). In terms of length of stay, the most common type of hospital is the short-stay or short-term hospital, in which most patients suffer from acute conditions requiring hospital stays of less than 30 days. The average length of stay in short-term hospitals is about 7 days and has declined significantly over the last 5 years. In long-term hospitals, most of which are chronic disease, psychiatric, or tuberculosis hospitals, the average length of stay ranges from 3 to 6 months (10).

The second method of classification is by type of service. Predominant is the general hospital, offering a wide range of medical, surgical, obstetric, and pediatric services. Specialty hospitals, on the other hand, provide care for a specific disease or population group. Examples of specialty hospitals are children's hospitals, maternity hospitals, chronic disease hospitals, psychiatric hospitals, and tuberculosis hospitals. During the first part of the twentieth century, a number of specialty hospitals were established as a result of philanthropists responding to the initiative of prestigious physician specialists who wanted to develop their own hospitals. Because of financial difficulties and advances in medical science that make general hospitals more appropriate and efficient, specialty hospitals are less common today. Most have either closed down or converted to general hospitals (11,13).

The third method of classifying hospitals is according to form of ownership: government or public ownership, private for-profit (proprietary) ownership, and private nonprofit (religious or voluntary) ownership.

PUBLIC HOSPITALS

Public hospitals are owned by agencies of federal, state, or local government. Federally owned hospitals are maintained primarily for special groups of federal beneficiaries: American Indians, merchant seamen, military personnel, and veterans. State governments have generally limited themselves to the operation of mental and tuberculosis hospitals, reflecting government's early role of protecting the healthy by isolating the mentally ill and persons with contagious diseases from the rest of society. Most local government hospitals are short-term general hospitals. These institutions constitute 28 percent of the nation's short-term hospitals and accommodate 18 percent of all admissions and 23 percent of all outpatient visits to short-term hospitals (Table 6-1). Local government hospitals can be divided into two types. The first is city, county, or hospital district institutions, mostly small or moderate in bed size, with medical staffs consisting of private physicians and serving both indigent and paying patients. These hospitals tend to be located in small cities and towns. Their costs are met primarily through third-party reimbursement, and they receive little tax support. For all practical purposes, they function the same as community-owned hospitals. The second type is large city or county hospitals in major urban areas. These hospitals serve mostly the poor, near-poor, and minorities. They are generally staffed by salaried physicians, mostly residents. Most are affiliated with medical schools. Their costs usually exceed their patient revenues, and so their deficits must be made up through tax subsidies.

Large urban public hospitals play an important role in the health care system. They are the place of last resort for the poor, both because they care for all patients regardless of ability to pay and because they provide services that private hospitals cannot finance or do not wish to offer: burn and trauma care, alcohol and drug abuse treatment, psychiatric services, care for persons with chronic and communicable diseases, abortion and family planning services, and so forth. They are located in areas where health resources, especially private physicians, are in short supply, and their outpatient departments are the only accessible source of ambulatory care for many inner-city residents. Large urban public hospitals average 10.3 outpatient visits per inpatient admission, compared to 6.3 outpatient visits per admission in privately owned hospitals over 500 beds (10). In addition, these hospitals play a major role in medical education; 70 percent are affiliated with a medical school and 75 percent offer residency training programs (32). More than half of all practicing physicians receive at least some of their training in public hospitals.

It was thought that enactment of the Medicare and Medicaid programs would greatly reduce the demand on public hospitals by giving the aged and the poor the means to purchase care from other sources. The expected exodus did not occur, however, probably because the gatekeepers of the community hospitals, private practitioners, are in short supply in inner-city areas. In addition, some of those who are located close enough to be accessible limited the number of welfare patients they would accept. Cultural and social barriers also discouraged the poor from approaching community hospitals. As a result, inpatient and outpatient use of public hospitals dipped only slightly in 1967, the first full year of operation of both Medicare and

TABLE 6-1. Hospitals, Beds, Admissions, and Outpatient Visits by Ownership and Type of Service, 1985

	Hospitals		Beds		Admissions		Outpatient Visits	
	Number	Percent	Number	Percent	Number	Percent	Number	Percent
Total—all hospitals	6872	100	1,318,000	100	36,304,000	100	282,140,000	100
Federal	343	5	112,000	8	2,103,000	6	52,342,000	19
Nonfederal								
Psychiatric	610	9	171,000	13	602,000	2	4,902,000	2
Tuberculosis	7	<1	6,000	<1	35,000	<1		
Long-term	128	2	31,000	3	92,000	<1	2,087,000	1
Short-term	5784	84	1,003,000	76	33,501,000	92	222,773,000	79
Short-term hospitals								
Nongovernmental								
Not-for-profit	3364	58	708,000	71	24,188,000	72	160,002,000	72
Investor-owned, for-profit	805	14	104,000	10	3,242,000	10	12,378,000	6
State and local governmental	1615	28	191,000	19	6,071,000	18	0,394,000	23

SOURCE: *Hospital Statistics.* Chicago, American Hospital Association, 1986.

Medicaid, and then continued a steady upward climb. Today a disproportionate share of charity care, nearly 90 percent, is provided by public hospitals (33).

Given the increasing demand that large urban public hospitals are called on to satisfy, their problems are great. Characteristically, these hospitals are old and outmoded. They tend to be underequipped, underfinanced, and understaffed. They have difficulty attracting physicians and rely heavily on interns, residents, and foreign-trained physicians. Their administration is constrained by the bureaucratic red tape and rigidity of city or county government. Public hospitals have responded to these difficulties in a variety of ways. Most are affiliated with medical schools to attract faculty as supervisory physicians and to facilitate the recruitment of residents. In some areas, a special agency or commission has been created to run the public hospital in order to buffer it from government bureaucracy. In some cases, the agency is completely separate from city or county government but is empowered by enabling legislation to borrow, issue bonds, and tax, much like a school district. In other instances, public hospitals have entered into contract management agreements with private organiza-tions most notably, investor-owned hospital systems. In fact, 45 percent of all hospitals under contract management are public hospitals (34). A number of public hospitals are attempting to improve their position by becoming the source of highly specialized tertiary services such as regional trauma services, burn care, neonatal intensive care, or kidney dialysis. Other aspects of this strategy include opening the medical staff to private physicians, adding amenities, and improving facilities to encourage physicians to bring their private patients to the public hospital, at least for more specialized services (35,36).

FOR-PROFIT HOSPITALS

For-profit, investor-owned, or proprietary hospitals are operated for the financial benefit of the individual, partnership, or corporation that owns the institution. Around the turn of the century, more than one-half of the nation's hospitals were proprietary. Most of these hospitals had been established by one or a small group of physicians who wanted a place to hospitalize their own patients, and most were quite small (37). Gradually, these institutions were closed or sold to community organizations. The number of proprietary hospitals declined steadily through 1972, although the number of beds in proprietary hospitals began to increase around 1960 as the better situated proprietary hospitals expanded to accommodate population increases and as new proprietary hospitals, typically larger than those that were closing, were built (see Table 6-2). As of 1985, proprietary hospitals comprised 14 percent of the nation's short-term hospitals, with 10 percent of the beds and 6 percent of the outpatient visits (see Table 6-1) (10).

The most significant trend over the past few years has been not the number of proprietary hospitals per se but the building or acquisition of a substantial number of hospitals by large, investor-owned corporations to form multiunit, for-profit hospital systems. In 1985 the five largest investor-owned corporations owned or leased about 450 hospitals, totaling 79,000 beds. These corporations manage another 265 hospitals, totaling 34,000 beds—most of which are nonprofit hospitals (38). After several years of spectacular increases, the rate of growth for investor-owned hospital chains slowed somewhat in 1985, although they continue to be the fastest growing sector of the hospital industry. Hospitals owned, leased, or managed by for-profit firms increased by 37.8 percent between 1980 and 1985 (39).

TABLE 6-2. Characteristics of Proprietary Short-Term Hospitals in the United States, Selected Years

Year	Number of Hospitals	Number of Beds	Admissions
1950	1218	42,000	1,661,000
1960	856	37,000	1,550,000
1970	769	53,000	2,031,000
1975	775	73,000	2,646,000
1980	730	87,000	3,165,000
1985	805	104,000	3,242,000

SOURCE: *Hospital Statistics.* Chicago, American Hospital Association, 1986.

Investor-owned hospital corporations claim that they are able to earn a profit by operating their hospitals more efficiently than nonprofit hospitals. They point to the availability of management specialists, the application of modern management techniques, cost savings in construction and maintenance, economies of scale, and group purchasing as the key factors enabling them to control costs sufficiently to make a profit and pay taxes without compromising quality. Investor-owned hospital systems have also been able to respond promptly to population shifts because of their ability to raise capital quickly (40). Critics of for-profit hospitals claim that they undermine traditional medical values and that their profits are attributable to the practice of "cream skimming"—admitting only patients with less serious medical conditions and patients who are able to pay the full costs of their hospitalization (41,42). By not admitting poorly insured patients, for-profit hospitals can avoid bad debts, which may run as high as 10 percent of total patient charges in nonprofit and public hospitals in certain locations. By not admitting seriously ill patients, for-profit hospitals can avoid providing expensive or unprofitable services. The quality of care in for-profit hospitals has also been criticized. The lower employee:bed ratio in these hospitals, for example, is pointed to as an indicator of lower quality and less sophisticated services rather than more efficient management. Another criticism is that even if for-profit hospitals are more efficient, their cost savings are not passed on to patients.

There is a growing body of research that focuses on the comparative analysis of for-profit and nonprofit hospitals. One recent study (43) that compared economic performance between eighty matched pairs of nonprofit and investor-owned chain hospitals concluded that total charges adjusted for case mix and net revenues per case were significantly higher in investor-owned chain hospitals, primarily as a result of higher charges for ancillary services. Investor-owned hospitals were found to be more profitable but incurred higher administrative costs; they also had fewer employees per occupied bed but paid higher salaries. The authors concluded that investor-owned chain hospitals realized greater profits primarily through more aggressive pricing and not through greater efficiencies. These results concur with the findings of earlier studies (44,45) but by no means reflect universal opinions within the health care industry. By contrast, another recent report (46) asserts that for-profit hospitals provide greater worth to society because they require virtually no social investment to keep them afloat, are more efficient, reinvest earnings in newer plants and equipment, and offer an equally broad range of services to patients, including the medically indigent.

Furthermore, it has been noted that the behavior of many nonprofit hospitals can barely be distinguished from that of their investor-owned competitors. As a result, the tax-exempt status of nonprofit hospitals may be challenged in the future (47). It is true that many nonprofit hospitals have adopted new legal structures that allow them to operate for-profit subsidiary corporations. Nonprofit hospitals are also evaluating and implementing numerous management techniques from the private sector (20).

In all fairness, the cream skimming that does occur in for-profit hospitals is likely to be attributed more to the location of the for-profit hospitals (e.g., in rapidly growing suburban areas) than to the actual turning away of patients who cannot pay. The refusal to admit patients with complex conditions requiring sophisticated services and the lack of high-cost, low-use specialized services are cited by for-profit hospitals as examples of the methods they use to avoid duplication by referring out patients requiring costly services—a longtime goal of those who would reform the health care system. Although the poor reputation of the small physician-owned, proprietary hospitals of the past was often well deserved, the new investor-owned hospital corporations are concerned about how the community views their institutions. A slightly higher proportion of for-profit hospitals are accredited by the Joint Commission on Accreditation of Hospitals (JCAH) than comparable-sized nonprofit hospitals. It seems appropriate to conclude that the implications of the recent growth of investor-owned hospitals are still unclear. A report by the Institute of Medicine (47) has remarked that the current debate about for-profit health care is fueled as much by values as by evidence. Perhaps the greatest challenge is to determine how for-profit and nonprofit hospitals can effectively and successfully coexist in a future that holds challenges for both of them. It is likely, however, that the increasingly competitive health care environment will make the relationship between the two quite strained.

NONPROFIT HOSPITALS

Fifty-eight percent of the nation's short-term hospitals are nonprofit or voluntary institutions owned and operated by community associations or religious organizations. These hospitals accommodate more than two-thirds of all short-term hospital admissions and outpatient visits (Table 6-1).

COMMUNITY HOSPITALS

Taken together, nonfederal short-term hospitals, whether for-profit, nonprofit, or public, are commonly referred to as "community hospitals" because they are typically available to the entire community and meet most of the public's needs for hospital services. Community hospitals represent more than 80 percent of the nation's hospitals. They provide care for more than 90 percent of all patients admitted to hospitals each year and accommodate 79 percent of all outpatient visits. In 1985 there were 5784 short-term community hospitals with about 1,000,000 beds (Table 6-1). The average length of stay in these hospitals is 7.1 days, down from 8.4 days in 1967 and 1968, shortly after Medicare and Medicaid went into effect. The steady decline in length of stay since then is due to changing styles of medical practice, the emphasis placed on utilization review in hospitals, and the shift to prospective per case reimbursement by Medicare.

The major role of community hospitals is to provide short-term inpatient care for patients with acute illnesses and injuries. However, their outpatient role has been growing in importance and accounted for 14 percent of gross hospital revenues in 1985. In that year there were 74,547,000 emergency room visits and 144,169,000 outpatient department visits and ancillary service visits by patients referred to departments such as laboratory, x-ray, or physical therapy for diagnostic or therapeutic procedures. Taken together, these three types of outpatient visit totaled 218,716,000 or 6.5 outpatient visits for every inpatient admission and represented a 3 percent increase over 1984 (10).

Community hospitals are experiencing pressures to expand their roles even more to become true community health systems (3,4). The fundamental rationale is that these hospitals represent their community's collective investment in health resources, assembled in one place and financially supported by all. Hence, access to these resources should not be limited to patients who happen to need inpatient hospitalization. More recently, diversification has also been undertaken for competitive and economic reasons.

Community hospitals are seeking to play a more central and substantial role in planning and coordinating the entire range of community health services. For a variety of reasons in the past, including a lack of physician interest, health insurance coverage biases, poor reimbursement for out-of-hospital services, the small size of the average community hospital, and resistance by nursing homes and other community health agencies to hospital encroachment, hospitals were slow to expand their roles. Now, however, the traditional role of the hospital as provider of inpatient care is changing rapidly. Many hospitals, especially the larger institutions, have added services in areas such as ambulatory care, which indicate a movement in the direction of a broadening role (Table 6-3). It appears that the persistent rise in the public's use of community hospitals has finally peaked, motivating many hospitals to search for new diversified services they might offer. Perhaps this development, more than the underlying rationale, will finally give impetus to the several-decades-old concept of the hospital as a community health center (48).

One-half of all community hospitals have fewer than 100 beds; in 1985 the average size was 174 beds (10). Small hospitals tend to care for less seriously ill patients than do larger hospitals. Their average length of stay is shorter and their care less intensive and less specialized. Small hospitals cannot support as broad a range of services as can larger hospitals and find it difficult to keep abreast with developments in medical technology. They also cannot support the range of management specialists found in larger hospitals (49). Several hundred smaller hospitals have closed since the early 1970s. During the 6-year period between 1980 and 1985, a total of 340 hospitals with 49,085 beds closed in the United States (50). Of these, 214 were community hospitals and all but 9 had less than 200 beds. An even greater number of small community hospitals have become part of multiunit hospital systems. In fact, the rapid growth of multihospital systems, both for-profit and nonprofit, is one of the most significant trends in the hospital field today.

MULTIHOSPITAL SYSTEMS

A total of 268 multihospital systems, defined as corporations that own, lease, or manage two or more acute care hospitals, accounted for 2477, or 43 percent, of the nation's community hospitals in 1985 (38). These 2477 system hospitals contain 364,837, or 36 percent, of the nation's community hospital beds. Of the 268 multihospital systems, 91, or 34 percent, are Catholic; 20, or 7 percent, have other religious affiliations; 105, or 39 percent, are secular nonprofit; and 52, or 19 percent, are investor owned (Table 6-4). Although they represent only 19 percent of the nation's multihospital systems, the investor-owned systems tend to be large, averaging 23 hospitals and 2110 beds per system, compared to only 6 hospitals and 1287 beds per nonprofit system. As a result, investor-owned systems contain 49 percent of all system hospitals, representing 35 percent of all system beds (38).

Multihospital systems are growing at a rate of about 5–7 percent more hospitals and 3–4 percent more beds each year. Growth rates of this magnitude add up quickly. It is projected that more than half of the nation's community hospitals, representing about 40 percent of the acute beds, will be part of multihospital systems by 1990 (51).

Two fundamental motives seem to underlie the multihospital system movement that is so dramatically changing the character of the hospital sector—organizational survival and organizational growth. Survival applies to the free-standing, single-ownership institution and explains why such a hospital decides to relinquish its autonomy and become part of a system. Organizational growth, on the other hand, applies to the system itself and explains why it seeks to build, buy, lease, or manage additional hospitals. For the single institution, today's increasingly complex, fast-changing, demanding, and even hostile health care environment has made survival of the fittest a stark reality. Competition, financial pressures, regulation, and other external forces so weaken or threaten many solo institutions that they turn to systems for the strength to survive, albeit under different ownership. For the established systems, acquisition of additional hospitals is a means to grow—to add new services, enter new markets, establish new referral patterns, or build more financial and political power (51–54).

Another associated trend is the recent proliferation of hospital alliances, which are defined as formally organized groups of hospitals or hospital systems that have come together for specific purposes, have specific membership criteria, and are controlled by independent and autonomous member institutions. In 1985 there were 13 hospital alliances ranging in size from 5- to 571-member institutions (38). Hospital alliances differ from multihospital systems in that they are generally voluntary affiliations of hospitals that have joined together to reap the benefits of joint activities such as group purchasing and shared product development, without relinquishing their independent identity and autonomy. Alliances lack the corporate control found in multihospital systems.

PATTERNS OF FINANCING AND OWNERSHIP

Patterns of hospital financing and ownership differ from country to country. Most countries recognize health care as an essential service in which government should have a major role. In Great Britain and many other industrialized nations, government owns and operates most of the hospitals and employs the physicians who work in them. In other countries, the government limits its role to financing care provided by private hospitals and private practitioners, but in countries such as Canada, where comprehensive national health insurance is in effect, hospitals operate primarily on public funds and hence are essentially controlled by the government even though many are not government owned. In the United States, by contrast, government's role has been generally limited to financing care for needy groups such as the aged, the poor, and the disabled. This role has grown, however, to the point where hospitals now receive 54

TABLE 6-3. Trends in Selected Hospital Facilities and Services (Community Hospitals), United States, 1960, 1985

Facility or Service	*Percent of Hospitals with Facility or Providing Service*		
	1960	*1985*	*1985*
		All hospitals	300–400-bed hospitals
Ambulatory care			
Emergency service	91	85	91
Outpatient department	54	55	73
Outpatient hemodialysis	NA[a]	25	63
Outpatient psychiatry	NA	21	37
Outpatient rehabilitation	NA	38	70
Outpatient volume	(70,700,000 visits) (2.9 visits/admission) (1962)	(218,716,000 visits) (6.5 visits/admission)	
Inpatient care			
Intensive care unit (all)	10	9	24
Neonatal care unit	NA	4	10
Pediatric care unit	NA	24	64
Cardiac care unit	NA	72	91
Mixed/other	NA	1	1
Self-care unit	3		
Home care program	3	27	39
Long-term care and rehabilitation			
Physical therapy	41	87	98
Occupational therapy	9	48	84
Skilled nursing care unit	NA	14	13
Inpatient rehabilitation unit	7 (1962)	8	22
Outpatient rehabilitation unit	NA	38	70

176

Mental Health care			
Inpatient unit	11	23	53
Outpatient unit	NA	21	37
Partial hospitalization program	NA	14	23
Emergency services	NA	36	62
Foster and/or home care	NA	4	6
Consultation and education	NA	33	59
Clinical psychologist	NA	39	62
Other			
Hospice	NA	12	23
Dental	27	53	75
Social work	15	84	99
Family planning	2 (1962)	13	25
Abortion service	NA	22	39
Alcohol/drug dependency	NA	20	34
Speech pathology	NA	47	75
Health promotion	NA	52	76
CT scanners	NA	49	62
Open heart surgery	NA	11	31

SOURCE: *Hospital Statistics.* Chicago, American Hospital Association, 1986.

[a]NA—not available, not applicable, or none.

TABLE 6-4. Hospitals and Beds in Multihospital Systems by Type of Ownership and Control, 1980 and 1985 (as a Percentage of All Systems in Parentheses)

Ownership Control	Number of Systems			Hospitals and Beds in Systems[a]						
	1980	1985	Percent Change 1980–1985	1980		1985		Percent Change 1980–1985		
				H	B	H	B	H	B	
Catholic Church related	124 (46.4)	91 (34.0)	−26.6	533 (29.7)	139,767 (40.9)	553 (22.3)	138,944 (32.4)	+3.8	−0.6	
Other church related	20 (7.5)	20 (7.5)	0	137 (7.6)	20,590 (6.1)	145 (5.9)	28,758 (6.7)	+5.8	+39.7	
Other not-for-profit	88 (33.0)	105 (39.2)	+19.3	426 (23.7)	91,356 (26.7)	571 (23.1)	110,339 (25.7)	+34.0	+20.8	
Investor owned	35 (13.1)	52 (19.4)	+48.6	701 (39.0)	89,635 (26.3)	1,208 (48.8)	151,326 (35.2)	+72.3	+68.8	
All systems	267 (100)	268 (100)	+0.4	1797 (100)	341,382 (100)	2,477 (100)	429,367 (100)	+37.8	+25.8	

SOURCES: Adapted from *Data Book on Multihospital Systems* 1980–1981, American Hospital Association, 1981 and the *The Director of Multihospital Systems, MultiState Alliances and Networks*, 7th ed., American Hospital Association, 1986.

[a]Includes hospitals (H) and beds (B) owned, leased, sponsored, or managed by multihospital systems.

percent of their income from government sources (primarily Medicare and Medicaid). The rest comes from private health insurance (36 percent), direct payments by patients (9 percent), and philanthropy (1 percent) (1). In short, the United States has a pluralistic public–private financing system with largely privately owned hospitals. However, as the portion of hospital income financed by government has increased (from about 25 percent in 1960 to 54 percent today), so has the amount of regulation.

The limited role of government in the ownership of hospitals in the United States has been shaped by four major forces. First, the government was still relatively weak in the 1800s, when the short-term hospital as it exists today was evolving as a result of advances in medical science. Innovations and progress generally came from the private sector. At that time, poverty was not so severe (or was not perceived as so severe) that the needy could not be cared for through charity and philanthropy in private hospitals. It was generally believed that the private sector could provide care for the poor as well as for those who could pay. The exception was in major cities with large concentrations of the poor. There, public hospitals were established to care for the needy.

Second, government responsibility for the public's health was viewed narrowly before the Depression of the 1930s and was limited mainly to public safety (i.e., protecting healthy citizens from persons with communicable diseases and mental illnesses); to providing care for special groups such as merchant seamen, military personnel, and veterans; and to assisting the needy. State government operated hospitals for its beneficiary groups, and city and county governments in large urban areas operated hospitals for the poor.

Third, our strong tradition of reliance on the private sector means that government becomes involved only when the private sector clearly fails to provide a critical service. For example, chronic disease, mental, and tubuerculosis hospital care would have been difficult to finance privately. The long stays that previously prevailed would have been expensive and not readily insurable. Hospitalization generally meant loss of one's job and income, especially since the incidence of hospitalization for these conditions was greatest among the poor. As a result, these areas of care have traditionally fallen to the public sector. The private sector proved better able to finance short-term hospital care through direct payments and private health insurance, and so the government's role has been supplementary. For example, the government helped to finance the construction of hospitals thorugh the Hill-Burton program beginning in 1946 and finance care for the groups that could not afford to pay, primarily the aged and the poor.

Fourth, government involvement has been resisted by the medical profession. Physicians represent a particularly powerful group in the United States and have long been concerned that government involvement in the health care system would compromise their economic and professional interests (55).

INTERNAL ORGANIZATION OF COMMUNITY HOSPITALS

From the outside, a community hospital appears as one organization with a clear goal of providing high-quality patient care to which the efforts of the professional and technical groups working there are devoted. However, from the inside, it is apparent that there are at least two different organizations with two distinct sets of goals: the administrative organization, which is responsible for the efficient management and operation of the institution as a whole; and the medical staff organization, which is responsible for the patient care provided by individual physicians.

Furthermore, there are three loci of authority within a hospital—the governing board, the medical staff, and the administration—and much balancing goes on between them (56,57). Each authority group has a distinct responsibility. The board is ultimately responsible for everything that goes on in the hospital, both administrative and professional. It oversees the operation of the hospital and carries out its responsibility by (1) adopting policies and plans to guide the hospital's operation; (2) selecting and delegating responsibility for the day-to-day management of the hospital administrator and supervising that person's performance; and (3) appointing physicians to the medical staff, approving the medical staff's organization for governing itself and for supervising the professional activities of its members, and delegating responsibility to the medical staff for the provision of high-quality patient care (58–60).

In practice, the three areas of authority are neither so clear nor so distinct. For example, it might seem that there is a clear distinction between governance and the medical staff's responsibility for patient care. Court decisions have made it clear, however, that the hospital as an institution has a corporate responsibility or legal liability for ensuring that patients receive high-quality patient care. Therefore, the governing board must make sure that only qualified physicians practice in the hospital and that quality review mechanisms are established and working (61). However, only the medical staff has the expertise to assess the qualifications and care provided by physicians. Although the medical staff is clearly subordinate to the governing board in terms of authority for the affairs of the institution, physicians are independent of strict control by the board because the board does not share their expert knowledge and special skill.

Employees of the hospital working in clinical areas often find themselves in the middle when physicians' actions conflict with hospital policy. Legally, they should follow hospital policy; however, professionally they are expected to follow the physicians' orders regarding patient care, and their day-to-day working relationships are with the medical staff. A substantial degree of physician independence from the hospital exists because most are in private practice and not employed by the institution. On the other hand, physicians must have access to a hospital to practice modern medicine, and only the governing board has the power to grant them the privilege of practicing there. This unique relationship between physicians and hospitals is not without stresses and strains, and it makes the governance and management of hospitals a challenging responsibility (62,63).

The distinction between adopting policies to guide hospital operations and managing operations on a day-to-day basis is not always clear, either. Problems arise when the governing board becomes involved in administrative matters, such as acting directly on employee grievances that come to their attention rather than referring them to the administrator. On the other hand, the administrator may make decisions that go beyond board policies. Thus the community hospital is not a united front, but rather an organization with at least two separate lines of authority—administrative and medical—and with some ambiguity between what is governance and what is management. Power at the top is shared, both because the board depends on the expertise of the medical staff and because of the independent contractor status of physicians. Administrators have also become very influential because of their expertise in dealing with the increasingly complex operational and regulatory issues confronting hospitals (64). Since the internal powers do not always agree among themselves on priorities and programs, hospitals often experience internal tensions and find it difficult to respond in a systematic way to environmental conditions and changing community needs.

THE GOVERNING BOARD

The governing board of the community hospital has evolved in function and structure as the hospital itself has developed new roles. During the late 1800s and early 1900s, when advances in medical science were transforming hospitals from custodial institutions for the sick poor to sources of effective and safe care for the entire community, board members were mostly wealthy benefactors who made substantial donations to establish and equip the hospital and meet its deficits. The primary function of the board at that time was trusteeship, that is, preserving the assets that they and others like them donated. The trustees' job was seen as providing the facilities and equipment the medical staff needed to care for their patients. There was little trustee involvement in medical matters. The administrator was essentially a clerk, and administrative duties were divided among the board members (11).

After World War I, the complexity and size of hospitals grew to the point where board members could no longer administer and financially support the hospital. Business managers were hired to handle administrative and financial matters; the business manager, along with the superintendent of nurses, reported to the board, and the board coordinated work between the two. As the complexity of the hospital and the competence of managers increased, the business manager gradually assumed responsibility for overseeing nursing and all other departments as well, so that only one person reported directly to the board. The manager's title became "superintendent." The board of trustees moved into an oversight role, relinquishing day-to-day management matters to the superintendent (65).

The governing board's role changed further as hospitals continued to grow, as management decisions took on greater complexity and significance, and as philanthropy yielded to patient revenue as the primary source of financial support. The board's role became one of overall policymaking and planning, and board membership was used to augment and supplement the skills of the administrative staff. Boards began to be composed of fewer philanthropists and more individuals with specific management skills, such as business executives, attorneys, bankers, architects, and contractors (65,66). Even so, community hospital boards remained relatively closed to external scrutiny, with their membership consisting essentially of self-perpetuating groups of community influentials (67–69). Board decisions were mostly in the areas of finance, personnel, and physical plant and their areas of expertise, and boards typically deferred to the medical staff on medical and patient care matters, delegating fully the responsibility for the qualifications and quality of care provided by the medical staff.

During the 1960s four major factors caused further changes in the governing board's role: (1) continuing advances in medical science, the proliferation of medical technology, and the rapid growth in the size and sophistication of hospitals gave rise to public concern about the cost of hospital care, while making even more central in the delivery of health care and valuable to the public; (2) public expectations regarding the hospital's responsibility to the community changed, so that hospitals began to be viewed as community resources with a definite obligation to respond to community needs; (3) regulation of hospital construction, costs, quality, and use, as well as labor relations, became more and more stringent, particularly following the establishment of Medicare and Medicaid; and (4) court decisions established the concept of corporate or institutional responsibility for ensuring the quality of patient care (62,70,71).

As a result of these forces, the governing board's role broadened and became even more demanding (72,73). Boards grew active in environmental surveillance, becoming knowledgeable about community concerns and external trends and interpreting their significance for the hospital (74,75). External pressures forced hospitals to reexamine their priorities and programs, and boards found it necessary to provide clearer direction and stronger leadership in long-range planning. Boards have also assumed an active role in seeing that community concerns and interests are brought into hospital decision making, and many have expanded community representation within their membership (76). The board has found itself in the role of balancing and mediating between the demands and pressures on the hospital from the community and external agencies, on one hand, and from the medical staff, employees, and other internal groups, on the other hand (59). Finally, boards have been forced to take a more active role in quality control, rather than abdicating this responsibility to the medical staff. Although the function of quality monitoring is still delegated to the medical staff, the board is now being held accountable for how well this function is carried out. The board is responsible for ensuring that the mechanisms for evaluating the credentials of physicians and monitoring the care they provide are established and working. Courts have held the board and the hospital responsible in malpractice cases in which reasonable precautions were not taken to ensure (1) careful selection of the medical staff; (2) establishment of high standards of care; (3) monitoring and supervision of care; and (4) enforcement of policies, rules, and regulations. In practice, board control over medical staff performance remains limited and depends more on the commitment of the medical staff, the character of hospital–medical staff relations, and moral sanctions than on formal sanctions such as suspending or terminating a physician's privileges, an action that is very rare.

As governing boards became more actively involved in medical and patient care matters, in both determining the hospital's role and relationships with other institutions and overseeing quality assurance mechanisms, physicians began to seek more involvement in hospital planning and policymaking. At the same time, boards felt a greater need for more direct physician participation in their deliberations to address issues related to quality, medical staff privileges, and changing medical technology and practice patterns (77,78). As a result, an increasing number of boards have added physicians to their membership. More than half of all community hospital boards now include physicians (79,80). Less frequent but emerging is the tendency of the administrator to serve on the board, generally with a change in title to "president" or "executive vice president," in a corporate type of structure (75).

A new issue for the hospital field concerns the structure and functions of governance within multiple hospital systems. Three models for structuring governance in multiple hospital systems have been described (81,82). In the parent holding company model, governing bodies exist at both the system and institutional levels. Some systems have adopted a variation of the parent holding company model in which there is a system-level governing board, but boards at the institutional level serve in only an advisory capacity. The responsibilities of the advisory boards are generally limited to community relations and monitoring quality of care (83). The third or corporate model occurs when only a system-level governing board exists to carry out all the governance activities of a multihospital system. A recent study of 159 multihospital systems revealed that 41 percent used the parent holding company model, 22 percent the modified parent holding company model, and 23 percent the corporate model (82). This study also revealed that regardless of the governance model, corporate-level boards are likely to retain responsibility for decisions regarding the transfer or sale of assets, the formation of new companies, purchase of assets greater than $100,000, changes in hospital by-laws, and appointment of local board members. For other activities, the governance model affects the locus of decision-making authority. In general, the more decentralized the governance model, the more likely it is that activities such as service development, strategic planning, capital and operating budget approval, medical staff privileges, and appointment and evaluation of the hospital chief executive officer will be under the authority of the local board. A major agenda item for future research on governance of multihospital systems pertains to the relationship between governance structure and operational efficiency and effectiveness. The corporate model has the advantage of structural simplicity and clear lines of authority while holding company models provide for greater input and involvement at the community level. Further examination of the advantages and disadvantages of these approaches to system-level governance will become more important as hospitals grow both horizontally and vertically in the future.

Today, governing boards are being challenged and scrutinized as never before. They are being called on to demonstrate their effectiveness in ensuring that the hospitals they govern meet community needs and provide high-quality care while at the same time function efficiently within a complex structure of guidelines and regulations, all in an environment of constant change. Not all boards are capable of performing this task. Boards have been criticized as too inward-looking, passive, uninformed, reluctant to become involved in medical matters, and unwilling to change the status quo. Recent legal decisions have found hospital board members personally liable for making hasty, ill-informed decisions (84). It appears, however, that the pressures discussed above are causing boards to take active steps to broaden and strengthen their membership, educate themselves more fully, and streamline their structure so that they will be better equipped to provide the strong leadership that will be required in the future (85–87).

HOSPITAL ADMINISTRATION

Hospital administration has grown in importance and status as hospitals have grown in size and sophistication (65,88,89). The job of implementing board policy and responsibility for the day-to-day management and supervision of the hospital is delegated by the board to the hospital administrator. The administrator has responsibility for managing the hospital's finances, acquiring and maintaining equipment and facilities, hiring and supervising hospital personnel, and coordinating hospital activities. The breadth of the administrator's responsibility is illustrated by a typical community hospital organization chart (Fig. 6-2). A key aspect of the administrator's job is to coordinate and serve as the channel of communication among the governing board, medical staff, and hospital departments. Another is strategic planning for the future development of the hospital's services. Large hospitals have several assistant administrators who are responsible for nursing, professional services, support services, and hospital finance.

In addition to financial, personnel, and physical plant matters, administration plays

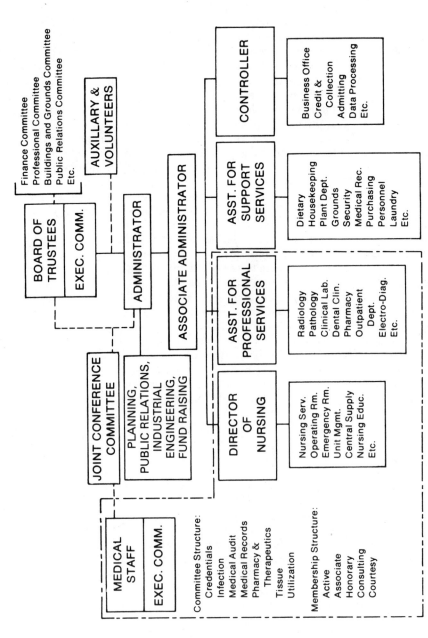

Figure 6-2. Prototypical hospital organization chart. (SOURCE: Reprinted with permission from Chamber of Commerce of the United States, *A Primer for Hospital Trustees*, Washington DC, 1974.)

184

an important role in patient care. For example, administration is responsible for coordinating the patient care departments with each other and with the support departments, ensuring that they are adequately equipped and staffed and technically up to date, and ensuring that they function smoothly. Administration must make sure that physician orders for the treatment of patients are carried out correctly and promptly by hospital personnel and also that orders do not conflict with governing board policies or hospital rules. The administrator is also actively involved in planning for new patient care services and in ensuring that the hospital meets accreditation, licensure, and other standards. Because the medical staff is not employed by the hospital, the administrator must establish a cooperative working relationship with the members in order to effectively handle the many tasks that involve both administration and medical questions. Finally, the administration acts as the liaison with the community and with external agencies, both bringing information from these sources into hospital decision making and planning and representing the hospital to these outside parties. Because of the increasing impact of external and regulatory pressures on hospitals, this boundary-spanning role has become one of the most important aspects of the administrator's job.

Hospital administration has advanced rapidly as a profession. Schulz and Johnson (90) describe the transition as moving from business manager (1920s–1940s), to coordinator (1950s–1960s), and now to corporate chief (with full authority for directing all aspects of the hospital's operation) and management team leader (promoting participative decision making by board, medical staff, nursing staff, and administrative representatives). Administrators are now full participants in the development of policies and plans, as well as in their implementation and in the external and internal affairs of the hospital (91,92). It has been suggested that in order to survive the challenges encountered by hospitals in the current competitive environment, the successful administrator must develop new skills and priorities, including the ability to innovate, value-based management, concern for patient satisfaction, and a willingness to accept entrepreneurial risk (93,94).

HOSPITAL MEDICAL STAFF

The governing board delegates responsibility for the provision of high-quality patient care to the medical staff, which is formally organized to carry out this responsibility and is accountable for it to the board (95). Unlike many advanced countries, where hospital medical staffs are composed of salaried physicians, the medical staffs of community hospitals in the United States are composed mostly of private practitioners who are not employees of the hospital. The relationship between the hospital and its medical staff is a mutually dependent and sometimes stressful one. The hospital is dependent on the medical staff to admit and care for patients and monitor the quality of patient care. In a sense, the clients of the hospital are the physicians, since it is they who admit patients, decide how long the patients will stay, and order hospital services. On the other hand, physicians are dependent on hospitals because, in order to practice modern medicine, they must have access to the diagnostic and therapeutic services of the hospital. This is particularly true of specialties such as obstetrics and surgery. Thus a quid pro quo relationship exists; physicians agree to abide by hospital policies and medical staff rules and to devote time to the medical staff's quality monitoring activities (in the past, they also contributed time to care for patients who could not pay), in return for the privilege of using the community's hospital to care for their private patients (96–98).

Different categories of appointment to the medical staff carry different privileges and responsibilities (99):

Active medical staff have full hospital privileges and provide most of the medical care in the hospital. They are responsible for the administrative activities of the organized medical staff. They can vote, hold office, and serve on committees.

Associate medical staff may consist of physicians and dentists who are being considered for advancement to the active medical staff. The period to be served in the associate medical staff status is defined in the medical staff bylaws. At the end of this period, frequently 1–2 years, the associate member is considered for advancement through the mechanism established in the bylaws.

Courtesy medical staff is composed of physicians who are eligible for active membership on the staff but who admit patients to the hospital only occasionally (usually because they are on the active staff of another hospital). They are not involved in any administrative functions.

Consulting medical staff includes physicians and dentists who are recognized for their professional expertise and who are willing to act as consultants to the hospital's medical staff, although they practice primarily in other hospitals.

Honorary staff consists of physicians or dentists who are recognized for their noteworthy contributions and/or outstanding service to the hospital. Honorary status is often attained at a certain age as defined in the medical staff bylaws.

Provisional status are initial appointments to the medical staff, except honorary and consulting, that are provisioned for a period of time designated in the medical staff bylaws. If at the end of the provisional period an individual has not satisfied the requirements for staff eligibility, provisional status automatically terminates.

House staff are interns and residents who form the house staff of a hospital. They function under the supervision of attending physicians but are employees of the hospital.

In carrying out its delegated responsibility for ensuring the quality of care, the medical staff governs itself, establishes qualifications for appointment to the staff and for clinical privileges, establishes standards of care and rules and regulations to guide the provision of care, and supervises the professional performance of its members. These duties are accomplished within the medical staff bylaws, which set forth the form, functions, and responsibilities of the medical staff. The bylaws must be approved by both the medical staff and the governing board (99–101).

The administrative head of the medical staff organization is the president or chief of staff. The chief of staff is responsible for (1) acting as a liaison between the governing board, the administrator, and the medical staff; (2) chairing the executive committee of the medical staff and serving as an ex-officio member of all committees and usually of the governing board; (3) establishing medical staff committees and appointing their members; (4) enforcing governing board policies; (5) enforcing medical staff bylaws, rules, and regulations; (6) maintaining standards of medical care in the hospital; and (7) providing for continuing education for the medical staff.

Although the chief of staff is usually elected by the medical staff for a 1 - or 2-year term, this position is also in a sense part of the hospital's administrative structure, directly accountable to the hospital's governing board. As such, the chief of staff is consulted by the board for advice on medical matters, as well as for assurance that the medical staff's responsibilities are being carried out. Administration of medical staff affairs can be a time-consuming job, but in most community hospitals the chief of staff fills this role in addition to pursuing a busy private medical practice. Larger hospitals often hire a full-time salaried medical director to carry out many of the administrative duties of the chief of staff; this trend is spreading although not without controversy (102).

Most of the organizational responsibilities of the medical staff are carried out by committees (99,103). The "executive committee" is the key administrative and policymaking body of the medical staff. It governs the activities of the medical staff, and all other committees are advisory to it. It is composed of the chief of staff, the chiefs of the clinical departments, and members at large elected by the active medical staff. The "joint conference committee" is the formal liaison between the governing board and medical staff and includes members from both groups plus the administrator. This committee is a forum for discussing medicoadministrative matters of mutual concern. The "credentials committee" reviews the qualifications of applicants to the medical staff and makes recommendations regarding appointments, annual reappointments, and clinical privileges. Recommendations are transmitted through the executive committee of the hospital's governing board, which has final decision-making authority regarding medical staff membership and privileges.

A second type of medical staff committee adivses or oversees specific functional areas or departments; examples include emergency room, nursing, pharmacy, special care, and disaster committees. A third type of committee is the evaluative or quality assurance committee responsible for monitoring the patient care provided by individual physicians. These include medical audit, utilization review, and tissue committees. Finally, a continuing education committee plans education programs for the medical staff. In larger hospitals, most of these committee functions are duplicated in each clinical department.

There is a small but growing body of empirical evidence in support of the presumption that the structure of the medical staff affects quality and other aspects of hospital performance (103–107). Roemer and Friedman (103) studied the extent to which the degree of structure of the medical staff influences the costliness, quality, and scope of hospital services and found that a relationship does exist. They concluded that a fairly highly structured medical staff organization functions better than a low or moderate structure. They found that effectiveness is enhanced by a core of full-time salaried physicians within the medical staff; a comprehensive department and committee structure; clearly specified policies, rules, and regulations; and thorough documentation of medical staff activities. This type of organization pattern offers the private physicians who use the hospital the benefits of full-time hospital-based physicians who provide administrative support and supervision and take the leadership in developing standards of care and educational programs. An interesting finding is that a core of full-time salaried physicians tends to stimulate the other physicians to take their quality monitoring responsibilities more seriously. The mix of both salaried and private practice physicians tends to provide an environment conducive for change and improvement. Another study (107) concluded that physician participation in hospital decision making was the single most important variable associated with lower patient mortality for acute myocardial infarction and that active physician participation in hospital wide decision-making bodies is strongly associated with overall quality of care.

It is apparent that hospitals are moving slowly, but surely, and not without conflict, toward more highly structured forms of medical staff organization that can be held more directly accountable for quality. At the same time, medical staff officers are being asked to participate more actively in governing board and management decision making. Recent shifts in reimbursement toward prospective payment methodologies have significantly changed the financial incentives for hospitals. To a greater extent than ever before, hospitals now must assure that hospital admissions are justifiable, that length of stay does not exceed accepted norms, and that treatment regimens are medically appropriate. The reality is, however, that much of the care provided to patients in hospitals is under the control of physicians. As a result, hospitals are faced with the formidable task of attempting to change physician practice patterns. Possible methods of changing physician behavior include education, peer review and feedback, administrative changes, participation in hospital activities, and penalties and rewards (108). It is clear that the need for hospitals to exercise greater control or influence over physician behavior represents a significant threat to physicians' traditional autonomy and may result in increased tension and conflict between hospital administration and medical staffs. Methods used by hospitals to influence physician behavior to achieve greater cost containment include direct appeals for assistance, joint ventures, limits on physician privileges, and employment of physicians (109). While direct appeals are the least threatening to physician autonomy and employment is the most threatening, all of these approaches are likely to be adopted by some hospitals in the future. There has been particular interest most recently in joint venture arrangements in which hospitals share the risks and benefits of new activities such as technology acquisition or clinic development with members of their medical staff. Joint ventures also provide a means of fostering hospital–physician bonding in an era of stress and competition. Clearly, the hospital–physician relationship of the future will be different than in the past.

TRENDS AND ISSUES IN THE HOSPITAL INDUSTRY

The high and persistently climbing cost of hospital care, combined with increasing disenchantment with regulatory efforts to reduce health costs, has led to a new emphasis on marketplace competition for hospitals. Although the overall annual rate of inflation for hospitals has declined from a high point of nearly 15 percent in 1982, health care costs in general and hospital costs in particular continue to increase at a rate far in excess of the Consumer Price Index (CPI). The obvious conclusions is that while inflationary pressures have been controlled for the general economy, hospitals have not been as successful in containing their costs. There are several reasons for this, including prior commitments to expensive building and construction projects by many hospitals, the growing role of sophisticated technology and computers in hospital care, the power of unions, and the hospital's limited ability to control the practice patterns of physicians. As a result of their continuing high costs, hospitals tend to be the prime target of the cost containment efforts of both public and private payors.

The mid-1980s have witnessed dramatic changes in hospital utilization patterns—changes strongly influenced by the introduction of prospective payment methodologies by Medicare and tremendous growth in managed health care plans such as HMOs and

PPOs. Average hospital occupancy rates declined by 13 percent between 1983 and 1985 (10). Lower occupancy has led to a widespread perception that hospitals are a mature, if not declining, industry. Declining occupancy combined with pressure to contain costs has resulted in a new competitive mind-set for hospitals that are actively pursuing diversification strategies, product-line management, marketing, and advertising. The long-term effects of this competitive approach to health care delivery continue to be debated with many deeply concerned about the impact it may have on hospitals' public service commitment to the poor.

These trends present special problems for small and rural hospitals whose difficulties in attracting resources, keeping up to date with advances in medical technology, and maintaining financial viability raise questions about their future survival and how they should relate to larger institutions offering the specialized services that they are not able to provide. Another challenge for hospitals concerns ethical issues, including those related to termination of life support services, nutrition and hydration for terminally ill patients, care for unsponsored patients, and allocation of resources to expensive and contested medical procedures such as artificial heart transplantation. These trends, their impact on hospitals, and the issues they raise are discussed in this section.

HOSPITAL COST CONTAINMENT

The nation's health expenditures have been increasing dramatically, with hospital spending leading the way. On a per capita basis, hospital expenditures increased from $50 per person in 1960 to $675 per person in 1985. This $675 was double the per capita spending for physicians' services, more than five times what was spent for nursing home care, and more than six times what was spent for drugs or dental services. Because the cost of hospital care has been increasing so much faster than other elements of health care, hospitals are consuming a larger and larger share of the nation's health expenditures. About 39 percent of our health expenditures now go for hospital care, compared to about 33 percent in 1960 (1).

In 1975, $39 billion was spent for care in community hospitals. By 1985, this figure had reached $130 billion, a 333 percent increase in 10 years. This increase occurred even though overall utilization of inpatient hospital services in 1985 (33,449 million admissions) was almost exactly the same as in 1975 (33,435 million admissions) (10). This leveling off of hospital admissions was a direct result of efforts to shift more care from an inpatient to an outpatient setting. Hospital admissions reached their lowest point in 10 years in 1985, although the overall population of the United States increased by 22 million from 1975 to 1985. Thus it is clear that the continuing high rate of inflation in hospital costs cannot be explained by increases in utilization. Instead, hospital cost increases are more likely attributable to changes in the nature of hospital output (i.e., in the intensity, scope, sophistication, and quality of hospital care) — which, in turn, cause hospitals to employ more and better labor inputs (accounting for 55 percent of all community hospital expenditures in 1985) and more and better nonlabor inputs.

Hospital services are continuously increasing in intensity, scope, and sophistication as a result of advances in medical science and community and physician demands for the widest possible range of the most up-to-date services. As a result, the cost per inpatient day increased over 15 times between 1960 and 1985, from about $30 per day to $460 per day. The average hospital stay now costs more than $3,000 (10).

Regarding intensity, patients today receive more laboratory, x-ray, and other diagnostic and therapeutic services than do patients treated for the same conditions a few years ago (23,110). Several factors have contributed to the increased intensity. Advances in medical science have made more diagnostic and therapeutic procedures available, and both patients and physicians want to take advantage of all that modern medicine has to offer. The nature of physician training in sophisticated hospitals may lead them to order more procedures. Another factor is the fear of malpractice suits, which leads to defensive medical practice. Physicians are inclined to order the extra laboratory tests or x-ray procedure "just to make sure." The shortening length of stay has resulted in patients receiving more services each day than if the same services were spread over a longer period of time. Many experts believe that a major factor is that physicians are not directly affected financially by the costs of the services they order on behalf of their patients. A most important factor again is hospital insurance, which has led patients to want the best of care regardless of costs. Only recently have insurance companies begun to implement tough utilization review protocols for hospital admissions and ancillary service use.

Regarding the broadening scope of services offered by community hospitals, advances in medical science have created new diagnostic and treatment technology not dreamed of a few years ago. Fetal monitoring, diagnostic radioisotope procedures, computed tomography, magnetic resonance imaging, lithotripsy, open heart surgery, organ transplants, laser and microscope surgery, radiation therapy, renal dialysis, and other complicated procedures require expensive equipment, expensive facilities, and skilled personnel. Communities and physicians alike have come to expect a wide range of services to be available in their local hospitals. As a result, there has been an increase in the scope and sophistication of services being offered by even relatively small community hospitals serving limited populations.

The increased investment by hospitals in equipment and facilities is reflected by a substantial increase in assets per bed. In 1960, the capital investment per bed in community hospitals was about $17,000. This figure is now well over $100,000. Expenditures for equipment, facilities, and supplies have been increasing faster than expenditures for personnel. As a result, nonpayroll expenses as a portion of total expenses increased from 38 percent in 1960 to 45 percent in 1985. However, the use of personnel has increased as well, from 2.3 employees per patient in 1960 to 3.9 in 1985, an increase of more than 70 percent. It is interesting to note that hospital full-time equivalent personnel (FTEs) have not declined as rapidly as patient admissions. From 1984 to 1985, admissions declined 4.9 percent, while FTEs decreased by only 0.7 percent. In addition, the skill levels of hospital personnel have increased, and more hospitals are employing physicians. The average hospital salary increased by 622 percent between 1960 and 1985, from $3239 to $20,139 (10).

Another cost increasing factor is debt financing of capital projects. In the past, hospital construction projects were financed mostly by community fund-raising drives, philanthropy, and government programs such as Hill-Burton. As these sources of capital declined in importance, hospitals have been forced to borrow a larger proportion of the funds needed for capital projects, adding interest expense to the cost of these projects (111).

A final and increasingly significant factor is the administrative cost of complying with regulations. Programs now exist to regulate hospital construction, rates, reimbursement, quality, use, plant safety, and labor relations, to name only a few. The array of complex and often conflicting requirements hospitals must comply with contributes substantially to increased costs. The current situation is approaching the point where the solution is becoming part of the problem: hospitals must spend money to comply with regulations, which adds to the costs that regulations are designed to control. As a result, there has been a marked shift away from regulatory controls over health care providers in favor of a competitive marketplace approach to cost containment. In 1986 the federal government terminated funding for the nation's health systems agencies (HSAs), the major source of regulatory review for hospital construction, services, and equipment, and it is expected that many states will follow the lead of California in all but abandoning certificate-of-need (CON) requirements for hospital services.

The prices hospitals charge private pay patients have increased even faster than total costs because of the difference between what hospitals charge to meet their full financial needs and what Medicare and Medicaid actually pay. These allowances, or discounts, along with the charity care and bad debts that hospitals incur but Medicare and Medicaid do not reimburse, are passed on to private pay patients and their insurance carriers in the form of higher prices. This "cost shifting" explains why hospital charges or prices have been increasing at a considerably faster rate than hospital costs. Private insurance carriers in recent years, however, have taken steps to limit the amount of cost shifting they have traditionally absorbed. Seizing the initiative inherent in PPOs, carriers have begun to initiate selective contracts with hospitals that grant them discounts or preferred rates. Individuals insured under such plans are given financial incentives for using the "preferred" hospitals. The hospitals are caught in a "catch-22" position, either they offer carriers discounted rates or face lower patient volume. Since hospital admissions have been declining, most hospitals are willing to compete for patients through competitive bidding on selective contracts. This is a dangerous scenario for many hospitals that could produce financial crisis in the future.

Clearly, the problem of hospital cost inflation is complex, and complex problems call for multifaceted solutions. It would seem that any solution must first encourage prudent hospital use consistent with good medical practice. There is empirical evidence that perhaps as many as one-fourth of all patient days provided by hospitals between 1974 and 1982 were not medically necessary (25). The public's use of hospitals may be constrained by building higher copayment and deductible provisions into health insurance policies and limiting benefits, although the arguments against shifting more of the economic burden to the consumer are many. Other strategies include (1) attempting to counterbalance the physicians' inclination to use the hospital by changing their financial incentives and developing more managed care plans such as HMOs and PPOs; (2) attempting to strengthen external review of the appropriateness of hospital use through public and private utilization review organizations; (3) encouraging the development of more ambulatory care, day care, home care, skilled and intermediate nursing care, and other out-of-hospital care programs and improving insurance coverage for them; and (4) interjecting greater marketplace competition into purchase of hospital services.

The question of how to deal with the increasing complexity and intensity of hospital care is equally difficult. It is physicians, not hospitals, who decide what diagnostic and therapeutic services to order for patients. Hence, changes in physician incentives and training must be part of the solution (109). Again, HMOs would seem to provide an appropriate set of incentives in this regard. Another approach would be to control malpractice insurance premiums and pressures that apparently cause physicians to practice defensive medicine. Finally, the financial incentives inherent in hospital reimbursement can be modified, as in the case with prospective payment, so as to discourage overuse of services.

Both public and private purchasers of health care services have recognized that prospective payment schemes as opposed to cost-based reimbursement introduce powerful incentives for health care providers to contain costs. The single most significant change in health care financing in the United States occurred when the Tax Equity and Fiscal Responsibility Act of 1982 (PL 97-248) established Medicare per case payment rates for hospitals based on 468 diagnosis-related groups (DRGs). Under this payment system hospitals are reimbursed a flat fee for the entire episode of hospitalization of a patient in a given DRG, regardless of the actual costs incurred in the care of that patient. DRG rates have moved from a blend of hospital-specific costs and national averages toward a national average over several years. If a hospital treats a patient for less than the DRG payment rate, it may retain the difference. If a patient requires more resources than allotted by the DRG, the hospital must absorb the loss. Adaptation to this new payment system has important implications for hospital organization and management including greater emphasis on efficient staffing, greater attention to discharge planning, and movement toward vertical integration (112).

HOSPITAL RESPONSES TO COMPETITION AND PROSPECTIVE PAYMENT

Hospitals are actively adapting to the new competitive environment. Prospective payment and price competition create a strong incentive for hospitals to achieve efficient staffing levels since labor represents approximately 55 percent of the average hospital's costs. It has even been suggested that by 1990, successful hospitals will have reduced their FTEs by 20–25 percent (20). Hospitals are looking at ways to utilize nurses more efficiently (113), considering substitution of licensed practical nurses for registered nurses or aides for practical nurses in some cases, or moving to an all R.N. staff in other instances. Hospitals are also attempting to increase productivity standards for hospital employees and investigating opportunities to cross-train employees to fill multiple positions. Unfortunately, this emphasis on cost containment and productivity is likely to create new conflicts between hospital administration and unions that are attempting to upgrade the professional status and salaries of their members.

Hospitals are also investigating other methods of increasing their profitability, including product-line management. The practice of analyzing hospital programs and services as strategic business units (SBUs) in order to identify and enhance profitable services and turnaround or eliminate unprofitable services is being advocated by many as a more businesslike approach to hospital management (114). The concern is that some hospitals may discontinue unprofitable services that are needed by the community. Many argue that defining health care as a commodity and rationing it based on ability to pay is unacceptable if our society holds that health care is a basic right (115). Still, a positive aspect of product-line management is the development and organization of services to meet the special needs of certain segments of the population. Examples include women's health centers and sports medicine clinics. It can be argued that competition is forcing hospitals to be much more sensitive to the needs and desires of people for convenient, specially tailored services.

Under the Medicare per case prospective payment system there is also a strong incentive for hospitals to discharge patients as soon as medically warranted; therefore, Medicare prospective payment has done a great deal to foster the effectiveness of discharge planning. The role of the discharge planner is critical in assuring that patients receive proper care after leaving the hospital. For elderly patients in particular, rapid rehospitalization may result unless proper discharge instructions and support services are received (116). In many instances the elderly patient cannot be discharged from the hospital until placement in a nursing home is secured or arrangements are made for home care. The necessity of assuring that patients receive proper postdischarge treatment has heightened the interest of many hospitals in operating their own skilled nursing units and home care programs. One major concern of the Medicare program and its Professional Review Organizations (PROs) is that hospitals may be discharging patients too soon in some instances. Hospitals are under great pressure to deliver exactly the right amount of care to Medicare patients since too much care may result in reimbursement denials and too little care can result in penalty assessments or lawsuits. As a result, hospitals are placing more emphasis on complete documentation of patient treatment records.

Vertical Integration

The increasing stringent economic environment has also spurred the interest of hospitals in vertical integration. Vertical integration represents a response by hospitals to capture and control more of the factors that lead to inpatient hospitalization. The ultimate goals of vertical integration include (1) increasing a hospital's market and financial position, (2) enhancing the hospital's overall cost effectiveness; (3) improving continuity of care, and (4) responding to changing consumer preferences. Vertical integration in a health enterprise involves linking together different levels of care and assembling the human resources needed to render that care. Vertical integration may be distinguished from diversification efforts in that vertical integration involves the development of new nonhospital services to support and enhance the hospital base while diversification involves the development of distinct new business lines that are independent from the hospital and have profit as their primary objective (117). Vertical integration has historically proceeded in two directions. As industrial firms integrated forward (toward the ultimate consumer of the firm's product), they either bought out the distributors of their goods or created their own distribution systems to bring their products to market. As they integrated backward (toward the supply of raw materials), they purchased either raw materials or the primary producers of the goods needed to manufacture their products (4).

Backward integration involves all of the activities in which a firm engages to secure an adequate supply of the raw materials needed to produce its particular product. In the health care setting, the product is a human service, patient care; therefore, backward integration involves the equipment, supplies, and human resources required to care for patients. The most critically scarce resources of a hospital are its professionals: physicians, nurses, technicians, and other health personnel. Efforts to secure adequate supplies of these individuals are essential to a health care provider's ability to function. Many hospitals have developed linkages with educational institutions, providing a source of new recruits by serving as training sites. Some hospitals have considered integrating backward into medical supplies and other goods needed to operate; however, these organizations may be entering very competitive markets dominated by large firms.

Since the hospital is the most highly organized form of production of health services, efforts by the hospital to provide those forms of care rendered to the patient prior to hospitalization can be considered forward integration—reaching out toward the patient. A major form of forward integration for a hospital involves development of ambulatory care systems. In health care a distribution or "feeder" system is that set of pathways which result in bringing the patient to the hospital. The feeder system of a hospital includes all of those settings in which the potential patient receives ambulatory services, or diagnosis, as well as the transportation systems and physician referral relationships that ultimately lead to hospitalization (4). The principal feeder system for most hospitals is a network of private physician offices and group practices. One way hospitals have moved to integrate physician practices is by providing office space on the hospital campus, assisting new physicians in starting practices, and helping to market physician services. Physician practice support services, such as office training, management, billing, and referral services, are also activities that build a feeder system and further develop forward integration.

Many hospitals have recognized the importance of a feeder system in building the name recognition of the facility and promoting patient accessibility. As a result, hospitals are engaging in more marketing and advertising activities that increase the visibility of their institutions including direct-mail advertising, use of billboards, and broadcasting on radio and television. There are three channels through which advertising may assist hospitals in increasing their market share: (1) hospitals may influence the choice of patients who are admitted through emergency departments or outpatient clinics; (2) patients may influence the choice of physicians with admitting privileges at multiple institutions; and (3) patients may actually choose a physician affiliated with a particular hospital, especially if they use a hospital referral service (118).

Vertical integration has particular significance for hospitals because it gives them the potential to package a broad range of health care services at a competitive price. There are distinct advantages to such integration if economies of scale result, and the hospital is able to control a broad range of referral services. Vertical integration focuses on hospitals being in the business of health rather than being oriented almost exclusively toward acute care services.

Vertical integration strategies for hospitals experiencing declines in census include several options (119). First, underutilized acute inpatient facilities can be converted to long-term care, substance abuse, mental health, or other services. Second, hospitals can focus on developing a coordinated and integrated delivery system whereby local residents can obtain most health care services through the programs, services, and facilities managed by one hospital. Third, many institutions have developed physicians' office buildings and ambulatory surgery, diagnostic, and primary care centers through joint ventures with their medical staff in order to improve their market penetration. Fourth, hospitals that are able to contract directly with HMOs, PPOs, third-party payors, and major corporate interests to provide a full range of preacute, acute, and postacute care services at a highly competitive price will place themselves in an excellent market position.

To date, there is relatively little empirical research that assesses the impact of vertical integration on hospital performance. There is one recent study that suggests hospital development of primary care group practice has a positive effect on hospital utilization and market share (120). During a 4-year period (1976–1982), hospitals that sponsored such group practices experienced a 9.0 percent increase in patient days, an 8.2 percent increase in admissions and an average increase in market share for patient days and admissions of 4.9 percent and 3.6 percent, respectively.

Despite these advantages, the movement toward vertical integration by hospitals may be slowed in the future because of difficulties such as a loss of institutional identity and autonomy, fear of domination by the larger players in the integrated system, uncertainty of roles within an umbrella corporation, and possible imbalances in political power at the governing board, medical staff, or management level (119). Furthermore, vertical integration presents additional problems for hospitals related to controlling the flow of patients between components of a coordinated system, acquiring the requisite expertise to manage new ventures, and maintaining traditional values and character. In order to remain viable and successful, individual institutions must examine the concept of vertical integration further and attempt to apply the knowledge attained in the business world to the health care industry.

Patient Satisfaction

As a result of growing competition, the satisfaction of hospital patients has become more salient to hospital administration in recent years. In the past, hospitals concentrated on satisfying members of their medical staffs in order to increase their market share, but now more attention is being given to the patient and patient preferences for care. Many suggest that hospitals should adopt a more market-oriented approach to providing services that actively considers the opinions and preferences of patients (121,122). In response, many hospitals have begun to routinely administer patient satisfaction surveys while others have initiated guest relations programs based on techniques used in hotels and other consumer-oriented service organizations. In many respects it is rather surprising that hospitals have paid so little attention to patient satisfaction in the past, particularly since in any other service situation the need to satisfy the customer is a foregone conclusion (123). It has been noted that the hospital environment can be very unpleasant and that patients are often fraught with apprehension and anxiety (124,125). Furthermore, negative aspects of hospital care have been linked with poor compliance with medical treatment protocols and even delayed physical recovery (126,127). Thus it is desirable to identify, and within reasonable limits, alter those factors that contribute to negative experiences within the hospital. Evaluation of patient satisfaction provides important information on the patients' perception of the quality of medical care and allows the patient as a consumer to have a greater voice in the design and delivery of health services.

SMALL AND RURAL HOSPITALS

In part because Hill-Burton priorities in the early years channeled funds to thinly populated rural areas, the United States is a nation of many small hospitals: about one-half of all community hospitals have fewer than 100 beds. These hospitals face a number of problems that threaten their future viability. First, they are losing patients. Admissions to community hospitals with fewer than 100 beds have declined, as has their average daily census (Table 6-5). Between 1975 and 1985, the number of community hospitals with fewer than 100 beds fell from 2,935 to 2,589 or almost 12 percent (10). Labor requirements are high in small hospitals for the services offered, and small hospitals tend to operate at less efficient levels of occupancy than larger hospitals (Table 6-6). These efficiency limitations, coupled with the limited financial means of some rural populations, have caused many small hospitals to incur substantial operating losses. Small hospitals offer a more limited range of services than larger institutions, because they have neither the patient volume nor the physicians or specialized personnel to support much beyond the basic essential services. Small hospitals are often located in areas where they have a difficult time attracting qualified personnel. Furthermore, the federal government's decision to adopt separate wage scales for urban and rural institutions under the Medicare prospective pricing system resulted in rural hospitals receiving about 20 percent less reimbursement than their urban counterparts (128). Together, these problems may lead to difficulty in achieving accreditation, and in meeting hospital certification and licensure standards, or may even threaten survival.

TABLE 6-5. Change in Average Daily Census by Hospital Size, United States, 1980–1985

Bed Size	Average Daily Census		Percent Change
	1980	1985	
6–24	2,308	1,400	−39
25–49	19,806	14,738	−26
50–99	67,630	52,643	−22
100–199	137,774	119,284	−13
200–299	133,391	118,290	−11
300–399	111,144	103,979	− 6
400–499	95,559	74,741	−22
≥500	179,254	165,817	− 9

SOURCE: *Hospital Statistics.* Chicago, American Hospital Association, 1986.

TABLE 6-6. Selected Indicators by Hospital Size, United States, 1985

Hospital Bed Size	Full-Time Equivalent Personnel per 100 Census	Percent Occupancy
6–24	429	37.4
25–49	393	42.9
50–99	342	55.0
100–199	344	61.9
200–299	369	61.8
300–399	369	70.2
400–499	407	72.5
·≥500	427	79.4

SOURCE: *Hospital Statistics.* Chicago, American Hospital Association, 1986.

Small hospitals also find it especially difficult to keep up with and respond to the increasingly complex and demanding regulatory environment without the range of management specialists common to larger institutions, and as a result, many are contracting with hospital systems or larger hospitals to take over their management (36). It would appear that the future viability of small hospitals will depend on adapting their mission and the services they offer to fit available resources, establishing relationships with other institutions, and seeking additional resources to support new programs to broaden their role in health care delivery in the communities they serve (129–131).

Because it is especially difficult for smaller hospitals to assemble the array of equipment and personnel or attain the patient volume needed to support a broad range of services, it is critical to consolidate around the small hospital to the greatest extent possible whatever health resources do exist in the community. Ideally, the hospital building or campus might include physicians' offices, facilities for public health nurses and health-related community organizations, a nursing home, and so forth. Consolidation would enable limited health resources to be stretched further and provide opportunities for jointly supporting personnel such as a home care nurse, laboratory technician, or physician assistant. The hospital need not own all of these facilities; merely grouping the community's health-related activities together would be an important step.

The key to the future of smaller rural hospitals still seems to lie in the concept of regionalization or networking, the much discussed but little implemented idea of formally relating small hospitals with larger urban hospitals (132–135). Regionalization begins with the concept that each level of hospital—small basic service hospitals, moderate-size community hospitals, and large regional referral center—should provide only those services that they can offer efficiently and at a high level of quality. Communities would be ensured access to a full range of services, not by each hospital attempting to provide every service, but rather by the development of closer relationships among networks of hospitals and their medical staffs to encourage the referral of patients to the institutional setting most appropriate to their needs. Such relationships could range from informal agreements to formal affiliations, jointly provided programs, or mergers of institutions into multihospital systems.

The specific objectives of regionalization include (1) a two-way flow of patients, with patients referred to larger hospitals for specialized services and returned to smaller hospitals for convalescent care, long-term care, follow-up care, and home care; (2) continuing education for physicians, nurses, and other personnel from the small hospitals through participation in the educational programs of the larger hospital; (3) assistance from administrative, nursing, and professional department heads and specialists from the larger hospital representing skills not available in the small hospitals; (4) consolidation (in the larger hospital) and sharing of services the small hospitals cannot provide as efficiently or at the same level of quality as larger hospitals; (5) regularly scheduled visits by physician specialists from the larger hospitals to conduct clinics and serve as consultants in the small hospitals; (6) sharing of personnel; and (7) joint purchasing (135).

The success of regionalization depends on the support of the community, the governing board, and the medical staffs of both the small and larger hospitals. There are few examples of effective regional relationships. In part, this situation reflects community and professional pride and a desire for independence. It also partially reflects the difficulty of working out the essential elements of regionalization: (1) the movement of referrals in both directions so that the small hospitals do not lose patients but maintain their census by providing basic, convalescent, and follow-up care; (2) reforming reimbursement to recognize a different distribution of patients among large and small hospitals; (3) granting physicians from the small hospitals privileges in the larger hospital and making them feel welcome to admit and treat their patients there when they need the specialized services of the larger hospital; and (4) broadening the role of the small hospital to include convalescent and follow-up care, long-term care, home care, and so forth. In the long run, regionalization may preserve rather than threaten the independence and viability of smaller hospitals.

UNIONIZATION OF HOSPITAL PERSONNEL

The number of health care unions has increased steadily in recent years, rising by 6 percent between 1980 and 1985 and bringing union representation to about 20 percent of all workers in health care institutions (136). This has occurred even through union representation in all industries dropped from 23 percent to 18 percent during the same period. These trends reflect both aggressive pursuit of white-collar service industries by labor unions and current upheavals in the health care field because of cost containment pressures (137). Prospective payment, downsizing and mergers have created new tensions for health care workers; as a result, their values are shifting such that they regard unions more favorably than in the past. Major issues for nurses and other hospital employees include job security, quality standards, and staffing levels as well as wages. Perhaps the most revealing change in the attitudes of health professionals toward unionization is the growing movement to establish collective bargaining capability for the house staff physicians in hospitals. California and the industrialized Eastern states have the greatest number of unionized hospitals, and unionization is most common in metropolitan areas. In addition, there tend to be more unionized hospitals in states that had labor laws before 1974.

When Congress began to consider bringing hospitals under Taft-Hartley, hospitals pressed for special protection against strikes, priority for National Labor Relations Board action on disputes, and mandatory mediation requirements. Hospitals also wanted to limit the number of bargaining units, with one each for professional, technical, clinical, and maintenance and service workers (138). In 1974 hospitals became subject to Taft-Hartley, but with special provisions. A hospital or union must give 90 days' notice to the other party of a desire to change an existing contract. The Federal Mediation and Conciliation Service (FMCS) must be given 60 days' notice, and 30 days' notice if an impasse occurs in bargaining for an initial contract after the union is first recognized. A cooling-off period of at least 10 days is required before a strike can occur to enable the hospital to plan for the care of patients. The FMCS may appoint a board of inquiry to mediate among the parties if it determines that a strike would impair delivery of health care to the community. Neither the hospital nor the union are required to accept the board's recommendation, although they must provide information and witnesses called for by the board (139).

With the exemption from Taft-Hartley removed, several factors have rendered the hospital industry more vulnerable to unionization. First, many hospitals lag behind industry in personnel practices. A substantial number have no professional personnel director, and policies for resolving grievances, discipline, promotion, seniority, overtime, and night-shift work are often poorly spelled out. Wages and fringe benefits in hospitals also appear to have lagged behind those of other industries.

Second, supervisory training is often insufficient. Department heads and supervisors are commonly promoted because of their professional or technical skills rather than their managerial or supervisory capabilities. In addition, supervisors and professional department heads may have divided loyalties between being part of hospital management, on one hand and members of professional associations that act as unions on the other hand.

Third, the reluctance of professional workers to unionize has diminished. The change in attitude is attributable, in part, to the fact that their professional associations act as their unions. Professional associations are more acceptable than national trade unions. In addition, the professional associations point to collective bargaining not only as a means of improving wages but also as a way to negotiate over staffing standards and work prerogatives that could affect the quality of patient care. The underlying issue of the balance between administrative and professional control regarding work and the work setting is especially important in institutions such as hospitals and adds a unique dimension to unionization in this industry. Also unique is the fear that a strike could cause harm to patients (140,141).

REGULATION OF HOSPITALS

In spite of the recent promotion of marketplace competition for health care providers, hospitals remain a highly regulated industry. External regulation of hospitals has grown rapidly since the mid-1960s. There are external controls over (1) institutional quality standards (licensure, certification, accreditation); (2) construction and expansion of facilities and services (Section 1122 of the 1972 Social Security Amendments, state certificate of need); (3) costs or rates (Blue Cross, Medicare, state rate regulation); and (4) use (Blue Cross, Medicare, Medicaid, PROs). Hospital regulations derive from both public agencies and private organizations. Many federal controls are tied to Medicare and Medicaid as conditions for participation or payment: certification, utilization review, and capital expenditure review, to name a few. The major private sector organizations that exert control over hospitals include Blue Cross plans and the Joint Commission on Accreditation of Hospitals (142). Regulations that most directly affect hospitals are discussed below.

Controls on Quality

The regulatory structure for controlling quality includes state licensure, federal certification, and voluntary accreditation (143–145). Licensure is a state function, generally carried out by the department of health, whereby minimum standards are established and enforced regarding the equipment, personnel, plant, and safety features an institution must have to operate. Licensing agencies are empowered to set standards, conduct inspections, issue licenses, close down facilities that cannot comply with the agency's standards, and provide consultation services. In many states, however, these agencies are underfinanced and understaffed; therefore, standards are not enforced stringently. In addition, there is a tendency to focus on fire, safety, and physical plant standards rather than standards for medical services.

Hospitals must be certified by the designated state agency in order to participate in Medicare and Medicaid. The purpose of certification is to ensure that care for beneficiaries of these programs is purchased only from institutions that can meet acceptable minimum quality requirements. In most states, the federal Department of

Health and Human Services (DHHS) contracts with the health department to carry out the actual inspection process. Virtually all community hospitals are certified, so it can only be concluded that the administration of this program is not very stringent.

Accreditation is a professionally sponsored, voluntary process carried out by the JCAH, a private organization formed in 1951 as a joint effort of the American College of Physicians, the American College of Surgeons, the American Hospital Association, and the American Medical Association. The JCAH establishes quality standards and surveys hospitals that choose to seek accreditation voluntarily. Standards relate to the structure and process aspects of quality, as well as outcome measures, and considerable emphasis is given to the organization of the medial staff. About three-fourths of the nation's community hospitals, and more than 95 percent of those with more than 200 beds, are accredited. Accreditation is designed to encourage institutions to maintain the highest possible levels of performance rather than just minimum standards. Accredited hospitals are deemed to meet DHHS's certification requirement. Although the relevance and rigor of the JCAH's standards and survey procedures are not above challenge, there is little question that from a historical perspective the JCAH has been a major force in elevating institutional standards.

Controls on Facilities and Services

Areawide hospital planning began with Hill-Burton in 1946 (146). States were required to define hospital service areas and inventory existing facilities, and identify the areas of greatest need as determined by bed:population ratios. Voluntary areawide planning was promoted by the American Hospital Association and the U.S. Public Health Service (PHS) beginning in 1959. In 1965, the Regional Medical Program was established to encourage regional planning in treatment of heart disease, cancer, and stroke. Federally sponsored health planning began in earnest in 1966 with the Comprehensive Health Planning Act. State planning agencies (A agencies) and areawide, private, nonprofit planning agencies (B agencies) were set up with federal aid to coordinate the development of health facilities and services and to discourage overbuilding and duplication. These agencies had little economic or political power, however, and no legal means of stopping capital projects, and it is generally agreed that few were effective (147).

The 1972 Social Security Amendments (Section 1122) added clout to facility and services regulation by authorizing denial of Medicare and Medicaid reimbursement for building and depreciation expenses for capital projects over $150,000 not approved by the designated state agency. Proposed projects were reviewed by area Comprehensive Health Planning (CHP) agencies, but approval powers remained with the state. There is some evidence that Section 1122 and state CON programs have contained the growth in beds but not in equipment and other capital investments (148). The National Health Planning and Resources Development Act of 1974 established a network of state and area planning agencies. This program linked federal funding more closely with state regulation and required states to establish certificate of need programs that require prior approval by state agencies of plans to build or modernize facilities or add new services (149). Findings of a study of certificate of need experience with computed tomographic scanners suggest that these programs have not been successful in either controlling the introduction of new technology or ensuring equitable distribution of equipment among hospitals (150). Evidence that CON review is costly, time-consuming, and only marginally effective in restraining hospital investments in new technologies and services led Congress to terminate funding for health planning beginning in 1986. Federal withdrawal from the health planning arena means that the fate of health planning agencies will now be a state issue. It is expected that many states will abandon CON review and rate regulation in favor of more competitive approaches to cost containment.

Cost Controls

Programs to control hospital costs or regulate hospital rates were introduced by federal and state agencies and by private third-party purchasers as a result of their concern over the rapid rise in their expenditures for hospital care (29). Public involvement in cost controls and rate regulation began in earnest after the rapid post-Medicare inflation in hospital costs in the late 1960s. Medicare had adopted cost-based reimbursement and, like Blue Cross, was directly affected by cost increases. Section 223 of the 1972 Social Security Amendments authorized Medicare to set upper limits on routine inpatient service costs for reimbursement purposes, and Section 1122 limited Medicare reimbursement for capital expenditures made without approval of the designated state planning agency.

The Economic Stabilization Program (ESP), which President Nixon imposed in 1971 to deal with economywide inflation, limited the amount by which hospitals could raise their rates from year to year. Hospitals were subject to ESP until 1974. It appears that this stringent program did slow rate increases and, to a lesser degree, cost increases during the 1971–1974 period, although costs soared dramatically as soon as the controls were removed. In the late 1970s, the Carter administration pushed without success for the reestablishment of federal cost and revenue controls for the hospital industry (151).

In addition to federal efforts, about a dozen states concerned with controlling their Medicaid expenditures have empowered state agencies or special public utility-type commissions to regulate hospital rates. In general, these agencies approve prospectively the rates hospitals may charge for their services based on budget review or formula methods for projecting hospital costs or financial needs for the coming year. Hospitals are then reimbursed at these rates rather than on the basis of the costs they actually incur. Thus hospitals are at risk to keep their costs below the prospectively set rates. Evidence regarding the effectiveness of state prospective rate-setting programs in containing costs is sparse but suggests that this strategy may have some potential. The critical question may well be whether this cost containment potential can be exploited with enough care and sensitivity so that the quality and financial viability of the hospital system are protected (152,153).

Recent federal cost containment efforts have been directed toward the Medicare program. Annual expenditures for Medicare increased from $3 billion in 1967 to $74.7 billion in 1985 and are projected to reach $99.1 billion by 1987 unless cost controls are added to the program (154). The Tax Equity and Fiscal Responsibility Act of 1982 established Medicare inpatient cost per case reimbursement limits based on DRGs. While prospective payment based on DRGs has been hailed by many as a new competitive approach to health care delivery, others suggest it is acutally a classic regulatory scheme (29). Within the hospital industry there is substantial controversy concerning the ability of DRGs to reflect true hospital costs since they do not adequately measure severity of illness or compensate for regional differences in costs or practice patterns (155). Since enactment of the Medicare prospective payment legislation, average length-of-stay and admission rates for Medicare patients have declined significantly. Hospitals have also acted to reduce staffing levels and overall expenses (156). Because prospective payment gives hospitals an incentive to provide less care, some have expressed concern regarding its possible effects on quality. From the hospital perspective there is also great concern regarding the inequities of a national payment rate and failure of DRG price increases to parallel increases in the cost of hospital operations. At this time Congress has not yet adopted a mechanism for incorporating capital costs into DRG payment rates, although a graduated system for including capital payments in prospective payment rates is anticipated in the near future. In spite of hospital complaints about the DRG system, a recent study of Medicare cost reports for 892 hospitals in nine states (Alaska, California, Connecticut, Florida, Illinois, Minnesota, Oregon, Texas, and Washington), found an average profit margin for Medicare services of 14.1 percent in 1984, although there is great controversy over the way Medicare-related costs were measured in this study (156). While hospital profits appear to be declining in subsequent years of the DRG program, it is clear that there will probably be extensive revisions and fine tuning of Medicare's prospective payment system in the years ahead to maximize its cost savings potential for the federal government.

Control of Utilization

The most recent form of regulation in the hospital industry is the attempt to control utilization (157–159). Medicare first required that hospitals and extended-care facilities establish utilization review programs as a condition for participation. Physician committees were to review the medical records of discharged Medicare patients to determine the necessity of the hospital care provided. This requirement was seen as a way to discourage inappropriate admissions and unnecessarily long lengths of stays and, hence, as a means of keeping Medicare and Medicaid expenditures down. However, utilization review raises a number of sensitive issues, because establishing standards and monitoring physician practices with regard to hospitals may be seen as infringing on professional judgment regarding patient care.

Building on the utilization review requirements, the 1972 Social Security Amendments established Professional Standards Review Organizations (PSROs) to strengthen the appropriate monitoring process. PSROs were established as non-profit organizations to review the quality and appropriateness of the care provided Medicare and Medicaid patients in all institutions under contract with DHHS. PSROs established standards of treatment against which utilization could be judged. Although the Reagan administration had originally targeted PSROs for extinction, the program was resurrected through the Tax Equity and Fiscal Responsibility Act of 1982, which requires implementation of Utilization and Quality Control Peer Review Organizations (PROs). PROs, which began operation in October 1983, are closely modeled after the original PSROs in terms of staffing and operational authority. One significant difference, however, is that the new PROs are private organizations and are capable of making utilization review contracts with the business community as well as Medicare and Medicaid.

Despite the widespread advocacy for greater competition in the hospital industry, a complex regulatory environment already exists. That environment is fragmented because a great number of individual regulatory programs have evolved as specific responses to specific problems. Attempts to coordinate and rationalize the multiplicity of regulatory programs to impact on the entire delivery system in a positive manner are relatively recent. Regulation has become expensive for hospitals as well, calling for more careful cost–benefit analysis of regulatory requirements. On the other hand, some argue that the forces currently giving rise to a much more competitive health care environment will make extensive regulation unnecessary.

ETHICAL ISSUES FOR HOSPITALS

Increasingly, hospital decision making is affected by administrative and biomedical ethical issues. Within the hospital setting these ethical concerns touch on a variety of administrative and patient care duties, including respect for patient privacy and confidentiality, informed consent, continuation of life support services to terminally ill patients, resource allocation decisions, and care for the poor (160). Many hospitals have constituted institutional ethics committees to provide ethical guidance on both clinical decision making and administrative problems. Because they are the focal point for the most complex applications of modern medicine, hospitals are naturally at the center of many of the most difficult and painful bioethical decisons of our generation. One of the most critical decisions relates to patient competency and the right to refuse treatment. While the right of competent patients to refuse medical care is well established, the desires of incompetent or comatose patients present a great ethical dilemma. Treatment decisions for terminally ill patients who are not able to express their own wishes are often shared among family members, legal guardians, and/or health care providers.

Understandably, health care providers are often reluctant to discontinue medical intervention because it violates their ethical commitment to sustaining life, and also because they fear legal repercussions. No less challenging is the ethical issue surrounding the definition of extraordinary or artificial medical intervention for the purpose of sustaining life. For example, medical and legal experts differ on the controversial issue of withdrawing nutrition and hydration supplied through artificial means to a dying patient (161). No less difficult are treatment decisions for severely handicapped newborns as illustrated by the federal government's "Baby Doe regulations," which attempted to establish procedures and guidelines for the care of such infants and to assure that they receive equal protection under the law (162). The challenge for hospitals is to assure that such decisions are made in a responsible manner, that family and physician viewpoints are exchanged, and that legal guidelines are understood and upheld. Frequently, it is the role of the hospital to serve as facilitator in the ethical decision-making process—a role that requires extreme sensitivity to the interests of all parties.

Current trends in health care, including the need to provide humane and respectful treatment for acquired immune deficiency syndrome (AIDs) patients, care for the growing elderly population, the health needs of unsponsored patients, and the application of new technological breakthroughs, particularly in the area of genetic engineering, will act to increase the hospital's central role in ethical decision making for health care in the years ahead. This challenge to provide compassionate, quality care that respects the privacy and dignity of all patients will be a critical focus for hospitals and their trustees.

REFERENCES

1. Waldo DR, Levit KR, Lazenby H: National health expenditures, 1985. *Health Care Financing Rev* 1986; 8:1–21.
2. Knowles J: The Hospital. *Sci Am 1973; 229:128–137.*
3. *Somers AR: Health Care in Transition: Directions for the Future.* Chicago, Hospital Research and Education Trust, 1971.
4. Goldsmith JC: *Can Hospitals Survive?* Homewood, IL, Dow Jones–Irwin, 1981.
5. Johnson EA, Johnson RL: *Hospitals Under Fire.* Rockville, MD, Aspen Systems Corp. 1986.
6. Schulz R, Johnson AC: *Management of Hospitals.* New York, McGraw-Hill, 1976, pp 33–36.
7. Shortell SM: Organization of hospital resources, in *Hospitals in the 1980s.* Chicago, American Hospital Association, 1977.
8. Burns, LA: A perspective on hospital ambulatory care, in Meshenberg KA, Burns LA (eds): *Hospital Ambulatory Care.* Chicago, American Hospital Association, 1983, pp 1–12.
9. Williams S, Shortell S, Dowling W, et al: Hospital sponsored primary care group practice: A developing modality of care. *Health Med Care Serv Rev* 1978; 1:1–13.
10. *Hospital Statistics.* Chicago, American Hospital Association, 1986.
11. MacEachern MT: *Hospital Organization and Management,* 3rd ed. Chicago, Physicians Record Company, 1957.
12. Rosenberg S: The hospital in America: A century's perspective, in *Medicine and Society.* Philadelphia, American Philosophical Society Library, publication 4, 1971.
13. Rosen G: The hospital—historical sociology of a community institution, in Freidson E (ed): *The Hospital in Modern Society.* New York, The Free Press, 1963, pp 1–36.
14. Corwin EH: *The American Hospital.* New York, Commonwealth Fund, 1946, pp 193–213.
15. Starr P: *The Social Transformation of American Medicine.* New York, Basic Books, 1982, pp 145–179.
16. Commission on Hospital Care: Expansion of hospitals, 1840–1900, in *Hospital Care in the United States.* Cambridge, MA, Commonwealth Fund, Harvard University Press, 1947, pp 454–526.
17. Davis K: The hospital's position in American Society, in Owen J (ed): *Modern Concepts in Hospital Administration.* Philadelphia, Saunders, 1962, pp 6–16.
18. Flexner A: *Medical Education in the United States and Canada,* Bulletin No. 4. New York, Carnegie Foundation for the Advancement of Teaching, 1910.
19. Berk AA, Chalmers TC: Cost and efficacy of the substitution of ambulatory for inpatient care. *New Engl J Med* 1981; 310:393–397.
20. Coile RC Jr: *The New Hospital: Future Strategies for a Changing Industry.* Rockville, MD, Aspen Publisher, 1986.
21. Somers AR: *Health Care in Transition: Directions for the Future.* Chicago, Hospital Research and Education Trust, 1971, pp 39–72.

22. Starr P: *The Social Transformation of American Medicine*. New York, Basic Books, 1982, pp 290–334.

23. Feldstein M: *The Rising Cost of Hospital Care*. Washington, DC, Information Resources Press, 1971.

24. *Trends Affecting the U.S. Health Care System*, DHEW publication (HRA) 76-14503. Bureau of Health Planning and Resource Development, Health Planning Information Service, 1976, pp 195–199.

25. Siu AL, Sonnenberg FA, Manning WG, et al: Inappropriate use of hospitals in a randomized trial of health insurance plans. *New Engl J Med* 1986; 315:1259–1266.

26. Davis K: Rising hospital costs: Possible causes and cures. *Bull NY Acad Med* 1972; 48:1354–1371.

27. McCarthy CM: Supply and demand and hospital cost inflation. *Med Care Rev* 1976; 33:923–948.

28. *Trends Affecting the U.S. Health Care System*, DHEW publication (HRA) 76-14503. Bureau of Health Planning and Resource Development, Health Planning Information Service, 1976, pp 124, 173–175.

29. Luft HS: Competition and regulation. *Med Care* 1985; 23:383–400.

30. Havighurst CC: Changing the locus of decision making in the health care sector. *J Health Politics, Policy and Law* 1986; 11:697–735.

31. Schulz R, Johnson AC: *Management of Hospitals*. New York, McGraw-Hill, 1976, pp 30–43.

32. Dumbaugh K, Bentkover J, Neuhauser D: Public hospitals: An evolution, in Levin A (ed): *Health Services: The Local Perspective, Proceedings of the Academy of Political Science*, Vol. 32. New York, The Academy, 1977, pp 148–158.

33. Ohsfeldt RL: Uncompensated medical services provided by physicians and hospitals. *Med Care* 1985; 23:1338–1344.

34. Alexander JA, Rundall TG: Public hospitals under contract management. *Med Care* 1985; 23:209–219.

35. Levin PJ: Public hospitals must adapt to changes in the delivery system. *Hospitals* 1977; 51:81–88.

36. *The Future of the Public General Hospital—An Agenda for Transition*. Report of the Commission on Public General Hospitals (R Nelson, chairman). Chicago, Hospital Education and Research Trust, 1978.

37. Stewart DA: The history and status of proprietary hospitals. *Blue Cross Reports*, Research Series 9, Chicago, Blue Cross Association, 1973.

38. Directory of Multihospital Systems, Multistate Alliances, and Networks. Chicago, American Hospital Association, 1986.

39. Annual survey of multihospital systems. *Mod Health Care* 1986; 16:49–193.

40. Kushman JE, Nuckton CF: Further evidence on the relative performance of proprietary and nonprofit hospitals. *Med Care* 1977; 15:189–204.

41. Relman AS: The new medical–industrial complex. *New Engl J Med* 1980; 303:963–970.

42. Relman AS: Selling to the for-profits: Undermining the mission. *Health Progr* 1985; 66:81–85.

43. Watt JA, Derzon RA, Renn SC, et al: The comparative economic performance of investor-owned chain and not-for-profit hospitals. *New Engl J Med* 1986; 314:89–96.

44. Lewin LS, Derzon RA, Maugulies R: Investor-owned and non-profits differ in economic performance. *Hospitals* 1981; 55:52–58.

45. Pattison RV, Katz HM: Investor-owned and non-for-profit hospitals: comparison based on California data. *New Engl J Med* 1983; 309:347–353.

46. Herzlinger RE, Krasker WS: Who profits from nonprofits? *Harvard Business Rev* 1987; 65:93–105.

47. Gray BH, McNerney WJ: For-profit enterprise in health care: The Institute of Medicine Study. *New Engl J Med* 1986; 314:1523–1528.

48. Somers AR: *Health Care in Transition: Directions for the Future.* Chicago, Hospital and Research and Education Trust, 1971, pp 99–126.

49. Spitzer WD: The small general hospital: Problems and solutions. *Milbank Mem Fund Quart* 1970; 48:413–477.

50. Mullner RM, McNeil D: Rural and urban hospital closures. *Health Affairs* 1986; 5:131–140.

51. Dowling WL: Multihospital systems—present status and future prospects. *Hosp Progr* 1983; 64:48–53.

52. Zuckerman HS: Multi-institutional systems: Promise and performances. *Inquiry* 1979; 16:291–314.

53. Brown M, McCool B (eds): *Multihospital Systems.* Germantown, MD, Aspen Systems Corp., 1981.

54. Ermann D, Gabel J: The changing face of American health care: Multihospital systems, emergency centers, and surgery centers. *Med Care* 1985; 23:401–420.

55. Starr P: *The Social Transformation of American Medicine.* New York, Basic Books, 1982, pp 79–144.

56. Coe R: *Sociology and Medicine.* New York, McGraw-Hill, 1970, pp 264–288.

57. Georgopoulos BA (ed): *Organizational Research in Hospitals.* Ann Arbor, University of Michigan Press, 1973.

58. Broehl WD: Policy formulation and implementation: The governing board, in Moss AB, Broehl WG, Guest RH (eds): *Hospital Policy Decisions: Process and Action.* New York, GP Putnam's Sons, 1966, pp 23–79.

59. Kovner AR: Hospital board members as policy-makers: Role priorities and qualifications. *Med Care* 1974; 12:971–982.

60. Melkonian D, Raichel T: Organization of a hospital. *Provider Rev Manual.* Chicago, Blue Cross Association, 1974, pp 18–50.

61. Southwick A: The hospital as an institution—expanding responsibilities change its relationship with the staff physician. *Calif West Law Rev* 1973; 9:429–467.

62. Perkins R: The physician's view of the hospital: A love–hate relationship. Parts 1 and 2. *Hosp Med Staff* 1975; 4:1–7; 1975; 4:10–14.

63. Scott WR: The medical staff and the hospital: An organizational perspective. *Hosp Med Staff* 1973; 1:33–38.

64. Perrow C: Goals and power structure: A historical care study, in Friedson E (ed): *The Hospital in Modern Society.* New York, The Free Press, 1963.

65. Johnson EL: Changing role of the hospital's chief executive officer. *Hosp Admin* 1970; 15:21–34.

66. Gilmore K, Wheeler J: A national profile of governing boards. *Hospitals* 1972; 46:105–108.

67. Blankenship LV, Elling RH: Organizational support and community power structure: The hospital. *J Health Hum Behav* 1962; 3:257–369.

68. Burling T, Lentz EM, Wilson RN: The board of trustees, in *The Give and Take in Hospitals*. New York, GP Putnam's Sons, 1956, pp 39–50.

69. Trends Affecting the U.S. Health Care System, DHEW publication (HRA) 76-14503. Bureau of Health Planning and Resource Development, Health Planning Information Service, 1976, pp 339–341.

70. *Darling vs. Charleston Community Memorial Hospital.* 33 Illinois, 2d. 236. 211 ME 2d. 253 (1965).

71. Springer E. The Darling case: Ten years later. *Hosp Med Staff* 1975; 4:1–7.

72. Shulz R, Johnson AC: *Management of Hospitals.* New York, McGraw-Hill, 1976, pp 47–67.

73. Willits RD: What boards of trustees do. *Trustee* 1974; 27:1–8.

74. Marmor T: Public accountability and consumerism, in *Hospitals in the 1980s.* Chicago, American Hospital Association, 1977, pp 189–202.

75. Pfeffer J: Size, composition and function of hospital boards of directors: A study of organization–environment linkage. *Adm Sci Quart* 1973; 18:349–364.

76. Cathcart HR: Including the community in hospital governance. *Hosp Progr* 1970; 51:72–76.

77. Guest R: The role of a doctor in institutional management, in Georgopoulos B (ed): *Organizational Research in Health Institutions,* Ann Arbor, University of Michigan Press, 1972.

78. Jorgensen CJ: Should doctors be on your board?, in Rakish JS, Darr K (eds): *Hospital Organization and Management.* New York, Spectrum Publications, 1978, pp 91–96.

79. Schulz R: Does staff representation equal active participation? *Hospitals* 1972; 46:31–35.

80. A profile of the hospital trustee. *Trustee* 1975; 28:21–23, 26.

81. Reynolds J, Stunden AE: The organization of not-for-profit hospital systems. *Health Care Management Rev* 1978; 3:23–36.

82. Morlock LL, Alexander JA: Models of governance in multihospital systems: Implications for hospital and system-level decision-making. *Med Care* 1986; 24:1118–1135.

83. Johnson RL: Boards are remodeled as hospitals merge. *Hospitals* 1980; 54:101–105.

84. Blues SM: New legal standards for trustee performance. *Health Progr* 1987; 68:60–63, 95.

85. Unbdenstuck RJ: Refinement of boards' role required. *Health Progr* 1987; 68:44–49.

86. Kovner A: Improving community hospital board performance. *Med Care* 1978; 16:79–89.

87. Prybil LD, Startweather DB: Current perspectives on hospital governance. *Hosp Health Serv Admin* 1976; 21:67–75.

88. Schulz R, Johnson AC: *Management of Hospitals.* New York, McGraw-Hill, 1976, pp 129–164.

89. Thompson J, Filerman G: Trends and developments in education for hospital administration. *Hosp Admin* 1967; 12:13–32.

90. Schulz R, Johnson AC: *Management of Hospitals.* New York, McGraw-Hill, 1976, pp 147–164.

91. Kovner A: The hospital administrator and organizational effectiveness, in Georgopoulos B (ed): *Organizational Research in Hospital Institutions.* Ann Arbor, University of Michigan Press, 1972, pp 355–376.

92. Kuhl IK: *The Executive Role in Health Services Delivery Organization.* Washington, DC, Association of University Program in Health Administration, 1977.

93. Brozovich JP, Shortell SM: How to create more humane and productive health care environments. *Health Care Management Rev* 1984; 9:43–53.

94. Coile RC, Jr., Pointer DD: The new age CEO. *Hospital Forum* (May–June) 1985; 28:39–41.

95. Williams KJ: Basic principles of medical staff organization. *Hosp Progr* 1970; 51:50–55.

96. Perkins R: The physician's view of the hospital: A love–hate relationship. Part 2. *Hosp Med Staff* 1975; 4:12.

97. Schulz R, Johnson AC: *Management of Hospitals.* New York, McGraw-Hill, 1976, pp 68–69.

98. Williams KJ: Medical staff issues—past and present. *Hosp Med Staff* 1972; 1:2–13.

99. *Accreditation Manual for Hospitals.* Chicago, Joint Commission on Accreditation of Hospitals, 1983, pp 89–104.

100. Blaes SM: Why and how should medical staff laws be revised? *Hospitals* 1973; 47:100–106.

101. Mills DH: Staffy bylaws: An internal code of conduct. *Hosp Med Staff* 1976; 5:7–9.

102. Harvey JD: The hospital medical director: an administrator's view, Rakish JS, Darr K (eds): in *Hospital Organization and Management,* Spectrum Publications, 1978, pp 132–136.

103. Roemer M, Friedman E: *Doctors in Hospitals.* Baltimore, Johns Hopkins University Press, 1971.

104. Shortell SM: Hospital medical staff organization: Structure, process and outcome. *Hosp Admin* 1974; 19:96–107.

105. Scott WR, Flood AB, Ewy W: Organizational determinants of services, quality, and cost of care in hospitals. *Milbank Mem Fund Quart* 1979; 57:234–264.

106. Shortell SM, Becker SW, Neuhauser D: The effects of management practices on hospital efficiency and quality of care, in Shortell SM, Brown M (eds): *Organizational Research in Hospitals.* Chicago, Blue Cross Association, 1976.

107. Shortell SM, LoGerfo JP: Hospital medical staff organization and quality of care: Results for myocardial infarction and appendectomy. *Med Care* 1981; 14:1041–1056.

108. Eisenberg J, Williams S: Cost containment and changing physicians' practice behavior. *JAMA* 1981; 246:2195–2201.

109. Glandon GL, Morrisey MA: Redefining the hospital-physician relationship under prospective payment. *Inquiry* 1986; 23:166–175.

110. *Trends Affecting the U.S. Health Care System.* DHEW publication (HRA) 76-14503. Bureau of health Planning and Resource Development, Health Planning Information Service, 1976, pp 162–181.

111. Grimmelman FJ: Are not-for-profit hospitals experiencing a revolution in capital sources? *Topics Health Care Financ* 1981; 7:45–55.

112. Newscomer R, Wood J, Sankar A: Medicare prospective payment: Anticipated effect on hospitals, other community agencies, and families. *J Health Politics, Policy and Law* 1985; 10:275–282.

113. Kovener RJ, Palmer M: Implementing the Medicare prospective pricing system. *Health Care Finan Mangement* 1983; 13:74–78.

114. Ruffner, JK: Product line management: How six healthcare institutions make it work. *Healthcare Forum* 1986; 29:11–14.

115. Nutter D: Access to care and the evolution of corporate, for-profit medicine. *New Engl J Med* 1984; 311:919.

116. Robinson BC, Barbaccia JC: Acute hospital discharge of older patients and extended control. *Home Health Care Serv Quart* 1982; 3:29–57.

117. Placella LE: Choosing a growth strategy: Diversification versus vertical integration. *Trustee* 1986; 39:26–28.

118. Folland ST: The effects of health care advertising. *J Health, Politics, Policy and Law* 1985; 10:329–345.

119. Weil TP: Vertical integration: The wave of the future? *Health Care Strategic Management* 1984; 4–11.

120. Wheeler JRC, Wickizer TM, Shortell SM: Hospital–physician vertical integration. *Hosp Health Serv Admin* 1986; 31:67–80.

121. Kotler P: *Marketing for Non-profit Organizations.* Englewood Cliffs, NJ, Prentice-Hall, Inc. 1975; pp 5–7.

122. Flexner WA, McLaughton CP, Littlefield JE: Discovering what the health consumer really wants. *Health Care Management Rev* 1977; 2:43–49.

123. MacStravic RS: Marketing health care: The manufacturing of satisfaction. *Health Marketing Quart* 1985; 3:157–170.

124. Taylor S: Hospital patient behavior: Reactance, helplessness or control? *J Soc Issues* 1975; 35:156–184.

125. Ben-Sira Z: The structure of a hospital's image. *Med Care* 1983; 21:943–954.

126. Wartman SA, Morlock LL, Malitz FE, et al: Patient understanding and satisfaction and predictors of compliance. *Med Care* 1983; 21:886–891.

127. Langer E, Janis I, Wolfer J: Reduction of psychological stress in surgical patients. *J Exp Soc Psychol* 1975; 11:155–165.

128. *Medicine and Health.* Washington, DC, McGraw-Hill, February 2, 1987; Vol. 41: p 2.

129. *Delivery of Health Care in Rural America.* Chicago, American Hospital Association, 1977, pp 38–61.

130. Murrin KL: Laying the groundwork: Issues facing rural primary care, in Bisbee GF Jr (ed): *Management of Rural Primary Care Concepts and Cases.* Chicago, The Hospital Research and Education Trust, 1982, pp 1–27.

131. Madison DL, Bernstein JD: Rural health care and the rural hospital, in Bryant J, Ginsberg A, Goldsmith B, et al (eds): *Community Hospitals and Primary Care.* Cambridge, MA, Ballinger, P 1976.

132. Phillips D: Reaching out to rural communities: Hospital's expanding role as a social agency, parts 1 and 2. *Hospitals* 1972; 46:33–38; 1972; 46:53–57.

133. Rannels HW, Ross DE, Waxman CR: The community hospital and regional health care responsibilities—how to do it! *Med Care* 1975; 13:885–896.

134. Grim SA: Win/Win: Urban and rural hospitals network for survival. *Hosp Health Serv Admin* 1986; 31:34–46.

135. McNerney WJ, Riedel D: *Regionalization and Rural Health Care,* Research Series 2. Ann Arbor, Bureau of Hospital Administration, University of Michigan, 1962.

136. McCormick B: Union activity on the rise, new AHA report states. *Hospitals* 1986; 60:73.

137. Schanie CF: Unionization and hospitals: Causes, effects, and preventive strategies. *Hosp Health Serv Admin* 1984; 29:68–78.

138. *Taft Hartley Amendments: Implications for the Health Care Field, Report of a Symposium.* Chicago, American Hospital Association, 1976.

139. Pointer D, Metzger N: *The National Labor Relations Act: A Guidebook for Health Care Facility Administrators.* New York, Spectrum Publications, 1975, pp 41–60.

140. Kilgor JG: Union organizing activity in the hospital industry. *Hosp Health Serv Admin* 1984; 29:79–90.

141. Wilmor IG: Management's viewpoint, in *Taft-Hartley Amendments: Implications for the Health Care Field.* Chicago, American Medical Association, 1976, pp 78–94.

142. Somers AR: *Hospital Regulation: The Dilemma of Public Policy.* Princeton, NJ, Princeton University, Industrial Relations Section, 1969.

143. Somers AR: *Health Care in Transition: Directions for the Future.* Chicago, Hospital Research and Education Trust, 1971, pp 101–131.

144. Schulz R, Johnson AC: *Management of Hospitals.* New York, McGraw-Hill, 1976, pp 185–201.

145. Schlicke CP: American surgery's noblest experiment: The story of hospital accreditation. *Arch Surg* 1973; 106:379–385.

146. Somers AR: *Health Care in Transition: Directions for the Future.* Chicago, Hospital Research and Education Trust, 1971, pp 132–161.

147. *Trends Affecting the U.S. Health Care System.* DHEW publication (HRA) 76-14503. Bureau of Health Planning and Resource Development, Health Planning Information Service, 1976, pp 91–109.

148. Salkever DS, Bice TW: Certificate-of-need legislation and hospital costs, in Zubkoff M, Raskin E, Hanft RS (eds): *Hospital Cost Containment: Selected Notes for Future Policy.* New York, Milbank Memorial Fund, 1978, pp 429–460.

149. Public Law 97-35. The Omnibus Budget Reconciliation Act of 1981. Washington, DC, U.S. Government Printing Office, 1981.

150. Pardini AP, Cohodes DR, Cohen AB: Certificate of need and high capital cost technology: The case of computerized axial tomographic scanners. Report to the Bureau of Health Planning, HRA, DHHS, HRA Contract 231-77-1004. Cambridge, MA: Urban Systems Research and Engineering, 1980.

151. Dunn W, Lefkowitz B: The hospital cost containment act of 1977: An analysis of the administration's proposal, in Zubkoff M, Raskin E, Hanft RS (eds): *Hospital Cost Containment: Selected Notes for Future Policy.* New York, Milbank Memorial Fund, 1978, pp 166–214.

152. Dowling, WL: Prospective rate-setting—concept and practice. *Topics Health Care Financ* 1976; 2:1–37.

153. Sloan F: Rate regulation for hospital cost control: Evidence from the last decade. *Milbank Mem Trust Quart* 1983; 61:195–217.

154. U.S. Senate, Special Committee on Aging, Health Care Expenditures for the Elderly: How much protection does Medicare provide? 97th Congress, Second Session. Washington, DC, U.S. Government Printing Office, April 1982.

155. Horn SD, Horn RA, Sharkey MS, et al: Severity of illness within DRGs: Homogeneity study. *Med Care* 1986; 24:225–235.

156. Iglehart JK: Early experiences with prospective payment of hospitals. *New Engl J Med* 1986; 314:1460–1464.

157. Chassin MR: The containment of hospital costs: A strategic assessment. *Med Care* 1978; 16(Suppl):27–35.

158. Goran MJ, Roberts JS, Kellogg M, et al: The PSRO hospital review system. *Med Care* 1975; 13(Suppl):1–33.

159. Congress of the United States, Congressional Budget Office. The impact of PSROs on health care costs: update of the Congressional Budget Office 1979 evaluation. Washington, DC, U.S. Government Printing Office, 1981.

160. Darr K, Longest BB Jr, Rakish JS: The ethical imperative in health services governance and management. *Hosp Health Serv Admin* 1986; 31:53–66.

161. Bresnohan JF, Drane JF: A challenge to examine the meaning of living and dying. *Health Progr* 1986; 67:32–37, 98.

162. Reiser SJ: Survival at what cost? Origins and effects of the modern controversy on treating severely handicapped newborns. *J Health Politics, Policy and Law* 1986; 11:199–214.

CHAPTER 7

The Continuum of Long-Term Care

Connie J. Evashwick

Long-term care is one of the greatest challenges facing the health care delivery system. In terms of population need, consumer demand, resource consumption, financing, and system organization, long-term care will be a dominant issue during the coming decades. In order for the limited resources available to meet increasing demand, the system that currently exists—an underfinanced disarray of fragmented services—must evolve into a well-organized, efficient, client-oriented continuum of care.

A case study illustrates the current issues and problems of long-term care.

> Mr. Jackson is a 61-year-old successful businessman who lives alone in a third-story suburban apartment. One night during the winter he slips on the ice while carrying groceries up the front steps of his building and breaks his hip. A neighbor calls the 911 emergency number, and eventually an ambulance arrives. The ambulance takes Mr. Jackson to the emergency room of the nearest hospital. Mr. Jackson cannot be admitted there because he does not have proof of insurance, credit cards, or even his checkbook on hand and his condition is determined not to be a life-threatening emergency. He is thus transferred to another hospital. Mr. Jackson's only physician is an internist who cannot handle a fracture, so Mr. Jackson is operated on by the surgeon on call.
>
> After the surgery, Mr. Jackson spends 4 weeks in the hospital, during which time he receives rehabilitation therapy. His insurance covers only the first 30 days of hospital care, so he is anxious to be discharged as quickly as possible. The physician recommends that Mr. Jackson go to a rehabilitation hospital. However, the nearest one is in the next town. Instead, Mr. Jackson agrees to spend a week or two at a nursing home until he is able to move about more easily. Mr. Jackson knows that he will be responsible for all payments, since there is no insurance for nursing home care, but he does not feel strong enough to go home alone. Mr. Jackson hates the nursing home because the staff are always irritable and hurried, and the pleasant ones seem to resign the day after he gets to know them. Most of the patients are quite elderly, and there is little spirit to encourage anyone to become more independent in hopes of going home.

At home, Mr. Jackson requires further recuperation before he is able to ambulate easily. He is not quite ill enough to qualify for home health care as defined by the regulations of his health insurance. Although technically not "home-bound," he nonetheless has no way to get down the stairs, let alone to the grocery store, post office, or pharmacy. A colleague from work offers to stop by the pharmacy and pick up a prescription for him. As a bachelor, he was accustomed to eating meals out and thus never cooked much for himself. A friend arranges for Meals on Wheels to deliver a hot meal at lunch and a cold snack for dinner. However, no food comes on the weekends. Mr. Jackson is supposed to return to the hospital outpatient department for rehabilitation therapy, but he is dependent on one of his neighbors being at home to help him get up and down the stairs. He cannot drive, so he must call a cab, which does not always come to the suburbs on time and is expensive.

Mr. Jackson struggles along for several weeks and eventually is able to return to work. He believes that the medical care and therapy he received have been of good quality. However, he also comes out of the experience with huge bills and negative feelings about the impersonality of the health care system, the high costs and low insurance coverage for long-term care, and the frustrating helplessness of even the professionals in mobilizing resources to facilitate even the simple functions of daily living. He realizes that if he were 20 years older, were no longer covered by his employer's insurance, had spent much of his savings, and lived in a house rather than in an apartment complex filled with friends and neighbors, his experience would have been far worse.

The implications? The existing formal system for providing care to persons with long-term, complex health problems is grossly inadequate: it is underfunded, highly regulated, too costly, and too disorganized—most of all, it does not meet the needs of consumers or providers. The demand for long-term care, as described below, will grow exponentially during the coming years. This growth, in turn, will exacerbate the forces that are already prompting change in organization and financing.

This chapter describes the various facets of long-term care as they exist in the late 1980s. It also presents a conceptual framework for understanding how the insufficient and ragged pieces can be molded into a rational system for the future. To begin with, the characteristics and the numbers of persons requiring long-term care are examined.

WHO NEEDS LONG-TERM CARE?

The primary consumers of long-term care are persons who have complex and/or chronic health care problems and functional disabilities. To quantify the long-term care population, it is necessary to analyze a mosaic of population segments. There are two basic types of clients.

The first group includes those who have relatively short-term problems but ones that require orchestration of a complex set of services. This group includes those with acute injury or illness who ultimately will regain complete recovery or independence but who require an extended period of convalescence or treatment. Persons with specific diseases, not necessarily characterized initially by functional disability, may also require complex, comprehensive care for a prolonged period of time. For example, those suffering with cancer, acquired immune deficiency syndrome (AIDS), cataracts, or hip fractures, may use, for a shorter period of time, some of the same long-term care services as those with permanent functional disabilities.

The second group is the traditional long-term care population. It is those who have ongoing ("chronic") and multiple health, mental health, and/or social problems and who are unable to care for themselves ("functionally disabled"). This includes the frail elderly persons with mental illness and/or mental retardation, those with developmental disabilities, victims of strokes and accidents, those with degenerative neurologic conditions or progressive systemic conditions such as kidney failure and diabetes, and infants and children with congenital abnormalities. Not all persons with complex, extended therapies, chronic conditions, or functional disabilities need the assistance of an organized system of care. Thus, determining the population requiring formal care mandates an understanding of the terms, the subsets of the population, and the portending growth.

"Chronic" usually connotes "permanent", or at least indefinite. For technical data collection purposes, "chronic" is defined by the National Health Interview Survey as any condition that lasts 3 months or more (1). Chronic conditions may be as life-threatening as coronary artery disease or as harmless as mild arthritis. Table 7-1 shows the prevalence of 10 chronic conditions. As is evident, the prevalence of chronic conditions increases with age. In addition, the majority of chronic problems are indeed permanent and thus accrue over time. Of persons age 65 and older, 80 percent have at least one chronic health problem, and the majority have multiple problems.

Functional ability has been described as a person's ability to perform the basic activities of daily living. Years of research have produced commonly accepted measures and scales of functioning. These are referred to as activities of daily living (ADL) (2) and instrumental activities of daily living (IADL) (3). Activities of daily living include the ability to eat, dress, perform personal care and grooming, bathe, walk, and maintain bowel and bladder continence. The instrumental activities of daily living include handling monetary affairs, telephoning, grocery shopping, housekeeping, doing chores, and arranging for transportation.

TABLE 7-1. Top Ten Chronic Conditions Affecting Persons ≥65 Years of Age, and Rate per 1000 Persons, 1981

Chronic Condition	Rate
Arthritis	495.8
Hypertensive disease	390.4
Hearing impairment	299.7
Heart conditions	256.8
Chronic sinusitis	151.7
Visual impairments	101.1
Orthopedic impairments	168.5
Arteriosclerosis	73.6
Diabetes	88.9
Varicose veins	77.7

SOURCE: U.S. Senate Special Committee on Aging, U.S. Senate: *Aging America, Trends and Projections.* Washington, DC, 1986, p 88.

Chronic illness and functional disabilities are interrelated. Both increase with age. Of persons under age 19, only 2.3 percent are limited in performing basic activities due to a chronic illness. Of those age 55–64, 22 percent are limited in activity to some degree. However, of those age 74 and older, 36 percent are limited in major activities due to chronic conditions, and an additional 3.5 percent have limitations in minor activities as well (4). Among those under the age of 65, many have some type of functional disability or chronic problem, and a small number may have needs for comprehensive, continuing care.

Additional population groups requiring long-term care include persons with mental conditions, those with neurologic diseases or degenerative neurologic conditions, victims of accidents resulting in paralysis or disfiguration, children with chronic congenital abnormalities, children with dyslexia and other similar problems, victims of paralyzing strokes, and the blind.

The National Center for Health Statistics has made several efforts to estimate the number of persons who require long-term care. Using 1977 data, Weissert and his colleagues estimated the total population in community settings in need of long-term care due to functional disabilities (5,6). They calculated the total number to be 6 million: 3.6 million community residents requiring personal care or mobility assistance; 0.6 million persons in board and care homes; and 1.8 million persons in nursing homes and long-term care facilities. To this are added 0.8 million mentally ill or retarded living in the community and 2.8 million developmentally disabled. In total, the estimate of persons requiring continuing care due to functional disabilities is more than 8 million (5,6). About two-thirds of these people are over the age of 65. Children and infants with birth defects or congenital abnormalities were not included in this study; thus, these population segments would be added to the total.

Table 7-2 shows the number of noninstitutionalized dependent persons by type of dependence and age. As is evident, those age 65 and over, while constituting only 11 percent of the population, represent about half of the dependent persons residing in the community.

More recently, Rice and Wick projected the number of persons with chronic conditions and disabilities on a state by state basis (7). As shown in Table 7-3, they estimate that the number of persons of all ages will increase by 31 percent between

TABLE 7-2. Number of Noninstitutionalized Dependent Persons, by Type of Dependence and Age

		Type of Dependence			
Age	Total	Personal Care	Mobility Assistance	Household Activity	Health Services
All	5455	1877	775	1969	833
<65	2626	820	240	937	629
65	2829	1057	535	1032	204
65–74	1064	345	196	415	106
≥75+	1765	712	339	617	98

SOURCE: Weissert, W: Estimating the long-term care population: Prevalence rates and selected characteristics. *Health Care Financ Rev* 1985; 6:

1980 and 2000. The number of persons age 75 and older limited in activity will increase by more than 75 percent.

The changing demographic composition of the United States will make long-term care an increasingly significant aspect of the health system. The number of people over the age of 65 will increase from 27.5 million in 1985 to 55 million in 2030 (8) (Table 7-4). The very old—those over age 85—will increase the most rapidly in terms of numbers and percent. As the number of old and very old people increases, the need for long-term care will rise. If even 20 percent of the older population requires assistance with basic activities of daily living, then in the near future more than 10 million people will need assistance.

WHAT IS LONG-TERM CARE?

"Long-term care" refers to health, mental health, social, and residential services provided to temporarily or chronically disabled persons over an extended period of time with a goal of enabling them to maintain as high as possible a level of independent functioning. There is no single regulatory or academic definition of long-term care.

TABLE 7-3. Projected Number of Persons with Limitation of Activity Due to Chronic Conditions and Percent Change by Age and Sex, 1980–2000

| | Number of Persons (in Thousands) | | | Percent Changes, |
Total	1980	1990	2000	1980–2000
All ages	33,235	38,013	43,472	30.80
<65	21,572	23,255	26,860	24.51
65–74	6,385	7,442	7,337	14.92
≥75+	5,279	7,315	9,275	75.71

SOURCE: Adapted from Rice D, Wick A: *Impact of an Aging Population on Health Care Needs, State Projections.* San Francisco, CA, University of California Institute for Health and Aging, 1985, Table 3.2, p 1-2.

TABLE 7-4. Actual and Projected Growth of the Older Population, 1900–2050 (Number in Thousands)

Year	Total Population	Age 65		Age 65–74		Age 75–84		Age 85+	
1900	76,303	3,084	4.0	2,189	2.9	772	1.0	123	0.2
1950	150,967	12,270	8.1	8,415	5.6	33,278	2.2	577	0.4
1980	226,505	25,544	11.3	15,578	6.9	7,727	3.4	2,240	1.0
2000	267,955	34,921	13.0	17,677	6.6	12,318	4.6	4,926	1.8
2040	308,559	66,988	21.7	29,272	9.5	24,882	8.1	12,834	4.2

SOURCE: 1900–1980 U.S. Bureau of the Census: Decennial Censuses of Population 1990–2050: U.S. Bureau of the Census. Projections of the Population of the United States, by Age, Sex, and Race: 1983 to 2080. Current Population Reports, Series P-25, No. 952, May 1984.

The several definitions below collectively convey the concept. Long-term care has been defined as:

A wide range of services which address the social, custodial, and medical needs of individuals who lack some capacity for self-care and whose continuing incapacity will necessitate the provision of care for a relatively long and indefinite period of time (9).

Support provided over an indefinite period of time to restore, maintain, retard, or prevent further deterioration of the ability to function for persons with conditions that are not likely to require immediate and intensive intervention by a highly trained health professional (10).

One or more services provided on a sustained basis to enable individuals whose functional capacities are chronically impaired to be maintained at their maximum level of health and well-being (11).

A range of services that addresses the health, personal care, and social needs of individuals who lack some capacity for self care. Services may be continuous or intermittent but are delivered for a sustained period to individuals who have a demonstrated need, usually measured by some index of functional dependence (12).

Health and social services provided within or outside institutions over extended periods to chronically ill, functionally impaired persons, most of whom are elderly (13).

A long-term patient is an individual who, because of physical or mental illness, deterioration, or disability, requires medical, nursing, or supportive health care for a prolonged period of time. Also included in this category is the individual who, because of severity of acute illness or injury, or resulting complications, requires an extended period of convalescence or treatment (14).

Those services designed to provide diagnostic, preventive, therapeutic, rehabilitative, supportive, and maintenance services for individuals of all age groups who have chronic physical and/or mental impairments, in a variety of institutional and noninstitutional settings, including the home, with the goal of promoting optimum levels of physical, social, and psychological functioning (15).

Throughout these differing definitions several themes are consistent. Long-term care is targeted at those with functional disabilities. The basis for the disabilities may be physical or mental, temporary or permanent. The goal is to promote or maintain independence in functional abilities. The services required, the professions involved, and the settings of care cover a broad spectrum and are orchestrated around the individual's unique needs.

HOW IS LONG-TERM CARE ORGANIZED?

The preceding definitions do not address the way in which long-term care is actually provided. About 90 percent of assistance comes from an informal network of friends and family (16). The formal means for providing long-term care has no uniform structure or financing. Rather, each community has its own combination of available resources, funding sources, and organization, and the latter is usually more informal than formal. A major dilemma in long-term care is the incongruence between what long-term care services should be and the way in which they currently operate.

As described above, long-term care is designed for people who require multiple and ongoing health, mental health, and social support services over an extended period of time and whose needs are likely to change. The ideal system of care for those who have multiple, multifaceted, and chronic illnesses is one that provides comprehensive, integrated care on an ongoing basis and offers various levels of intensity that change as a client's needs change. The goal is to provide the medical and related support services required to enable the person to maximize functional independence. This contrasts with the goal of acute care, which is to "cure" the patient of an illness. Many clients may use only select components of the system and may remain involved with the organized system of care for a relatively short period of time; others may use only a limited and stable set of services over a prolonged period of time.

This ideal system of long-term care is referred to throughout the remainder of this chapter as the "continuum of care." There is no universal definition of a continuum of care. The definition used here, which is described in more detail below, is as follows: "A continuum of care is an integrated, client-oriented system composed of both services and integrating mechanisms that guides and tracks patients over time through a comprehensive array of health, mental health and social services spanning all levels of intensity of care" (17). According to this definition, the continuum of care is a comprehensive, coordinated system of care designed to meet the needs of patients with complex and/or ongoing problems efficiently and effectively. The continuum of care concept extends beyond the traditional definitions of long-term care. It is more than a collection of fragmented services. The continuum of care concept includes mechanisms for organizing those services and operating them as an integrated system.

The needs of the clients of the continuum of care are multiple and multifaceted and change over time. It is thus essential that the services available to assist the clients represent a comprehensive range of health, mental health, and social support services. Moreover, service delivery must be reorganized and modified as the client's needs change. One of the underlying assumptions of a continuum of care is that, through an organized system, one can access appropriate assistance quickly and efficiently. Ideally, a continuum of care:

- Facilitates the client's access to the appropriate services at the appropriate time
- Monitors the client's condition and changes services as the needs change
- Coordinates care of many professionals and disciplines, thus producing high quality, as well as efficient care
- Integrates care provided in a range of settings
- Is cost-effective, matching resources to the patient's condition

There are over 60 distinct services that might be included in the ideal continuum of care. For simplicity here, the services are grouped into seven categories: extended inpatient, acute inpatient, ambulatory care, outreach, wellness, and housing. A list of services within these categories is given in Table 7-5. A more detailed description of the services is given in Table 7-6.

In brief, the basic categories represent the basic types of assistance that a person would need over a given period of time, through periods of both wellness and illness. Extended inpatient care is for persons who are so sick or functionally disabled that they require ongoing services provided in a formal health care institution but who are not so acutely ill that they require the technological and professional intensity of a hospital.

TABLE 7-5. Continuum of Care Services

Extended
  Skilled nursing
  Intermediate care
  Psychiatric intermediate care
  Swing beds
  Nursing home follow-up
  Respite care
Acute
  Medical/surgical inpatient
  Psychiatric inpatient
  Rehabilitation inpatient
  Comprehensive assessment
  Consultation service
Ambulatory
  Physician care
  Outpatient clinics
  Geriatric assessment clinics
  Day hospital
  Adult day care
  Mental health clinic
  Satellite clinics
  Psychosocial counseling
  Alcohol and substance abuse
Home care
  Home health—Medicare
  Home health—private
  Hospice
  High technology
  Durable medical equipment
  Home visitors
  Home-delivered meals
  Homemaker and personal care
Outreach/linkage
  Screening
  Information and referral
  Telephone contact
  Transportation
  Emergency response system
  Support groups
Wellness/health promotion
  Educational programs
  Wellness clinics

(Continued)

TABLE 7-5. (Continued)

Recreational and social groups
    Senior volunteers
    Congregate meals
    Meal discounts
Housing
    Continuing care retirement communities
    Senior housing
    Congregate care
    Adult family homes

TABLE 7-6. Continuum of Care Services

Extended inpatient

Skilled nursing care—provides medical and continuous nursing care services to patients who are not in the acute phase of illness and require primarily convalescent, rehabilitative, and/or restorative services

Intermediate care—provides nursing, supervisory, and supportive services to patients who do not require the degree of care or treatment that a skilled nursing unit is designed to provide

Psychiatric intermediate care—provides medical care, nursing services, and intensive supervision to the chronically mentally ill, mentally disordered, or other mentally incompetent persons

Swing beds—usually in small or rural hospitals; may be used flexibly to serve long-term care or acute patients

Nursing-home follow-up—a program whereby geriatric specialists from the hospital or home health program follow patients during their stay in a nursing home; this is arranged with the administrator of the nursing home and legally may be done on a formal or informal basis

Respite care—facilities and services that assist care givers by providing short-term care for frail or disabled individuals to help meet family emergencies, planned absences (e.g., vacations or hospitalization), or allow for family care givers to shop or do errands

Acute inpatient

Medical/surgical—provides acute care to patients in medical and surgical units on the basis of physicians' orders and approved nursing care plans

Psychiatric—provides acute care to emotionally disturbed patients, including patients admitted for diagnosis and/or treatment of psychiatric problems, including substance abuse, on the basis of physicians' orders

Rehabilitation—therapies include physical, occupational, and speech; provides coordinated multidisciplinary physical restorative services to inpatients

Comprehensive geriatric assessment—also Geriatric Evaluation Unit (GEU), Geriatric Assessment Unit (GAU); a multidisciplinary team of professionals, which may include physicians, nurses, social workers, pharmacists, and therapists, assesses the elderly patient's medical, psychological, functional, and social status and recommends a comprehensive plan of treatment and/or care

Geriatric consultation service—consultation by an individual or a team of health professionals specializing in geriatrics; provided upon request of the patient's physician or mental health professional

---

(Continued)

TABLE 7-6. (Continued)

Ambulatory

Physician care—medical care for individual patients provided by primary care and specialist physicians in their office or a clinic setting

Outpatient clinics—organized services (or clinics) for provision of nonemergency medical and/or dental services for ambulatory patients based in hospitals or free-standing facilities

Geriatric assessment clinics—usually organized by hospitals, out-patient clinics staffed by geriatric specialists who provide a comprehensive interdisciplinary assessment and plan of care for older patients; in some instances, the clinic is the patient's source of primary care; in others, the results of the assessment are referred back to the patient's regular physician

Day hospital—a program that provides intensive medical, psychiatric, nursing, and/or rehabilitation services to individuals who spend the day at the hospital and return home in the evening, who do not need 24-hour nursing care, but who would need to be inpatients of the hospital were the day program not available

Adult day care—centers providing health, recreation, and social services to adults during daytime hours, usually Monday through Friday; may include intake assessment, health monitoring, rehabilitation therapies, minimal nursing care, drug supervision, personal care, a noon meal, and transportation; health services may be provided but are not as intense as those provided in a day hospital—there are typically two models: the "social" model that concentrates on socialization and supervision and serves primarily those with mental conditions, and the "medical" model that cares for those with a more severe degree of physical impairment

Mental health clinic—outpatient mental health clinic that provides services such as mental status assessment, alcohol, drug abuse control, psychosocial counseling, and psychotherapy

Satellite clinics—outpatient clinics, usually at some distance from the hospital or physicians' offices, that provide limited care to ambulatory patients; with regard to geriatrics and long-term care, such clinics are often located in senior housing complexes or in conjunction with senior centers

Psychosocial counseling—provision of medical care, including diagnosis, treatment, and counseling, for psychiatric outpatients by psychiatrists, psychologists, social workers, and other health care professionals

Alcohol and substance abuse assistance—services for the provision of medical, psychiatric, rehabilitative treatment, and counseling for patients with a primary diagnosis of alcoholism or other chemical dependence

Home care

Home Health, Medicare—a program that provides, under a physician's orders, medical, nursing, rehabilitation, and social services to patients in their homes; clients are those who are recovering from hospitalization, are homebound, and require only intermittent care. Service, staffing, and payment are tightly regulated by Medicare

Home Health, private—an organized program that provides medical, nursing, other treatment, social services, personal care, and homemaker services to the patients in their place of residence

Hospice—a program providing palliative care—primarily medical relief of pain and symptom management—and support services to terminally ill patients and assistance to their families in adjusting to the patient's illness and death

High Technology—therapy provided in the home for patients requiring antibiotic infusion, chemotherapy, enteral or parenteral nutrition; the therapy mechanisms involves infusion of liquid solutions by pumps and related equipment

Durable Medical Equipment (DME)—products designed to assist individuals needing medical care at home. It includes items such as wheelchairs, canes, walkers, electric beds, and respira-

(Continued)

TABLE 7-6. (Continued)

Home care (Continued)

tors; equipment may be purchased or rented; many DME items are paid for by the Medicare and Medicaid programs if prescribed by a physician

Home Visitors—volunteers who act as "friendly visitors" and provide companionship on a regular basis to those who are homebound, especially to those who live alone

Home-delivered meals—a service for the preparation and delivery of nutritionally balanced meals, including special diets, to those who are not able to provide or prepare meals for themselves; "Meals on Wheels" is a nationwide program sponsored by the Older Americans Act; the cost of meals to the patient is $2–2.50, with subsidies through government and private programs

Homemaker and personal care—services include housekeeping, homemaking, personal care, reporting significant observations, teaching clients to perform various tasks, and performing limited nursing duties for which the aide has been trained

Outreach/linkage

Screening/Outreach—health education and screening programs offered to the public directly within their communities, sometimes in collaboration with groups such as neighborhood associations or community clinics

Information and Referral—a special program to provide information about and referral to services available in the community; a formal "Information and Referral" program is sponsored by the Older Americans Act; many senior centers and related community programs offer this service

Telephone Contact—a 24-hour hotline that may provide one or all of the following: counseling, information, referral, and checkup services or monitoring for all kinds of health and health-related problems

Transportation—providing or arranging for transportation to meet daily needs and to make accessible a broad range of services for the disabled

Emergency Response System—a program for frail or disabled individuals whereby subscribers have a portable emergency response unit in their apartments that will automatically secure a phone line and call for help in an emergency; the program is intended to give older persons who live alone the security that they can get help if needed, and thus the program contributes to enabling the older person to maintain independent living in their own homes

Support groups—education, therapy, and socialization groups for patients or their caregivers having similar health problems; such groups include those for family members who are caregivers for stroke victims, spouses of patients with Alzheimer's Disease, and parents of children with multiple sclerosis

Wellness/health promotion

Educational programs—programs for patients, families, and community members to provide information on health or social problems; a series may be on different aspects of a single illness or on multiple topics; education may be provided through community forums, one-on-one teaching, through videocassettes, or other means

Wellness clinics—health maintenance, disease prevention and management, as well as exercise programs for social, psychological and physical well-being; examples include risk reduction (e.g., smoking cessation and weight reduction programs), health and nutrition education, exercise and stress management programs

Recreational and social groups—activity programs and social groups sponsored by health care or social service agencies, usually targeted at persons with common interest or problems (e.g., healthy seniors, the developmentally disabled)

(Continued)

TABLE 7-6. (Continued)

Wellness/health promotion (Continued)

Senior Volunteers—a hospital volunteer program making particular efforts to recruit and involve older adults

Congregate Meals—group meals provided by a social service agency, health organization, or housing complex designed both to facilitate socialization and ensure healthy eating

Meal discounts—many hospitals and nursing homes invite seniors in the community to eat in the cafeteria during off-hours; meals are usually provided at a discount

Housing

Continuing Care Retirement Communities—a program through which older adults commit to reside in a community complex for the remainder of their lives; the site has the physical facilities and services to provide a spectrum of care, including apartments for independent living, accommodations with personal care, and nursing home care; services may be paid for on a fee-for-service basis, may be included in a monthly fee, or a combination thereof; an entry fee and monthly fee are common

Senior Housing—housing accommodations designed specifically to meet the physical and security needs of elderly persons who are capable of living independently without assistance; senior housing ranges from publicly supported buildings intended for low-income seniors to elite retirement complexes for the wealthy; senior residential facilities may be licensed by the state

Congregate Care—special housing for physically handicapped, mentally disabled, or frail individuals of any age, but particularly the aged, which includes meals provided in a common area and may provide varying degrees of supervision and personal care assistance; nursing care is rarely provided; such facilities may be licensed by the state under health or social service laws

Adult Family Homes—a program where adults who require supervision or assistance with the basic activities of daily living go to a family in the community either during a transition from the hospital to their own home or as a permanent arrangement; adult homes may be licensed by the state under health or social service laws

---

The majority of extended care facilities are referred to as "nursing homes," although this is a broad term that includes many levels and types of programs. Acute inpatient care is provided for those who have a major and acute health care problem. For the majority of persons, a typical hospital stay of 5–7 days is the intensive aspect of a longer spell of illness, preceded by diagnostic testing and succeeded by follow-up care. Ambulatory care services are provided within the formal health care facility, whether a physician's office or the outpatient clinic of a hospital, and provide a wide spectrum of preventive, maintenance, and recuperative services for persons who manifest a variety of concerns, from those who are entirely healthy and simply want an annual checkup to those with major health problems who are recuperating from hospitalization. Home care represents a variety of nursing, therapy, and support services provided to persons who have some degree of illness but who are able to satisfy their needs by bringing services into the home setting. Home health programs range from formal organizations providing skilled nursing care to relatively informal networks of peers who maintain telephone contact on a regular basis.

Outreach programs make health services readily available in the community rather than within the formidable walls of a large institution. Health fairs and cancer screening, for example, are targeted at the healthy or mildly ill who want to take preventive measures to stay healthy. Wellness programs are provided for those who are basically healthy but actively participate in exercise and health screening programs. Housing might be a complex designed specifically for seniors or the handicapped, with call-buttons built into the apartments and a nurse on call in event of an emergency.

Over time, a person might use any or all categories of service. The levels of care match the client's needs based on his condition at the time and the resources available to meet those needs. The services may, and typically are, provided by different organizations. However, it is also evident that if a single organization provides multiple services, a person who uses one is likely to call on the same organization when seeking other services. Moreover, although a person might have only a single problem, such as Mr. Jackson's broken hip, over time, a series of services are required. Continuity of care is enhanced when the provision of care is coordinated by a single organization.

The categories are for heuristic purposes only. The order of the categories and the services comprising them can vary. The categories can appropriately be reordered on the basis of the dimension being considered: duration of stay, intensity of care, stage of illness, disciplines of professionals, type of facility, and availability of informal support. Within each category are health, mental health, and social services, potentially provided by professional clinicians, provider organizations, families, and/or patients themselves. A more accurate diagram would be a multidimensional matrix showing the interrelationship of all of these factors in caring for a single individual and family. Such a matrix would be dynamic, not static, for the relationships would change over time and for each individual client.

Within the categories, the services of the continuum are distinct. Each has different regulatory, financing, target population, staffing, and physical requirements. A primary reason for organizing services into a continuum is to achieve integration; yet a major inhibiting factor is the differences among services that make unified planning and operations quite difficult. One dilemma faced by administrators in the initial creation of a continuum of care in the current climate is that each service must be dealt with separately.

One of the major complaints of those involved in providing long-term care throughout the years has been that services are highly fragmented. This fragmentation results in poor quality and high costs. The trend in the 1980s has been for organizations to start or acquire many services but to allow each service to operate independently. A major thesis of the continuum of care is that the benefits do not occur automatically with the addition or aggregation of many services. Rather, integrating management structures are critical to realizing the potential of the continuum to improve quality and cost effectiveness of patient care.

By definition, the continuum of care is more than a collection of fragmented services. It is an integrated *system* of care. The basic concept of the continuum of care is to provide a cost effective way to meet the full range of health, mental health and social support needs a person would have over a period of time, including periods of wellness or illness. The organization orchestrating the continuum takes responsibility for coordinating and arranging access to all services for its clients and for maintaining contact with the clients so that services can be changed as the client's needs change. An organization need not have all services under its direct control; rather, it may have a variety of formal and informal relationships with other providers in the communities.

To gain the system benefits of efficiencies of operation, economies of scale, and quality of product, integrating mechanisms are essential. Four integrating management systems are required: structure, information systems, case management/care coordination, and financing. Figure 7-1 presents a schematic diagram of the services and integrating mechanisms of the continuum.

Intraorganization and interentity planning and administration must be structured. Patient services are not likely to be coordinated unless the units that are providing the services are coordinated administratively, particularly when budgeting and financial issues arise. Practicing in a continuum of care also creates changes in the traditional roles of health, mental health, and social service professionals. New roles and responsibilities develop in relation to patients and families, provider and payor organizations, and other professionals. The human component is the single most important aspect of the continuum of care for the patient and practitioner, and thus the human dimensions must be managed as well as the financial and structural aspects. Administrative structures are necessary to (1) ensure channels of communication and cooperation; (2) establish clear lines of authority, accountability, and responsibility for patient care services; (3) negotiate budgets and financial trade-offs; and (4) present a cohesive, consistent message in interactions with external agencies and the community. Administrative mechanisms include committees that crosscut service areas, a designated senior administrator responsible for decisions that affect several different departments, interdisciplinary team conferences for clinicians, clinical liaisons assigned to service programs that have frequent patient referrals, multidepartment planning teams, and multidisciplinary and multidepartmental task forces focusing on specific short-term issues.

Integrated information systems are necessary for efficient management of the continuum. Many health and social service organizations still maintain separate clinical, financial, and utilization data systems; many, particularly social service

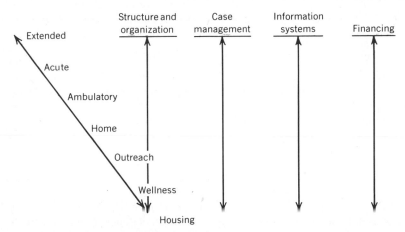

Figure 7-1. Continuum of care services and integrating mechanisms. The seven categories and 60 plus services of the continuum of care can be ordered on several dimensions; the order thus can vary. The integrating mechanisms are management systems which encompass and coordinate services at all levels (SOURCE: Evashwick C, Weiss L: *Managing the Continuum of Care: A Practical Guide to Organization and Operations*. Reprinted with permission of Aspen Publishers, Inc., © 1987.)

agencies and small health care companies, are not computerized. Very few health care organizations have data systems set up to track patients as they move from one type of service to another, such as from acute hospital care to home care. Yet, financing of health care and social services is increasingly dependent on prepaid and/or capitated systems encompassing a comprehensive service package. In order to implement quality assurance and utilization review programs, assess efficiency of operations and economies of scale, and track and aggregate patient experiences, comprehensive and integrated data systems and accompanying management reporting systems are imperative.

Care coordination, also referred to as *case management*, is becoming formally established as a result of the evolution of the continuum of care. In instances where there are multiple service programs under the same organization, patient referral and tracking and continuity of care do not necessarily occur automatically. The more comprehensive and complex the service organization, the more important it is to have a mechanism for client referral and tracking and a means of maintaining personal contact with clients as they move from one clinical provider to another. Continuity of care, with changes in types of care as the client's needs change, requires ongoing contact with clients, even when they are well. Case management is gaining understanding and acceptance in the health care field. The basic steps include client identification, assessment, care planning, service arrangement, monitoring, and follow-up. When dealing with a continuum of care, the role of the case manager is to facilitate access by clients to the various services comprising the continuum. Some of the services might be owned and operated by the primary organization; some may be arranged through contracts or informal agreements. The authority of the case manager varies: in a brokerage model the case manager facilitates access to services; in a total control model the case manager can also authorize payment for services.

Comprehensive and capitated financing systems are proliferating. On the basis of third-party payers' efforts to limit total expenditures for health care, government and private insurers are moving away from fee-for-service medical care and developing programs whereby providers agree to accept a single payment for caring for a client. The provider then decides what and how many services to order and assumes the financial consequences. Providers are forming coalitions in order to be able to provide the spectrum of services that a client might need. Concomitantly, consumers are joining health plans that may limit the range of providers they can choose from but predetermine and limit the amount that they must pay.

Capitated financing not only enhances the operation of a continuum of care but also provides incentives to develop such a continuum. The clinical provider seeking to offer services tailored to a client's needs requires the flexibility to order the most appropriate services without inhibitions driven by financial rather than clinical considerations. Capitated financing, when it covers a comprehensive range of services, has the potential to offer this flexibility.

Capitated financing also encourages organizations to operate more efficiently. In the absence of payer-required billing and reporting by a fee-for-service cost center, health care institutions do not have the incentive to maximize reimbursement by cost-shifting among services. Under the present situation, many health care organizations are still able to operate multiple services as distinct entities, receiving capitation for basic inpatient care and cost reimbursement for other services. In addition, capitated payment enables an efficient organization to keep any surplus that it makes. As capitated financing grows more common, the health care organization cognizant of reimbursement will want to position itself to maximize capitated payment across a wide range of services.

Capitated financing is accelerating the development of comprehensive health care delivery systems, or continuums of care. In particular, the enrollment of Medicare beneficiaries in HMOs and Competitive Medical Plans (CMPs) is causing many health care organizations, both provider-based and insurer-based, to offer a broader range of services at a competitive price in order to attract or retain Medicare clients. When such an offering is marketed, the provider and the insurer share (at least ideally) a common commitment to the efficient delivery of services. Success is more likely when internal incentives encourage the delivery of high-quality health care services in the most appropriate setting, and when data processing systems are effective in tracking and reporting cost and utilization levels.

Diversification, too, contributes to the trend toward comprehensive financing. As health care organizations offer a wider array of services, they want to be certain that the payment will be forthcoming for all services. They also prefer to minimize the billing and collection effort. Thus insurance that covers a wide array of services and other arrangements that enable and entice consumers to pay for a "package" of service are growing in type and number.

A word on the financing of the continuum of care is in order. The financial assumptions underlying the continuum include savings due to economies of scale, efficiencies of operation, increased market share, and revenue from new lines of business. Each of these may occur, and the success of each has been documented. The model continuums of care that exist, such as On-Lok and Mt. Zion Hospital Medical Center, both in San Francisco; ACCESS in Rochester, New York; and Connecticut Community Care Program, in Connecticut, have conducted research that shows that the clients of a continuum of care be cared for at a cost less than clients with similar needs in the community—under certain circumstances. Nonetheless, to achieve the potential financial advantages of a continuum, the system must be organized and operated with the financial objectives in mind and with ongoing data collection that enables that organization to monitor financial performance and revise operations accordingly.

In brief, the assumptions underlying the continuum of care are as follows: (1) because of the complex ongoing needs of many clients, comprehensive, integrated care is more beneficial (i.e., of higher quality) than fragmented care; (2) an organized system of care is more efficient and makes better use of scarce resources than fragmented, disorganized services; and (3) an integrated set of services has both market and financial advantages that are not offered by individual services. The goals and objective of the continuum of care are to meet consumer demand, enhance quality, maintain and increase market share, and improve financial viability.

For many people, families and friends serve as the structure orchestrating the continuum of care. However, as the population requiring continuing care grows, and as the health care system comes under multiple and increasing pressures, it becomes evident that informal sources alone will not be able to meet the demand for coordinating care. More significantly, there is growing awareness that the fragmentation of the formal structure is inadequate and inappropriate for meeting the future needs of clients, providers, or payers of health care. The following sections describe the major services and integrating mechanisms.

SERVICES OF THE CONTINUUM

From the 60 or more discrete services constituting the continuum of care, those that contact the greatest number of consumers and use the greatest amounts of health care resources are described in detail below. Other services are presented briefly in Table 7-6.

HOSPITALS

The hospital captures the spotlight of the health care delivery system because of the large number of people it cares for and employs, the size of the physical plant, the number of dollars spent, and the visibility of its high technology. The common vision is of the acute hospital activities: complicated machines, bustling staff, and patients arriving and departing quickly, cured of their ailments. In reality, the hospital plays a significant role in providing the continuum of long-term care (18–21).

Of the 6676 hospitals in the United States in 1983, 6148 were short-term. The remaining 528, however, are long-term (22). The distribution of these is shown in Table 7-7. By definition, these hospitals care for patients who have an average length of stay greater than 30 days. A high proportion of long-stay hospitals are psychiatric and are integral parts of the continuum of care for the mentally ill.

In addition to long-term hospitals, community hospitals provide many of the services of the continuum of care (23). A nationwide survey conducted to ascertain the activities of hospitals in long-term care and geriatrics demonstrated that hospitals provide a wide array of programs and services that reach patients and families before and after a stay in the inpatient unit (24).

Many hospitals also own, contract with, or operate long-term care facilities that

TABLE 7-7. Long-Term Hospitals and Beds, According to Type of Hospital Ownership, United States, 1983

Hospital Type	Number	Beds
General	22	11,464
Federal	13	9,978
Nonfederal	9	1,486
Psychiatric	377	183,843
Federal	22	18,549
State–local government	240	151,266
Nonprofit	50	6,814
Proprietary	65	7,214
Tuberculosis/respiratory	5	547
Other	124	29,578
Federal	2	578
State–local government	54	19,424
Nonprofit	58	8,363
Proprietary	10	1,213

SOURCE: American Hospital Association, *Hospital Statistics.* Chicago, IL, American Hospital Association, 1984.

offer skilled nursing and/or intermediate care. This enables the hospital to continue to care for patients who are not yet ready to be discharged into the community but whose needs can be met in an institutional setting less intense than that of the acute hospital unit. In 1984, the 6250 hospitals reporting to the American Hospital Association had 811 skilled nursing units with 55,571 beds and 433 other long-term care units with 35,481 beds (25).

Rehabilitation tends to be a long-term service, regardless of the setting. Even patients who are discharged quickly from a short-term community hospital often continue to receive therapy for months afterward. Rehabilitation is provided by many community hospitals and takes three institutional forms: as a separate hospital, as a hospital that is part of a medical complex, and as a unit within an acute hospital. Inpatient rehabilitation services are usually linked with outpatient services and often with home health as well. The growth of rehabilitation programs and their organizational forms are shown in Table 7-8 (26).

Federal hospitals, short-stay as well as long-stay, include Veterans Administration (VA) facilities. The VA operates its own continuum of care for veterans. VA complexes often include short-stay hospitals, long-stay hospitals or units within the acute hospital, skilled nursing facilities or units, adult day care, and home health programs. The VA has also been on the forefront of developing geriatric research, education, and clinical programs for physicians, and several VA hospitals have special centers for geriatrics.

The rationale for hospitals to be involved in long-term care is clear (27–29). Nationally, 38 percent of hospital discharges and 45 percent of hospital inpatient days are for persons age 65 and older (30). One in four older adults is admitted to the hospital each year, and of those admitted, more than 50 percent are readmitted at least once (31). As noted above, the health problems of seniors are characterized as chronic and multifaceted. For hospitals to provide high-quality care to seniors, they must address the needs of these patients beyond the few days spent in the hospital. As the older population grows in number and proportion, the hospital will be faced with an increasing demand for comprehensive, coordinated, continuing care by senior consumers and their families.

A second trend prompting hospitals' involvement in the continuum of care is capitated financing. As comprehensive and capitated payment systems grow, the acute hospital finds it advantageous from a financial standpoint and essential from a marketing standpoint to provide a spectrum of services.

Beginning in 1984, the Robert Wood Johnson Foundation sponsored a nationwide demonstration, the Program for Hospital Initiatives in Long-Term Care (32). This program funded 24 hospitals of varying characteristics to develop comprehensive and coordinated long-term medical care and social services to elderly individuals. The

TABLE 7-8. Growth and Organizational Distribution of Rehabilitation Programs, United States, 1980–1985

Year	Hospitals Reporting	Rehabilitation Hospitals	Rehabilitation Beds	Rehabilitation Units	Rehabilitation Beds	Total Beds
1980	6,407	68	5,902	303	8,772	14,674
1985	6,253	73	6,210	512	14,372	20,582

SOURCE: Section for Rehabilitation Hospitals and Programs. Chicago, IL, American Hospital Association, 1986.

requirements included developing not only a continuum of services, but in addition, systems for case management, integrated management information systems, and clinical education. The experiences and concrete products resulting from this program are likely to further encourage and facilitate the participation of hospitals in providing a continuum of long-term care.   .

For quality of care, consumer demand, market competition, and financial reasons, it can be expected that the acute hospital will continue expanding its activities in the field of long-term care.

NURSING HOMES

In 1980 more than 1.4 million persons had physical, mental, and functional disabilities sufficiently severe such that they had to reside in an institution where they could receive formal care on a regular basis. Projections indicate that this number may rise to 2.3 million persons by the year 2000 (33). These persons are cared for in more than 24,000 long-term care facilities (34).

"Nursing home" is a broad term that encompasses a wide spectrum of facilities, ranging from three-bed, privately owned adult residential care homes to small units of acute community hospitals to 1200-bed government-operated institutions. Each state licenses long-term care facilities, and each has its own licensing requirements, reimbursement policies, governing regulations, classification systems, and terminology. Thus, as part of the regulatory process, each state establishes its own definitions of long-term care institutions.

For national data collection purposes, the National Center for Health Statistics defines a nursing home as, "an establishment that provides nursing or personal care to the aged, infirm, or chronically ill" (35). The American Health Care Association defines a nursing home as "an institution, licensed by the state in which it is located, that provides long-term health care services according to the needs of its patients and/or residents. Nursing homes are staffed by trained professionals who provide the elderly, the chronically ill, and the convalescent with essential health and social services according to standards designed to assure quality care" (36).

Once licensed by the state, facilities meeting specified criteria can be "certified" by the federal Medicare program and/or state Medicaid program to care for the patients whose care is paid for by these programs. Federal terminology and regulations pertain to long-term care facilities to the extent that they are linked to Medicare and Medicaid payment systems. Federal definitions distinguish four general types of care.

A Skilled Nursing Facility (SNF) is defined by the National Center for Health Statistics (NCHS) as a nursing home in which 50 percent or more of the residents receive nursing care during the week and in which at least one full-time registered nurse or licensed practical nurse is employed. The emphasis in SNFs is on providing 24-hour per day nursing care, as well as restorative, physical, occupational, and other therapies. Patients eligible for SNF care under Medicare are those who are recovering from acute episodes of illness and who have just been discharged from an acute hospital. To receive certification and reimbursement from Medicare, the facility must not only be licensed by the state but also meet stringent federal requirements for staffing, operations, and physical facility. Of all the nursing homes in the United States, in 1985, only 6451 were certified as Medicare SNFs (37).

An Intermediate Care Facility (ICF) is defined by NCHS as a nursing home in which less than 50 percent of the residents receive nursing care during the week but that employs at least one full-time registered nurse or licensed practical nurse. The emphasis is on providing regular, although not 24-hour per day, nursing care, and social and rehabilitative services, in addition to room and board, for people not fully capable of independent living. ICFs that meet federal standards may elect to participate in their state's Medicaid program.

An Intermediate Care Facility for the Mentally Retarded (ICF/MR) provides supervision, socialization, and assistance in activities of daily living for the mentally retarded and those with other mental conditions. No particular nursing staff requirements are specified.

Personal care homes, residential care homes, domicilliary homes, and board and care homes provide sheltered living and one or more meals to persons who do not need nursing care or therapies. Residents may receive assistance with administration of medications, special diets, limited supervision for functional activities of daily living, and assistance in arranging for health care services. Recreation and social activities may also be offered. However, no health care professionals are on staff. Precise definitions and licensing requirements vary by state.

The terms "subacute" and "step-down" came into use during the early 1980s. They refer to a level of intensity of nursing care greater than the skilled nursing facility but less than the acute hospital. As of 1987, these terms have no standard definitions. Individual states have defined these services and authorized payment for them under state programs.

"Convalescent home," "retirement center," "nursing home," and other similar terms have no specific meaning. Nursing homes may be free-standing, units of hospitals, or integral parts of a campus of care retirement center. Many facilities have a combination of skilled nursing care, intermediate care, and/or personal care beds.

The National Master Facility Inventory Survey compiles data on nursing and related care homes, excluding hospital-based long-term care units. (In 1980, the latter totaled 1056 with 76,024 beds.) As shown in Table 7-9, the 1980 survey included 23,065 nursing homes having a total of 1,537,338 beds. In size, the homes range from 3 to over 1200 beds. Of all nursing home beds, 40 percent are in homes with 100–199 beds. Half of the homes had 50 beds or fewer, and 95 percent had less than 200 beds. In the entire United States, only 77 nursing homes have over 500 beds, and 38, or nearly half of these, are in New York and Pennsylvania.

Geographically, nursing homes are distributed unevenly. State bed:population ratios range from 21 to 95 per 1000 population age 65 and older. In 1980, the national average of beds per 65+ population was 60.2/1000. Regardless of geographic location, nursing homes have occupancy rates of 90–98 percent, indicating a widespread demand.

Nursing homes tend to be for-profit; 80 percent of the homes and 70 percent of the beds are proprietary (Table 7-10). Prior to the 1966 passage of Medicare, nursing homes were primarily local operations owned by independent operators. Increasingly, nursing homes now belong to large corporations and have highly standardized operations.

The health services provided in a nursing home include nursing care, personal care, medications supervision, activities programming, counseling, supervision, and general assistance with activities of daily living. The amount of nursing care varies considerably with the type of facility and the needs of the individual patient. Some homes also

TABLE 7-9. Number of Nursing and Related Care Homes and Beds, by Bed Size, United States, 1980

Size	Homes	Percent	Beds	Percent
All	23,065	100.00	1,537,338	100.00
3–9	5,492	23.8	29,238	1.9
10–24	3,006	13.0	47,965	3.1
25–49	3,030	13.1	112,093	7.3
50–74	3,332	14.4	199,673	13.0
75–99	2,375	10.3	208,995	13.6
100–199	4,737	20.5	617,165	40.1
200–299	766	3.3	177,581	11.6
300–499	250	1.1	90,584	5.9
500+	77	0.3	54,044	3.5

SOURCE: National Center for Health Statistics; Sirrocco A: Nursing and related care homes as reported from the 1980 NMI survey, *Vital and Health Statistics*, Series 14-No. 29, Table 7. DHHS Publ. No. (PHS) 84-1824. Washington, DC, Public Health Service, U.S. Government Printing Office, December 1983.

TABLE 7-10. Number of Nursing and Related Care Homes and Beds, by Bed Size, According to Type of Ownership, United States, 1980

	Homes		Beds		Average Size
Government	936	(4%)	126,907	(8%)	136
3–49	223		7,300		33
50–99	322		21,706		67
100+	391		97,901		250
Proprietary	18,669	(81%)	1,072,243	(68%)	57
3–49	10,232		152,503		15
50–99	4,229		304,290		72
100+	4,208		615,450		146
Not-for-profit	3,460	(15%)	338,188	(22%)	98
3–49	1,073		29,493		27
50–99	1,156		82,672		92
100+	1,231		226,023		183
All	23,065		1,537,338		67

SOURCE: National Center for Health Statistics; Sirrocco A: Nursing and related care homes are reported from the 1980 NMI survey, *Vital and Health Statistics*, Series 14-No. 29, Table 6. DHHS Publ. No. (PHS) 84-1824. Washington, DC, Public Health Service, U.S. Government Printing Office, December 1983.

provide rehabilitation, respiratory illness care and therapy, and high-technology infusion therapies. In addition, nursing homes provide secure, supportive environments, with regular, well-balanced meals and socialization opportunities.

Consistent with the services provided, the staffing in nursing homes is primarily by nurses aides and licensed vocational or practical nurses. In Medicare-certified homes, regulations require one Registered Nurse (R.N.) during the day shift for every 99 beds. Required staffing levels vary by state. Homes do not have full-time rehabilitation, medical, pharmacy, dietary, psychiatric, or social services staff unless they are large or specialize.

In broadest terms, the residents of nursing homes are:

- Persons requiring extended convalescence or rehabilitation following an acute episode of illness or trauma
- Persons with chronic and permanent physical conditions requiring nursing care on a daily basis
- Persons with functional disabilities, whether physical or mental, which make it impossible or difficult for them to function and remain independent
- Persons with chronic or permanent mental conditions who require constant supervision
- Persons of all ages

Table 7-11 highlights the salient characteristics of nursing home residents. The typical resident is white, female, and unmarried. Four out of five nursing home residents are over the age of 65; more than one-third are over the age of 85. Major causes for admission include mental dysfunctioning, incontinence, night wandering, ADL or IADL dysfunctioning, and lack of informal support systems.

It is important to note that for every person residing in a nursing home, there are two to four times as many persons equally disabled residing in the community (38). Physical illness is less often a major cause for admission than an inadequate social support system.

TABLE 7-11. Selected Characteristics of Nursing Home Residents

Patient Characteristics	Percent of Residents
Female	71.2
Age 85+	34.5
Married	11.9
Clinical characteristics	
Bedfast	37.3
Incontinent of bladder or bowel	45.3
Chronic brain syndrome/senility[a]	56.9
Congestive heart failure[b]	4.0
Stroke[b]	7.9
Cancer[b]	2.2
Arteriosclerosis[b]	20.3

SOURCES: Characteristics of Nursing Home Residents, Health Status and Care Received: National Nursing Home Survey, United States, May–December 1977, Publ. (PHS) 81-1712 (*Vital and Health Statistics*, Series 13, No. 51, Tables 5, 8, and 10), Hyattsville, MD, National Center for Health Statistics, 1979. Discharges from Nursing Homes: 1977 National Nursing Home Survey, Publ. (PHS) 81-1715 (Vital and Health Statistics, Series 13, No. 54, Tables 3–5). Hyattsville, MD, National Center for Health Statistics, 1981.

[a]Listed as a chronic condition or impairment.

[b]Listed as a primary diagnosis.

At any given time, 5 percent of those age 65 and older reside in nursing homes. Of those over age 85, 20 percent reside in nursing homes. However, the chance of spending at least some time in a nursing home is far higher—from 25 to 40 percent of all older persons enter a nursing home at least once (39,40). As the older population increases, the demand for nursing home care will grow correspondingly.

Rice and Wicks have analyzed the distribution and demand for nursing home beds based on current utilization rates and population growth (41). They project that by the year 2000, 2.3 million persons will need nursing home care (Table 7-12). The number of seniors requiring nursing home care is projected to increase 71 percent; the number of persons age 85 and over requiring care will increase by 119 percent.

The financing of nursing home care is supported by two primary sources: individuals pay for nearly half; Medicaid pays for about half (42). Contrary to public knowledge, Medicare does not pay for most nursing home care; it pays for only 2–3 percent. In 1986 the annual cost of care in a nursing home was $25,000 (43). The majority of persons enter nursing homes as private-pay clients. If their stay is long, they rapidly exhaust their resources and become eligible for Medicaid. This "spend down" phenomenon is a major policy issue for federal and state governments and individuals.

HOME HEALTH

During the 1980s, home health became one of the most rapidly growing areas of health care. This trend reflected the convergence of three major factors: the financial pressures on hospitals to diversity and to control patient flow under capitated reimbursement systems, an increase in demand due to the growth of the older population, and the desire by both consumers and payors to minimize health care costs by substitution of less intense alternatives to institutional care. As shown in Table 7-13, the demand for home health care is expected to continue to growth, with a projected increase of 43 percent between 1980 and 2000.

Home health agencies are of two major types: Medicare-certified and private. These are described separately.

Medicare-Certified Home Health Agencies

Home health agencies that meet stringent federal standards can be certified by Medicare to care for clients enrolled in Medicare Part A or Part B. The agency is shaped

TABLE 7-12. Projected Number of Nursing Home Resident and Percent Change, by Age and Sex, 1980–2000

Age	1980	2000	Percent Change
All	1,409,577	2,307,936	63.7
<65	203,011	249,978	23.1
65–84	1,206,565	2,057,958	70.6
≥85+	493,767	1,083,514	119.4

SOURCE: Rice D, Wick A: *Impact of an Aging Population on Health Care Needs: State Projections.* San Francisco, CA, University of California Institute for Health & Aging, 1985, Table 3.5, p III-6.

TABLE 7-13. Projected Number of Persons Receiving Home Health Services and Percent Change by Age and Sex, 1980–2000

Age Group	Number of Persons		Percent Change 1980–2000
	1980	2000	
<65	759,680	947,205	24.7
Males	357,099	454,019	27.1
Females	402,580	493,186	22.5
Age 65–84	722,133	1,176,338	62.9
Males	248,395	384,165	54.7
Females	473,739	792,173	67.2
≥85	197,276	450,362	128.3
Total	1,481,813	2,123,542	43.3

SOURCE: Rice D, Wick A: *Impact of an Aging Population on Health Care Needs: State Projections.* San Francisco, CA, University of California Institute for Health & Aging, 1985, Table 3.6, p III-7.

by federal requirements and serves almost exclusively Medicare, workers' compensation and private insurance clients. Home health agencies are licensed by most states, and a few states require a certificate of need.

To be eligible for home health coverage by Medicare, a client must be homebound and require short-term, intermittent nursing care or physical therapy. Services must be prescribed by a physician.

Home health agencies may also provide occupational therapy, speech therapy, medical social work, and home health aide services. These can be reimbursed by Medicare, but only if the client first meets the preceding criteria. Additional services, such as nutrition counseling, pharmacy consultation, respiratory care, ostomy therapy, chemotherapy, intravenous care and infusion therapy, may be provided in conjunction with the other services or provided separately and paid for directly by the client.

Durable medical equipment, ranging from walkers to electric beds, is often provided in conjunction with home health care. The home health agency may have formal or informal arrangements with a local durable medical equipment company to provide the needed equipment. If the equipment is to be paid for by Medicare, it must be prescribed by the patient's physician.

The number of home health agencies mushroomed during the mid-1980s. In 1980, the non-for-profit, community-based Visiting Nurse Association was the predominant type of agency. Medicare-certified home health agencies numbered 2858. As of 1985, the number had increased to 5755. From 1982 to 1984 the total number of Medicare home visits increased from 31.3 million to 39.8 million, the average per visit charge increased from $39.85 to $45.94, and the total charges increased from $1.3 billion to $1.9 billion (44).

Home health agencies productivity and size are measured by visit. Nationally, approximately 2 million people received home health care in 1985 (45). Of these, each person received an average of 28 visits per person over a period of 10–12 weeks. Individual agencies provided a range from 10,000–300,000 visits per year, with a mode of 50,000 per agency. The majority of the clients of Medicare-certified agencies are over the age of 65; for many agencies seniors comprise 80-90 percent of their clients.

The charge for a home health visit varies according to the type of professional service and the geographic area. In 1985 the mean charge for a visit was $53 (46).

Medicare-certified home health agencies typically receive the majority of their funding from Medicare. However, Medicaid, Workers' Compensation, local government programs, and private insurance also subsidize home health services and often require that the providing agency be Medicare-certified. As of 1987, Medicare-certified agencies are paid by Medicare on a cost-reimbursement basis. Thus there is no particular financial incentive to establish services or clients beyond the Medicare program. Nationally, in 1985, Medicare paid $2.3 billion under Part A and $48 million under Part B for home health care for Medicare enrollees (47).

Private Home Health Agencies

Private home health agencies provide a wide array of services to the homebound. Private home health agencies are not certified for payment by Medicare, and, concomitantly, are not bound by Medicare regulations. Although in some states they must be licensed as health care providers, in many states, these agencies operate under the auspices of only a business license.

The services provided include the same professional services as Medicare-certified agencies plus numerous others. Services include skilled nursing, physical therapy, occupational therapy, speech therapy, medical social work, home health aides, homemakers, high-technology home infusion therapy, and ventilator care. Agencies also arrange for durable medical equipment to be provided to their clients. In contrast to the Medicare-certified agencies, which can only provide intermittent and brief visits, private home health agencies provide 24-hour care, daily care, and specialty services such as personal grooming, bathing and shaving, housekeeping, transportation, shopping, meal preparation, and home repair.

Clients comprise a broader group than those served by Medicare-certified agencies. While the latter receive the majority of their referrals directly from hospitals for patients who are being discharged, private home care agencies must engage in active marketing to secure clients. Clients range from new mothers and infants who elect for early discharge after childbirth to young accident victims who require 24-hour nursing care to Workers' Compensation clients who need rehabilitation before returning to work to seniors living alone who have no severe health problems but do have functional disabilities. Private home care does not require a physician's prescription (except for private insurance and Workers' Compensation cases), and thus clients come from many sources. Social service agencies, Medicare-certified home health agencies, relatives, and friends all make referrals.

Because private home care agencies are not reimbursed or certified by any federal agencies, there is so single source of national statistics, and data may be more representative than accurate. The great majority are proprietary; a few operated by churches or social service agencies are not-for-profit.

Private home care agencies charge by the hour, rather than by the visit; often a minimum number of hours is required. Charges are considerably less than Medicare-certified agencies, even for the same service, because private agencies are not required to have comparable staffing, which adds to overhead. Thus a 1-hour visit from an R.N. may be half of the charge of one visit (which may range from 45 minutes to 2 hours) from a R.N. of a Medicare-certified agency. The trade-off is that some professional services, such as medical social services, may not be available from a private agency, and quality control may not receive the same attention as that enforced by government regulation.

Payment is by private insurance companies, through Workers' Compensation, or directly from the individual. Public programs, specifically Title XX of the Social Security Act, the Older Americans Act, and block grant monies, may be used to contract with a local home care agency to care for the clients eligible for the particular program. Such contracting is often done with the not-for-profit private home care agencies.

Like Medicare-certified home health agencies, private home care services have grown in number during the mid-1980s (although there are not irrefutable national statistics due to the reason mentioned above), and the demand for both is likely to continue to increase. Until the early 1980s, private and Medicare agencies tended to be separate and, hence, to compete with each other for some types of cases. The current trend is for companies to offer both services. Because of Medicare regulations, even if housed in the same office, the two programs must be operated very strictly as separate businesses.

HOSPICE

"Hospice" is a concept of providing care for the terminally ill. It began as a formal program in Great Britain and spread to the United States during the 1970s. The philosophy of hospice is that terminally ill persons should be allowed to maintain life during their final days in as natural and comfortable a setting as possible (48). Every attempt is made to enable the person to remain at home, including use of palliative drug therapy. An interdisciplinary team cares for the patient in both home and institutional settings. Psychosocial and spiritual counseling, for both the patient and the family, is included as an integral facet of the health care services. Bereavement counseling with the family continues after the patient's death.

Hospice programs vary in their organization. They may be offered by hospitals, home health agencies, or nursing homes, or they may be free-standing. Hospices may also be informal or may meet federal Medicare regulations to be formally certified. Ten elements common to all hospices have been identified by Lack and Buckingham (49):

- Service availability, including medical and nursing care, to home care patients and institutional inpatients on a 24-hour per day, 7-day per week, on-call basis
- Home care service in collaboration with inpatient facilities
- Control of symptoms (physical, psychological, social, spiritual)
- Provision of care by an interdisciplinary team
- Physician-directed services
- Central administration and coordination of services
- Use of volunteers as an integral part of the health care team
- Acceptance into the program based on health needs, not ability to pay
- Treatment of the patient and family together as a unit
- Bereavement follow-up service

These activities represent the philosophy of hospice. The Joint Commission for the Accreditation of Hospitals (JCAH) has established specific criteria for accrediting hospices. The federal Medicare program also has delineated programmatic requirements for hospices that seek certification to be reimbursed for services by Medicare.

The number of persons cared for by hospices annually is estimated to be 100,000 (50). To participate in a hospice program, a person must generally have a diagnosis of terminal illness fatal within 90–180 days. The client and family must be willing to acknowledge the imminence of death and desire palliative care. The majority of hospice patients are victims of cancer. Some hospice programs require the clients to have a care giver; others care for patients who live alone and have no designated care giver.

The idea of the hospice and its implementation received considerable national attention (51). During the 1970s, demonstration projects to test the impact on quality of life for clients and cost effective use of resources were funded by the federal government. Ultimately, service criteria and payment authorization for hospice under Medicare were included in the Tax Equity and Fiscal Responsibility Act of 1982 and extended in 1986.

In 1986, 1500 programs throughout the nation considered themselves to provide hospice care (52). There are several free-standing hospice facilities, although these are very few in number. Neither the organizational setting nor the physical location determines recognition as a "hospice." Rather, it is the approach to care.

Hospice services may be funded by Medicare, some private insurance companies, and private individuals. To be certified to receive payment by Medicare, a hospice must meet federal regulations and the patients must express formal intent to participate in the hospice program. As of 1986, 275 hospices had been certified for participation in Medicare (53). Hospice services not organized as a special program may nonetheless be paid for as separate home health, hospital, or nursing home care.

ADULT DAY CARE

Adult day health is a daytime program of nursing care, rehabilitation therapies, supervision and socialization that enables frail (usually elderly) people to remain in the community. The purpose of adult day health is to enable persons who are functionally disabled and/or moderately ill but not in need of 24-hour nursing care to remain in their homes at night with their families and friends while receiving the care that they need during the day. The goal is to foster the maximum possible health and independence in functioning for each client as well as the optimum combination of care giving and respite for each family. For many, if a supportive home environment and day health care are not available, the only alternative is to enter a nursing home.

Adult day care programs serve a range of clients, from people just recovering from acute trauma who need rehabilitation, to those with permanent physical disabilities requiring daily nursing care, to those with no major physical limitations but mental functioning impairments. Most day care programs identify a particular type or types of clients whom they can care for effectively and then target that segment of the patient population (54). More than 70 percent have some type of mental or behavioral problem.

The majority of day care clients are elderly and average nearly 75 years of age. More than two-thirds are female, and about two-thirds live with a spouse, family, or friends. Nearly half of the participants are eligible for Medicaid. The functional and personal client characteristics suggest that day care is, indeed, an alternative to nursing home care for those who would be unable to function alone but who are able to live with family or friends, provided respite and daily supervision are available.

Participants of adult day health come to the center for 4–8 hours during the day and then return home at night. Most programs operate Monday through Friday only. Services provided include nursing care, medical care if needed, medication regulation, pharmacy counseling, physical therapy, occupational therapy, speech therapy, psychosocial counseling, medical social services, nutrition counseling, a balanced diet, socialization opportunities, and transportation. Some services are provided by employed staff, and some are provided by private professionals through contract or referral. Patients keep their own physicians, and the staff of the adult day health program maintain regular contact with the physician about the client's condition.

Day care programs have proliferated during the 1980s. There is no comprehensive reporting mechanism that captures programs in the entire United States. However, the National Institute on Adult Daycare (NIAD) of the National Council on Aging (NCOA) report only one center operating in 1985 that was open before 1970. Table 7-14, which is taken from a nationwide survey, shows the recent rapid increase in the number of programs. NIAD estimates that in 1986, there were at least 1200 adult day centers in the United States (55).

Adult day programs are sponsored by a variety of organizations, including hospitals, nursing homes, community social service agencies, church groups, and senior centers. Average enrollment is 37, with 50 the maximum capacity for most centers. The average daily attendance is 19; most participants come 2 or 3 days per week. Based on a national survey that had a 71 percent response rate, NIAD estimated that on an average day in 1986, 14,750 persons of a total 27,200 enrollees attended 772 adult day centers (56). If the total number of operating centers is approximately twice this, then about 50,000 persons per year participate in adult day health programs. This is half the 100,000 persons annually receiving hospice care and 2.5 percent of the 2 million receiving home health care.

Adult day care programs have most often developed as "grass-roots efforts" to meet community need (57). Most are not-for-profit. There are no national certifications or regulations for adult day care. Some states govern adult day care with licensing and other regulations, but these vary widely. At this point in the evolution of adult day care, the primary source of information and programmatic guidance is the National Council on Aging National Institute on Adult Day Care (58).

Funding for adult day care programs is usually accomplished by pooling funds from

TABLE 7-14. Growth of Adult Day Center Programs, Dates of Opening ($N = 845$)

Date	Number	Percent
1981–1986	496	59
1976–1980	249	29
1970–1975	88	10
Before 1970	12	1

SOURCE: Von Behren R: *Adult Day Care in America: Summary of a National Survey.* Washington, DC, National Council on the Aging National Institute on Adult Daycare, October 1986, Table 7.

a variety of public and private programs. There is no single source that routinely covers day care. In most states, Medicaid funds, social service block grant monies, and state public health or welfare monies may be used for adult day care. Despite the fact that the majority of participants are seniors, Medicare does not authorize adult day care per se.

Medicare will pay for specific outpatient services, such as rehabilitation therapies, which may be provided by an adult day care center. In 1986 charges to patients and/or third-party payers averaged $22–32 per person per day (59). The costs of adult day care range from $35–50 per person per day, and most programs depend on subsidy by foundations, grants, private contributions, and parent organizations.

OTHER SERVICES

The continuum of care includes at least 60 distinct services. Hospitals, nursing homes, and home health represent the largest numbers of health care organizations serving the greatest number of clients. The many other services, however, should receive due consideration in planning, managing, and analyzing a continuum of care. Table 7-6 includes a brief description of additional services.

INTEGRATING MECHANISMS

For a continuum of care to function as a *system of care* rather than as a collection of fragmented services, integrating mechanisms are essential. As described above, these include an internal organization that coordinates the operations of various services; a financing mechanism that enables pooling of funds across services; a management information system that integrates clinical, utilization, and financial data and follows clients across settings; and a case management/care coordination program that works with clients to arrange services. These integrating mechanisms are in various stages of development, and in few instances there are mature examples of comprehensive systems that include all of these components. Case management and financing are discussed in more detail below.

CASE MANAGEMENT/CARE COORDINATION

Care coordination is also referred to as *service coordination, case management*, and various other terms. The purpose of care coordination is to work directly with clients and families over time to assist them in arranging and managing the complex set of resources that the client requires to maintain health and independent functioning. Care coordination seeks to achieve the maximum cost effective use of scarce resources by helping clients get the health, social, and support services most appropriate for their needs at a given time.

Care coordination is a process (60–62). The components are assessment, care planning, arrangement of services, monitoring, and reassessment. Assessment is usually done by a multidisciplinary team that includes a nurse, a social worker, a physician, and other professionals as required by the particular client. When possible, assessment includes evaluation of the home environment and family situation. Based on the results of the assessment, the team concurs on a specific plan of action and recommends an array of appropriate services. The care coordinator (case manager) is responsible for arranging the services ordered by the team and then maintains contact with the client and with the service providers to confirm that services are being delivered and meeting the client's needs. Reassessment of the client's status occurs either according to a regularly scheduled checkup with the clinicians or when the care coordinator detects a change that warrants reevaluation.

Two basic models of care coordination/case management are prevalent: the brokerage model, under which the case manager arranges for providers to deliver services to a client but has no direct control over payment; and the full-service model, under which the case manager can authorize payment for certain services.

Care coordinators are typically nurses, social workers, or health care professionals trained explicitly as case managers. The role is still evolving, and until recently, the care coordination functions have been performed by various disciplines without recognition of a separate and distinct role. A care coordinator can handle 20–80 active clients, depending on the breadth and intensity of the model, the dependence level of the clients, and the organizational resources supporting the care coordination operations.

Care coordination/case management is not a function reimbursed by Medicare, private insurance, or other traditional health care payment sources. An individual care coordination/case management program may be paid for entirely or partially by certain state government programs, such as Medicaid, Title XX, mental health or Medicare/Medicaid/Older Americans Act demonstration grants; by private monies, such as grants, foundations, donations; or through private pay of the clients. Care coordination is usually paid for by organizations, not patients. However, there is growing recognition of the value to families, and a few direct pay programs are beginning to emerge. Clients (or families) pay $50–$100 for an initial assessment and then pay a lesser fee for ongoing monthly consultation.

Only lately has care coordination gained widespread recognition for its contributions to the quality and financial viability of continuing care. Historically, most formal care coordination/case management programs have been based in public sector and social service agencies, and many have been operated as demonstrations (63,64).

During the past few years, the providers and payers of health care have recognized the need to develop a cost effective means of dealing with the complexity of patients' ongoing needs for comprehensive care. Care coordination has the potential to coordinate an array of resources, both internal to a given organization and available in other community agencies, and to make astute use of a variety of financial resources to maximize the care affordable by the client. The trend to recognize the distinct role of a case manager/care coordinator is further enhanced by the expansion of health care organizations into continuums of care, with more than a single type of service available within the same organization and with a pool of funds for health and social support services that can be spent at the discretion of the provider.

The cost effectiveness of care coordination/case management has been examined and documented by a number of demonstration projects (65,66). However, the cost of such a program is still fairly high, and with no direct and widespread reimbursement source, many organizations are reluctant to initiate care coordination programs, despite recognizing their value.

Care coordination/case management is likely to become more prevalent in the future. As part of this expansion, continued examination of the cost effectiveness of the program and refinement, and streamlining of the models, are likely to occur.

FINANCING

Financing is one of the primary problems inhibiting the provision and organization of long-term care on a coordinated, continuing basis. The definition of a continuum of care assumes (1) adequate financing available to provide clients with an array of needed health, mental health, and social services and (2) access to such financing. At national and local levels, the current mechanisms of financing inhibit the operation of a continuum of care in three fundamental ways. First, adequate funds are not available. Second, the financing streams are highly fragmented, with the various streams having different eligibility criteria, service coverage, reporting and operating requirements, and payment policies (Table 7-15). Third, most organizations do not have control over all the pertinent financing streams, thus limiting their ability to pool financing and allocate funds from an internal process.

In 1984 the nation spent $387.4 billion on health care. Of this, 59 percent was paid by private sources, and 42 percent was spent by federal, state, and local governments. Distribution by service shows that hospital care is the largest single source of care, accounting for 41 percent of the expenditures. Approximately 19 percent of expenditures was spent each on physician and other personal care, and 8 percent was spent on nursing home care.

Medicare funding is targeted at acute health care. Medicare accounted for $63.1 billion of the $387.4 million 1984 expenditures. Only $545 million, less than 1 percent, was spent on nursing home care. Home health care received $1898 million, or 3 percent of expenditures. Hospice care allocations were $2 million.

In contrast, Medicaid pays heavily for nursing home care. The 1984 expenditures for Medicaid totaled $32.4 billion; 42 percent went for nursing home care.

Of the total $32 billion spent on nursing home care in 1984 by all payers, nearly half was paid by state Medicaid programs, and nearly one-half was paid by private individuals. Private insurance, the VA, and a variety of other sources accounted for the remaining few percent. In a number of states, payment for nursing home care is the largest single item in the state's Medicaid budget. As the number of older persons increases, there is likely to be a concomitant increase in the demand for nursing home care. The budget implications for the nation and for the states are overwhelming. Thus the public sector is exploring means to limit expenditures for nursing home care. These have included preadmission screening, substitution of home care and community-based services, and placing certificate of need restrictions to prevent the construction of additional nursing home beds.

The financial implications for the individual are also severe. Very few people, including the age 65+ population, which is at greatest risk, have the personal funds to afford complex, community-based, or institutional care over a prolonged period of time. Currently, nearly one-half of the expenditures for nursing home care are made by individuals. At an average cost of $2000 per month, very few people can afford an extended stay in a nursing home. The result is a phenomenon referred to as "spend down." Once older persons have used all of their personal resources for themselves or a spouse, they become impoverished and qualify for Medicaid. To many older people and their families, the emotional cost of becoming an impoverished ward of the government, as a result of the government's own regulations, is as great as the financial cost.

Within the private sector, the potential of long-term care insurance is being cautiously examined (67). Because of the changes in life expectancy and health status of the current and upcoming cohorts of seniors, insurance companies have had difficulty in projecting realistic life tables and thus have been reluctant to offer long-term care insurance. Now, the recognition of the growing demand for such insurance, by both the government and individuals, has sparked new attention. By 1986, a number of private companies offered some type of insurance for nursing home care (68). Unfortunately, many of these policies did not cover home health care. This thus perpetuates the phenomenon that occurred in the hospital arena, providing incentives to care for people in institutions instead of in their home or on an outpatient basis, to the possible detriment of both cost and quality.

Capitated financing programs and ones that include acute, long-term, and supplemental care are also on the increase. Health Maintenance Organizations (HMOs), described in detail in Chapters 5 and 11, have experienced a resurgence during the 1980s. In efforts to be competitive, HMOs have expanded the range of services they cover. HMO financing of a wide array of services approaches a continuum of care, where funding from multiple sources is pooled, and services can be ordered based on the client's needs, not segmented according to payors' regulations.

Social Health Maintenance Organizations (S/HMOs) were funded by the federal government in 1982 as an experiment to test the concept of a broad package of health and social support services provided to older adults through an HMO-like organization (69,70). The four federal demonstration projects include the Senior Care Action Network (SCAN), Long Beach, California; Kaiser Permanente Medical Care Program, Portland, Oregon; Ebenezer Society, Minneapolis, Minnesota; and Metropolitan Jewish Geriatric Center, Brooklyn, New York.

The S/HMOs contributed to the advancement of the continuum of care concept by publicizing the benefits to quality and the organizational feasibility of providing an integrated range of health and social services. They also advanced the thinking about comprehensive financing by preparing actuarial estimates of and documenting experience in the use of services in a comprehensive, coordinated system of care. By the time that the S/HMO experimental programs got underway, Medicare had proceeded with authorization of capitated payment to federally certified HMOs and Certified Medical Plans (CMPs).

As of October 1, 1985, the federal government permitted HMOs to enroll Medicare clients on a shared-risk basis. Federally certified programs are required to offer all the services covered under Medicare Part A and Part B. These requirements, and the financial benefits to be gained, have resulted in contracts among combinations of hospitals, physician groups, home health agencies, and HMOs. Medicare HMOs initially received mixed reactions across the country by both consumers and providers. In some areas such as Southern California and Minnesota, Medicare HMOs have grown rapidly. In other areas of the nation, senior HMO development has been quite slow.

HMOs for the younger population have continued to grow. The number of HMOs grew from 243 in 1981 to 480 by December 1985 (71). Enrollment during the same time period increased from 10.3 to 21 million. HMO membership increased by 25 percent in 1985 alone—an indication of the upsurge in capitated finance programs experienced during the mid-1980s. Further growth is expected throughout the remainder of the decade.

Such programs aid the development of comprehensive, continuum of care delivery systems by enabling the individual health care organization to acquire control over financing streams that will pay for several types of services.

Recognition is growing of the need to change the financing of health and social

TABLE 7-15. Major Federal Programs Supporting Long-Term Care Services: Services Covered, Eligibility, and Administering Agency

Program	Services Covered	Eligibility	Administering Agency	
			Federal	State
Medicaid/Title XIX of the Social Security Act	Skilled nursing facility[a] Intermediate care facility[b] Home health[c] Adult day care[b]	Aged, blind, disabled persons receiving cash assistance under SSI; others receiving cash assistance under AFDC; at state option, persons whose income exceeds standards for cash assistance under SSI/AFDC (i.e., the "medically needy")	Health Care Financing Administration/HHS	State medical agency
	2176 "waiver" services (e.g., case management, homemaker, personal care, adult day care, habilitation, respite, and other services at state option)[d]	Aged, blind, disabled, or mentally ill Medicaid eligibles (including children) living in the community who would require nursing home level care; at state option, persons living in the community with higher income than normally allowed under a state Medicaid plan		In some case the 2176 "waiver" program may be administered by another agency (e.g., state agency on aging)
Medicare/Title XVIII of Social Security Act	100 days of skilled nursing facility care; Home health; hospice	Generally Social Security status; persons 65 years and over; persons under 65 years entitled to federal disability benefits; and certain persons with terminal renal disease	Health Care Financing Administration/HHS	Not applicable

244

Program	Services	Eligibility	Federal agency	State agency
Social Services Block Grant/Title XX of Social Security Act	Various social services as defined by the state, including homemaker, home health aide, personal care, home-delivered meals	No federal requirements; states may require means tests	Office of Human Development Services/HHS	State social services/human resources agency; in some cases other state agencies may administer a portion of Title XX fund for certain groups (e.g., state agency on aging)
Older Americans Act/Title III	Variety of social services as determined by state and area agencies on aging, with priority on in-home services; also case management, day care, protective services; separate appropriation for home-delivered meals	Persons ≥60 years; no means tests, but services are to be targeted on those with social or economic need	Administration on Aging/Office of Human Development Services/HHS	State agency on aging
Supplemental Security Income/Title XVI of Social Security Act	Federal income support; maximum federal payment for persons with no income is $325 per individual and $488 per couple in 1985; supplemental payment for nonmedical housing and/or in-home services, as determined by state	Aged, blind, disabled persons who meet federally established income and resources requirements; states may make payments to other state-defined eligibility groups	Social Security Administration/HHS	State supplemental payment program may be state or federally administered

SOURCE: O'Shaughnessy C. Price R, Griffith J: Financing and Delivery of Long-Term Services for the Elderly. Washington, DC, Congressional Research Service, Library of Congress Publ. No. 85-1033 EPW, October 17, 1985.

[a]Required for individuals over age 21.

[b]At option of the state.

[c]Required for individuals entitled to skilled nursing home care.

[d]May be offered under a waiver of Medicaid State plan requirements, if requested by the state and approved by HHS. May include waiver of Medicaid eligibility requirements and stipulation that services be offered on a statewide basis.

services in order to accommodate clients' needs for specific services and for a continuum of care approach to care. However, dramatic changes will be necessary, and they are likely to occur slowly over time, rather than in one major change. Thus the financing of comprehensive, coordinated care will continue for some time to require creativity on the part of all health and social service organizations.

THE LONG-TERM CONTINUUM OF THE FUTURE

Do continuums of long-term care exist? Is it possible to overcome the problems of fragmentation, financing, and access to create an effective, efficient, consumer-oriented, high-quality system of care? Few, if any, complete continuums of long-term care are now in operation in the late 1980s. However, the feasibility of a continuum of care has been ably demonstrated. Select programs throughout the nation provide encouragement for the future. These include:

At the national level: the National Long-Term Care Demonstration Project sites, the federal Channeling Grant Projects, the Social HMOs
At the state level: California's Multi-Service Senior Program and Linkages, Connecticut's Community Care program, Oregon's FIG
At the private level: The Robert Wood Johnson Foundation Program for Hospital Initiatives in Long-Term Care, various continuing care retirement communities

Each of these has multiple components of the continuum of long-term care, including integrating mechanisms and an array of services. Streamlined management and the consistent impact of these systems on quality and cost effectiveness remain to be achieved. Clearly, the challenge to health care organizations of the future will be to formulate and refine the operations of the continuum of care so that comprehensive systems incorporating both long-term and acute care become the norm (Table 7-6).

In contrast to Mr. J's experience, how do extant and future continuums provide long-term care? The following scenario already occurs in exemplary organizations:

> Mrs. Smith is an 80-year-old widow who lives alone. She slips in the bath tub and breaks her hip. She uses her voice-activated emergency response system necklace to call for help. When received, the call automatically asks what the problem is, then calls both a neighbor and emergency assistance. The neighbor comes over to be with Mrs. Smith, having agreed in advance to help in times of emergency. The paramedics also arrive within minutes, stabilize Mrs. Smith, and take her to the hospital. Mrs. Smith belongs to a hospital-initiated senior program, Senior Services (SenSer), which was notified automatically via computer when the call came in. A decal in Mrs. Smith's front window also alerted the paramedics that Mrs. Smith is a SenSer member. By the time that Mrs. Smith arrives at the hospital's emergency department, her admission information is already processed and her internist has been contacted.
> While in the hospital, a case manager, with whom Mrs. Smith talked when she enrolled in SenSer, visits her and reassures her that whatever services she needs

will be arranged. When Mrs. Smith has recovered enough to be discharged from the acute service, she is transferred to a rehabilitation-oriented skilled nursing facility operated by the hospital. Mrs. Smith never liked the idea of being in a "nursing home," but she does not feel negative about this one because the ambience is positive, the staff are pleasant and encouraging, and she is confident that her physician and case manager will arrange her transfer home.

Indeed, several weeks later Mrs. Smith goes home with home health nursing and rehabilitation follow-up. Meals on Wheels brings a hot meal daily for 4 weeks, and a homemaker comes in twice a week to help with personal care, shopping, mail, and housekeeping. The emergency response system gives Mrs. Smith the security to remain alone at night, and she knows that she can call the Senior Services number at any time if she has questions or needs nonemergent assistance. Mrs. Smith also knows that her physician is regularly informed of what is happening to her.

Mrs. Smith's total spell of illness cost her very little out of pocket. The health care services she used were all participants in the Medicare HMO in which she was enrolled. She paid regular monthly payments in addition to Medicare Parts A and B, which covered a variety of long-term care services. As long as Mrs. Smith did not exceed the lifetime allowance, she could use whatever levels of institutional or community-based services her physician and case manager felt necessary. Mrs. Smith also had the peace of mind of knowing that she had organized her legal and financial affairs well in advance—just in case anything serious happened to her. A social worker from SenSer had helped her to prepare a will, designate a sibling to handle temporary durable power of attorney, and express her preferences to her physician about desire to have life-sustaining measures.

POLICY ISSUES

The public policy issues pertaining to long-term care are complex, and most can be approached from several different perspectives (72–79)—making a conclusive assessment, or a definitive discussion, difficult. This section outlines the major policy issues that should be considered by those involved in creating or managing a continuum of care. The ultimate resolution of the problems is likely to take place gradually. Thus the specifics of the issues may be different in any given year, but the overriding concerns are likely to remain for some time.

FRAGMENTATION

As is evident from the preceding discussion, the continuum of care consists of a myriad of different services, each provided by different organizations and each funded by several different public and/or private sources. To provide any type of comprehensive, continuous care requires achieving cohesion. At the same time, flexibility must be maintained in order to tailor the program to the unique needs of each individual. Individual service providers and agencies must cooperate—and, although this is readily acknowledged, establishing the mechanisms to do so requires overcoming history and learned preference.

Funding for long-term care services comes from health, mental health, social service, public welfare, social security, and housing programs, to mention only a few. Each payer, whether private or public, has distinct requirements. Fragmentation of delivery is likely to continue as long as the funding streams remain separate. The intent of the continuum of care is to be able to pool funding streams in order to provide the services required by any individual. However, putting in place the mechanisms to do this is ahead of the field.

QUALITY

Quality is one of the nation's major concerns about health care, and about long-term care in particular. Nursing homes are notorious for questionable quality, even though the majority provide adequate care (80,81). Rigorous standards have been imposed by Medicare and Medicaid, as well as by state licensing and certification programs, to try to ensure a minimum level of quality. Professional organizations and consumer groups are also active in establishing criteria and programs to enhance quality (82,83).

The issues, however, are likely to remain. The majority of persons requiring care over a prolonged period of time have basic functional disabilities, and the care provider other than family or friends is likely to be an unskilled aide. Such persons are paid very low wages, often have difficult and unpleasant work, and have little incentive to remain on the job, let alone excel.

The financing of long-term care affects more than the personnel issue. With minimum financing, long-term care services simply cannot afford the physical or technological luxuries that acute care services or families can offer. Quality must be balanced with the amount of demand and resource allocation. These become issues for society, as well as individual patients and organizations.

FINANCING

The financing of the continuum of care is extremely complex, and numerous books have been written on the problems (84–87) and potential resolutions of various segments. In general, however:

- The level of fundings for long-term care is disproportionately less than that for acute care (most would say too little, regardless of the relationships to spending for other purposes).
- Despite low levels of funding, long-term care in the aggregate is extremely expensive for the individual as well as society. The annual cost of nursing home care is roughly the same as the annual income for a family of four. The cost of long-term care can cause an individual or family to become impoverished. One-half to one-third of state Medicaid budgets are spent on long-term care.
- Funding is also highly fragmented, as noted above. This inhibits economies of scale and efficiencies of operation.

- Funding sources also restrict flexibility of care by specifying in detail the services that can and cannot be paid for by a given payer.
- A confusing assortment of payment systems have evolved under Medicare, Medicaid, HMOs, and private insurance. Each state has its own financing and administrative system for long-term care and related services. Dealing with various funding systems results in consumption of regulatory and operator resources, to no particular benefit for the consumer.

As the older and disabled populations grow in number over the coming decades, the need and demand for health care have the potential to bankrupt the Medicare trust fund and jeopardize the financial viability of state governments, as well as impoverish patients and their families. The continuum of care offers potential benefits in handling the financing of both acute and long-term care. However, these problems constrain the ease with which a continuum can maximize its potential to achieve financial viability.

PROVIDER ATTITUDES AND KNOWLEDGE

Long-term care is traditionally the stepchild of health care professionals, as well as funders (88). Many providers find that acute care, with its high technology and patient goals of curing, is far more exciting than the comparatively low technology and functional goals of long-term care. Biomedical knowledge about geriatrics has expanded rapidly during the 1970s and 1980s. As a result, the health profession's educational programs now give greater attention to geriatrics and long-term care than in the past. However, professional rewards and compensation still favor acute care. In the final sense, the provision of professional care is dependent on the individual practitioner's attitudes and skills.

CONSUMER DEMAND AND CHOICE

Most consumers do not want to think about long-term care in any form. When the American Association for Retired Persons (AARP) launched a new program of long-term care insurance, nearly 0.25 million flyers were sent out. The response was only 1200 (89). Similarly, a nationwide survey by the AARP found that the majority of persons age 65 and older did not know what services Medicare actually covered. Furthermore, most believed that Medicare covers nursing home care (90). It is difficult for policymakers or health care providers to change the system for long-term care when consumers do not support this as a priority. Increasing consumer understanding about the organization and financing of the continuum of long-term care is thus essential.

Federal and state governments, employers, and insurance companies are placing constraints on consumers' choice of health care. Some state Medicaid programs, for example, limit the providers that enrollees can go to. As demand grows and resources become tight, greater constraints might be enacted. As systems such as the continuum of care are implemented, with the intent to produce economies of scale and efficiencies of operations, the freedom of choice for the consumer must be considered.

AVAILABILITY AND ACCESSIBILITY

Despite the growth of health, mental health, and social support programs during the past decades, there are still services that are not universally available or accessible. Adult day care centers, for example, numbered about 1000 nationally in 1985, and most serve only 20–50 persons per day. Nursing home beds are in short supply in some parts of the country because the state, in an attempt to limit Medicaid spending, has not allowed the construction of new facilities. For some services, availability and accessibility remains an issue and one that is closely tied to amount of public program money allocated to long-term care. The operation of a continuum of care assumes access to the key services. Thus, to the extent that public policy (and funding) limits service access or availability, the continuum of care will be abbreviated and patient flow inhibited accordingly.

Long-term care in the United States has undergone major changes in the last 20 years and will continue to change very markedly in the future. It has gone from an insular, isolated system of care located mostly in nursing homes to a broader, more extensive network of many services available at many locations throughout the community. Its financing sources, its coordinating mechanisms, and its general attitude and atmosphere have changed greatly, as has public awareness of its increasing importance in the future. The future for the continuum of care, while challenged by all of the various forces facing health care in general today, is impressive and exciting.

REFERENCES

1. Perrott G St J, et al: *Care of the Long-Term Patient: Source Book on Size and Characteristics of the problem.* PHS Publ. No. 344, Washington, DC, U.S. Government Printing Office, 1954.
2. Katz S, Ford AB, Moskowitz RW, et al: Studies of illness in the aged. The index of ADL: A standardized measure of biological and psychosocial function. *JAMA* 1985; 185:94.
3. Lawton P, Brody E: Assessment of older people, self-maintaining and instrumental activities of daily life. *The Gerontologist* 1969; 9:179–186.
4. Manton K, Soldo B: Dynamics of health changes in the oldest old: New perspectives and evidence. *Milbank Mem Fund Quart* 1985; 63:206–285.
5. Weissert W: Size and characteristics of the non-institutional long-term care population. *Project to Analyze Existing Long-Term Care Data, Final Report,* Vol. II. U.S. Department of Health and Human Services, July 1983.
6. Weissert W, Scanlon W: Estimating the long-term care population: National prevalence rates and selected characteristics. *Project to Analyze Existing Long-Term Care Data, Final Report,* Vol. II. U.S. Department of Health and Human Services, July 1983.
7. Rice D, Wick A: *Impact of An Aging Population of Health Care Need. State Projections.* Institute for Health & Aging, San Francisco, University of California, 1985.

8. U.S. Bureau of the Census: *Projections of the Population of the United States by Age, Sex, and Race: 1983 to 2080.* Current Population Reports, Series P-25, No. 952, May 1984.

9. Arthur Young: *Long Term Care: An Industry Composite, 1985.* New York, Arthur Young International, 1985, p 3.

10. Winn S: Course on Long-Term Care. Department of Health Services Administration, School of Public Health and Community Medicine, University of Washington, Seattle, WA, 1978.

11. Brody E: *The Long-Term Care of Older People: A Practical Guide.* New York, Human Sciences Press, 1977, p 14.

12. Kane R, Kane R: *Values and Long-Term Care.* Lexington, MA, Lexington Books, 1982, p 2.

13. Pollack W: *Expanding Health Benefits for the Elderly.* Vol. I, *Long-Term Care.* Washington, DC, The Urban Institute, 1979, p 2.

14. U.S. Department of Health, Education and Welfare: *Areawide Planning for Facilities for Long-Term Treatment and Care.* Report of the Joint Committee of the American Hospital Association and Public Health Service. PHS Pub. No. 930-B-1, Washington, DC, U.S. Government Printing Office, 1963, p 8.

15. Weissert W: Long-term care: An overview, *Health, United States, 1978,* USDHEW Publ. No. 78-1232, Washington, DC, U.S. Government Printing Office, 1978, p 93.

16. Doty P, Liu K, Wiener J: An overview of long-term care. *Health Care Financ Rev* 1985; 6.

17. Evashwick C, Weiss L: *Managing the Continuum of Care: A Practical Guide to Organization and Operations.* Rockville, MD, Aspen Publishers, 1987.

18. Evashwick C: Long-Term Care Becomes Major New Role for Hospitals. *Hospitals* 1982; 56.

19. The Hospital Research and Educational Trust: *The Role of the Hospital in Caring for the Elderly.* Chicago, The Hospital Research and Educational Trust, 1983.

20. Persily N, Brody S: *Hospitals and the Aged: The New Old Market.* Rockville, MD, Aspen Publishers, 1984.

21. Rochleau B: *Hospitals and Community-Oriented Programs for the Elderly: Innovations in Health Care.* Ann Arbor, MI, AUPHA Press, 1983.

22. American Hospital Association: *Hospital Statistics, 1984.* Chicago, American Hospital Association, 1985.

23. Evashwick C, Rundall T, Goldiamond B: Hospital services for seniors: Results of a national survey. *The Gerontologist* 1985; Vol:631–637.

24. *Emerging Trends in Aging and Long-Term Care Services.* Chicago, Hospital Research and Educational Trust, 1986.

25. American Hospital Association, op cit (Ref. 22).

26. Mullner R, Nuzum F, Matthews D: Inpatient medical rehabilitation: Results of the 1981 Survey of Hospitals and Units. *Arch Phys Med Rehab* 1983; 64:354–358.

27. Evashwick C: *Hospitals and Older Adults: Current Actions and Future Trends.* Chicago, The Hospital Research and Educational Trust, 1982.

28. Campion E, May M: Why acute care hospitals must undertake long-term care. *New Engl J Med* 1983; 308.

29. Evashwick C, Read W: Hospitals and LTC: Options, alternatives, implications. *J Healthcare Financ Management,* 1985; 52–58.

30. American Hospital Association, Hospital Data Center, direct communication, 1986.

31. Evashwick C: Long-Term Care Becomes Major New Role, *op cit* (Ref. 18), pp 50–55.

32. Robert Wood Johnson Foundation Program for Hospital Initiatives in Long-Term Care: Program Brochure, 1984.

33. Rice, Wick: op cit (Ref. 7).

34. National Center for Health Statistics; Sirrocco A: Nursing and related care homes as reported from the 1980 NMFI survey. *Vital and Health Statistics,* Series 14, No. 29, DHHS Publ. No. (PHS) 84-1842, Public Health Service, Washington, DC, U.S. Government Printing Office, December 1983.

35. Ibid.

36. American Health Care Association pamphlet, Washington, DC, American Health Care Association, no date.

37. Health Care Financing Administration, direct communication, January 1987.

38. Kane R, Kane R: Long-Term Care, in Williams S, Torrens P (eds): *Introduction to Health Services,* 2 ed. New York, Wiley, 1984.

39. Palmore E: Total chance of institutionalization among the aged. *The Gerontologist* 1976; 16:504–507.

40. Vincent L, Wiley JA, Carrington RA: The risk of institutionalization before death. *The Gerontologist* 1979; 19:

41. Rice, Wick: op cit (Ref. 7).

42. O'Shaughnessy C, Price R, Griffith J: *Financing and Delivery of Long-Term Care Services for the Elderly.* Library of Congress Publ. No. 85-1033 EPW, Washington, DC, Congressional Research Service, October 17, 1985.

43. Kerschner P: Keynote Address. Long-Term Care Conference, Los Angeles, CA, January 26, 1987.

44. Health Care Financing Administration: Medicare Data, Table No. AA12. *Outreach* 1986; 5.

45. National Association for Home Care: Facts about home care: The Numbers. *Homecare,* March 26, 1986.

46. Ibid.

47. Health Care Financing Administration: Medicare Statistics Division, personal communication, January 1987.

48. Zimmerman J: *Hospice: Complete Care for the Terminally Ill.* Baltimore-Munich, Urban and Schwarzenber, 1981.

49. Lack SA, Buckinghma RW: *The First American Hospice—Three Years of Home Care.* New Haven, CT, The Connecticut Hospice, 1978.

50. National Hospice Organization: Fact Sheet. Arlington, VA, National Hospice Organization, 1986.

51. Torrens P: *Hospice Programs and Public Policy.* Chicago, American Hospital Association, 1984.

52. National Hospice Organization, op cit (Ref. 50).

53. Health Care Financing Administration, Medicare Statistics Division, personal communication, January 1987.

54. Tedesco J, Oberlander DeW: *Adult Day Care.* Chicago, The Hospital Research and Educational Trust, 1983.

55. Von Behren R: *Adult Day Care in America: Summary of a National Survey.* Washington, DC, National Council on Aging National Institute for Adult Day Care, 1986.

56. Ibid.

57. Pfeiffer E (ed.): *Daycare for Older Adults: A Conference Report.* Durham, NC, Duke University Center for the Study of Aging and Human Development, 1977.

58. National Council on the Aging National Institute for Adult Day Care: *Standards for Adult Day Care,* Washington, DC, National Council on the Aging, 1984.

59. Tedesco, Oberlander, op cit (Ref. 54).

60. Steinberg R, Carter G: *Case Management and the Elderly,* Lexington, MA, DC Heath & Co., Lexington Books, 1983.

61. Evashwick C, Ney J, Siemon J: *Case Management: Issues for Hospitals.* Chicago, Hospital Research and Educational Trust, 1985.

62. Weiss L: Care coordination, in Evashwick and Weiss, op cit (Ref. 17).

63. Zawadski R: *Community-Based Systems of Long Term Care.* New York, The Haworth Press, 1983.

64. Bennet R, Frisch S, Gurland B, et al: *Coordinated Service Delivery Systems for the Elderly.* New York, The Haworth Press, 1984.

65. Hamm L, Kickham T, Cutler D: Research, demonstration and evaluations, in Vogel R, Palmer H (eds): *Long-Term Care: Perspectives from Research and Demonstrations.* Rockville, MD, Aspen Publishers, 1985.

66. O'Shaughnessy et al op cit (Ref. 42).

67. National Chamber Foundation: *Catastrophic and Long-Term Health Care: Private Sector Alternatives.* Washington, DC, National Chamber Foundation, 1986; Lane L: The potential of private long-term care insurance. *Pride Inst J Long-Term Home Health Care* 1985; 4: ICF Inc., *Private Financing of Long-Term Care: Current Methods and Resources,* ICF Inc., January 1985.

68. Meiners M: The case for long-term care insurance. *Health Affairs* 1983; 2:

69. Leutz W, Greenberg J, Abrahams R, et al: *Changing Health Care for an Aging Society: Planning for the Social Health Maintenance Organization.* Lexington, MA, DC Heath & Co, 1985.

70. Greenberg J, Leutz W, Abrahams R: The national social health maintenance organization demonstration, *J Ambulatory Care* 1985; 8:135–142.

71. InterStudy: *National HMO Census, 1985.* Excelsior, MN, InterStudy, 1986.

72. Harrington C, Newcomer R, Estes C: *Long-Term Care of the Elderly: Public Policy Issues.* Beverly Hills, CA, Sage Publications, 1985.

73. Meltzer J, Farrow F, Richman H: *Policy Options in Long-Term Care.* Chicago, The University of Chicago Press, 1981.

74. LaPorte V, Rubin J: *Reform and Regulation in Long-Term Care.* New York, Praeger, 1979.

75. Oriel W: *The Complex Cube of Long-Term Care.* Silver Spring, MD, American Health Planning Association, 1985.

76. Federal Council of the Aging: *The Need for Long-Term Care:* Information and Issues. DHHS Publication No. (OHDS) 81-20704, Washington, DC, Department of Health and Human Services, 1981.

77. Health Care Financing Administration: *Long-Term Care: Background and Future Directions: Discussion Paper.* DHHS Publ. No. (HCFA) 81-20047, Washington, DC, Department of Health and Human Services, 1981.

78. National Council on the Aging: *Public Policy Agenda.* Washington, DC, National Council on the Aging, 1986.

79. Callahan J, Wallack S: *Reforming the Long-Term Care System.* Lexington, MA, DC Heath & Co., 1981.

80. Vladeck B: *Unloving Care: The Nursing Home Tragedy.* New York, Basic Books, 1980.

81. Moss F, Halamandaris V: *Too Old, Too Sick, Too Bad: Nursing Homes in America.* Germantown, MD, Aspen Systems Corp., 1977.

82. National Institute on Medicine, Committee on Nursing Home Regulation: *Improving the Quality of Care in Nursing Homes.* Washington, DC, National Institute of Medicine, March, 1986.

83. Smith D: *Long-Term Care in Transition: The Regulation of Nursing Homes.* Ann Arbor, MI, AUPHA Press, 1981.

84. Davis K, Rowland D: *Medicare Policy: New Directions for Health and Long-Term Care.* Baltimore, MD, The Johns Hopkins University Press, 1986; Healthcare Financial Management Association: Long-Term Care: Challenges and Opportunities. Oakbrook, IL, Healthcare Financial Management Association, 1985; Tedesco J (ed): *Financing Quality Care for the Elderly.* Chicago, IL, The Hospital Research and Educational Trust, 1985.

85. Davidson S: *Medicaid Decisions: A Systematic Analysis of the Cost Problem.* Cambridge, MA, Ballinger, 1980; Congressional Budget Office: *Medicaid: Choices for 1982 and Beyond.* Washington, DC, Congressional Budget Office, June 1981.

86. National Task Force on Long-Term Care Policies, Health Care Financing Administration, Department of Health and Human Services: Series of Task Force Working Papers. Washington, DC, Health Care Financing Administration, 1986.

87. Congressional Research Service: *Long-Term Services for the Elderly: Background Materials on Financing and Delivery of Long-Term Care Services for the Elderly.* Washington, DC, U.S. Government Printing Office, 1986; Feinstein P, Gornick M, Greenberg J: *Long-Term Care Financing and Delivery Systems: Exploring Some Alternatives.* HCFA Publ. No. 03174, Baltimore, MD, Department of Health and Human Services Health Care Financing Administration, June 1984.

88. Evashwick, Weiss: Section IV: Human Resources. *Managing the Continuum,* op cit (Ref. 17).

89. Personal communication, American Association of Retired Person, 1986.

90. Cafferata G: Knowledge of their health insurance coverage by the elderly. *Med Care* 1984; 22:835–847.

CHAPTER 8

Mental Health Services: Growth and Development of a System

Mary Richardson

Mental health services have experienced considerable growth and change over the last several decades. Who is treated, and the problems they are treated for, have altered with changing definitions of mental illness, changing viewpoints about the appropriate response to mental health problems, and increasing social recognition and acceptance of mental health services as a treatment rather than a custodial function. This chapter describes the development of mental health services in this country, the users and reasons for use, the organization and financing of services, recent trends, and the problems of providing care. Although related issues of utilization and financing are discussed in other chapters, the unique nature of mental health services are presented in detail in this chapter.

HISTORICAL PERSPECTIVES ON DEFINITIONS OF MENTAL ILLNESS

Societies have always defined and classified human behavior in ways that differentiated between what was acceptable and what was not. Description of the more subtle maladaptations of human beings to society involves attention to social and cultural values; as value systems change, so do conceptions of deviant behavior. Societal tolerance of deviant behavior partially determines what constitutes mental illness. In more recent times, psychiatric or emotional disability has been defined within biologic, sociologic, and cultural frameworks. However, scientific definitions have philosophical roots in a history that predates much current scientific thought.

During the Middle Ages, aberrant behavior was attributed to demonic influences, evil spirits, and the like. In an agrarian feudal society, deviance relates to the ability to work and sustain oneself. People regarded as "mad" were allowed to wander about if they were not too troublesome (1). Communities were able to offer them some basic support; if they became troublesome, they were driven away.

With the rise of a mercantile society in Europe and a breakdown of feudal estates, major social and political upheavals occurred. Many people were left homeless, with no means of support. Groups of unemployed people and disbanded soldiers drifted around the countryside. Persons who had previously been defined as mad or insane were classified together with those who were poor or homeless. They were grouped together in a much larger category of people considered to be socially destitute. Small communities quickly lost the ability to offer even minimal support to these people.

In England, the Elizabethan Poor Laws of 1601 heralded a recognition of the responsibility of government, and society as a whole, in addressing the problems of the destitute and the ill. In each community parish, overseers were assigned to provide care for these sick and disaffected members of society. Later, lunatic hospitals were opened throughout England. These hospitals existed more to protect the citizenry by isolating social misfits than to provide even a minimum of care. Conditions in these institutions were generally abominable. Inmates were often chained and provided only the barest essentials of survival.

In 1656 the French Parliament authorized the construction of the Hôpital Generale. The poor, the sick, and the insane were confined in circumstances much like those of the English lunatic hospitals. However, with the eighteenth century came the Age of Enlightenment and a revolution in scientific thought. In France, Philippe Pinel introduced the idea of mental illness with a medical framework (2). Pinel was initially the physician of the Infirmaries at the Hospice de Bicêtre in Paris. Although he was historically given credit for unchaining the inmates and introducing humanistic treatment, writings discovered more recently reveal that it was actually Jean-Baptiste Pussin, the governor of mental patients, who had actually begun this more humane treatment (2). The ideas of both Pinel and Pussin, who had once been a patient at Bicetre, spread throughout Europe and later to the United States.

In the late 1800s, Kraepelin, a German physician, outlined a concise system of classification establishing mental illness as a separate and distinct disease entity subject to the rules that applied to physical or somatic diseases. His work legitimized psychiatry as a branch of medicine. Kraepelin described in detail the symptoms, course of the disease, and prognosis of dementia praecox and manic–depressive psychoses. Sigmund Freud, the father of psychoanalysis, described neuroses in a deterministic fashion by proposing that all events could be traced to a specific origin. He described mental illness as related to disturbances and distortions from unconscious developmental difficulties in psychic growth and maturation and traumatic experiences and conflicts over sexual and self-destructive instincts. Although psychotherapy came to be regarded as a medical and psychiatric specialty, Freud established the psychological viewpoint.

Continuing biomedical research in the twentieth century produced evidence that supported the concept of organic causations for mental illness. The discovery of the spirochete that causes syphilis and general paresis and discoveries of chromosomal aberrations in mental retardation were cited as such evidence. Studies of schizophrenia, defined as a diagnosis by Bleuler in the early 1900s (replacing dementia praecox) and manic–depressive syndromes have suggested possible familial tendencies. For example, 10 percent of siblings and children of schizophrenic patients are also diagnosed as schizophrenic, possibly indicating a biogenetic basis for this illness. Transcultural studies of mental illness have demonstrated remarkably uniform prevalence rates for schizophrenia in different countries and cultures. However, modern techniques for the study of chromosomal aberrations do not isolate genetic differences, and even with clinical evidence suggesting a biologic component, critics would argue that a diagnosis of schizophrenia is highly subjective, and that the perception of behavior as being schizophrenic is relative to the environmental context. Studies of other illnesses such as the neurotic or drug abuse syndromes have so far been unable to identify biogenetic factors.

SOCIAL PSYCHIATRIC AND BEHAVIORAL DEFINITIONS

During the twentieth century there has been increasing acceptance of pluralistic determinants of mental illness, including biologic, sociologic, and social factors. Harry Sullivan was the first American psychiatrist to develop a theory stressing the importance of interpersonal relations in disease etiology. Concurrent with the development of social psychiatric definitions were new psychological and behavioral concepts of mental illness. Carl Jung broke away from the Freudian approach and formed the field of analytic psychology. Erich Fromm, a psychoanalyst never trained in medicine, and others applied anthropologic and sociologic concepts to Freud's theories. Later, John B. Watson discarded Freudian theory and developed behaviorism, which recognized only observable behavior as critical to the diagnosis of mental illness. He believed that all behavior was predictable on the basis of environmental stimuli. Psychologists introduced classic conditioning and learning theory to psychiatrists and other psychopathologists.

Social psychiatric and behavioral definitions of mental health reduced reliance on the disease concept of mental illness as internally manifested by the client; rather, social and cultural relativity and personality development were emphasized as significant factors in mental health. The development of humanistic psychology also had origins in the behavioral movements. The Freudian approach was considered too pessimistic and the behavioral approaches too mechanistic. Carl Rogers developed the technique of client-centered therapy, which recognized the clients' roles in affecting their own rehabilitation. According to this approach, client behavior is compared to expected behavior for the culture or environment of the patient. Differences between adaptive and maladaptive functioning vary from culture to culture and are more or less acceptable according to one's economic or social status. The validity of these broader environmentally based approaches are supported by transcultural psychiatric research that documents mental illness in all cultures and suggests that outward manifestations of these illnesses are shaped by the childrearing practices, indoctrinations, sanctions, encouragements, and discouragements of each culture.

Definitions of mental illness may also be predicated on the social and cultural values of the care provider and may be in conflict with the accepted norms of the recipient. This problem can be difficult if care providers are representative of the majority group within a population and the potential recipient is a member of a minority group. Behavior that is tolerated, accepted, or even encouraged within the minority group may be seen as deviant or sick behavior by the majority group. For example, an epidemiologic study of psychiatric disorders in a Pacific Northwest coastal Indian village revealed differing symptom patterns in men and women (3). Women, suffering more from psychoneuroses, were viewed as ill within this society, whereas men, generally suffering from alcoholism, not only did not seek treatment but were not even considered ill by their community. Hence treatment for women was accepted and even encouraged, whereas treatment of men was not. Finally, defining the overlap between social problems and mental illness is difficult. Are deviations such as delinquency or criminal behavior a mental health problem? What about poverty, discrimination, and unemployment? Mental health professionals must determine the extent of their roles as caregivers and as agents of social change.

EXTENT OF MENTAL DISORDERS

The American Psychiatric Association classifies mental illness within three general categories: impairment of brain tissue, mental deficiency, and disorders without a clearly defined clinical cause. Most disorders treated by mental health professionals fall in the third category, but diagnosis of these problems is subjective in actual clinical practice. The Diagnostic and Statistical Manual (DSM III), published by the American Psychiatric Association, contains this classification system, which is used extensively in diagnosing mental illness (4). These classifications are generally used in studies of incidence and prevalence of mental disorder.

Recently, the National Institute for Mental Health (NIMH) sponsored a multisite epidemiologic and health services research study, entitled the "Epidemiologic Catchment Area (ECA) Program," that assesses mental disorder prevalence, incidence, and service use rates in about 20,000 community and institutional residents (5). An interview schedule, called the "Diagnostic Interview Schedule (DIS)," was developed for use by lay interviewers to assess the presence, duration, and severity of symptoms in study participants according to DSM III diagnostic criteria. Interviews were subsequently scored by computer according to diagnostic algorithms specified by DSM III and other diagnostic systems.

INCIDENCE AND PREVALENCE OF MENTAL ILLNESS

There are an estimated 29.4 million Americans who suffer from mental illness (6). An ECA study of the 6-month prevalence of 15 mental disorders in the United States revealed between 16.4 and 23.1 percent of the population to have diagnosable mental disorders (6). Phobias were found to be the most common mental disorder, affecting from 5.1 to 12.5 percent of those surveyed. Substance abuse disroders, including alcohol abuse/dependence, is the second most common category, found in 4.8 to 7.5 percent of Americans. Affective disorders, including major depression, were found in 4.1 to 6.6 percent of those surveyed. Schizophrenia was reported for 0.6–1.2 percent of Americans.

Prevalence rates vary for men and women and according to age. The most frequent diagnosis for men aged 18–64 is alcohol abuse/dependence, with severe cognitive impairment becoming the most prominent diagnosis for men ages 65 and over. Phobias are the most common diagnosis reported for women of all ages. Drug abuse/dependence is cited as the second most prevalent mental health problem for women ages 18 to 24, while major depression is more often cited by women ages 25 to 44.

The rates of mental disorders, except for cognitive impairment, dropped after age 45 for both men and women. Among substance abuse disorders, alcohol-related disorders were two to three times as prevalent as drug-related disorders.

DEVELOPMENT OF MENTAL HEALTH SERVICES IN THE UNITED STATES

EARLY MENTAL HEALTH SYSTEM

The development of American psychiatry in the nineteenth century was strongly influenced by Dr. Benjamin Rush, long considered the father of American psychiatry, who was also a pioneer in hospital reform. Before the nineteenth century, formal treatment centers were nonexistent. Private physician services were available to those with money. The rest faced imprisonment or hospitalization, with one not much different from the other. Ths hospital reform spearheaded by Pinel in the late 1700s in France was paralleled in this country by Rush's activities. The American Psychiatric Association was started through the efforts of affiliated hospital superintendents who, like Rush, were concerned with hospital conditions. Even into the early twentieth century, treatment of mental illness based on medical/clinical approaches occurred in state-supported hospitals, which were often located in remote areas and functioned as large human warehouses.

The disease concept of mental illness implies that the patient can become "well" and generally assumes that the therapist, historically a psychiatrist, will diagnose the illness and define subsequent treatment. The Freudian model has led to long-term and intensive psychotherapy and to therapeutic and personal requirements that are beyond the resources available to the state hospitals. Mental illness was also highly stigmatized and subject to funding limitations by state legislatures, with the primary purpose of providing public protection from "crazy people," rather than providing a public good for people with psychiatric problems.

The National Mental Health Act of 1946 (PL 79-487) signified an increased federal interest in the plight of the mentally ill. The law created the National Institute of Mental Health and increased appropriations for therapy and research. In addition, recognition of the psychological problems of soldiers during World War II motivated Veterans Administration (VA) hospitals to provide expanded mental health services.

DEINSTITUTIONALIZATION AND THE GROWTH OF OUTPATIENT SERVICES

The development of psychopharmacology in the 1950s had a profound impact on the field of mental health. Psychotropic drugs led to dramatic breakthroughs in the treatment of mental illness and enabled thousands of patients previously considered incurable to be effectively treated on an outpatient basis. The use of these drugs also created a climate that encouraged the development of various innovative therapeutic approaches.

Before World War II, few outpatient mental health facilities existed. With growing federal interest, the number of outpatient facilities increased. At the same time, the prognosis for the thousands of patients in mental hospitals—many of whom suffered from schizophrenia, depression, and mania—remained dismal. However, the use of antipsychotic medications for schizophrenia, antidepressants for depression, and more recently, lithium in the treatment of mania, rapidly improved the prognosis for these patients. With the development of psychotropic medications, medical/clinical models of treatment continued to be the major influence on hospital treatment of mental illness. Psychotropic drugs also led to a radical decline in hospital lengths of stay for patients with psychiatric diagnoses. Patients now could control their behavior through the use of these drugs and, it was hoped, function within the community. Thus, a mental health system previously based primarily on inpatient facilities had to develop new approaches to serving patients who no longer needed to be hospitalized.

Although mental health professionals continued to expand their understanding of mental and emotional disorders, the general public was still distrustful of, and misinformed about, the nature of mental illness, and there was little advocacy for improvement except from the mental health community. Nevertheless, there was a dramatic increase in outpatient clinics from 400 before World War II to 1234 by 1954 (7).

Finally, in 1955 the National Mental Health Study Act (PL 84-182) was passed, which authorized $750,000 for a 3-year study of the entire mental health system. The result was the Action for Mental Health Report, published in 1961. Although this report covered many issues in the provision of mental health services, the primary emphasis of the legislation that followed, during the Kennedy Administration, was on outpatient services. Concern was increasingly focused on providing comprehensive mental health services to people not requiring hospitalization as well as to those not previously having access to mental health services. The Mental Retardation Facilities and Community Mental Health Centers Construction Act of 1964 (PL 88-164) provided construction monies for community mental health centers that were to serve designated catchment areas of 74,000–200,000 people. The five basic services that the centers were required to provide included inpatient, outpatient, emergency, day treatment, and consultation and education services. Significantly, the legislation mandated that services be provided regardless of the patient's ability to pay.

Many centers were built with the newly available funding for construction, but money for staffing and operations continued to be scarce. Finally, in 1967, an amendment to the legislation provided the necessary operations money on a matching basis, with funding for each center declining over an 8-year period. This was the "seed money" concept, and it was hoped that the construction and development of a community mental health center would encourage the community to gradually assume financial responsibility for services. Since catchment areas varied in their ability to provide matching funds, the subsidy for services in different areas also varied considerably. And although there was an allowance for the poorer communities, the capability to readily obtain local matching funds was a distinct advantage for some centers.

In retrospect, the whole notion of matching local funds ignored the inability of some communities to assume the associated financial burden, especially in areas of greatest need. Since many centers faced closure or significant reduction in services, additional legislation (PL 94-63) was passed in 1975. This law included provision for a 1-year distress grant at the end of the 8 years of operational support if alternate funding was not obtained. This legislation was designed to overhaul the community mental health center network and also to increase the original five required services to 12, including care for drug abuse problems, children, and the aged, as well as screening, follow-up, and community living services. Planning and evaluation of local community mental health services was mandated; 2 percent of each center's budget was to be used for these purposes.

Community mental health centers are also required to operate under the authority of a board of directors that represents the local community. These boards, however, are often composed of well-educated, upper-middle-income poeple who are frequently health care providers despite the location of many mental health centers in lower-income communities.

Concern for the inadequacies of the mental health system led President Jimmy Carter to establish the President's Commission on Mental Health in 1977. The President's wife, Rosalynn, served as honorary chairperson, indicating her active interest in mental health services in Georgia during Carter's tenure as governor. The report produced by the commission went on to influence policy formation and in many ways became the heart of the Carter Administration's Mental Health Systems Act, passed by Congress in 1980 (PL 96-398) (1). Although the Systems Act authorized continuation of provision to establish additional Community Mental Health Centers and authorized spending for many new initiatives, it was never implemented. Under the conservative administration of President Ronald Reagan, monies authorized were never appropriated.

ORGANIZATION AND USE OF MENTAL HEALTH SERVICES

MENTAL HEALTH SERVICE SETTINGS

According to NIMH records (6), there is an inventory of 3289 mental health organizations in the United States. Of the total, 2546, or 77.4 percent, were state operated or funded. Types of facilities included 841 providing inpatient care, 816 residential treatment care, 801 residential supportive care, 1485 partial care, and 2353 outpatient care. An NIMH ECA study of 5.6 million episodes of care revealed that 18 percent were for inpatient or residential treatment, 77 percent for outpatient care, and 5 percent for partial care. This reverses the 1955 figures, when 77 percent were inpatients or residents, and 23 percent received outpatient care.

In the past decade, the national philosophy toward deinstitutionalization has been responsible for a dramatic reduction in the census of state mental hospitals and the equally dramatic emergence of programs and facilities to transform both the nature and focus of psychiatric care. Between 1955 and 1980 the resident census of state and county mental hospitals has declined from 559,000 to 138,000, or to one-quarter of the previous census (8). There were 279 state mental hospitals reported in operation in the United States in January 1983 (9). By January 1984, this number decreased to 277. Of the state mental hospitals in operation during 1983, 30 were exclusively for children, 12 were security hospitals for the criminally insane, and 9 were teaching hospitals. The remaining 226 were not limited to a special program goal or specific clientele.

State and county mental hospitals, however, remain the predominant type of facility used, but the number of inpatients and residents served in them continue to decline.

Comparisons of 1983 data with 1981 data show that the number of beds has decreased from 140,140 to 128,626. Inpatient days decreased from 44,558,000 to 42,270,000, and the end-of-the-year hospital census decreased from 125,246 to 117,084.

Despite vigorous efforts at deinstitutionalization, state and county mental hospitals continue to be a locus of care for a wide variety of patient populations. In many respects, they serve as the "floor" of the mental health service system. Often they are the "source of last resort" and provide acute inpatient care to patients who have been unresponsive to treatment in other settings or who have exhausted their financial or other resources.

A study of the changes in one state hospital's clientele between 1972 and 1980 showed a 50 percent reduction in long-stay patients and a 27 percent increase in admissions (10). In addition, the authors report a new long-stay population. Over an 8-year period, the hospital has shifted from serving a largely homogeneous population of long-stay schizophrenics plus a smaller short-stay group of patients with similar characteristics to serving a smaller proportion of the original clientele plus larger numbers of patients with differing characteristics. While the old long-stay patients are predominantly middle-aged and elderly schizophrenics, the new patients fall into several categories, including young male schizophrenics, female schizophrenics distributed more evenly across age groups, and elderly female patients with organic brain syndromes.

The contemporary roles of state hospitals are now being reanalyzed. While it is true that state and county hospitals provide the majority of inpatient days of care, largely because of their role in long-term care, they also provide a multiplicity of other inpatient care functions to a large and especially disadvantaged and disturbed patient population (8).

Deinstitutionalization was to have shifted patient care from long-term care hospitals to short-stay hospitals and/or community mental health centers. Community mental health centers were launched with a philosophy that included responsibility to a total population, as defined within a catchment area, and a mission to serve as the base of community care for people leaving mental hospitals. They were also designed to bring mental health services to previously unserved or underserved populations. Problems beset the community mental health movement as some found fertile ground in some areas of the country and inhospitable ground in others. The availability of community-based services stimulated an increase in utilization of mental health services by many people who had never previously sought services, while the major segment of the targeted population, chronically mentally ill individuals, did not always find their way to the mental health center doorstep.

More recently, community mental health centers have experienced a shift in control of policy from federal to state authority and have undergone considerable change in staffing, array of services, and sources of revenue. Many centers are experiencing a period of organizational decline. The broad service mandate of old has been replaced by a more limited array of services. Some argue that there will soon be a revitalization of the community mental health movement, but with significant changes (11). They suggest a movement of community mental centers into the corporate private sector, maintaining the central concepts of community mental health, but becoming a corporate medicine creation such as the Preferred Provider Organization (PPO), Health Maintenance Organization (HMO), Employee Assistance Program (EAP), or other similar managed medical system, as discussed in other chapters of this book.

Of all the organized health care settings, only the nursing home (Chapter 7) can be demonstrated clearly to have become a substitute for the long-term custodial care function of the state and county mental hospital (8). Of an estimated 1.7–2.4 million chronic mentally ill Americans, approximately 150,000 have been residents of psychiatric hospitals for one year or longer, 750,000 reside in nursing homes, and the remainder live at home or in a variety of community residences, including board and care homes. The number of beds in, and the admissions to, psychiatric units of general medical hospitals increased during the period 1955–1980. However, survey data reveal no evidence that many or most of these patients were former or potential state and county hospital patients (12). On the other hand, general hospitals, especially public hospitals, do treat a segment of the chronic mentally ill population. Many would argue that current trends regarding people with chronic mental illness represent "reinstitutionalization" rather than deinstitutionalization.

An outgrowth of deinstitutionalization has been the recent appearance of scores of homeless people in urban centers across the country. In New York City, for example, an estimated 36,000 homeless inhabit the streets, shelters, subways, and abandoned buildings. A study of 100 homeless individuals treated at Bellevue Psychiatric Hospital's emergency service revealed that 96.6 percent of the sample had been hospitalized for psychiatric disabilities previously (13).

A survey of 68 homeless adults in eight urban emergency shelters in Hennepin County, Minnesota indicated significant rates of mental illness, alcoholism, minor criminality, and chronic medical and dental problems (14). Many factors, in addition to deinstitutionalization, contribute to the increase of homeless individuals. Social agencies are often unresponsive to individuals with little sophistication or tolerance for frustration, as mentally ill people are likely to be. The availability of single room occupancy hotels has decreased substantially and government cuts in various entitlement programs have drastically depleted the meager allotments available for chronic mentally ill people living in the community.

Another significant trend in the organization of mental health services has been the rapid growth of the private sector. The private psychiatric hospital is generally categorized as either nonprofit or for-profit. Few, if any, nonprofit hospitals have been founded in decades. Their financing comes from a variety of sources, including fees, endowments, grants, governmental contracts, and private donations. As of 1980, there were 184 private psychiatric hospitals in the United States, two-thirds of which were for-profit. Of these for-profit hospitals, 109 of 121 (90 percent) were owned by corporations (15). The for-profit groups have been characterized by the development of corporate chains. Admissions to private psychiatric hospitals increased toward the end of the period 1955–1975 (8). This increase, however, may reflect the expansion of private hospital insurance and a trend on the part of the federal government to be less involved in the regulation and provision of health care (16).

Outpatient care expanded rapidly in the private sector as well, accounting for most of the twelvefold increase in outpatient care episodes (8). During the period 1979–1981, the number of outpatient visits to private psychiatric hospitals more than doubled from 30,004 to 69,660 while outpatient visits, overall, decreased (12). Yet most outpatients today have had no prior inpatient experience and have not shifted their locus of care. They are simply availing themselves of a relatively new service.

UTILIZATION OF MENTAL HEALTH SERVICES

Mental health services are utilized at differing rates depending on such factors as race, age, and sex. The concepts of utilization variables and data assessment presented in

Chapter 3 are relevant to understanding and interpreting mental health data; specific aspects of use of mental health services are presented in this section.

Where people seek services differs depending on patient characteristics and payment source. Figure 8-1 indicates admission rates per 100,000 civilian population by age and type of inaptient psychiatric service. During 1980, persons in the age group 25–44 accounted for the largest percentage of admissions to the inpatient psychiatric services of state and county mental hospitals (48 percent), private psychiatric hospitals (39 percent), VA medical centers (51 percent), and nonfederal general hospitals (45 percent). When age-specific admission rates per 100,000 civilian population are compared within inpatient services, the middle age groups (18–64) generally showed higher rates than did the young (under 18) or elderly (65 and over).

Persons under 18 years of age represented 25 percent of outpatients in free-standing psychiatric outpatient clinics and 23 percent of outpatients in private psychiatric hospitals (6). Of patients receiving outpatient care, 7 percent were over 65 years of age.

Utilization of inpatient services according to sex and race is illustrated in Figure 8-2. The percentage of male admissions significantly outnumbered females in state and

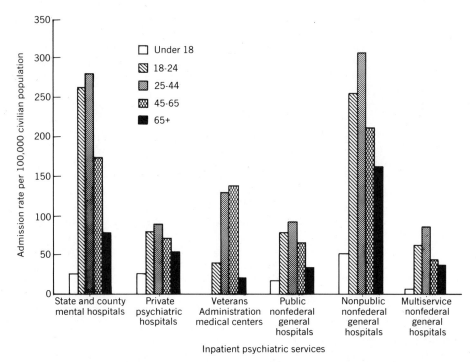

Figure 8-1. Admission rates per 100,000 civilian population, by age and type of inpatient service, United States, 1980. (SOURCE: National Institute of Mental Health; Taube CA, Barrett SA (eds): *Mental Health, United States, 1985.* Department of Health and Human Services Publishing Number (ADM) 85-1378. Washington, DC, Superintendent of Documents, U.S. Government Printing Office, 1985.)

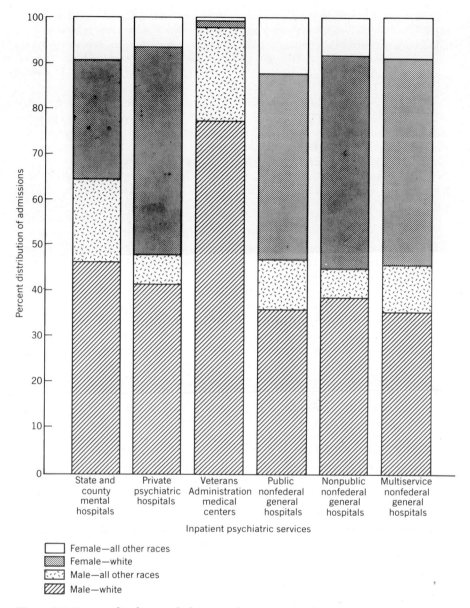

Figure 8-2. Percent distribution of admissions, by sex, race, and type of inpatient psychiatric service, United States, 1980. (SOURCE: National Institute of Mental Health; Taube CA, Barrett SA (eds): *Mental Health, United States, 1985*. Department of Health and Human Services Publishing Number (ADM) 85-1378. Washington, DC, Superintendent of Documents, U.S. Government Printing Office, 1985.)

county mental hospitals (64.9 percent vs. 35.1 percent) and, as expected, in VA medical centers. The slightly greater percentage of female admissions relative to male admissions for each of the remaining inpatient psychiatric services is consistent with the percentages of males and females in the civilian population of the United States. The highest admission rates for both males and females occurred in nonfederal general hospitals.

Comparisons among the various types of inpatient psychiatric services show that admission rates per 100,000 civilian population for whites and persons from all other races differ most widely within public mental health organizations; that is, state and county mental hospitals, public nonfederal general hospitals and VA medical centers. Persons from all other races were admitted to the inpatient psychiatric services at rates ranging from more than double to one-third more. In multiservice nonfederal general hospitals, the admission rate for persons from all other races was slightly higher than the rate for whites.

An analysis of admissions to private psychiatric hospitals reveals that most are white and over half are female. Patients are typically in their mid-thirties and are fairly well educated. Private practice psychiatrists were the major referral source for these patients on admission and discharge. They received diagnoses of affective disorders more frequently than other diagnoses.

Schizophrenia was the most frequent primary diagnosis for admission to state and county mental hospitals. It was the second most frequent diagnosis to VA medical centers, nonpublic nonfederal general hospitals, and private psychiatric hospitals (Figure 8-3). Affective disorders were the primary diagnosis for only 14 and 13 percent of admissions to VA medical centers and state and county mental hospitals, respectively. These data are consistent with the fact that chronically and severely mentally ill persons are more likely to be dependent on the public system of care. However, private settings do serve this population as well.

The percentage of admissions with primary diagnosis of alcohol-related disorders varied considerably by type of inpatient psychiatric service. They represented the most frequent primary diagnoses among admissions to VA medical centers and a significant number of admissions to state and county mental hospitals. Less than 10 percent of admissions to remaining types of inpatient psychiatric service had a primary diagnosis of alcohol-related admissions. More recent trends signify a change in regard to alcohol and drug abuse. Society, and especially employers, have begun to fully understand the major role alcohol and drug abuse/dependence plays in a wide range of physical and mental illnesses. The potential for successful early intervention in mediating the effects of abuse has been the cause for increased efforts to restructure reimbursement mechanisms and allow for improved coverage of drug and alcohol-related problems. As a result, there has been a significant increase in the number of alcohol and drug treatment programs in a variety of organizational types.

Comparisons among the inpatient psychiatric services show considerable variation in length of stay by type of diagnosis (6). State and county mental hospital admissions with organic disorders had the longest inpatient stay, followed by admissions related to schizophrenia. Length of stay is also affected by principal source of payment. State and county mental hospitals had the longest median inpatient stays for each expected principal source of payment, with the exception of commercial insurance. Admissions expected to use commercial insurance had the longest median stay (21 days) in private psychiatric hospitals. These data support the notion that restructuring of mental health benefits by third-party resources has had a profound impact on the increase of private psychiatric hospitals.

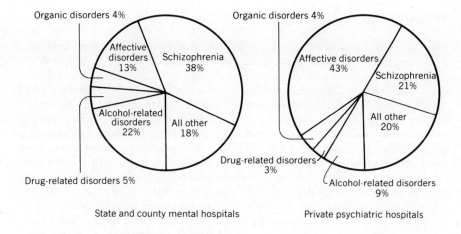

State and county mental hospitals

Private psychiatric hospitals

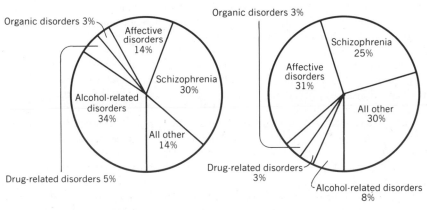

Veterans Administration medical centers

Nonfederal general hospitals

Figure 8-3. Percent distribution of admissions, by selected primary diagnosis and type of inpatient psychiatric service, United States, 1980. (SOURCE: National Institute of Mental Health; Taube CA, Barrett SA (eds): *Mental Health, United States, 1985*. Department of Health and Human Services Publishing Number (ADM) 85-1378. Washington, DC, Superintendent of Documents, U.S. Government Printing Office, 1985.)

MENTAL HEALTH PERSONNEL

There are many different types of professionals providing mental health services. They involve a number of interesting and complex issues, mostly unique to the mental health field and discussed in this chapter, but often also similar to other personnel issues discussed in Chapter 10.

PSYCHIATRISTS

Psychiatry is the medical specialty dealing with mental disorders. Traditional psychiatry offers medical/clinical definitions of mental illness. Social psychiatry, in contrast, is concerned with the environmental and societal phenomena involved in mental and emotional disorders and the use of social forces in the treatment of such disorders. Much of the scientific work of social psychiatry has been in the area of epidemiology, particularly estimation of the incidence and prevalence of mental illness in community and hospital settings. Growing concern for the environment in large mental hospitals during and after World War II also added impetus to the social psychiatric movement, and as early as 1946, the American Psychiatric Association adopted a rigid set of standards for mental hospitals and appointed a Central Inspection Board for enforcement of these standards. Social psychiatry, in an effort to transform these large institutions from custodial care to treatment centers, developed the concept of the therapeutic community, the fundamental tenet of which is that patients can assist in their own rehabilitation as well as in the rehabilitation of other patients.

Social psychiatry also includes transcultural and community psychiatry. Transcultural psychiatry studies the incidence and prevalence of mental disease across societies and delineates the social forces that affect the manifestations of these illnesses. Community psychiatry has been described as "social psychiatry in action" (13) and is involved in the development, planning, and organization of community mental health programs and consultation to local agencies.

The number of psychiatrists in the United States increased from approximately 7000 in 1950 to more than 32,000 by 1985, including those working primarily in administration (17). The Graduate Medical Education National Advisory Committee (GMENAC) panel on psychiatry estimated a need for 38,500 psychiatrists by 1990, based on population trends (15). A shortfall of approximately 20 percent, or 8500 psychiatrists is predicted, with the greatest shortage expected in child psychiatry.

Increased competition from other disciplines may, however, reduce the impact of this shortfall. In 1975–1976, for every 100,000 U.S. citizens there were only 12.4 psychiatrists, but there were 19.5 psychologists and 32.2 social workers. Trends such as the granting of hospital admitting privileges to licensed psychologists and increased third-party reimbursement for nonphysician providers may further increase the number of other mental health providers who may offset the proposed shortage in psychiatry. Furthermore, internists, family practitioners, behavioral pediatricians, and neurologists may further encroach on psychiatric territory (15).

PSYCHOLOGISTS

Psychology, which struggled to create its own professional identity in the early years of this century, has emphasized scientific research in academic settings. Beginning as a philosophy, psychology has become firmly established as a social science, and psychologists have promoted and conducted research on the functioning of the human mind, especially through development of scientific testing instruments. Beginning in the early twentieth century, psychological testing began to be used in conjunction with psychiatric treatment. Research by psychologists in classic conditioning and behavior theory also aided psychiatrists, who still provided most therapeutic care.

During World War II, psychologists began to be seen in an increased role in clinical practice. With the expansion of mental health services in Veterans Administration hospitals, the training of clinical psychologists began in earnest. In 1946 the Veterans Administration, in conjunction with the American Psychological Association, began the Veterans Administration Psychology Training Program, which is still a major source of training for clinical and counseling psychologists. The professional application of psychology received further endorsement in the American Psychological Association Vail Conference of 1973, which emphasized the continued training of clinicians and scientists in psychology.

Psychologists are licensed or certified in all states and the District of Columbia. In almost all states, the training required for licensure is a doctoral degree, although a few states allow limited licensure for graduates of master's degree programs; however, independent private practice is prohibited. Licensure is not required for practice in some settings, however, and unlicensed psychologists most often practice in school or community mental health facilities. The American Psychological Association reports a 1986 membership of 63,000; there may, in fact, be over 70,000 master's- and doctorate-level psychologists (18). The numbers of psychologists, social workers, and Registered Nurses (R.N.s) working in all mental health organizations increased significantly between 1976 and 1982 (19).

SOCIAL WORKERS

The history of social work dates back to the late nineteenth century and the volunteer mothers who provided disadvantaged persons with charitable aid through the Charity Organization Societies. Social work began to develop as a profession during the early twentieth century. Reform-minded women struggling for equality became social workers and began working in medical and psychiatric settings, schools, and correctional institutions. The development of social psychiatry also prompted the formation of a professional identity for social workers. Adopting the Freudian psychoanalytic model of many psychiatrists, social workers struggled for increasing responsibility in the treatment of mental and emotional disorders. The practice of psychotherapy expanded the social worker's domain from providing charitable assistance to the poor to providing a therapy that was viewed as legitimate by middle- and upper-class people. Since psychoanalysis and psychotherapy remained medical specialties, social workers were not too successful in developing a separate professional identity, and their practice continued in the shadow of psychiatry.

Social work continues to struggle for an independent identity and a more equal role in the delivery of mental health services. Training includes 2-year associate degree programs graduating human service workers, baccalaureate programs in social work currently recognized as the beginning professional level, master's-level degrees in social work, and doctoral programs. In addition to the basic training of the discipline, social work education offers specialized training in mental health and in human services administration. The National Association of Social Workers lists about 70,000 members, but there may be as many as 300,000 social service workers (18). Social workers are licensed in more than 23 states, and efforts toward social work licensure are under way in many other states.

PSYCHIATRIC NURSES

The professional training of nurses in this country began in the 1860s and consisted primarily of apprenticeships. The first training program that prepared nurses to care for the mentally ill was started in 1882 at McLean Hospital, a private psychiatric facility in Waverly, Massachusetts. Although there was a growing appreciation of nurses who received this type of training, poorly funded psychiatric hospitals continued to employ lesser-trained aides at very low pay. Whatever nursing care did exist in these hospitals consisted mainly of custodial care focusing on the physical needs of the patient, and the nurse continued to practice in a dependent relationship with a physician.

The development in the 1930s of somatic treatments for mental illness, such as insulin shock therapy, psychosurgery, and electroshock therapy, required the services of highly skilled nurses and established a more significant role for nurses in psychiatric treatment. The advent of the therapeutic community in psychiatric hospitals broadened the role of the nurse even further. As the 24-hour care necessary for developing and maintaining the therapeutic milieu was recognized, the nurse became a valuable member of the therapeutic team. The involvement of nurses in group psychotherapy after World War II resulted in federal appropriations for training nurses. However, despite the recognition of psychiatric nursing as a legitimate nursing role, the exact function of the nurse in mental health care remained only vaguely delineated.

Nursing education has become much more academically based over the past 20 years as the need for college-level training programs and nursing research was recognized. Graduates of nursing schools obtained an increasingly strong professional and academic education, often training side by side with psychiatrists, psychologists, and social workers. Nurses who earned advanced degrees were often recruited for teaching, however, and the 2-year associate degree and diploma nurses were more prevalent in clinical practice. As nurses began to move into the role of psychotherapists, partially in response to the shortage of psychiatrists in most hospitals, interprofessional conflicts developed. But the exploding demand for psychotherapists further legitimized the nurse's role in therapy, and, by the late 1960s, the clinical specialty of psychiatric nursing was firmly established. The first organization to certify clinical specialists in psychiatric nursing, in 1972, was the New Jersey State Nurses Association.

Nursing education includes training in psychiatric nursing at all academic levels. The associate degree nurse with 2 years of training in an academic program and the diploma nurse trained in a hospital program most often provide clinical services. The baccalaureate- and master's-level nurses often work in supervisory positions or in teaching, and doctorate-level nurses usually teach rather than provide clinical services. The majority of clinically active psychiatric nurses work in hospital settings.

Clinical psychiatric nurses have not been received with overwhelming enthusiasm by other mental health professionals, partially as a result of controversies regarding professional status and duties within the nursing profession itself. Nursing has yet to define clearly the appropriate roles of nurses and their relation to other mental health professionals. In addition, paraprofessionals such as mental health workers and psychiatric aides prefer nurses to perform supervision and management roles so as to leave a wider territory for their own struggle for psychotherapeutic practice rights. In community settings social workers want to perform psychotherapy and have psychiatric nurses perform more in the tradition of the public health nurse. Currently, many psychiatric nurses in mental health settings do not have the specialized graduate-level training that the title implies. There are over 1 million nurses in the United States (18);

of the 187,000 nurses in the American Nurses Association, 12,000 are categorized as psychiatric nurses.

OTHER MENTAL HEALTH PERSONNEL CONCERNS

The roles of the various mental health service providers vary with the setting in which they practice. Inpatient psychiatric services are oriented toward the more traditional medical/clinical model, with the psychiatrist assuming the primary role and nurses, psychologists, and social workers offering support services. The growth of community services provided some impetus for change toward a more egalitarian role for all mental health professionals, particularly in the community mental health centers, which were intended to operate within the social and behavioral models of treatment. However, the more traditional therapies persist even in these centers, and all professionals practice similarly. Differences in professional training are reflected more in incomes than in professional activity, and most mental health professionals jockey for the same narrow therapeutic territory. Psychiatrists frequently also assume consulting and supervisory roles in addition to providing care and supervising medications.

Administration in mental health has been largely performed by psychiatrists in mental hospitals. Community mental health centers, although originally envisioned to have psychiatrists as directors, tend to use primarily psychologists and social workers as administrators. Since clinical skills alone are inadequate for administration, educational programs have been developed to offer some training in administration and management for mental health professionals, especially in social work and community psychiatry. In addition, there is a growing trend toward professionally trained mental health administrators without a clinical background.

Table 8-1 presents the supply and distribution of personnel among mental health facilities, excluding VA medical centers. Growth in personnel occurred beginning approximately in 1950 and reflects the increase in mental health concerns and increased appropriations for training. Equally important to note is the increase in personnel with baccalaureate degree or lower levels of education during this time. The mental health system experienced an explosion in the demand for practitioners as increased federal funding was authorized by Congress. In addition to increased demand for psychiatrists, psychologists, social workers, and psychiatric nurses, a number of allied mental health fields developed; these fields represent 12 percent of all mental health personnel (5). In 1982 more than 390,000 full-time equivalent (FTE) staff were employed in mental health organizations in the United States (19). This was substantially more FTE personnel than were reported for 1976 and 1978.

Professionals with expertise in mental health concerns are practicing an increasingly wide range of disciplines. Schools of education are training counseling and guidance personnel as well as special education teachers who work in schools and other settings. The special needs of people recovering from mental and emotional disabilities have been recognized by such professional groups as occupational and recreational therapists and vocational counselors. Practitioners in marriage counseling, art, music, dance therapy, and religion provide counseling and therapy in many mental health settings. Training for these allied professionals varies tremendously. These personnel serve as mental health workers, alcohol and drug abuse counselors, day care workers, board and homecare providers, foster parents, patient advocates, and hospital

TABLE 8-1. Number and Percent Distribution of FTE Staff Positions in Mental Health Organizations (Excluding VA Medical Centers), by Discipline, United States, Selected Years 1976–1982[a]

Staff Discipline	Percent		
	1976	1978	1982[a,b]
All staff	100.0	100.0	100.0
Patient care staff	67.8	67.8	69.5
Professional patient care staff	31.1	33.1	N.A.
Psychiatrists	3.5	3.2	3.5
Other physicians	0.8	0.7	0.7
Psychologists[c]	2.8	3.1	4.3
Social workers	5.2	5.8	7.6
Registered nurses	8.8	9.3	11.1
Other mental health professionals (B.A. & above)	7.8	8.9	
Physical health professionals and assistants	2.2	2.1	42.3
Other mental health workers (less than B.A.)	36.7	34.7	
Administrative, clerical, and maintenance staff	32.2	32.2	30.5

SOURCE: National Institute of Mental Health; Taube CA, Barrett SA (eds): *Mental Health, United States, 1985.* Department of Health and Human Services Publication Number (ADM) 85-1378. Washington, DC, Superintendent of Documents, U.S. Government Printing Office, 1985.

[a]For the most recent year shown in this table, some organizations were reclassified as a result of changes in reporting procedures.

[b]Since 1982 data were not available for nonfederal general hospital psychiatric services, 1980 data were used; data for all other organization types are for 1982.

[c]For 1976–1978, this category included all psychologists with a B.A. and above; for 1982, it includes only psychologists with an M.A. and above.

psychiatric aides. In some mental health centers, half of the positions are filled by these individuals.

Indigenous healers are rarely recognized by traditional mental health service providers but have an important role in caring for physical and emotional disturbances in many minority cultures. Community volunteers are also an important component of the mental health work force. Thousands of people offer their time and services, performing tasks ranging from assisting with clerical needs to working directly with patients.

Issues of access to care raise concerns over the racial and economic mix of mental health professionals and the predominance of male practitioners. Speculation about the capability of many providers to respond to different cultural groups, and especially the poor, fosters much of this concern, particularly since the poor and minorities often have lower use rates for mental health services. Psychiatry, in particular, includes few minority practitioners, and foreign medical graduates often staff state and county hospitals. Foreign graduates may have difficulty adapting to the culture and language of their American clientele. Psychology also has few minority practitioners, but graduate programs are now increasing the number of minority and women students. About 10 percent of graduate students currently are minorities, and 33 percent of psychology doctorates in 1976 were awarded to women (5). Social work has long recognized the importance of training in different social and cultural systems, has many minority practitioners, and, indeed, has traditionally been considered a woman's field. Men have now been increasingly entering social work and, to a lesser extent, nursing.

FINANCING MENTAL HEALTH CARE

From 1965 to 1981 health expenditures increased from 6 percent to 9.8 percent of the gross national product (GNP) (15). Americans spent $387.5 billion on health care in 1984, accounting for 10.6 percent of the U.S. GNP (20). Approximately 29¢ of every health care dollar is spent by business in the form of health insurance premiums. This portion continues to rise as the cost of medical care increases. Chapter 11 discusses these trends, while this section of this chapter focuses specifically on unique issues related to mental health care.

In 1984 the estimated cost of alcohol, drug abuse, and mental illness was $237.6 billion. This includes the direct, indirect, and crime-related economic costs to society. They are as follows:

Direct costs	$39 billion (18%)
Indirect (lost productivity, unemployment, mortality)	$157 billion (66%)
Other (crime related)	$36 billion (16%)

Hospitals account for about 53 percent of the direct treatment costs. Specialized treatment facilities for alcoholism, drug abuse, and mental illness account for 37 percent of the total direct costs.

Most Americans do not pay for all of their own health care. They are covered under some type of third-party reimbursement, whether it is publicly funded such as through Medicaid and Medicare, or through insurance companies. Government has responded to the cost explosion in health care by legislating an end to the cost-reimbursement system for Medicare providers and establishing that federal payment be based on payer-determined prices. In addition, both government and industry have fostered a climate encouraging competition among organized providers of care.

To date, psychiatry has been excluded from the capitated reimbursement plan under Medicare—diagnosis-related groups (DRG), which was phased in starting in 1983 (Chapter 11). Hospitals defined as rehabilitation, long-term, pediatric, or psychiatric continue to be paid under a cost-based reimbursement system with limits on rates of growth. The exemptions were based on uncertainty about how well a DRG-based payment system would work for specialized facilities and units. Exemptions for psychiatry, however, are not likely to last.

One study of the impact of prospective payment on hospital charges and mix of services provided to a group of Medicare patients treated for mental disorders focused on per case reimbursement and its effect on hospital charges (21). The results suggest that per case reimbursement provides incentives to reduce the cost of the hospital stay, but the cost savings may be offset by a higher readmission rate, and the reimbursement structure may ultimately influence the pattern of care. Researchers are attempting to create an alternative diagnostic matrix that demonstrates how length of stay is influenced by severity of psychiatric illness, level of disability, and the nature of the psychosocial support system (22).

Psychiatric insurance under other forms of insurance is inconsistent, as well. Traditionally, coverage for mental illness has been characterized by limitations in the form of caps on total coverage available and higher coinsurance and deductibles than for general medical coverage. However, since the 1970s major U.S. employers have become increasingly aware of the need to give greater priority to emotional problems (23). Mental health benefits are experiencing new definitions, designs, and structures for corporate programs. The image of the American worker as being able to cope with any problem is being drowned in a sea of alcoholism, drug abuse, and legal, marital, and financial problems (23). Simultaneously, insurance is focusing more on prevention as a means of increasing efforts to reduce absenteeism and to increase worker productivity.

The importance of prevention is further illustrated by increased knowledge of mind and body interactions and the role that mental health services play in the overall health care system. A review of 25 studies regarding the effect of treatment for alcoholism, drug abuse, and mental illness on the subsequent reduction of general medical care utilization indicated reduced utilization and a median cost of medical care savings of 20 percent 1 year after treatment (24).

One organizational type to emerge in response to economic pressures and need for greater integration of the differing parts of the health care system has been HMOs (Chapter 5). Insurers and employers have also collaborated with fee-for-service practitioners and hospitals to create PPOs and Exclusive Provider Organizations (EPOs) intended to offer care at a discounted rate. Comprehensive prospective payment systems such as these will play an increasingly important role in the future of psychiatric services. Psychiatric practice in HMOs, concurrently the most common model of prospective payment, has been shown to be cost effective, and differing models of mental health service delivery have emerged. Psychiatric services are often included in other alternative provider organizations as well. However, they are likely to have modest coinsurance payments and strict limits on the duration of services. Employee Assistance Programs, originally focused on alcohol treatment, are expanding in scope, and corporate mental health programs are moving in-house through the employment of staff psychiatrists, psychologists, and social workers.

TRENDS AFFECTING THE MENTAL HEALTH SYSTEM

Policy regarding mental health issues has been affected profoundly by case law in previous years. Three areas of legal change have had major effects on the chronic mentally ill. They include substantive and procedural alterations in civil commitment laws, the limited implementation of a constitutionally based right to treatment, and the partial recognition of a right to refuse treatment (25).

Deinstitutionalization and the way it was implemented was a significant factor in the development of civil commitment laws. The influx of previously hospitalized mentally ill people into the community and the lack of consistent residential and treatment services created a significant group of people whose life styles varied significantly from those of the general population. Philosophical debates raged as to the right of an individual to choose this "alternative life style," and the responsibility of society to ensure that persons who appeared unable to care for themselves had protection under the law. Civil commitment laws, initially general in definition, became more definitive and embodied criteria specifying dangerousness or the incapacity to care for self with the presence of mental illness as a requisite for commitment. Laws also became specific as to the duration of commitment, and the time length was generally brief. Finally, individuals committed under these laws had rapid access to courts, public defenders, and other elements of the judicial system which ensured due process.

Implementation of laws in most states became quite literal, and dangerousness often became the deciding criterion. Yet, findings suggest that irrespective of commitment criteria, 85 percent of persons committed are not dangerous. This emphasis may significantly reduce the number of people who could be helped by commitment and, some would argue, contribute to the increase of urban homeless people (25).

The right to treatment was first addressed in 1952 in civil commitment cases relating to sexual psychopaths. *Rouse v. Cameron* in 1966, based on arguments of cruel and unusual treatment and the right to due process, found that people judged criminally insane had the right to treatment (26). Since the early cases did not define criteria for treatment, but merely stated that some effort was required, there was little immediate impact. A decision by Judge Frank Johnson of Alabama in 1972, based on a class action suit (*Wyatt v. Stickney*) related to conditions in state hospitals, required that right to treatment be enforced and implemented (27). Various courts have subsequently specified minimum standards for treatment. In 1975 the Supreme Court cast significant doubt on a constitutionally derived right to treatment by deciding the case of *O'Connor v. Donaldson* (28) on the narrowest possible grounds. Donaldson, a patient in a Florida hospital for 14 years, sued for damages and demanded his release. The narrowness of the ruling limited the potential impact of the right-to-treatment litigation on increased support for the chronically mentally ill (25).

The right to refuse treatment raises often conflicting interests between the society, the therapist and the patient. The implications of behavior control through the use of behavior therapies, drug therapy, and psychosurgery create problems that have been addressed by the judicial system and by mental health professionals. The first of two right to refuse cases considered by the court was *Mills v. Rogers* (29), a class action suit brought by patients at Boston State Hospital. In the years since, clinicians have been confronted with a bewildering set of pronouncements from the courts (30). Evidence suggests that the right to refuse treatment has significantly increased both use of seclusion and transfers to maximum-security hospitals (25) for chronically mentally ill individuals. In one case, *Stensvad v. Reivitz* (31), the court ruled that the purpose of commitment is custody, care, and treatment, and that such treatment reasonably includes psychotropic medication.

Another significant and growing factor in the development of policy regarding mental health services is the increase in patients' rights advocacy movements. Most recently, the federal government has passed legislation requiring states that accept federal funds for mental health services to create programs for protecting and advocating the rights of the mentally ill. This legislation is patterned after similar legislation in the field of developmental disabilities. Protection and advocacy agencies for developmentally disabled individuals are mandated in each state and funded through federal appropriation. Although meeting mixed enthusiasm among professionals and others in the field of developmental disabilities, advocates for the developmentally disabled have generally been regarded as the pioneers in advocacy movements. They remain a significant and powerful force. Legislation establishing similar advocacy organizations within mental health builds on the developmental disabilities programs by overlaying the new system on the existing one. On the basis of the success of protection and advocacy systems for the developmentally disabled, there is considerable opportunity for mental health advocates and professionals to work together for the betterment of the service system.

Our society is slowly working toward a better understanding of the nature of mental health. Much of what is currently known and believed is predicated on a mixture of fact and untested theory. The mental health system is working vigorously to catch up with current knowledge and philosophy, but its efforts are warped by a confusing mixture of economic and political constraints. Previous philosophy that heralded the ability of all people to live in the community has not been realized. Many people who need mental health services and have no financial or social resources find only limited, or possibly no, services. Mental health services for those who do have resources have expanded and changed considerably, leaving even greater evidence of a two tiered system of care.

Despite the many problems that remain in the system, mental health professionals, citizen advocates, and consumers continue to labor toward greater access to financial resources, more and improved services, and less stigma for mental illness. Custodial treatment still exists, but we are learning how to better use all of our treatment resources. Many people do go unserved or inappropriately treated, but the problems of the mentally ill continue to receive attention and concern. In short, the mental health system continues to gain credence and legitimacy as a significant and important part of health care.

REFERENCES

1. Levine M: *The History and Politics of Community Mental Health.* Oxford, Oxford University Press, 1981.

2. Weiner DB: The apprenticeship of Philippe Pinel: A new document, "Observations of Citizen Pussin on the Insane." *Psychiatry* 1979; 136:1128–1134.

3. Shore JH, Kinzie JD, Hampson JD, et al: Psychiatric epidemiology of an Indian village. *Psychiatry* 1973; 36:70–81.

4. Diagnostic and Statistics Manual. Washington, DC, American Psychiatric Association, Task Force on Nomenclature Statistics, 1981.

5. Regier D, Myers J, Kramer M, et al: The NIMH epidemiologic catchment area (ECA) program: Historical context, major objectives and study population characteristics. *Arch Gen Psychiatr* 1984; 41:934–941.

6. Facts and Figures from the Alcohol, Drug Abuse and Mental Health Administration. U.S. Department of Health and Human Services, July 1986; No. 4.

7. Rumer R: Community mental health centers: Politics and therapy. *J Health Politics, Policy and Law* 1978; 3:531–558.

8. Goldman H, Adams N, Taube C: Deinstitutionalization: The data demythologicalized. *Hosp Commun Psychiatr* 1983; 34:129–134.

9. Green S, Witken M, Atay J, et al: State and County Mental Hospitals, United States, 1982–83 and 1983–84, Statistical Note 176, ADAMHA, July 1986.

10. Craig T, Laska E: Deinstitutionalization and the survival of the state hospital. *Hosp Commun Psychiatr* 1983; 34:616–622.

11. Panzetta A: Whatever happened to community mental health: Portents for corporate medicine. *Hosp Commun Psychiatr* 1985; 36:1175–1179.

12. Rosenstein M, Mellazzo-Sayre L: Characteristics of admissions to selected mental facilities: An annotated book of charts and tables; Statistical Note 174, NIMH, November 1985.

13. Lipton F, Sabatini A, Katz S: Down and out in the city: The homeless mentally ill. *Hosp Commun Psychiatr* 1983; 43:817–821.

14. Knoll J, Carey K, Hagedorn D, et al: A survey of homeless adults in urban emergency shelters. *Hosp Commun Psychiatry* 1986; 37:283–286.

15. Bittker T: The industrialization of American psychiatry. *Am J Psychiatr* 1985; 142:149–154.

16. Robbins L: The private psychiatric hospital: The impact of current trends. *Psychiatr Hosp* 1983; 14:13–16.

17. Telephone Communication, American Medical Association, January 9, 1987.

18. President's Commission on Mental Health: Final Report, Vol. II, Task Panel Reports. Washington, DC, U.S. Government Printing Office, 1978.

19. National Institute of Mental Health: *Mental Health, United States, 1985.* Taube CA, Barrett SA (eds): DHHS Publ. No. (ADM) 85-1378. Washington, DC, U.S. Government Printing Office, 1985.

20. Trends in health insurance coverage for mental illness. National Association of Private Psychiatric Hospitals, Washington, DC, 1985.

21. Rupp A, Steinwachs D, Salkever D: The effect of hospital payment methods on the pattern and cost of mental health care. *Hosp Commun Psychiatr* 1984; 35:456–459.

22. Biegal A: Planning psychiatry's future. *Hosp Commun Psychiatr* 1986; 37:551–554.

23. Goldbeck W: Psychiatry and industry: A business view. *Psychiatr Hosp* 1983; 13:11–14.

24. Jones K, Vischi T: Impact of alcohol, drug abuse and mental health treatment on medical care utilization: A review of the research literature. *Med Care* 1979 (Suppl) 17:

25. Lamb H, Mills M: Needed changes in law and procedure for the chronically mentally ill. *Hosp Commun Psychiatr* 1986; 37:475–480.

26. *Rouse v. Cameron,* 373 F2d 451 (DC Cir 1966).

27. *Wyatt v. Stickney,* 344 F SSupp 383 (MD Ala 1972).

28. *Donaldson v. O'Connor,* 493 F2d 507 (Stu Cir 1974).

29. *Mills v. Rogers,* 50 USLW 4676 (June 18, 1982).

30. Appelbaum P: Refusing treatment: The uncertainty continues. *Hosp Commun Psychiatr* 1983; 34:11–12.

31. *Stensvad v. Reivitz* et al., No. 84-C-383-S (W D Wis January 10, 1985).

PART FOUR

Resources for Health Services

CHAPTER 9

Medical Technology
and Its Assessment

Bryan R. Luce

Technology is credited with the benefits of American medicine as well as what ails it. It is the hope for a long, productive life for millions of people, a primary reason for the spiraling costs of care, and the source of many social and ethical dilemmas such as the rationing of health care and the harvesting of human organs for transplants. It has even given rise to new definitions of death. At different times and places and by different analysts it has been accused of not being accessible to all members of the population, being overused, misused, and misunderstood. It has been said to have diffused too rapidly without adequate assessment or regulation, yet today some express a concern of innovation being stifled, capital being unavailable for technology acquisition, and reimbursement being inadequate.

This chapter is intended to shed light on many of these issues. It will attempt to explain how medical technology fits into the American health care system, what the public policy issues are, and how these issues are being addressed by different elements of society.

The chapter discusses two major issues: medical technology and medical technology assessment. The development and innovation process of medical technology that demonstrates how innovations build on prior knowledge and the amount of investment that is required in terms of both money and time is presented first. Next, the reader is provided with a picture of the process of diffusion of medical technologies from an innovative idea to widespread use to obsolescence. The relevance of any particular technology is often related to the stage of its life cycle. Later, it will be seen that the assessment process is also related to the life cycle stage. Then, the appropriate use of medical technologies, presently the subject of a raging controversy within both the medical and health policy communities, is discussed. As will be clear from this discussion, it is not possible to fully discuss medical technology without addressing the appropriate practice of medicine. Although the section on appropriateness ends the first section of this chapter, it is a fitting way to introduce the discussion of medical technology assessment, since the assessment process largely involves determination of the appropriate application of medical technology.

This section first describes the many organizations, public and private, which conduct technology assessments. They include the Food and Drug Administration (FDA), the Congressional Office of Technology Assessment (OTA), and other Department of Health and Human Services (DHHS) activities. Within the private sector many organizations such as the American Medical Association, the American Hospital Association, and the American College of Physicians are also active in formal assessment activities.

An overview of some of the more widely used and important methods of assessment—randomized clinical trials, case studies, group judgment methods, quality-of-life measurement, and finally, cost-benefit and cost-effectiveness analyses— is then presented. The chapter concludes with some thoughts about the future of technology and its assessment.

The concept of technology is a very broad one: the application of organized knowledge to practical ends (1). Thus technology connotes much more than either a widget or a machine. Similarly, medical technology is a broader concept than might otherwise be assumed. A comprehensive definition of medical technology in common use today is: techniques, drugs, equipment, and procedures used by health care professionals in delivering medical care to individuals, and the systems within which care is delivered (1). From a practical standpoint, however, the discussion in this chapter generally centers on drugs, medical devices, and medical and surgical procedures: that is, the practice of clinical medicine and its tools.

INNOVATION, DEVELOPMENT, AND DIFFUSION

In many ways, the history of medicine is intricately tied to the history of advances in medical technology. Much of modern medicine practice can be traced to the origins of the stethoscope in the early nineteenth century, the thermometer and roentgen rays in the late nineteenth century, and the sphygmomanometer and the electrocardiogram (ECG) recorders in the early twentieth century, all of which allowed the physician to better understand the internal workings of the human body. Twentieth-century anesthesia permitted surgery to blossom, and the miracle of antibiotics did not occur until well into the twentieth century.

Not only is the practice of medicine highly influenced by technological advances; so is the location of that practice. As technology became more sophisticated, complicated, and expensive, it served as a catalyst for centralizing medical care in the hospital. Major surgery such as coronary artery bypass graft (CABG) requires a sophisticated team approach; major diagnostic machines such as the computerized tomography (CT) scanner and the magnetic resonance imaging (MRI) machine require large capital outlays; intensive care units require sophisticated monitoring equipment as well as highly trained integrated staff.

In contrast, today, because of a number of technological innovations as well as financial pressures, technology is allowing patients to be cared for and treated in outpatient settings and at home. Much of ophthalmologic surgery is now being performed in outpatient settings, as are many other surgical procedures and diagnostic testing prior to entering hospitals. Technology permits handicapped people to see, hear, speak, and move. Monitoring devices can permit cardiac implants to transmit vital information over telephone lines; respirators maintain breathing in the home; kidney dialyzers are commonly used at home as is parenteral nutrition, an intravenous technology for patients who cannot swallow or digest food. In fact, technology is a prime reason that home health care expenditures are one of the fastest growing sectors in American health care today. In 1983 expenditures for home health care were over $5 billion; they are expected to top $16 billion by 1990 (2).

Technology also profoundly influences who practices medicine. No longer does the general practitioner do everything. The extreme specialization in medicine has been due to not only the increasing volume of medical knowledge but also to sophisticated technological advances, much of which is controlled by specializing subgroups of physicians. For instance, as technological advances occurred in obstetrics, including cesarean section, electronic fetal monitoring, and neonatal intensive care, encouraging births to be located in hospitals, physicians replaced midwives and obstetricians replaced general practitioners. Advances in surgical techniques such as microsurgery, organ implantation, and coronary artery bypass procedures have had similar effects on both general practitioners and general surgeons. Thus technology has helped to transform medicine from primarily an art to a blend of art and science and, in turn, required that physicians become more technologically trained scientists.

The following section discusses the nation's investment in biomedical research and development that has served as the fuel for these technological advancements.

FUNDING BIOMEDICAL RESEARCH AND DEVELOPMENT

Biomedical research and development is funded by both the federal government and the private sector. From 1975 to 1985, funding has grown steadily from $4.7 billion to $12.8 billion. During this time, however, there has been a shift in relative support, with industry increasing its share and government decreasing its share (see Fig. 9-1). The U.S. pharmaceutical industry itself reports that it has recently been increasing its investment for developing new drugs, from 11.7 percent of sales in 1980 to 15.1 percent of sales in 1985 (3). Nevertheless, health research and development spending as a percentage of total national health expenditures has decreased substantially over the past 15 years. In 1984 health research and development accounted for 3.1 percent (see Table 9-1), down from 3.9 percent in 1972, a 21 percent drop. Although that proportion is a little higher than the average for all industry in the United States, it is relatively low for technologically dependent industries (4). Thus, since health care is technologically sophisticated, yet highly labor-dependent, the present level of investment may be unreasonable if the downward trend continues. However, serious concern is being expressed today that changing reimbursement patterns and budgetary pressures due to cost-containment initiatives will significantly dampen industry's investment in new product development (5).

THE DIFFUSION OF TECHNOLOGIES

The spread of a technology into society once it is developed is known as *diffusion*. It includes entry, adoption, widespread use, and final obsolescence of an innovation—the life cycle of a technology.

Diffusion is an important concept to study because it is both affected by and, in turn, affects many important socioeconomic processes. Industry is interested in the demand for its products, and that demand is affected by the relative costs and benefits of the

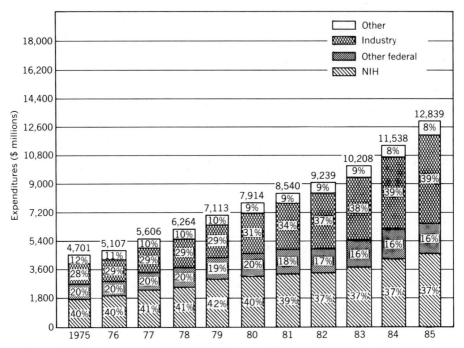

Figure 9-1. National support for health R&D by source, 1975–1985 (dollars in millions). (SOURCE: National Institutes of Health, *NIH Data Book, 1985.*)

TABLE 9-1. National Health Expenditures (1984)
(Dollars in Billions)

National health care	$384.3
Health research and development	11.8
All health technology assessment	1.3
Clinical trials	1.1
Health services research	<0.2
Other technology assessment	<0.05

SOURCE: *Assessing Medical Technologies,* copyright 1985 by the National Academy of Sciences.

innovation, regulatory constraints, reimbursement rules, pricing, and medical acceptance. Whereas the public is concerned with having access to new beneficial procedures, devices, and drugs such as heart transplants and cyclosporin (a new drug that inhibits the body's natural rejection mechanisms), payers—including private insurers and federal and state governments—are concerned with adoption of a technology before it has been adequately assessed. Figure 9-2, depicts the life cycle of a technology from basic research to obsolescence. Included in this diagram are some of the many environmental factors such as regulation, evaluation, and reimbursement policies that affect the diffusion process.

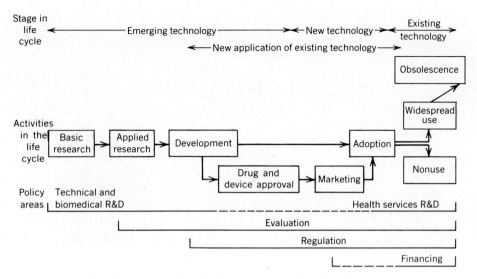

Figure 9-2. Life cycle of a medical technology. (SOURCE: Office of Technology Assessment.)

The diffusion curve of an innovation is typically described in an S-shaped fashion (Fig. 9-3), with an initial slow introduction, and a take-off phase characterized by an increasing rate of adoption that slowly levels off as it matures and, perhaps, decreases as it approaches obsolescence. Several empirical studies have plotted such a course (6,7). For instance, in a 1981 publication the Congressional Office of Technology Assessment (OTA) plotted the course of adoption of the CT scanner in the United States (Fig. 9-4). The CT scanner was introduced into the United States in the early 1970s. In 1974 there were 45 scanners in operation. Within 2 years there were 475 operational scanners or a tenfold increase. By 1977, scanners were being bought and installed at a rate of about 40 per month. Although total volume continued to increase, a year later the rate of increase was cut in half and continued to decline later. During this time, there was a great deal of public debate over control of capital expenditures in health care. Congress enacted the Health Planning and Resources Development Act of 1974 (PL 93-641), which covered the nation with a system of local health planning agencies. If any single technology was specially targeted for regulatory control with the intentions of creating a more orderly process of diffusion, it was the CT scanner. Later in that decade (1978), the National Guidelines for Health Planning were issued, which attempted to establish utilization guidelines and standards that planning agencies could use for 11 technologies, including the CT scanner. Nevertheless, as Figure 9-4 suggests, these and other efforts had little or no effect on diffusion of CT scanning into the U.S. health care system. This widespread diffusion occurred before there was hard evidence of efficacy or cost-effectiveness from well-designed studies (8).

Today, researchers are watching diffusion of a similar expensive and dramatic diagnostic technology, magnetic resonance imaging (MRI). By 1985 it was reported to be in its take-off phase of diffusion. But despite the weakening of planning and certificate-of-need (CON) regulations in the 1980s, these regulatory programs are reported to have retarded diffusion in the United States (9). In addition, new

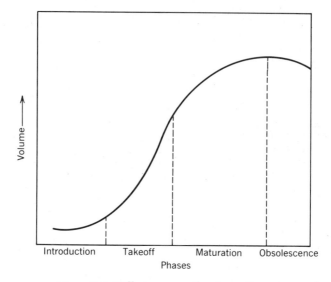

Figure 9-3. Diffusion curve of an innovation.

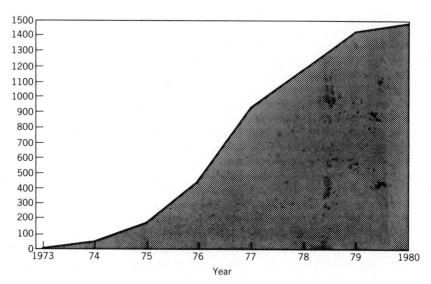

Figure 9-4. Cumulative number of CT Scanners installed (1973–1980). (SOURCE: Office of Technology Assessment.)

reimbursement policies such as the Medicare prospective payment system may also be delaying its diffusion. As with the CT scanner, there is similar concern that adequate testing of the technology's relative value was not systematic prior to widening adoption of the machine.

CABG, an open heart surgical procedure to correct coronary artery vessel blockage, has diffused very rapidly in this country at great expense but with generally inadequate scientific evidence of safety, efficacy, and cost-effectiveness. In 1972, 2600 patients had such an operation; by 1981, that figure had grown to almost 53,000 patients, at a total cost of about $500 million (10).

The CT scanner and coronary artery bypass surgery are good examples of technologies that have influenced public health policy development. From the middle 1960s to the end of the 1970s, debate raged over increasing costs due to rapid acceptance of untested and overused technologies. Rising from this debate were health planning and hospital utilization review legislation and increased calls for technology assessments. Because of its perceived ineffectiveness by the 1980s, the regulatory approach began to give way to a more market oriented approach for controlling diffusion. Payment policies were being changed from cost-based policies to policies being set propsectively, placing the purchaser at increased financial risk for the adoption and use of technology. Today, for instance, Medicare pays a set amount of money per hospital admission [i.e., per diagnosis-related group (DRG)], rather than guaranteeing cost recovery. Concern immediately shifted from that of overadoption to one of underadoption (5), although a significant shift in diffusion rates has yet to be demonstrated. Nevertheless, there is evidence that new, expensive technologies may not be adequately reimbursed. For instance, a recent survey of hospitals that have purchased the extracorporeal shock wave lithotripter (ESWL), an imaginative, but expensive, noninvasive method for crushing kidney stones through shock waves, reveals that Medicare's DRG prospective payment system pays only 57 to 82 percent of the costs of the therapy. Since the DRG payment in this case is based on the patient's condition rather than the procedure performed, hospitals are paid the same amount regardless of whether the hospitals have ESWL or whether it is used. Thus, ironically, in 1987, hospitals without ESWL stand to gain an estimated $4.5 to $8.8 million in Medicare payments. Similarly, hospitals with MRIs had a total reported Medicare loss of $31 million (11).

The ultimate effect of these reimbursement policies on technology diffusion—that is, the providers' willingness and ability to purchase technology—is yet to be determined. But little doubt remains that technology continues to diffuse before adequate assessment is conducted.

THE APPROPRIATE USE OF TECHNOLOGIES

Studies have shown that there is enormous variation in medical practice, contrary to the general belief of the public (12–15). Where one lives, who one's practitioner is, and in which setting or hospital that physician practices often determine how one will be treated. This may seem counterintuitive since medical education in this country—indeed, in most of the Western world—has been nearly standardized since the early days of this century, state medical and nursing licensure standards are similar across the states, hospitals conform to standards of the Joint Commission on Accreditation of Hospitals (JCAH), and nationally read professional medical journals disseminate state-of-the-art knowledge of medical practice. Much of this knowledge stems from the many millions of dollars of clinical research findings funded by NIH and the private sector as well as results of medical technology assessments to be discussed in a later section of this chapter. Yet large variations in medical practice persist.

In 1978 the Congressional Office of Technology Assessment (OTA) estimated that only 10 to 20 percent of all procedures currently used in medical practice had been shown to be efficacious by controlled (clinical) trial. OTA concluded that "Given . . . examples of technologies that entered widespread use and were shown later to be inefficacious or unsafe, and the large numbers of inadequately assessed current and emerging technologies, improvements are critically needed in the information base regarding safety and efficacy and the processes for its generation" (16).

The concerns expressed in 1978 persist and have been argued to represent a threat to the autonomy of the medical profession. In 1983 the National Academy of Sciences' Institute of Medicine convened a conference on the subject of variations in medical practice. Participants generally agreed that unless the medical profession came to grips to resolve this issue, it risks a future where external pressures from government, insurers and the public will dictate priorities in the practice of medicine (17).

John Wennberg, the most active researcher in the area of medical practice variation, has shown that one's chance of having a major surgical procedure varies dramatically according to where one lives (Fig. 9-5 demonstrates this point quite clearly). In 1975, within three New England states (Rhode Island, Maine, Vermont), an individual was six times more likely to undergo a tonsillectomy in one location over another and four times more likely for a hysterectomy and prostatectomy (12). He observed in Maine, for instance, that a woman's chance of having a hysterectomy by the time she reached age 70 was 20 percent in one area and 70 percent in another.

These differences cannot be attributed to characteristics of patients, access to service, or insurance protection. Rather, the variation seems to be related primarily to practice styles of physicians. Wennberg's and others' studies indicate that such variation is found throughout the Western world. Disturbingly, the variation is not linked to patient outcomes. Wennberg's explanation of these findings is that scientific evidence of the value of much of medical practice is lacking, ambiguous, or unheeded.

Public policy concern ranges from inefficiencies, to trauma to patients and unnecessary surgical risk, to matters of pure economics. For instance, over 2500 "extra" hysterectomies were performed in one Maine market area over another, resulting in a potential avoidable cost in excess of $10 million (13). Nationwide implications of this are staggering. Another study by the Rand Corporation has shown that large and significant variation of medical and surgical procedures persist across large areas in the United States. Of 123 procedures, 67 showed at least threefold differences between sites (14). Both Wennberg and Robert Brook of Rand have estimated that if physicians in high practice style areas changed their styles to those of their colleagues in low practice style areas, national health expenditures could be reduced by up to 30 to 40 percent (15). This potential for saving money has recently captured the political attention of both Congress and the Department of Health and Human Services. In 1986 Congress allocated several millions of dollars for further research in this area.

Not only medical and surgical procedures are misused. In 950 B.C., Homer is reported to have stated "many (drugs) were excellent and when mingled, many fatal." A study by the American Hospital Association has estimated that 7 percent of all hospital admissions are related to the misuse of prescribed pharmaceuticals, and in 1983, such drug-induced illnesses led to an estimated 2.7 million admissions costing up to $5 billion (18).

There is similar evidence of the widespread diffusion of medical devices without adequate evidence of efficacy. CT and MRI have already been mentioned. A case study

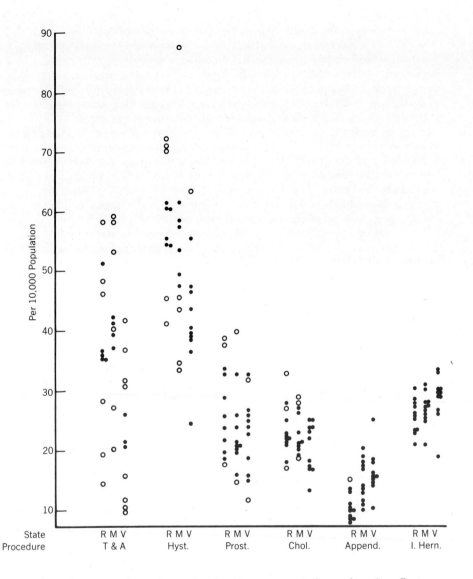

Figure 9-5. Age-adjusted rate of procedure for six common surgical procedures (tonsillectomy–adenoidectomy, hysterectomy, prostatectomy, cholecystectomy, appendectomy, and inguinal hernia) in Rhode Island (R), Maine (M), and Vermont (V) (1975). Rates of surgical procedures vary greatly among hospital areas. The rates shown are for the six most common surgical procedures for the repair or removal of an organ in the 11 most populous hospital areas of Maine, Rhode Island, and Vermont (1975). The rate of tonsillectomy varies about sixfold among the 33 areas; the rates of hysterectomy and prostatectomy vary about fourfold. Moreover, many of the extreme rates for these procedures differ from the average rate for the state by an amount that is statistically significant (open circles). There is much disagreement among physicians on the value of the high-variation procedures. Similar patterns of variation for these procedures have been observed in Iowa, England, and Norway. (source: Wennberg JE: Dealing with medical practice variations: A proposal for action. *Health Affairs* 1984; 3:6–32.)

commonly cited in the literature is that of gastric freezing to cure ulcers (19). This medical device was introduced in 1962. Before it was tested for safety and efficacy, 2500 machines were sold in the United States and an estimated 25,000 operations were performed, causing patients considerable harm. All this was due to erroneous results of a few uncontrolled case studies that were purported to show dramatic benefit in curing ulcers without medication or surgery. Several years later, gastric freezing was shown by controlled randomized trials to have no benefit whatsoever (19,20).

Gastric freezing is an extreme example of the diffusion of a worthless technology. Mostly, the Food and Drug Administration (FDA) ensures that prescription drugs and certain medical devices are safe and efficacious when applied under prescribed conditions. However, no agency ensures that medical or surgical procedures pass an initial safety and efficacy test prior to diffusion into the general population.

Once any technology is available, whether it is a drug, a device, or a medical or surgical procedure, physicians are constrained in their use solely by their training, ethics, economic considerations, their estimate of patient benefit, and threat of malpractice suits. Thus the appropriate use of all available medical technologies are, in the main, left to physician and patient discretion. Testing for appropriateness is a principal purpose of medical technology assessment and is presented in the following section.

ORGANIZING FOR TECHNOLOGY ASSESSMENT

Today a number of organizations in government and the private sector have assumed responsibilities for assessing medical technologies. These organizations attempt to address many of the issues and concerns discussed earlier in this chapter. As a rule, these organizations have been created over time as a response to the perceived needs of society.

REGULATION: AN HISTORICAL OVERVIEW

In 1906 the Food, Drug and Cosmetic Act established the new Food and Drug Administration (FDA) to regulate the marketing of drugs and foods for safety. It was passed in response to unsafe and falsely advertised products, primarily of the home remedy or "patent medicine" type. In 1938 an amendment requiring safety of drugs to be demonstrated through more rigorous and sophisticated testing was enacted, largely as a result of public catastrophes such as the Elixir of Sulfanilamide deaths (21). In 1962 further drug amendments extended regulatory authority of the FDA to require that drugs be tested for efficacy as well as safety prior to marketing. Passage of this legislation was due, in large part, to the thalidomide tragedy (22).

FDA authority over the marketing of medical devices has lagged behind that of drugs. The 1938 amendments sought truth in labeling and provided some marketing control, but only if devices were "adulterated" or "misbranded." By the 1970's, adverse affects of unsafe medical devices had been documented (23), leading to further amendments to the Food, Drug and Cosmetic Act in 1976 empowering the FDA to regulate the marketing of medical devices for safety and efficacy.

In the period following the 1965 Medicare and Medicaid Amendments to the Social Security Act, there arose a number of other legislative attempts to regulate the adoption and use of medical technologies due mainly to concerns about the ever-increasing cost of medical care. In the late 1960s health planning legislation was passed that helped to spur state-CON legislation around the country. These laws were intended to guide the diffusion of capital-intensive technologies (as well as to guide hospital bed capacity). In 1974 the federal planning legislation was greatly strengthened. (See the earlier discussions of the diffusion of the CT scanner.)

Other legislative routes were followed to regulate hospital utilization such as the requirement of Medicare that hospitals have utilization review committees and the enactment of the national Professional Standards Review Organizations (PSRO) program.

Also during this period, Congress created the Office of Technology Assessment (OTA) to guide itself in the increasingly technological world in which it was operating. OTA's Health Program issued its first major report in 1976 outlining opportunities and needs for assessing medical technologies (24). Two years later, Congress established the National Center for Health Care Technology (NCHCT), whose mission was to "set priorities for technology assessment, and encourage, conduct, and support assessments, research demonstrations, and evaluations concerning health care technology" (25). NCHCT was also to advise the Health Care Financing Administration (HCFA) on Medicare specific coverage policy issues. Before the Center could mature, it was defunded in 1981 largely as a result of the medical professions' and the medical device and pharmaceutical industries' belief that its technology assessment activities unduly threatened the innovation process.

Today, there continues to be concern that technologies are not adequately and fully assessed prior to their diffusion and use in medical practice as discussed earlier in this chapter. The more prominent organizations whose mission includes the control or assessment of medical technologies are discussed below. Figure 9-6 shows the relationships of the principal organizations engaged in technology assessment in the United States.

THE FOOD AND DRUG ADMINISTRATION

The FDA can be considered the backbone of the government's medical technology assessment activities. It regulates entry into the U.S. market of all drugs and relevant medical devices, requiring manufacturing firms to demonstrate that their products are safe and efficacious. Thus FDA *requires* rather than *conducts* assessments. Specifically, it develops product standards, regulates testing, develops and/or approves clinical protocols, and evaluates technical and clinical evidence provided to it by manufacturers and carefully regulates product labeling. It does no clinical testing itself.

FDA generally requires that companies demonstrate safety and efficacy only as claimed in their labeling, not relative to other products or procedures. Thus, testing is usually done compared to a placebo.

Drug Regulation

In order for drugs to enter the U.S. market, the manufacturer must proceed through two major steps established by the FDA: (1) the investigational new drug (IND)

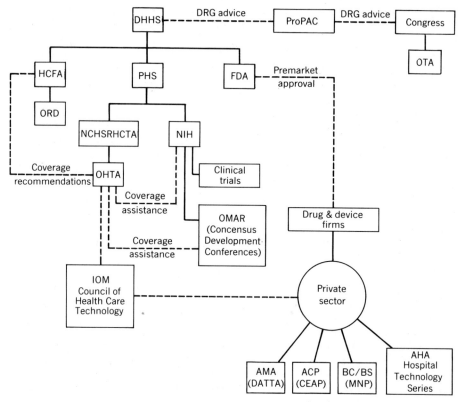

Figure 9-6. Relationships of technology assessment organizations in the United States, 1987. (ACP, American College of Physicians; AHA, American Hospital Association; AMA, American Medical Association; BC/BS, Blue Cross and Blue Shield; CEAP, Clinical Efficacy Assessment Project; DATTA, Diagnostic and Therapeutic Technology; DHHS, Department of Health and Human Services; FDA, Food and Drug Administration; HCFA, Health Care Financing Administration; IOM, Institute of Medicine; MNP, Medical Necessity Program; NCHSRHCTA, National Center for Health Services Research and Health Care Technology Assessment; NIH, National Institutes of Health; OHTA, Office of Health Technology Assessment; OMAR, Office of Medical Applications of Research; ORD, Office of Research and Demonstrations; OTA, Office of Technology Assessment; PHS, Public Health Service; ProPAC, Prospective Payment Assessment Commission.)

application process and (2) the new drug application (NDA) process (26). The IND process normally precedes testing in humans in the United States. The firm describes the proposed clinical studies, the qualifications of the investigators, the chemical properties of the drugs, and the results of all pharmacologic and toxicity testing gained from laboratory animals as well as results from any available human studies, usually from other countries. If FDA approves the IND application, the firm may proceed with the NDA step, normally a three-phase clinical testing program in humans, culminating in relatively large (usually 700–3000 patients) multisite randomized controlled trials. The results of these studies are then presented to FDA for market approval. In some instances, additional "Phase 4" postmarketing surveillance studies are required.

The entire drug development process leading to FDA approval reportedly takes as long as 7–10 years and is extremely expensive. When one includes the development costs of unsuccessful efforts, as much as $90 million is needed for each new chemical entity that reaches the U.S. market (27).

Device Regulation

The 1976 Medical Device Amendments to the Food, Drug and Cosmetic Act require that all medical devices be classified into one of three groups: Class I, general controls; Class II, performance standards; and Class III, premarket approval.

In general, the approval process for medical devices is less onerous than that for drugs. Class I devices (e.g., medical and surgical supplies) essentially require only FDA notification of intention to market and are not closely regulated; Class II devices (e.g., noninvasive diagnostic test equipment) must pass general performance standards; however, Class III devices (e.g., pacemakers, total hip prostheses) are regulated for safety and efficacy and must pass through a clinical testing phase more similar to those mandated for drugs (although much less demanding).

A manufacturer of a Class III device is required to file an investigational device exemption (IDE) application (which is similar to the IND drug process). The IDE permits the firm to test the device in controlled settings on humans in order to establish its safety and efficacy. The resulting evidence is then submitted to the FDA in the form of a premarket approval application (PMAA).

THE NATIONAL INSTITUTES OF HEALTH

The National Institutes of Health contribute to medical technology assessment by sponsoring clinical trials and by conducting consensus development conferences on specific medical practice issues.

NIH's principal mission is to support basic and applied biomedical research in the United States. Although only 5 percent of its total budget is spent on clinical trials, this amounted to $275 million in 1985 (28). The National Cancer Institute is by far the largest sponsor of such research, accounting for 59 percent of all NIH monies spent on clinical trials (29). Although funded by NIH, most trials are investigator-initiated by research clinicians from medical centers all over the United States.

The Office of Medical Applications of Research

Another major technology assessment activity of NIH is the consensus development program organized by the Office of Medical Application of Research (OMAR). Whereas the NIH sponsored clinical trials are typically conducted on medical and surgical procedures in a very early phase of development, the consensus development conferences typically concern medical practice that is in a much more advanced stage of diffusion. Some topics (e.g., CT scanner) are chosen because they are important or controversial new technologies; others (e.g., screening for cervical cancer) are chosen because they are widespread and controversial issues.

These conferences are meetings of experts to arrive at consensus regarding the appropriate use of a given medical technology. The experts are brought together in an open forum to review evidence of safety and efficacy/effectiveness° of the technology under study. The panel then secludes itself for a short period of time in order to reach consensus on a statement of what is known about the application of the technology and what they agree is appropriate state-of-the-art practice.

NIH's objective in sponsoring these conferences is to transfer knowledge to the medical community rather than to create knowledge. The latter is the purpose of the clinical trials. Thus special attention is paid to disseminating the results of the conferences, first by holding a news conference, then by publishing the results in the *Journal of the American Medical Association* (JAMA) and by wide distribution of booklets summarizing the findings.

As of the end of 1986, over 60 conferences had been held. Table 9-2 contains a selection of topics chosen to emphasize the diversity of subjects addressed.

THE OFFICE OF TECHNOLOGY ASSESSMENT

OTA is Congress' technology research and advisory body. Established by Congress in the early 1970s to assist it in better understanding complex technological issues, OTA is divided into a number of programs, including the Health Program within the Health and Life Sciences Division.

The main thrust of the OTA Health Program is to assist Congress in developing policies concerning medical technologies and their assessment. Its reports tend to be general in nature, drawing conclusions from evidence and expert opinion rather than specific assessments of individual technologies. For instance, OTA was instrumental in educating Congress and the country concerning the lack of safety, efficacy, and cost-effectiveness information of medical technologies.

Although general in scope, OTA's reports are often accompanied by one or many case studies of individual technologies. Even these case studies, however, are often syntheses of information rather than evaluations of primary data. Many assessments include not only cost, efficacy/effectiveness, and cost-effectiveness, but legal and

TABLE 9-2. NIH Consensus Development Conferences: Selected Topics

Date	Conference Title
1977	Breast cancer screening
1979	Intraocular lens implantation
	Removal of third molars
1981	CT scan of the brain
1983	Critical care medicine
	Liver transplantation
1984	Lowering blood cholesterol to prevent heart disease
1986	Smokeless tobacco
	Magnetic resonance imaging

SOURCE: NIH, Office of Medical Application of Research, 1986.

°*Efficacy* generally refers to the assessment of a technology under ideal conditions of use; *effectiveness*, under average conditions of use.

ethical implications as well. By 1986, the OTA Health Program had generated 24 main reports of technology assessment issues plus 37 case studies and other background papers and technical memoranda (30). Its 1987 budget is approximately $1.6 million.

Following a specific request from a major standing Congressional Committee, OTA normally conducts its studies by forming an advisory panel for each major topic, gathering evidence from the literature and expert opinion, writing a report on its findings, and circulating drafts of the report to a wide audience for criticism. It then releases its published report to the requesting committee.

OTA is credited with having guided Congress in a number of major technology issues, including legislation establishing the National Center for Health Care Technology in 1978 (which was defunded in 1981). OTA appoints both the Prospective Payment Assessment Commission (ProPAC) and the Physician Payment Review Commission (PhysPRC) and was instrumental in passage of the law establishing the Institution of Medicine's Council on Health Care Technology.

THE HEALTH CARE FINANCING ADMINISTRATION

The Health Care Financing Administration (HCFA) is responsible for administering Medicare and the federal aspect of state Medicaid programs. Its medical technology activities are mainly associated with coverage and reimbursement policies and, to a lesser extent, research and demonstrations.

New procedures are evaluated for coverage determination at as local a level as possible and generally must pass a rather loosely defined test to determine whether they are reasonable and necessary (31). When coverage cannot be resolved at the local or regional level, HCFA's central office initiates a more formal process, first by referring the issue to its internal physician panel and then, if still unresolved, referring it to the Office of Health Technology Assessment (OHTA) within the Public Health Service (PHS) for a more structured review and recommendation.

The HCFA Office of Research and Demonstrations (ORD) conducts and sponsors some studies associated with medical technology and its assessment, but these studies are generally aimed at more general delivery and reimbursement of services than at individual technologies. An exception was the National Heart Transplant study in which HCFA sponsored a study to help to determine its coverage policy. ORD devotes no more than 10 percent of its $31 million research and development budget to technology assessment. A selection of ORD topics include heart transplant, kidney dialysis and transplantation, cyclosporin, magnetic resonance imaging, and implantable devices (32).

NATIONAL CENTER FOR HEALTH SERVICES RESEARCH AND HEALTH CARE TECHNOLOGY ASSESSMENT

The National Center for Health Services Research and Health Care Technology Assessment both sponsors extramural monies for the study of technologies and their assessment and conducts assessments intramurally mainly through its OHTA in support of HCFA coverage policy.

The extramural program consists of investigator-initiated research across all areas of health services research, including topics in health services financing, organization, quality, utilization; health information systems; the role of market forces in health care delivery; and health promotion and disease prevention as well as research related more directly to medical technology issues. Although the National Center's total extramural research budget ($11.3 million in 1987) is considerably smaller than ORD's budget, a much higher percentage of its monies is devoted to technology assessment. In addition, the Center conducts intramural research on many of the topics noted above.

Office of Health Technology Assessment

Located within the National Center, OHTA is primarily responsible for advising HCFA on coverage policy, assuming this role from the now defunct National Center for Health Care Technology (NCHCT). The Public Health Service (PHS) had previously assisted the Medicare program in guiding coverage policy; however, when NCHCT was created, that process became more formalized. In 1981, when NCHCT was deactivated, the then National Center for Health Services Research (NCHSR)—now called the National Center for Health Services Research and Health Care Technology Assessment—created OHTA to continue that coverage advisory function for HCFA.

As stated earlier, when HCFA cannot resolve a coverage issue within its own system, it formally requests the Public Health Service to advise it. PHS refers that request to OHTA, which then publishes a notice to that affect in the Federal Register, requesting information and advice from interested and knowledgeable parties.

OHTA assessments are normally concerned with safety and efficacy/effectiveness, not cost-effectiveness, and generally address the acceptability and appropriateness of a procedure. In the past, PHS advice was to either cover or not cover a procedure, without explicitly providing guidance as to the appropriate conditions of recommended use. More recently, however, OHTA is addressing the conditions under which a technology should be covered. For instance, in 1986, OHTA recommended to HCFA that heart transplants be covered, but only for persons age 55 and under and only when performed in facilities meeting certain criteria (e.g., high volume, high success rate).

OHTA reviews and synthesizes existing data, literature, clinical trial evidence, and expert opinion rather than collecting primary data. It also relies heavily on consultation with the relevant medical specialty societies and federal agencies such as FDA and NIH. Between 1981 and 1986, OHTA prepared over 100 coverage recommendations, nearly all of which were accepted by HCFA in its coverage policy determination.

In 1984 Congress passed the Health Promotion and Disease Prevention Act, which required the National Center to set aside monies for technology assessment ($3.0, $3.5, $3.5 million in 1985–1987, respectively) and to earmark a portion of these monies ($0.5, $0.75, $0.75 million in 1985–1987, respectively) as matching funds for support of the Institute of Medicine's Council on Health Care Technology (see discussion below).

OHTA technology assessments efforts are guided by its National Advisory Council on Health Care Technology Assessment.

PROSPECTIVE PAYMENT ASSESSMENT COMMISSION

As part of the 1983 Amendments to the Social Security Act, Congress established ProPAC to advise and assist both Congress and the Secretary of DHHS in maintaining and updating Medicare's Prospective Payment System (PPS). Appointed by OTA, ProPAC has two primary responsibilities: (1) recommending to the secretary the annual economic update factor for the entire system that includes an adjustment for changes in technology and (2) recommending changes in the relative weights to the DRGs. The latter responsibility requires ProPAC to study individual technologies as they apply to hospital inpatient care.

When a new technology begins to diffuse into the hospital environment, it must fit within some DRG that has been calibrated based on previous methods of practice. If the new technology either decreases or raises costs of providing care, the DRG may no longer reflect the relative resource intensity of providing care and thus may inappropriately compensate the hospital for that case. ProPAC's responsibility is to assist in determining when a DRG needs to be created or recalibrated and what that change should be. Two examples illustrate the issues involved and the potential impact of the diffusion of important new technologies.

Magnetic resonance imaging was assessed in the 1980s. MRI is an expensive technology that can apply to a growing number of types of hospitalized cases (i.e., DRGs). The question becomes whether—and, if so, how—the Medicare prospective payment system (PPS) should be modified to reflect the additional costs of providing care. If no change is made, hospitals that adopt MRI will lose money on such cases (11). If all relevant DRGs are increased to reflect the additional costs to the entire system, hospitals that are slow to adopt MRI will be overcompensated and hospitals that adopt MRI will be undercompensated (since the additional payment is spread across all cases). If an additional DRG "add-on" is made for ony those hospitals that adopt MRI or for only those case where MRI is used, payment may be more equitable on a case-by-case basis, but such a method begins to resemble the previous inflationary cost-based system that PPS was designed to reform. ProPAC's recommendation was to pay an add-on to the DRG for each scan. However, HCFA has been reluctant to adopt such a policy and as of early 1987 has not made any change to the DRG system for MRI.

Extracorporeal shock wave lithotripsy (ESWL) provides another example of the new technology–existing DRG dilemma. Prior to the lithotripsy technology, the treatment of kidney stones in a hospital could be managed either medically or surgically, depending on clinical indications, with the surgical DRGs being roughly three times more expensive than the medical DRGs. Although the lithotripster is an expensive machine to buy and install (approximately $2 million), it crushes kidney stones noninvasively and thus tends to be more expensive per case than medical management but considerably less expensive than surgery. Fitting the lithotripsy into either category could either under- or overpay a hospital for adopting the technology. After studying hospital cost data, ProPAC recommended that HCFA temporarily utilize the higher of the two medical DRGs that it calculated would just cover costs if the machine were used efficiently. HCFA decided to simply pay ESWL within the existing medical DRGs (33).

Both MRI and ESWL are examples of the importance of ProPAC's role and the potential far-reaching effects of reimbursement policies on the adoption, diffusion, and, ultimately, innovation and development of new technologies.

OTHER GOVERNMENT ACTIVITIES

A number of other governmental agencies conduct activities related to medical technology assessment. For instance, the National Center for Health Statistics of the Public Health Service collects and disseminates information on health services utilization and health status of the U.S. population and funds relevant methodologic work such as the measurement of health status versus quality of life. The Veterans Administration (VA) funds clinical and health services research, much of it related to technology, throughout its system. The Centers for Disease Control (CDC) supports assessments of technologies related to clinical laboratories and disease prevention and health promotion. The Department of Defense conducts some clinical trials, but most of its other medical technology assessment activities are limited to military applications.

PRIVATE SECTOR TECHNOLOGY ASSESSMENT ACTIVITIES

Although public policies and agencies tend to dominate discussion of medical technology assessment issues, the private sector is also very active in this area by contributing funding and generating information.

Pharmaceutical and Device Industries

The pharmaceutical industry devotes enormous resources to the assessment of its products, as mentioned earlier in the discussion of FDA's job in regulating drug entry into the marketplace. The industry estimates that in 1985 $4 billion was spent on research and development activities and that each new clinical entity requires 7 to 10 years and an average investment of over $90 million (34). This investment includes all the preclinical and clinical trial research required for FDA premarket approval.

The medical device industry also spends large amounts of money on assessments of its products, although on a much smaller scale than the pharmaceutical industry. A very rough estimate is that 5 percent of sales are devoted to research and development, which may total $1 billion annually (30). In addition, the medical device industry probably devoted only about 4 percent of its research and development (R&D) expenditures, or $35 million to clinical trials (35), in part because it generally takes less time to bring devices to the market and FDA evidence of performance standards, safety and efficacy is usually less rigorous than that required for drugs.

Recently, due to increased pressures from the more competitive marketplace exhibiting greater price sensitivity to costly new technologies, drug and device firms are beginning to invest in cost-effectiveness analysis (CEA) of their products (36). In some cases, firms are beginning to integrate economic analysis into premarket clinical trials as well as to sponsor retrospective CEAs using existing literature and data sources such as claims files. These cost-effectiveness studies also differ from more traditional clinical studies by being comparative studies. That is, rather than being compared to placebo, the technologies are being examined for cost-effectiveness compared to competing choices of therapy; for example, coronary artery bypass surgery compared to percutaneous transluminal coronary arteriography (PTCA), a procedure that uses a balloon catheter used to open restricted coronary arteries.

Insurers, Medical Associations, and Providers

Most of the remaining technology assessement activities sponsored by private sector organizations rely on synthesizing existing information in order to assist technology policymaking. Very seldom are new data collected. In addition, most of these activities assess safety and efficacy issues rather than broader socioeconomic concerns such as cost-effectiveness and legal and ethical implications. Sponsoring such activities are several of the more prominent health care organizations, including the Blue Cross and Blue Shield Association, American Hospital Association, American Medical Association, American College of Physicians, and Institute of Medicine.

All insurers must have some system to determine its coverage policy, just as Medicare must, although private insurers often take a "follow the leader" approach. The leader may be HCFA (for Medicare), or possibly the Blue Cross and Blue Shield Association. In other cases, such as in organ transplantation issues, HCFA has been slower than commercial insurers in making coverage decision. Just as HCFA relies on the Public Health Service, many insurers rely on the appropriate medical societies for guidance as well as having their own internal medical advisory panels.

A prominent and well-defined private insurer assessment activity is the Blue Cross and Blue Shield Association's Medical Necessity Programs (MNP). Established in 1977, MNP attempts to assist in formulating coverage policy by selectively reviewing existing technologies in order to eliminate or reduce coverage for outmoded, ineffectual, and/or misused medical and surgical procedures. By 1985, the program had identified over 90 procedures that were classified as outmoded, had called for the elimination of routine laboratory and x-ray testing, and developed guidelines for respiratory therapy (30). MNP uses BCBS' Medical Advisory Panel and requests the cooperation from such medical societies as the American College of Physicians and American College of Radiology to guide its assessments.

The American College of Physicians (ACP) sponsors the Clinical Efficacy Assessment Project (CEAP), an expansion of MNP. This program relies on literature review and expert opinion from among its membership to review the appropriate application of established technologies used in the practice of internal medicine.

The American Medical Association (AMA) sponsors the Diagnostic and Therapeutic Technology Assessment (DATTA) program, which is similarly designed to educate its memberships of the value and appropriate use of technologies. DATTA tends to concentrate more on new and emerging diagnostic and therapeutic technologies. For each topic, the DATTA program reviews existing evidence, formulates relevant questions, and surveys a panel of experts within AMA's membership ranks.

The American Hospital Association's (AHA) Hospital Technology Series is a program that focuses on hospital devices and equipment from the hospital administrator's point of view. The evaluations are concerned primarily with the cost and service implications of technologies that are entering clinical practice. Evaluations are based on synthesis of technical reports and the professional literature as well as selected and focused interviews with technical and hospital experts.

THE INSTITUTE OF MEDICINE

The latest entry into the field of medical technology assessment in the United States is the Institute of Medicine's (IOM) Council on Health Care Technology. As was stated earlier, Congress earmarked matching funds through the auspices of the National Center for Health Services Research and Health Care Technology Assessment. IOM was thus given a charter to establish an organization that is cosponsored by both private and public monies to help to guide and coordinate technology assessment policy. The Council is made up of leaders throughout private industry and the academic community and has set an agenda to develop a clearinghouse for technology assessment literature and reports, assist in guiding the development of methods for assessment, identify information and data for assessments, and develop guidelines for evaluation. The new Council is mandated to sponsor, coordinate, and/or commission assessments.

CONCLUSIONS

As this overview of several of the major organizations included in medical technology assessment in the United States indicates, the predominant activity is that of assessing existing information. The principal exceptions are the pharmaceutical and medical device firms who must generate primary data for FDA premarket approval, clinical trials sponsored by NIH, and to a much lesser degree other federal agencies.

As was indicated earlier in this chapter, little is known concerning the appropriate use of many technologies. The final section of this chapter addresses some of the methodological issues of assessing medical technologies.

METHODS FOR ASSESSMENT

A number of different techniques and methodologies are used in the assessment of medical technologies. Some of the more common ones have already been mentioned: the randomized clinical trials (RCT), group judgement methods, literature review, and cost-effectiveness analysis.

A helpful way to discuss the methods for evaluating technologies is to use a four-step framework for assessment: identification, testing, synthesis, and dissemination (Fig. 9-7).

This process is applicable even to later stages in the life cycle of a technology. Because technologies may diffuse prematurely without adequate assessment, they are often used for new indications or for different groups of patients, and their relative efficacy may change as new competing technologies are developed.

IDENTIFICATION

It is difficult to determine which technologies should be assessed. Of course, by law, drugs and medical devices can be marketed only with FDA approval, so the industry systematically identifies these technologies for assessment early in their life cycle. Later, these same technologies may face a market test due to price sensitivity of the insurer, the hospital, the Health Maintenance Organization (HMO) or even the physician or the consumer. In such a case, the market itself is identifying the technology—requesting, in effect, that cost effectiveness be assessed.

In the previous section we discussed the substantial role of the insurer (HCFA, Blue Cross, etc.) in identifying technologies for assessment during the coverage policy determination of a new technology. In other cases, such as with OTA, a technology is chosen for assessment as a case study either for the purpose of illustrating a policy issue or because it has assumed national significance, such as the CT scanner. Other bodies such as the old National Center for Health Care Technology (NCHCT) or BCBS'

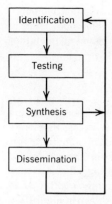

Figure 9-7. Process of assessing medical technologies. (SOURCE: Office of Technology Assessment, U.S. Congress: *Strategies for Medical Technology Assessment,* Washington, DC, 1982.)

Medical Necessity Program rely on advisory councils to develop priorities for assessment using criteria such as high per unit cost, high volume, potential safety issues, and uncertainty concerning efficacy and appropriate use.

TESTING

Safety and Efficacy

Testing refers to primary data being generated systematically for analysis. The gold standard for testing technologies is the *randomized clinical trial (RCT)* since it provides the most valid and reliable information. Human subjects are randomly assigned to the experimental and comparison and/or control groups, blinded, if possible, as to which group they are in and followed over time to determine efficacy, safety and, possibly, cost-effectiveness. When possible, even the clinicians and evaluators are blinded as to which subjects are in which group. Randomization and blinding helps to minimize any bias in the findings.

Many times, blinding or random assignment are impracticable or even impossible. For instance, one cannot blind surgeons and patients when testing surgical techniques . . . sham surgery is unethical. Similarly, once a treatment is thought to be efficacious, it may be unethical to withhold treatment as would be necessary in random assignment.

Various observational methods are used when randomization cannot be done in order to minimize bias. For instance, a matched control study attempts to match pairs of patients in both groups on all-important variables that could have an impact on therapeutic outcome such as age, sex, symptoms, and severity of disease.

A very common method found in the medical literature is the *case study*. In fact, individual clinicians develop their own particular practice style based in large part on observations of their own cases. Although the case study method has its place in informing medical practice, its role may be better served as a method of identifying when a formal assessment is warranted rather than serving as evidence that a technology is or is not efficacious.

Another useful method of study is the *clinical data bank* or *registry approach*. These types of historical files are set up to follow patients who have certain medical conditions (e.g., cancer) or have undergone a certain procedure (e.g., cardiac catherization).

They can be helpful in studying long-term epidemiologic trends and clinical outcomes. Cancer registries are the oldest and most common example of this method. Thus, in themselves, the clinical data bank and registry is not a method of assessment, but rather a way to organize and gather data for assessment.

Cost-Effectiveness Analysis (CEA)

Although most of the technology assessment methods are primarily used for testing safety and efficacy, CEA is becoming increasingly popular since it is clear that when technology decisions are made there are economic constraints that require trade offs (37). Unlike *cost-benefit analysis (CBA)*, which values all outcomes in terms of dollars, thus necessitating the explicit valuing of life, limb, pain, and suffering, CEA is used to calculate the net cost of acquiring some health outcome. A convenient way to conceptualize the cost-benefit and cost-effectiveness approach is shown in Figure 9-8.

The medical or health treatment (see box *A* in Fig. 9-8) can lead to changes in both health services resource use (e.g., open heart surgery—*B*) and health status (e.g., years of life saved—*C*). Changes in health status (*C*) in turn, can lead to a change in productive output (*D*). Box *E* shows the economic value that can be placed on that health status change. A CBA calculates the net economic value in boxes *B, C, D,* and *E*. Cost-effectiveness analysis generally compares the net economic changes in health resource use (*B*) with the net change in health status (*C*). Table 9-3 provides comparisons of the cost per year of life saved (or cost per quality-adjusted year of life saved) as reported in a number of cost-effectiveness studies in the literature.

Lately cost-effectiveness analysis has sometimes been added to clinical and observational studies. Typically, patients in the study are followed for standard safety and efficacy evaluation but also monitored for economic outcomes, such as health care utilization patterns and work loss. In addition, special patient survey questionnaires that assess overall health status change are sometimes used. For example, HCFA funded the National Heart Transplant Study, which followed a series of heart

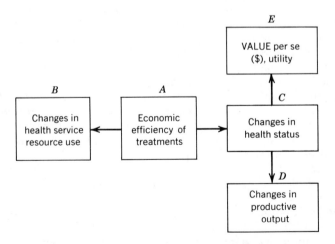

Figure 9-8. Measuring efficiency in health care. (SOURCE: Drummond MF: *Principles of Economic Appraisal in Health Care.* Oxford, England, Oxford University Press, 1980.)

TABLE 9-3. Costs per Year of Life Saved for Some Health Investments

Investment	Cost per Year of Life Saved (1986 U.S. $)[a]
Neonatal intensive care, 1000–1499 g	$ 5,500
Coronary artery bypass surgery (*three-vessel*)	$ 7,200°
T4 (thyroid screening)	$ 7,700
Treatment of severe hypertension (diastolic > 105 mmHg) in males age 40	$11,400
Treatment of mild hypertension (diastolic 95–104 mmHg) in males age 40	$23,200
Heart transplantation	$26,854°
Estrogen therapy for postmenopausal symptoms in women without a prior hysterectomy	$32,900
Neonatal intensive care, 500–999 g	$38,800
Coronary artery bypass surgery for *single-vessel* disease with moderately severe angina	$44,200
School tuberculin testing program	$53,100
Continuous ambulatory peritoneal dialysis .	$57,300
Hospital hemodialysis	$65,600

SOURCE: Adapted from Drummond MF: Economic evaluation and the rational diffusion and use of health technology. *Health Policy* in press.

[a]Each figure, except for those marked with an asterisk (°), refers to cost per *quality-adjusted* life year saved.

transplant patients, assessing effectiveness, quality of life, and direct and indirect economic costs, as well as other social and legal issues (38).

SYNTHESIS

The third component of the process of assessment is the synthesis of information, a practice that is widely used and perhaps overly relied on. Many technology assessments found in the literature today are developed using a technique falling under the general heading of synthesis. The most common and simple method of synthesis is the standard literature review. One person surveys what is written about a procedure, discards that which is deemed unimportant, and draws conclusions regarding the value of the procedure. The quality of a literature review depends on the ability and diligence of the reviewer, that individual's personal biases, and the quality and consistency of the evidence found in the literature. This last point can be a particularly difficult problem because multiple independent clinical studies of a given technology often reveal conflicting results, partially because they are conducted at different times, with different patients using different methods of design and different techniques of analysis.

Today, formal quantitative synthesis techniques, collectively termed *meta analysis*, have been devised to assist in resolving many of these difficulties. Meta analysis permits a reviewer to consolidate the results of multiple, unrelated studies on a given issue, differentially weighting studies depending on the rigor of research design, sample size, and so forth. Thus, an RCT may be weighted more heavily than an observational study; a large trial more heavily than a small one.

A less quantitative but particularly popular method for synthesizing information is a family of techniques termed "group judgment" or "consensus" methods (39). The Consensus Development format used by the NIH was described earlier. There are other variations such as the Delphi and Nominal Group Process techniques, which are more structured methods of eliciting group judgments. The AMA's DATTA program and the American College of Physicians' CEAP, both of which were described in the previous section, are examples of less structured group judgment methods. DATTA is more of a poll than a group judgment method. Some techniques systematically combine clinical trial evidence with the group judgment (40,41); other techniques assume that the experts being polled already are aware of the existing evidence (Delphi, DATTA).

DISSEMINATION

The dissemination phase of the assessment process is arguably the most underrated of the four phases being discussed here. Relatively little attention has been paid to how information about clinical practice is disseminated, how it is received once the information arrives, and whether—and why—change really takes place (1). Stated differently, we do not understand very well to what doctors pay attention. We simply know that there is clearly much misunderstanding of evidence that both does and does not exist concerning the efficacy, safety, cost-effectiveness, and other social, legal and ethical implications of the use of technologies. Practicing clinicians rely on their own store of knowledge from their training, personal experience, colleagues, the literature, and other educational materials and programs, perhaps roughly in that order of importance.

Many organizations attempt to make technology assessment information available. There are numerous medical journals, often sponsored by medical societies; the National Library of Medicine catalogs and indexes medical and health journals; and many of the organizations discussed in this chapter sponsor assessment activities specifically for the purposes of disseminating the results to their membership and the medical community at large. Yet little is known of the effectiveness of these efforts.

FUTURE CONSIDERATIONS

The United States is leaving the era of health care expansion, leaving the era of laissez-faire payment policies that pay—seemingly without questions—for whatever is ordered by physicians and whatever is charged for their services. These past payment policies have fueled technological innovation, adoption, and use. Since costs were not much of a constraint, high tech medicine could soar, as could quality of care to the extent that the two are linked. It is well known that medicine in the United States is the most technologically advanced system in the world, and believed by many to be the best care in the world.

However, there have been many excesses as well, excesses that are certainly not limited to the United States.

The major threat to the wondrous technological innovations that could be ours in the future probably lies in the hands of the politicians who must control the deficit and of the medical and health services communities who will have to convince an increasingly skeptical public that their own house is in order. The threat is not in the hands of the innovators of health care technology and other venture capitalists, both of whom will respond to the signals that society sends them.

This chapter has attempted to describe medical technology—its development, diffusion, adoption, use, and assessment. Although the United States probably has the most sophisticated technology generating and assessment systems in the world, much still needs to be done. The basic tools are available, however. Sufficient capital and innovative capabilities exist in private industry. Public agencies and private organizations are in place and assessment methods are useful and available. Basic and applied research monies are available. The country does have an effective system to ensure that drugs and devices are not marketed prior to safety and efficacy being established. However, there is no such system for medical and surgical procedures. Nor is there sufficient information about the appropriate use of any of the classes of technologies in the inventory.

Today, we are seeing more organizations launching assessment activities and existing ones being further developed. This is true of the federal government, medical societies, and insurers. Also, assessment programs are coming under greater scrutiny by policymakers. For instance, OHTA is under the microscope of both Congress and the manufacturers' associations. In general, the assessment enterprise gains greater attention as assessment becomes a gateway to payment and marketing success. Manufacturers are looking beyond safety and efficacy of their products to broader implications such as quality of life and cost-effectiveness. They are also sponsoring more comparative studies.

Nevertheless, despite the gains made to date, the challenge of the future is to learn to use the tools we have in order to better understand the technology and its use within the practice of medicine.

REFERENCES

1. Office of Technology Assessment, U.S. Congress: *Strategies for Medical Technology Assessment.* Washington, DC, 1982.

2. Reiser SJ, Anbar M (eds): *The Medicine at the Bedside: Strategies for Using Technology in Patient Care.* New York, Cambridge University Press, 1984, p 11.

3. Pollard MR, Persinger GS, Perpich JG: Technology innovation in health care. *Health Affairs* 1986; 3:86.

4. Institute of Medicine: *Assessing Medical Technologies.* Washington, DC, National Academy Press, 1985, p 37.

5. Bessey EC: "Innovation in an era of cost containment," in Southby RMCK, Greenberg W, Luce BR (eds): *Health Care Technology Under Financial Constraints.* Columbus, OH, Battelle Press, 1987.

6. Russell LB: *Technology in Hospitals: Medical Advances and Their Diffusion.* Washington, DC, The Brookings Institution, 1979.

7. Office of Technology Assessment, U.S. Congress: *Policy Implications of the Computed Tomography (CT) Scanner: An Update.* Washington, DC, 1981.

8. Office of Technology Assessment, U.S. Congress: *Policy Implications of the Computed Tomgraphy (CT) Scanner.* Washington, DC, 1978.

9. Steinberg EP, Sisk JE, Locke KE: The Diffusion of Magnetic Resonance Imagers in the United States and the World. *Internati J Technol Assess Health Care* 1985; 1:537.

10. Valvona J, Sloan F: Rising Rates of Surgery Among the Elderly. *Health Affiars* 1985; 4:108–118.

11. Chu F, Cotter D: PPS policies should reflect payment adjustments for new technologies. *Business and Health* 1986; 4:60.

12. Wennberg JE: Dealing with medical practice variations: A proposal for action. *Health Affairs* 1984; 3:6–32.

13. Wennberg JE: Dealing with medical practice variations: A proposal for action. *Health Affairs* 1984; 3:15.

14. Chassin MR, Brook RH, Park R et al: Variations in the use of medical and surgical services by the Medicare population. *New Engl J Med* 1986; 314:285–309.

15. Wennberg JE, Brook RH: Addressing medical practice variations: A challenge for pros and private review agencies, paper presented to the National Health Policy Forum. Washington, DC, 1985.

16. Office of Technology Assessment, U.S. Congress: *Assessing the Safety and Efficacy of Medical Technologies.* Washington, DC, 1978, p 7.

17. Iglehart JK: Editor's note. *Health Affairs* 1984; 3:

18. Morse LM: Therapeutic drug use review reduces incidence of drug related illness. *Business and Health* 1986; 3:58.

19. Fineberg HV: Gastric freezing. A study of diffusion of a medical innovation, in *Medical Technology and the Health Care System: A Study of the Diffusion of Equipment-Embodied Technology.* Washington, DC, National Academy of Sciences, 1979, p 173.

20. Hiatt HH: *America's Health in the Balance: Choice or change.* New York, Harper & Row, 1987, p 173.

21. Lambert EC: *Modern Medical Mistakes.* Bloomington, Indiana, Indiana University Press, 1978.

22. Lawless EW: *Technology and Social Shock.* New Brunswick, NJ, Rutgers University Press, 1977.

23. Banta D, Brown S, Behney C: Implications of the 1976 Medical Devices Legislation. *Man and Medicine* 978; 3:131–143.

24. Office of Technology Assessment, U.S. Congress: *Development of Medical Technologies: Opportunities for Assessment.* Washington, DC, 1976.

25. U.S. Department of Health, Education and Welfare, Office of the Assistant Secretary: *NCHCT Fact Sheet,* n.d.

26. Food and Drug Administration, U.S. Department of Health and Human Services: *General Considerations for the Clinical Evaluation of Drugs.* Washington, DC, U.S. Government Printing Office, 1977.

27. Pharmaceutical Manufacturers Association: *PMA Statistical Factbook*. Washington, DC, 1984.

28. National Institutes of Health, Office of the Director: *Report on the Patterns of Funding Clinical Research*. Bethesda, MD, 1985.

29. National Institutes of Health: *NIH Data Book*. Bethesda, MD, 1985.

30. Institute of Medicine: *Assessing Medical Technologies*. Washington, DC, National Academy Press, 1985.

31. Lewin and Associates: *A Forward Plan for Medicare Coverage and Technology Assessment*, Final Report, Contract No. 282-45-0062. Prepared for the Assistant Secretary for Planning and Evaluation, DHHS, Washington, DC, 1986.

32. Health Care Financing Administration: Unpublished data, 1986.

33. Office of Technology Assessment, U.S. Congress: *Health Technology Case Study 36: Effects of Federal Policies on Extracorporeal Shock Wave Lithotripsy*. Washington, DC, May 1986.

34. Institute of Medicine: *Assessing Medical Technologies*. Washington, DC, National Academy Press, 1985, p 46.

35. Institute of Medicine: *Assessing Medical Technologies*. Washington, DC, National Academy Press, 1985, p 52.

36. Luce BR: Cost-Effectiveness Studies of Medical Technologies by Private Industry. Paper presented to the Association for Health Services Research, Annual Meeting, Chicago, IL, 1985.

37. Warner KE, Luce BR: *Cost-Benefit and Cost-Effectiveness Analysis in Health Care: Principles, Practice and Potential*. Ann Arbor, MI, Health Administration Press, 1982.

38. Health Care Financing Administration, Office of Research and Demonstration: *National Heart Transplant Study*. Battelle Final Report, Vols. I–VII, 1985.

39. Fink A, Kosecoff J, Chassis M, et al: Consensus Methods: Characteristics and guidelines for use. *Am J Publ Health* 1984; 74:979.

40. Park RE, Fink A, Brook RH, et al: Physician ratings of appropriate indications for six medical and surgical procedures. *Am J Publ Health* 1986; 76:766.

41. Jacoby I: The Consensus Development Program of the National Institutes of Health: Current Practices and Historical Perspectives. *Internat J Technol Assess Health Care* 1985; 1:420.

CHAPTER 10

Health Care Professionals

Ira Moscovice

Health care professionals play an important role in the provision of services to meet the health needs of the population. This chapter highlights health care professional trends and discusses issues of provider supply, education/training, distribution, specialization, and the role of the public sector in the production of health care professionals.

EMPLOYMENT TRENDS IN THE HEALTH CARE INDUSTRY

The twentieth century has witnessed a dramatic growth in the number and types of personnel employed in the health care industry. Table 10-1 shows the rapid gains in health sector employment in the United States, starting with a pool of fewer than 500,000 employees in 1910 and growing to more than 5 million by 1980. These figures include primarily those individuals with training and skills unique to the health care industry and exclude clerical staff, artisans, laborers, and others who have supporting roles in the delivery of health services. It has been estimated that almost one-third of all health sector employees fall into this supporting category (1). The importance of these approximately 1.5 million nonclinical workers should not be overlooked.

The health care industry is the largest single employer of all the industries monitored by the Department of Labor (2). It has maintained a steadily increasing proportion of all persons employed, and currently includes more than 5 percent of the U.S. labor force. Thus, employment in the health sector has outpaced overall employment in our economy as well as total population growth. This growth is accentuated by the fourfold increase in the rate of health care personnel per 100,000 population, from a low of 518 in 1910 to a high of 2209 in 1980 (Table 10-1).

More extraordinary than the increased supply of health care personnel has been the emergence of a wide variety of new categories of personnel, including physicians' assistants (PAs), nurse practitioners (NPs), dental hygienists, and laboratory technicians, nursing aides, orderlies and attendants, home health aides, occupational and physical

TABLE 10-1. The Health Sector as a Proportion of All Employed Persons, by Decade: 1910–1980

	1910	1920	1930	1940	1950	1960	1970	1980
Employment in health sector (1,000s)[a]	479	624	859	972	1,394	1,966	3,130	5,030
Total number of persons employed (1,000s)[b]	38,167	41,614	48,829	44,888	56,225	64,639	78,627	97,270
Health sector as a proportion of all occupations	1.3%	1.5%	1.8%	2.2%	2.5%	3.0%	4.0%	5.2%
Total U.S. population (1,000,000s)	92.4	106.5	123.1	132.6	152.3	180.7	205.1	227.7
Rate of health personnel per 100,000 population	518	586	698	733	915	1,088	1,428	2,209

SOURCE: Adapted from Mick, S. Table 7, Understanding the problems of human resources in health, 1925–77: Recommendations from the CCMC and current realities, paper prepared for a conference at Georgetown University, May 1977.

[a]These figures do not include secretarial and office workers, craftsmen, laborers, and other personnel such as cooks, janitors, and so on who work in supporting roles in the health care industry.

[b]Figures for 1980 include employed persons 16 years of age and over; figures from 1940 to 1970 include employed persons 14 years of age and over; earlier data are based on persons 10 years of age and over.

therapists, medical records personnel, x-ray technicians, dieticians and nutritionists, social workers, and the like. The Department of Labor currently recognizes almost 700 different job categories in the health industry (2). The most rapid growth in the supply of health care personnel has occurred in these recently developed categories.

The traditional health care occupations of physicians, dentists, registered nurses, pharmacists, and optometrists generally have experienced dramatic declines in their relative proportion of all health care personnel as compared to the marked increase in recent decades in the supply of medical, nursing, and dental allied health personnel. One exception is registered nurses, who continue to comprise the largest single group of health care personnel. More than two-thirds of all personnel employed in the health care industry are in nontraditional allied health or support services positions (3).

The primary reasons for the increased supply and wide variety of health care personnel in the twentieth century were the interrelated forces of technological growth, specialization, and the emergence of the hospital as the central focus of the health care system. The hospital became the setting where new technology could be implemented and where medical, nursing, and other health professional students could be educated. The technological revolution has led to the increased use of hospitals, with a corresponding concentration there of health care personnel. However, current concerns with escalating health care costs have led to a substantial increase in the use of health care facilities outside the hospital (4). These facilities include urgent care centers, ambulatory surgery centers, free-standing diagnostic centers, Health Maintenance Organizations (HMOs), and the like. The hospital sector is not likely to have increased employment in the near future.

Technological innovation has also led to increased specialization of health care personnel, primarily during the last 30 years. This specialization has resulted in the formation of new categories of health care providers within the traditional professions (e.g., pediatric nephrologists and gastroenterologists in medicine, periodontists in dentistry) and the advent of new types of allied health professional (e.g., occupational therapists, radiologic technicians, speech pathologists).

These health care personnel trends will be discussed in greater detail by focusing on three of the more traditional groups of professionals—physicians, dentists, and nurses—and two of the recently developed categories of personnel—PAs and NPs.

THE EXPANDING SUPPLY OF PHYSICIANS

THE PHYSICIAN SURPLUS

The number of physicians in the United States has increased rapidly in the last two decades, with 466,600 active physicians practicing in 1982 (Table 10-2). Between 1965 and 1982, there has been a 62 percent increase in the supply of physicians, resulting in an average of approximately one physician per 500 population. The increase in physician supply has been due primarily to two important trends—the rapid increase in the number of graduates from medical schools since 1965 and the substantial immigration of foreign-trained physicians into the United States (5).

Table 10-3 shows the substantial increase in both the number of medical schools and the number of enrolled medical students over the past two decades. By 1985, the yearly number of graduates from medical schools had more than doubled in just 20 years. This

TABLE 10-2. Number of Active Physicians: 1965, 1970, 1975, 1980, 1982

Health Occupation	1965		1970		1975		1980		1982	
	Number	Personnel per 100,000 Population	Number	Personnel per 100,000 Population	Number	Personnel per 100,000 Population	Number	Personnel per 100,000 Population	Number	Personnel per 100,000 Population
Physicians	288,700	145.5	326,200	156.0	384,500	174.4	457,500	197.0	466,600	198.8
MDs	277,600	139.9	314,200	150.0	370,400	167.9	440,400	189.5	448,600	191.0
DOs	11,100	5.7	12,000	6.0	14,100	6.5	17,100	7.5	18,000	7.8

SOURCE: *Fourth Report to the President and Congress on the Status of Health Personnel in the United States,* U.S. Department of Health and Human Services, Publ. No. (HRS)-P-0084.4, U.S. Government Printing Office, May 1984.

increase can be directly attributed to the massive federal outlays for training, research, and construction in the 1960s and 1970s. By the early 1970s, 40 to 50 percent of medical school support came from federal sources (6). However, the retreat of the federal government from an active role in the financial support of medical education has been initiated in the mid-1980s as a result of the overall pressures to reduce federal spending and the perception that there is an adequate overall supply of physicians in the United States. At present, the federal government provides approximately 25 percent of medical school financial support (7).

The second important factor in the increased supply of physicians has been the influx of foreign medical graduates (FMGs) into the United States. By the mid-1960s, favorable immigration policies for physicians had encouraged this movement. By the early 1970s, FMGs accounted for more than 40 percent of new physician licentiates, 30 percent of filled residency positions, and 20 percent of active physicians in the United States. One-third of the growth in the supply of physicians in the 1970s was due to increases in the number of physicians trained outside the United States (8).

The vast majority of the increase in FMG supply occurred before 1976 (Table 10-3).

TABLE 10-3. Number of Medical Schools, Students, and Graduates: Academic Years 1964–1965 Through 1984–1985[a]

Academic Year	Number of Schools	Number of Students		Number of Graduates
		Total	First Year	
1964–1965	88	32,428	8,856	7,409
1965–1966	88	32,835	8,759	7,574
1966–1967	89	33,423	8,964	7,743
1967–1968	94	34,538	9,479	7,973
1968–1969	99	35,833	9,863	8,059
1969–1970	101	37,669	10,401	8,367
1970–1971	103	40,487	11,348	8,974
1971–1972	108	43,650	12,361	9,551
1972–1973	112	47,546	13,726	10,391
1973–1974	114	50,886	14,185	11,613
1974–1975	114	54,074	14,963	12,714
1975–1976	114	56,244	15,351	13,561
1976–1977	116	58,266	15,667	13,607
1977–1978	122	60,456	16,134	14,393
1978–1979	125	62,754	16,620	14,966
1979–1980	126	64,195	17,014	15,135
1980–1981	126	65,497	17,204	15,667
1981–1982	126	66,485	17,320	15,985
1982–1983	127	66,886	17,230	15,824
1983–1984	127	69,443	17,175	16,327
1984–1985	127	67,090	16,992	16,347

SOURCE: Crowley A, Etzel S, Petersen E, et al, "Undergraduate medical education," *JAMA* 1985; 254:1565–1572.
[a]Includes schools of basic medical sciences.

That year marked the passage of PL 94-484 (the Health Professions Education Assistance Act of 1976), which stated, "there is no further need for affording preference to alien physicians and surgeons in admission to the United States under the Immigration and Nationality Act." The enactment of PL 94-484 noticeably limited the emigration of FMGs to the United States. The number of FMGs filling residency positions decreased from 18,395 in 1972–1973 to 12,477 in 1985–1986. This figure has stabilized in the 12,000–13,000 range during the past 5 years (see Table 10-4). FMGs are currently filling less than 17 percent of all residency positions, compared to a peak of 33 percent in 1970. A recent major change is the dramatic increase in the proportion of FMGs who are U.S. citizens who received their medical training outside the United States (55 percent in 1985 as compared to 35 percent in 1979). Further growth in the number of U.S. physicians will not be influenced as much as it has been in the past by the influx of FMGs; however, FMGs will remain an important factor in the U.S. health care system.

In summary, there has been a marked increase in the supply of U.S. physicians in the last two decades due to an increased number of medical school graduates and the immigration of FMGs. An obvious question is, why was it necessary to use this dual strategy for increasing the physician supply? The answer is twofold. First, before the 1970s, policymakers strongly believed that there was a serious shortage of physicians in the United States, with several studies estimating the shortage in 1975 to be in the range of 10,000 to 50,000 (9). Second, our country has not had a coordinated physician personnel policy; undergraduate and graduate medical education systems have operated independently of each other (5). Historically, the students graduating from U.S. medical schools have filled only two-thirds of the available residency positions, leaving the less desirable positions (both for residencies and permanent employment) for FMGs. FMGs have helped to staff U.S. hospitals and have been more willing than U.S. medical school graduates to practice in relatively unpopular geographic and/or specialty areas.

It is not surprising, then, that the twofold strategy for increasing the physician supply more than met the perceived physician shortages of the 1960s and early 1970s. The final report of the Graduate Medical Education National Advisory Committee (GMENAC) estimates there will be a surplus of 70,000 physicians by 1990 (10). How the public and private sector reacts to this perceived surplus will influence future physician training, supply, and practice.

TABLE 10-4. Foreign Medical Graduates (FMGs) in Residency Positions

	1979	1982	1983	1984	1985
Total FMGs	12,070	13,123	13,221	13,525	12,477
Percentage of total residents	18.7	19.0	18.4	18.0	16.8
U.S. citizen FMGs	4,229	6,388	6,990	7,386	6,868
U.S. citizen FMGs as a percentage of all FMGs	35.0	48.6	52.8	54.6	55.0

SOURCE: Anne E. Crowley, "Foreign Medical Graduates in U.S. Graduate Medical Education," *JAMA* 1986; 256:1551–1554. Copyright 1986, American Medical Association.

TRENDS IN SPECIALTY DISTRIBUTION

The significant increase in the supply of physicians described above had led to major concerns about the specialty and geographic distribution of physicians. Simply increasing the supply of physicians did not guarantee that necessary medical services would be readily available to the general population. Of particular interest was the availability of primary care—the entry level into the health care system where basic medical services are provided. Primary care includes the diagnosis and treatment of common illnesses and diseases, preventive services, home care services, and uncomplicated minor surgery and emergency care.

The increased supply of physicians has not resulted in major changes in the proportion of physicians in the primary care specialties—general practice, family practice, general internal medicine, and general pediatrics (Table 10-5). Within the primary care specialties, the number of family practitioners, internists, and pediatricians grew faster than the overall physician supply in the 1970s. However, these gains were offset by the declining number of general practitioners due to death or retirement. The strong growth in surgical specialities that characterized the specialty distribution up to 1970 ceased in the following years. Despite efforts to increase support for primary care residencies and decrease support for surgical residencies, less than 40 percent of physicians are in primary care specialties providing basic medical services, and almost 30 percent are surgeons. The final report of the GMENAC projects significant surpluses of surgical and medical specialties, with a near balance of supply and demand for primary care specialties in 1990 (Table 10-6).

The real goal of any physician supply policy should be to provide appropriate medical services that are readily accessible to the general population. Knowledge of the physician specialty distribution does not provide information on physician productivity, practice case mix, or the scope of services provided. The controversy over the extent of primary care provided by specialists and specialty care provided by primary care physicians highlights this point (11,12). Future needs for physicians cannot be based solely on knowledge of the number and types of physicians in our country.

GEOGRAPHIC DISTRIBUTION OF PHYSICIANS

One of the assumptions underlying federal health personnel policy in the 1960s and early 1970s was that a significant increase in the overall supply of physicians would both resolve the problem of a serious shortage and improve the geographic distribution of physicians. Clearly, there is no longer a shortage of physicians in the United States. Nevertheless, the chronic shortage of physicians in rural and inner city areas continues to persist (13).

With the output of physicians from medical schools outpacing the growth of the U.S. population, the population/physician ratio declined from one physician per 840 people in 1960 to one per 524 people in 1983 (Table 10-7). From 1960 to 1970, the vast majority of these physicians located in urban areas. However, the supply of physicians increased in both Standard Metropolitan Statistical Areas (SMSAs) and non-SMSAs after 1970. Among people living in SMSAs and non-SMSAs, there was a 28 percent decrease in the population/physician ratio in the period 1970–1983. However, the

TABLE 10-5. Number of Active Physicians (MDs) and Percentage Distribution by Specialty Groups

Specialty	1963 Number	1963 Percent	1968 Number	1968 Percent	1976 Number	1976 Percent	1981[b] Number	1981[b] Percent	1990[b] Number	1990[b] Percent
All specialties	261,728	100.0	296,312	100.0	348,443	100.0	430,745	100.0	566,930	100.0
Primary care specialties[a]	110,071	42.1	116,760	39.4	135,881	39.0	163,383	37.9	239,830	42.3
Other medical specialties	12,291	4.7	15,762	5.3	18,955	5.4	29,242	6.8	41,080	6.8
Surgical specialties	67,745	25.8	81,820	27.6	98,667	28.3	113,704	26.4	129,610	22.9
All other specialties	71,621	27.4	81,970	27.7	94,940	27.3	124,416	28.9	156,410	27.6

SOURCES: Rosenblatt R, Moscovice I: *Rural Health Care*. New York, Wiley, 1982, Table 4.2 and *Fourth Report to the President and Congress on the Status of Health Personnel in the United States*, U.S. Department of Health and Human Services, Publ. No. (HRS)-P-0084.4, Government Printing Office, May 1984.
[a]Includes general practice, family practice, general internal medicine, and general pediatrics.
[b]Projections.

315

TABLE 10-6. Ratio of Projected Supply to Estimated Requirements, 1990

		Ratio (%)	Requirements	Surplus (Shortage)
Shortages	Child psychiatry	45	9,000	(4,900)
	Emergency medicine	70	13,500	(4,250)
	Preventive medicine	75	7,300	(1,750)
	General psychiatry	80	38,500	(8,000)
Near Balance	Hematology/oncology-internal medicine	90	9,000	(700)
	Dermatology	105	6,950	400
	Gastroenterology-internal medicine	105	6,500	400
	Osteopathic general practice	105	22,000	1,150
	Family practice	105	61,300	3,100
	General internal medicine	105	70,250	3,550
	Otolaryngology	105	8,000	500
	General pediatrics and subspecialties	115	36,400	4,950
Surpluses	Urology	120	7,700	1,650
	Orthopedic surgery	135	15,100	5,000
	Ophthalmology	140	11,600	4,700
	Thoracic surgery	140	2,050	850
	Infectious diseases-internal medicine	145	2,250	1,000
	Obstetrics gynecology	145	24,000	10,450
	Plastic surgery	145	2,700	1,200
	Allergy immunology-internal medicine	150	2,050	1,000
	General surgery	150	23,500	11,800
	Nephrology-internal medicine	175	2,750	2,100
	Rheumatology-internal medicine	175	1,700	1,300
	Cardiology-internal medicine	190	7,750	7,150
	Endocrinology-internal medicine	190	2,050	1,800
	Neurosurgery	190	2,650	2,450
	Pulmonary-internal medicine	195	3,600	3,350
Estimated	Physical medicine and rehabilitation	75	3,200	(800)
	Anesthesiology	95	21,000	(1,550)
	Nuclear medicine	N/A	4,000	N/A
	Pathology	125	13,500	3,350
	Radiology	155	18,000	9,800
	Neurology	160	5,500	3,150

SOURCE: *Third Report to the President and Congress on the Status of Health Professions Personnel in the United States*, U.S. Department of Health and Human Services Publ. No. (HRA) 82-2. U.S. Government Printing Office, January 1982.

TABLE 10-7. Population/Physician Ratios by SMSA, 1950–1983

SMSA or County Size Classification	Population/Physician Ratio									Percent Decrease
	1950	1960	1970	1972	1974	1976	1978	1980	1983	1970–1983
U.S. total	845	840	728	687	658	617	578	556	524	28.0
SMSA	707	721	622	584	558	522	489	469	447	28.1
Non-SMSA	1412	1443	1416	1378	1328	1250	1165	1117	1026	27.5

SOURCES: Reprinted, with permission of the Blue Cross and Blue Shield Association, from *Inquiry*, Vol. 19 (1982), p. 46. All rights reserved; Bureau of Health Professions, *Supply and Characteristics of Selected Health Personnel, U.S. Department of Health and Human Services*, Publ. No (HRA)-81-20, U.S. Government Printing Office, June 1981; Roback G, Randolph L, Mead D, et. al: *Physician Characteristics and Distribution in the U.S.*, American Medical Association, Chicago, 1985.

recent increase in physician supply has not been enjoyed by all counties. Rural counties with the smallest populations have gained few new physicians during this period (13).

The impact of specialization on the geographic distribution of physicians is not surprising. Until recently, general practitioners were the majority of physicians in rural areas. The supply of general practitioners has since dwindled, to be replaced in the late 1970s and 1980s by recently trained family practitioners and other specialists. Graduates of family practice residency programs have located in non-SMSAs more frequently than have other specialists, with half of 1982 graduating family practice residents locating in towns of less than 50,000 people (14). Family practitioners will undoubtedly be the core of the future rural physician supply.

Large metropolitan areas are rapidly becoming physician-saturated. Policymakers have traditionally assumed that physicians, particularly specialists, would not locate in rural areas as their supply increased. These views have been challenged by research that concluded that economic or market forces have caused major changes in the distribution of board-certified specialists (15). By the late 1970s, communities with more than 20,000 residents often had board-certified specialists. Board-certified specialists who moved to nonmetropolitan areas settled in regional centers that already had a sufficient number of physicians (16). Thus, those areas in greatest need of physicians (counties with populations under 25,000) still have great difficulty in attracting family practitioners or specialists.

Physicians have been reluctant to locate in rural areas for such reasons as lack of adequate medical facilities, professional isolation, limited support services, inadequate organizational frameworks including lack of group practices, excessive workloads and time demands, economic disincentives, lack of social, cultural, and educational opportunities, and spouse influence (17). Efforts to improve the distribution of physicians have tried to address these factors.

Federal efforts to improve the distribution of physicians have included loan forgiveness, the National Health Service Corps, Area Health Education Centers, and extensive support for the development of family practice training programs (18,19). These programs have been largely dismantled in recent years due to the Reagan administration's efforts to contain federal health care costs.

Other efforts to improve physician distribution include the attempts of Offices of Rural Health in states such as North Carolina, North Dakota, and Nevada to increase the recruitment and retention of health care providers in rural areas, and cooperative ventures of consortiums of states to decentralize medical education programs and coordinate the placement of graduates (17). Examples of cooperative programs include the WAMI program (Washington, Alaska, Montana, and Idaho) and WICHE (Western Interstate Commission for Higher Education).

Despite the variety of approaches that have attempted to alter the urban/rural location of physicians, maldistribution persists. Market forces have started to alter the distribution of physicians, yet many rural communities still find it difficult to recruit and retain physicians. Those communities with the greatest need continue to have the biggest problems in attracting physicians.

Developing policies to alter the physician distribution requires knowledge of which areas are underserved, plus the reasons for this problem and the amount and type of resources necessary to address it (20). The limited impact of previous attempts suggests that broader policy options should be considered. The possibilities include changing reimbursement systems to provide a financial reward for physicians practicing in underserved areas; modifying the medical school admissions process to place emphasis on applicants interested in primary care practice; or changing the undergraduate and graduate medical education system to ensure that the curriculum, counseling, clinical setting, and role models presented to medical students are related to the health needs of society.

Physician maldistribution persists in the United States, despite the oversupply of physicians. Inefficient policies that continue to produce an excess of specialists in return for a small number of primary care physicians who locate in rural areas need to be carefully examined. Future policies that influence the training and reimbursement of physicians should be compatible with goals for improved physician distribution.

THE MEDICAL EDUCATION PIPELINE

The past 15 years has been a period of change for both undergraduate and graduate medical education. The stereotype of the typical medical student—a white urban male who will eventually practice a medical or surgical specialty in a large urban setting—has changed.

On the undergraduate level, medical school class size increased by more than 50 percent, with 1980–1981 entrance class totaling more than 17,000 students during the 1970s (21). First-year enrollments have decreased slightly during the past 5 years but remain in the 17,000 range (7). The number of applicants to medical school has declined approximately 15 percent from its peak in the mid-1970s. This decline has been caused by the reduced number of reapplicants, the skyrocketing costs of medical school tuition, cutbacks in federal grants and loans for medical students, and the societal perception of a current physician oversupply.

The undergraduate medical curriculum remains broad-based, with the first 2 years consisting of lectures and laboratory work in the basic sciences, followed by 2 years of work in the clinical sciences through seminars and work in hospital wards and clinics. The role models and values in most medical schools continue to emphasize acute care for hospitalized patients (22). However, the recent increase in noninstitutional services due to cost containment pressures could lend to the development of new medical role models outside the hospital. The professional socialization of the medical student has shown signs of changing, with increased emphasis on preceptorships in primary care settings and shifts in the focus of a growing number of medical school faculty from research to service. The latter has occurred due to recent changes in the distribution of medical school funding that have resulted in a deemphasis of federal support and greater reliance on state and local support as well as revenues from faculty practice income (8).

Another important issue affecting the medical education system has been the number of women and minority students in medical schools. Concerted efforts have been made to increase their enrollment, resulting in a sizeable increase over the past 15-year period from 11 to 34 percent of female first-year medical students and a moderate increase from 9 to 17 percent of minority first-year students (Tables 10-8 and 10-9). The proportion of black medical first-year students has recently declined and Asian and Pacific Islanders have surpassed blacks as the largest minority group among first year medical students.

The graduate medical education pipeline has also undergone major changes in the

TABLE 10-8. First-Year Students in Medical Schools, by Sex: Selected Academic Years 1970–1971 to 1985–1986

Academic Year	All First-Year Students	Male Students	Female Students	Percent Female of First-Year Students
1970–1971	11,348	11,695	3,656	23.8
1980–1981	17,204	12,234	4,970	28.9
1985–1986	16,929	11,141	5,788	34.2

SOURCE: Iglehart J: Trends in Health Personnel. *Health Affairs* 1986; 5:128–137.

past 15 years. The total number of residency positions increased significantly to approximately 75,000 positions by 1985, with the percentage of filled first-year positions increasing to over 90 percent (8). The increase in fill rate was due to an increased demand for first-year residency positions by graduates of U.S. medical schools. In fact, the proportion of residencies filled by FMGs has significantly decreased since 1970.

The specialty distribution of residencies changed dramatically with greater emphasis being placed on primary care specialties. By 1980, almost one-half of all first-year residency positions were in the primary care specialties of family practice, internal medicine, and pediatrics. The growth in these specialties has stabilized since the mid-1970s and will not increase further unless stimulated by new federal and state policies (23).

Policymakers have recently recognized the importance of the availability of residency positions in the distribution of physicians by specialty and geographic location. Serious concerns have been raised about the growing imbalance between applicants and available residency positions. In 1983 the National Resident Matching Program had 24,900 applications for 17,952 residency positions (24). There will clearly be increased competition for residency positions in the near future as hospitals are forced to respond to the financial pressures induced by restrictions on third-party reimbursement (25). This competition will be particularly acute for FMG applicants and could eventually lead to inability of some U.S. medical school graduates to train in their first specialty choice.

In summary, graduate and undergraduate medical education has changed in the past 15 years. The final report of the GMENAC recommended: decreasing the size of medical school classes by 10 percent by 1984; no longer using capitation payments merely to influence specialty choice; and selectively using special-purpose grants to accomplish specific goals such as continued growth for family medicine and general medicine programs, support for primary care preceptorships, and renovation and construction of improved ambulatory training facilities.

These recommendations have been implemented slowly, if at all. For example, the reduction in medical school class size has been less than 1 percent per year during the past 5 years. Despite the current oversupply of physicians, federal and state decision makers must continue their efforts to develop effective policies that influence physician training.

TABLE 10-9. Minority Students in the First Year of Medical School[a]

Academic Year	All First-Year Students	Racial/Ethnic Category					Total Minority	Percent Minority of First-Year Students
		Black	Hispanic	Asian or Pacific Islander	American Indian	Other Minority[b]		
1970–1971	11,255	697	100	190	11	—	998	8.9
1975–1976	15,216	1,036	336	282	60	73	1,787	11.7
1979–1980	17,014	960	766	512	55	—	2,293	13.5
1985–1986	16,929	854	869	1,139	53	—	2,915	17.2

SOURCES: *Third Report to the President and Congress on the Status of Health Professions in the United States*, U.S. Department of Health and Human Services Publ. No. (HRA) 82-2. Government Printing Office, January 1982; Iglehart J: Trends in Health Personnel, *Health Affairs* 1986; 5:128–137.

[a]Excludes students at the University of Puerto Rico for academic years 1970–1971 through 1976–1977.

[b]Data were not provided for the category "Other minority" for certain years. Where such data are provided, they include a number of persons now counted under "Hispanic."

321

DENTISTRY: A PROFESSION IN TRANSITION

By 1985, there were approximately 140 thousand active dentists practicing in the United States. Although the supply of dentists has increased during the past decade, the ratio of active dentists to population has increased only slightly from 47.0 per 100,000 population in 1970 to 54.9 per 100,000 population in 1982 (Table 10-10). As in medicine, the increases that occurred can be attributed to federal legislation passed in the 1960s eand early 1970s that directly attempted to remedy a perceived shortage of dentists. This legislation resulted in increases in the number of dental schools from 47 to 60 in the period 1960–1980 and an increase in the number of first-year dental students from 3,600 to more than 6,000 in the same period (Table 10-11).

Some of the recent trends that have affected medical schools have also influenced dental schools. The percentage of female first-year students in dental schools increased significantly in the past decade, with one-fourth of 1984 first-year dental school students being female (26). The proportion of minority first-year dental students increased moderately over the same period, from 9 percent in 1970 to 17 percent by 1984 (26). Dental schools have started to deemphasize their support from federal sources and have increased their state support, dental clinic revenues, and fees from tuition. An extremely important recent trend has been the sizeable decrease in the number of applicants to dental schools. Dentistry has experienced a steeper decline in its number of applicants than any other health profession in recent years. During the past decade, the number of dental school applicants decreased by more than one-half, resulting in an increase in the acceptance of dental school applicants from 37 to 78 percent during the same period (7). The declining applications and smaller class sizes and increased costs have forced three dental schools to announce their closing since 1984. In addition, first-year enrollments have steadily declined in the 1980s with a 15 percent decrease in the period 1980–1984 (26).

Unlike their physician counterparts, dentists typically work in solo private general dental practices. However, the current economic pressures on the dental profession have initiated some changes in the delivery of dental services. During the 1980s, a variety of nontraditional practice settings have emerged for dentists, including HMOs and retail locations in malls, stores, and plazas. Although only a small proportion of dental services are currently provided in these settings, this innovation is an indication of the more competitive environment in dentistry in the 1980s.

The vast majority of dentists are in general practice. Only one of every seven dentists are specialists, and the proportion of specialists has remained relatively stable during the 1980s. Orthodontists constitute almost two-fifths of all dental specialists, with oral surgeons totaling an additional one-fourth of the specialist population (Table 10-12).

There is significant variation in the distribution of dentists across regions of the United States and metropolitan/nonmetropolitan areas. This variation is caused by the same factors that have led to physician maldistribution, as well as by the lack of reciprocity in the licensing of dentists across states. More than half of all dentists practice in the state where they trained, yet 18 states do not have a school of dentistry (8). The northeastern and western portions of the country have the highest dentist/population ratios, and the South, with its increased rural area, has the lowest ratio (Table 10-13). In 1980 metropolitan areas had 60 dentists per 100,000 population compared to 37 per 100,000 in nonmetropolitan areas. These figures do not reveal the

TABLE 10-10. Total and Active Dentists and Dentist/Population Ratios: Selected Years, December 31, 1950–1982

Year	Number of Dentists[a]		Total Population (Thousands)	Dentists per 100,000 Population		Active Civilian Dentists[b]	Civilian Population (Thousands)	Active Civilian Dentists per 100,000 Civilian Population
	Total	Active		Total	Active			
1950	89,730	79,190	153,622	58.4	51.5	75,310	151,238	49.8
1960	105,200	90,120	182,287	57.7	49.4	84,500	179,742	47.0
1970	116,250	102,220	206,466	56.3	49.5	95,680	203,499	47.0
1975	126,590	112,020	217,095	58.3	51.6	106,740	214,957	49.7
1980	147,280	126,240	228,831	61.7	55.2	121,240	226,715	53.5
1982	147,250	132,010	233,194	63.1	56.6	126,810	231,004	54.9

SOURCE: *Fourth Report to the President and Congress on the Status of Health Personnel in the United States*, U.S. Department of Health and Human Services Publ. No. (HRS)-P-0084.4. U.S. Government Printing Office, May 1984.

[a]Includes dentists in federal service.

[b]Dentists in the Veterans Administration and U.S. Public Health Service are counted as civilian dentists.

TABLE 10-11. Number of Dental Schools, Students, and Graduates: Academic Years 1960–1961 Through 1982–1983

Academic Year	Number of Schools	Number of Students		Number of Graduates
		Total	First Year	
1960–1961	47	13,580	3,616	3,290
1970–1971	53	16,553	4,565	3,775
1980–1981	60	22,842	6,030	5,550
1982–1983	60	22,235	5,498	—[a]

SOURCE: *Fourth Report to the President and Congress on the Status of Health Personnel in the United States,* U.S. Department of Health and Human Services Publ. No. (HRS)-P-0084.4, U.S. Government Printing Office, May 1984.

[a]Data are not available at this time.

TABLE 10-12. Number of Active Dental Specialists by Specialty: December 31, 1982.

Type of Specialist	All Dental Specialists	
	Number	Percent Distribution
All specialists	18,370	100.0
Orthodontists	6,742	36.7
Oral surgeons	4,220	23.0
Periodontists	2,502	13.6
Pedodontists	2,230	12.1
Endodontists	1,420	7.7
Prosthodontists	1,007	5.5
Public health dentists	128	0.7
Oral pathologists	121	0.7

SOURCE: *Fourth Report to the President and Congress on the Status of Health Personnel in the United States,* U.S. Department of Health and Human Services Publ. No. (HRS)-P-00,84.4. U.S. Government Printing Office, May 1984.

even larger supply of dentists practicing in the biggest metropolitan areas and nonmetropolitan areas with large cities. Thus, the smallest, poorest rural communities continue to have the greatest need for dentists. The likelihood of improving this situation in the near future is not good, as previous efforts to broaden the distribution of dentists have generally been ineffective (17).

AUXILIARY PERSONNEL

The practice of dentistry has undergone major technological and organizational changes in the past two decades. Of particular importance has been the increased use of dental auxiliary personnel. The three major types of dental auxiliaries are dental hygienists, dental assistants, and dental laboratory technicians. Dental hygienists provide oral prophylaxis services and dental health education and are the only group of

TABLE 10-13. Dentist/Population Ratios According to Geographic Region, United States, 1983

Geographic Region	Number of Active Civilian Dentists per 100,000 Population
United States	55.7
Northeast	67.5
New England	68.0
Middle Atlantic	67.4
North Central	56.5
East North Central	56.1
West North Central	57.4
South	44.7
South Atlantic	47.1
East South Central	44.0
West South Central	41.3
West	60.9
Mountain	54.0
Pacific	63.4

SOURCE: *Health United States, 1985.* Hyattsville, MD, U.S. Department of Health and Human Services, Public Health Service, December 1985.

dental auxiliaries that is licensed. Dental assistants have generally supported the dentist at chairside and have had the opportunity in some states to perform expanded functions under the supervision of the dentist. Dental laboratory technicians make oral appliances following the written prescription of a dentist.

Nearly all dentists have at least one auxiliary and more than half currently employ hygienists (25). The government has supported the training of expanded-function dental auxiliaries (dental hygienists or dental assistants who receive additional education and training that enables them to perform a broader range of clinical functions), as well as the training of dental students to help improve their administrative and organizational skills in managing multiple auxiliary team practices (27). Support for the auxiliary concept has been due largely to an observed increase in the productivity of dental practices that employ auxiliaries. An earlier study found that solo general practice dentists without auxiliaries averaged 42 visits per week in 1979; productivity monotonically increased with the number of auxiliaries employed, with 103 visits per week for those dentists employing four or more auxiliaries (28).

The dental profession is in transition. There has been a relative increase in the supply of dental services in recent years, resulting in a potential surplus of dentists unless there is a significant decrease in dental school enrollments (8). The role of the expanded-function dental auxiliary is unclear, given this potential surplus and depends on the state of the economy. The demand for dental care is particularly sensitive to economic conditions, despite the significant growth in third-party payment for dental services (almost 45 percent of the U.S. population had some form of dental insurance coverage in 1983) (29). The substantial gains made in the prevention of dental disease through community water supply fluoridation will tend to reduce the demand for dental services in the future. All of these factors support the hypothesis that dental practice will be increasingly competitive. The impact of this increased competition on the price of dental care, the distribution of dentists, and the diffusion of innovations, such as the use of expanded-function dental auxiliaries, will shape the practice of dentistry in the coming years.

NURSING: SHORTAGES AND FUTURE ROLE CHANGES

THE PARADOX OF INCREASED SUPPLY BUT CONTINUED SHORTAGE

Registered nurses are the largest group of licensed health care professionals in the United States. The supply of nurses increased from 316,000 in 1950 to 1,404,000 in 1983, resulting in a more than twofold increase in the nurse/population ratio during the same period. The supply of nurses has grown at a rate twice that of the population for the period 1950–1980 (30). The yearly number of nursing graduates has also doubled from 35,000 in 1966 to 74,000 in 1982 (25).

Table 10-14 presents a profile of the registered nurse supply from a survey in 1980 that was sponsored by the federal Bureau of Health Professions. Almost one-fourth of nurses were not employed in nursing positions. Most nurses were women; almost three-fourths were married, and only 7 percent were from minority groups. In 1980 two-thirds of registered nurses were diploma school graduates and almost one-fourth were baccalaureate or advanced-degree graduates. The shifting educational pattern of registered nurses, with increased emphasis on a 4-year baccalaureate degree and continued significant reductions in hospital-based diploma school graduates, is discussed in greater detail below.

Despite the overall gains in registered nurse supply, for many years the shortage of nurses seemed to worsen (30). Understanding the causes for the imbalance between the supply and demand is not easy. Some have pointed to the large number of inactive nurses as the main reasons for the perceived shortage. Although a 24 percent inactive rate may seem high, the labor force participation of nurses is similar to that of women in comparable professions. Personal characteristics and the role of women in society appear to be as important as job characteristics in influencing nurses to work (16). Only 8 percent of unemployed nurses are actively seeking nursing employment; the vast majority of unemployed nurses are over 50 years of age or married with children at home (31). One job characteristic that appears to influence the nurse employment rate is salary. Nurses are not paid well relative to their training and responsibilities, and the nurse shortage has been termed a shortage at a price due to lagging salaries (32).

Approximately one-third of employed nurses work part-time (30). The majority of part-time nurses are married with children at home. Although concern has also been focused on nursing attrition due to burnout and/or poor working conditions, surveys indicate only a small increase in the number of nurses working in other professions (30). Thus, the possible shortage of nurses cannot be attributed to increases in the number of part-time workers or attrition from the profession.

The reason for the perceived shortage of nurses is not clear. The most likely explanation appears to be increased demand for nursing services from several sectors

TABLE 10-14. Statistical Profile of Registered Nurses, November 1980[a]

Characteristic	Total Registered Nurses, 1980	Total Employed in Nursing, 1980	Total Not Employed in Nursing, 1980
Total number	1,615,846	1,235,152	379,712
Median age	38.4	36.3	47.1
Percentage male	2.7	3.0	1.6
Percentage minority	7.0	8.2	3.4
Percentage married	70.8	68.1	79.8
Percentage married with children at home	47.5	46.3	51.6
Percentage whose basic nursing education was			
Diploma	63.4	59.6	75.7
Associate degree	18.5	21.2	9.7
Baccalaureate or higher degree	17.3	18.5	13.6
Percentage whose highest nursing related education was			
Diploma	54.6	50.9	66.4
Associate degree	17.7	20.0	10.1
Baccalaureate	22.1	23.2	18.4
Masters or doctorate	5.1	5.3	4.4

SOURCE: Levine E, Moses E: Registered nurses today: A statistical profile, in Aiken L (ed): *Nursing in the 1980's: Crises, Opportunities, Challenges,* (L. Aiken, ed.) Philadelphia, Lippincott, 1982, Table 26.1.

[a]Percentages included on this table are derived from the segment of the total population indicating the particular characteristic being studied.

of the health care system—acute hospital-based care, long term care for the growing number of chronically ill people, home-based care, and preventive care. Two-thirds of all registered nurses worked in hospitals in 1985 (24). This proportion should decrease as more health services shift from inpatient to ambulatory settings.

The demand for nursing services should continue to grow. More hospitals will continue to have nursing vacancies on evening shifts and in their intensive care and coronary care units. The expected growth in the supply of nurses will not be able to meet all the demand for nursing services in the future. To achieve an improved balance between the supply and demand for nursing services, institutional and other employers must become more sensitive to the special needs of working women.

Like many other health care professionals, nurses are not distributed evenly throughout the United States. The maldistribution appears to be due to the geographic immobility of women who are married and second wage earners in a family, as well as the inability of rural and inner city hospitals to offer an adequate range of incentives (e.g., flexible hours, increased salaries, and fringe benefits) to attract nurses (16).

Rural institutions have found that urban-based education and training programs are often not relevant to rural needs. Rural hospitals must frequently hire recent nursing graduates with limited skills and often resort to depending on pool nurses from temporary employment agencies (16). This problem is of particular concern due to the increased responsibilities and range of skills required of rural nurses. In the near future, rural providers are not likely to improve their chances of attracting well-trained nurses with a broad range of skills.

NURSING EDUCATION AND ROLE CHANGES

The federal government provided almost $2.0 billion for nursing education during the period 1965–1985. This support, as well as market forces, helped to increase the number of nursing graduates entering the profession. Table 10-15 shows the more than twofold increase in the number of admissions to registered nursing programs over the past 2 decades. Of particular interest is the shift that has occurred in the control of nursing education from the hospital to nursing educators in colleges and universities.

There are three forms of training that lead to licensure as a registered nurse: 3-year diploma programs that are hospital based, 2-year associate degree programs that are generally community college based, and 4-year baccalaureate nursing programs in universities or 4-year colleges. In 1960, 83 percent of all nursing graduates were trained in hospitals; in 1980, 83 percent were trained in colleges and universities (33). The number of graduates from diploma programs has decreased rapidly since 1965 as baccalaureate and associate programs have grown.

Leading nurse educators have proposed that a baccalaureate degree be required for licensure as a registered nurse (34). The 1985 New York State Nursing Association's proposal (1985 NYSNA) attempts to create a distinction between professional nurses with baccalaureate degrees and nurse technicians with associate degrees; diploma school graduates and licensed practical nurses would no longer be relevant (35). The legislative response to this controversial proposal has been mixed to date. A synthesis of the potential problems associated with the proposal suggests that it would result in increased costs and length of nurse training and restricted access to the nursing profession, and would exacerbate the nursing shortage in many areas of the United States (36). Nurse training has changed dramatically in recent years, with the potential for even greater change in the future. The decisions made concerning the baccalaureate requirement issue will have important implications for the future supply of registered nurses.

The nursing profession is attempting to change its role in the health care system. The leaders of the profession have called for an expansion of the independent role of

TABLE 10-15. Admissions to Schools Offering Initial Programs in Registered Nursing by Type of Program, Selected Years 1960–1982

	Registered Nursing Programs			
Year	Baccalaureate	Diploma	Associate Degree	Total
1960–1961	8,674	38,460	2,085	49,219
1970–1971	20,299	28,792	29,433	78,524
1980–1981	35,808	17,494	56,899	110,201
1981–1982	35,928	18,928	60,423	115,279

SOURCE: *Fourth Report to the President and Congress on the Status of Health Personnel in the United States,* U.S. Department of Health and Human Services, Publ. No. (HRS P-00,84.4), May 1984.

the nurse within the hospital and the creation of new professional roles outside the hospital (33). Hospitals will remain the major employer of nurses due to continued technological advances and increased insurance coverage for the general population. Nurses are seeking to clarify their relationship to physicians, particularly within the context of clinical decision making in the hospital (33). They have developed new delivery modes, such as primary nursing, in which the nurse assumes direct responsibility for comprehensive care for a group of patients over a given time period.

A variety of new roles has emerged for the registered nurse. Included are positions such as clinical nurse specialist, nurse practitioner, nurse anesthetist, and nurse clinician. These positions involve employment in new ambulatory care settings (HMOs, ambulatory surgery centers), nursing homes, and home care programs providing care for the elderly and others with chronic illnesses, as well as positions in hospitals.

Nursing professionals want to control their future. They are trying to shed the traditional stereotype of the nurse as an underpaid female hospital laborer. In the process, considerable controversy has been created both inside and outside the profession. Associate degree and diploma graduates want to continue to function in viable roles within the nursing profession. Institutions desire to employ combinations of nursing personnel suitable for their particular environments. These forces, as well as the current restrictive interpretation of state nurse practice acts, suggest that there will be no easy solutions to changing, and hopefully strengthening, the future relationships of nurses, physicians, and health care institutions.

NEW CATEGORIES OF HEALTH CARE PERSONNEL: PHYSICIAN ASSISTANTS AND NURSE PRACTITIONERS

The perceived shortage of physicians in the mid-1960s led to the development of two new types of health care providers—PAs and NPs. The first PA training program was established at Duke University in 1966; the initial NP program was started at the University of Colorado in 1965.

PAs are persons qualified by academic and practical training to provide patient services under the direction and supervision of a licensed physician who is responsible for the performance of the PA (37). PAs are able to diagnose, manage, and treat common illnesses, provide preventive services, and respond appropriately to common emergency care situations. The typical PA training program consists of 2 years of didactic study followed by clinical training. However, training programs vary widely in terms of admission requirements, curriculum, and site of educational training. There were 57 programs training PAs in the United States in February 1983 (25).

NPs are registered nurses who have completed formal programs of study preparing them for expanded roles and responsibilities (38). These expanded roles include obtaining comprehensive health histories, assessing health status, performing physical examinations, formulating and managing a care regimen for acute and chronically ill patients, teaching, and counseling (39). There are a range of training programs for different types of NPs, including pediatric, nurse midwife, family, adult, psychiatric, and geriatric programs. Slightly more than half of the more than 200 NP training programs are certificate programs that generally last for 8–12 months; the remainder are master's programs lasting from 1 to 2 years.

GMENAC estimated that approximately 16,000 NPs would graduate from formal training programs by 1980, and more than 2000 new NPs are now expected to graduate each year (38). The Association of Physician Assistant Programs estimates a PA supply of 15,000 at the beginning of 1983, with approximately 12,500 active (25). The PA totals include formal PA training program graduates and others who have passed the PA certifying examination. Approximately 1500 new PAs graduate from PA training programs every year.

Almost three-fourths of PAs work in primary care specialities, with the majority in family practice (25). Surgical specialities account for 13 percent of all PAs, with general surgery and orthopedic surgery having the largest number. PAs have located in nonurban areas more frequently than physicians or the general population (17). Many PA programs were designed to train assistants to rural physicians and have succeeded in placing graduates in rural areas.

Several estimates are available on the specialty distribution of NPs. GMENAC estimates that 30 percent are family NPs, 25 percent are pediatric NPs, 20 percent are adult NPs, 10 percent are maternity NPs, 10 percent are midwives, and 5 percent are other types. NP graduates have been more likely than PAs to locate in urban areas. Research suggests that the structure of training programs is an important factor affecting the geographic distributions of NPs and PAs (38).

There are important differences in the perceived roles of PAs and NPs (40). PAs are viewed by the medical profession as physician extenders who can perform many of the usual functions completed by physicians. Nurses view the NP as a registered nurse in an expanded role. The expanded role includes greater supervision of and responsibility for primary patient care, with extra emphasis on the traditional nursing values of prevention and counseling. Despite these differences in perceived roles and in education and training requirements, PAs and NPs appear to be similar in many of their performance characteristics.

Several issues related to the performance of NPs and PAs are generally considered as resolved. The research literature provides sufficient evidence that NPs and PAs are well accepted by patients, provide similar quality of care as physicians for basic health care problems, increase the availability and accessibility of health services, increase physician productivity in small primary care practices by up to 50 percent, and are generally cost effective from an employer's perspective (40–42). The individual effectiveness of a PA or NP is strongly related to environmental characteristics of the practice, including size, organizational structure, and location, as well as the physician's work style and willingness to delegate responsibility to the PA or NP.

ISSUES IN PA AND NP USE

Among the issues that need to be resolved before PAs and NPs can be used fully are legal restrictions to practice, reimbursement policies, and relationships with physicians. The legal status of PAs and NPs is uncertain and varies considerably across states. Some states permit considerable delegation of tasks and responsibilities to the PA, including drug prescriptions when a physician countersigns within 24 hours. State legislation governing expanded medical delegation has been unduly restrictive with respect to the scope of practice of qualified nonphysicians (43).

Laws and regulations governing the expanded role of the nurse are changing rapidly but inconsistently. Although the majority of states have altered their nurse practice acts to facilitate expanded roles, the constraints on the scope of practice of NPs varies from state to state. The restrictions appear to be fewer for NPs than for PAs, but changes in legal authority must take place before NPs will be able to practice independently. The nonphysician health care provider technical panel of GMENAC recommended that state laws and regulations should not require physician supervision of NPs and PAs beyond that needed to assure quality of care (38).

Third-party reimbursement imposes another constraint on the use of PAs and NPs. Current policies generally link the reimbursement of PAs and NPs directly to the employing physician or institution. Most insurers do not recognize PAs and NPs as legitimate providers of medical care. Private fee-for-service physician practices or other ambulatory settings have had difficulties in securing reimbursement for nonphysician services. Reimbursement may be even greater than legal restrictions. Policymakers must carefully review inconsistent public policies that fund the training of PAs and NPs but then deny reimbursement for the services they provide.

A third area of concern is future relationships of PAs and NPs with physicians. In the past, physicians have shown reasonable acceptance of these personnel (40). The current surplus of physicians could result in reduced employment opportunities for PAs and NPs. Nonphysician health providers may be forced to compete with new physician graduates for available jobs.

The future of NPs and PAs is uncertain. Past employment of these providers was motivated by the shortage and geographic maldistribution of physicians. The shortage has now turned into a surplus, and physicians have started to locate in previously underserved areas. These trends may cause problems for future employment of NPs and PAs, who will need to adapt to the changing health care environment (44). Emerging roles for NPs and PAs include providing primary care to underserved areas and populations, such as the elderly and the mentally ill, providing preventive care, and providing specialty services in hospitals in lieu of house staff. New practice settings for NPs and PAs include schools, industrial settings, prisons, nursing homes, and HMOs. Resolution of problems regarding legal restrictions, reimbursement policies, and relationships with physicians will undoubtedly influence the ability of NPs and PAs to meet these new challenges. NPs and PAs will thrive in the future only if they are cost effective from both an employer's and a social policy perspective.

FUTURE ISSUES FOR HEALTH CARE PROFESSIONALS

This chapter has summarized trends in health professional supply. Federal and state support has resulted in large increases in the number of graduates from health professions schools. The significant increase in the supply of health personnel has created a surplus of many types of health care professionals.

The federal and state investment in health care personnel has improved access to health services, helped health professions schools to remain fiscally viable, and increased opportunities for careers in the health professions for women and minorities (45). Federal and state support for health professional training programs has been reduced in the 1980s. Budgetary pressures have caused a reallocation of funds that have been targeted for health professions programs to other portions of federal and state budgets. It will be important to monitor the impact of future cutbacks on enrollments in health professions schools. Many of the major trends currently affecting the U.S. health care system—aging of the population, restrictive public and private sector reimbursement, growth in alternative delivery systems, and restructuring of the health care industry, including the increased corporate practice of medicine—will have a significant impact on the future employment opportunities available for health professionals (46).

The health care system has exhibited an extraordinary capacity to expand. Federal and state decision makers have focused their efforts on constraining, or at least stabilizing, overall health care expenditures. Approaches that could be used to help contain expenditures range from fostering competition between health care providers to improve the efficiency of service delivery, to using the reimbursement mechanism to influence provider behavior, to limiting the supply of health care professionals.

Health care cost containment strategies need to be developed in concert with health care personnel policies. The health care system offers strong resistance to fiscal cutbacks. Major system changes—competition between health providers, alterations in reimbursement policies, and the like—can best be implemented if constraints on the flexible use of health personnel are reduced. Alternatives to the existing methods of training, licensing, regulating, and reimbursing health care personnel should be seriously considered.

The surplus of personnel has been identified as one of the factors that have led to increased health care expenditures. Future health care personnel policies, at both the federal and state levels, will need to be targeted to meet specific goals. Modifications in the number and types of health professionals that are trained must be considered in light of the current focus on cost containment.

REFERENCES

1. Sorkin A: *Health Economics.* Cambridge, MA, Lexington Books, 1984.
2. Torrens P, Lewis C: Health care personnel, in Williams S, Torrens P (eds): *Introduction to Health Services.* New York, Wiley, 1980.
3. U.S. Bureau of the Census: *Statistical Abstract of the United States.* U.S. Government Printing Office, 1981.
4. Blendon R: In Ginzberg E (ed): *Policy Choices for the 1990's: An Uncertain Look Into America's Future in the U.S. Health Care System.* Totowa, NJ, Rowman & Allanheld, 1985.
5. Stevens R: The muddle over medical manpower. *Prism* 1975; 3:10–63.
6. Reinhardt U: *Physician Productivity and the Demand for Health Manpower.* Cambridge, MA, Ballinger, 1975.
7. Iglehart J: Trends in health personnel, *Health Affairs* 1986; 5:128–137.
8. *Third Report to the President and the Congress on the Status of Health Professions Personnel in the United States,* Publ. No. (HRA) 82-2. U.S. Department of Health and Human Services, 1982.
9. Hansen W: An appraisal of physician manpower projections. *Inquiry* 1970; 7:102–114.

10. *Report of the Graduate Medical Education Advisory Committee to the Secretary,* DHHS, Vol 1: *GMENAC Summary Report,* Publ. No. (HRA) 81-653. U.S. Department of Health and Human Services, 1980.

11. Aiken L, Lewis C, Craig J, et al: The contribution of specialists to the delivery of primary care. *New Engl J Med* 1979; 300:1363–1370.

12. Rosenblatt, R, Cherkin D, Schneeweiss R: The structure and content of family practice: Current status and future trends. *J Family Pract* 1982; 15:681–723.

13. Fruen M, Cantwell J: Geographic distribution of physicians: Past trends and future influences. *Inquiry* 1982; 19:44–50.

14. American Academy of Family Practice: *Report on Survey of 1982 Graduating Family Practice Residents,* Chicago, July 1982.

15. Schwartz W, Newhouse J, Bennett B, et al: The changing geographic distribution of board-certified physicians. *New Engl J Med* 1980; 303:1032–1037.

16. Moscovice I, Rosenblatt R: *The Viability of the Rural Hospital.* Rockville, National Center for Health Services Research, 1983.

17. Rosenblatt R, Moscovice I: *Rural Health Care.* New York, Wiley, 1982.

18. Rosenblatt R, Moscovice I: The National Health Service Corps: Rapid growth and uncertain future. *Milbank Mem Fund Quart* 1980; 58:282–309.

19. Gessert C, Smith D: The national AHEC program: Review of its progress and consideration for the 1980's. *Publ Health Rep* 1981; 96:116–120.

20. Hadley J: Alternative methods of evaluating health manpower distribution. *Med Care* 1979; 17:1054–1060.

21. Ginzburg E, Brann E, Hiestand D, et al: The expanding physician supply and health policy: The clouded outlook. *Milkbank Mem Fund Quart* 1981; 59:508–541.

22. *Report of GMENAC to the Secretary, DHHS:* Vol 5: *Educational Environment Technical Panel,* Publ. No. (HRA) 81-655. U.S. Department of Health and Human Services, 1980.

23. Steinwachs D, Levine D, Elzinga J, et al: Changing patterns of graduate medical education. *New Engl J Med* 1982; 306:10–14.

24. LeRoy L, Ellwood D: Trends in Health Manpower. *Health Affairs* 1985; 4:77–90.

25. *Fourth Report to the President and Congress on the Status of Health Personnel in the United States,* Publ. No. (HRS)-P-OO 84:4. U.S. Department of Health and Human Services, 1984.

26. *Health United States, 1985,* Publ. NO. (PHS) 86-1232. U.S. Department of Health and Human Services, December 1985.

27. Machlin S: Dental manpower, in *Health, United States, 1981,* Publ. No. (PHS) 82-1232. U.S. Department of Health and Human Services, 1981.

28. *The 1979 Survey of Dental Practice.* Chicago, American Dental Association, 1980.

29. *Sourcebook of Health Insurance Data: 1984–1985.* Washington, DC, Health Insurance Association of America, 1986.

30. Levine E, Moses E: Registered nurses today: A statistical profile, in Aiken L (ed): *Nursing in the 1980's: Crises, Opportunities, Challenges.* Philadelphia, Lippincott, 1982.

31. Moses E: *The Registered Nurse Population: An Overview,* Report No. 82-5. Hyattsville, MD, Bureau of Health Professions, U.S. Department of Health and Human Services, 1981.

32. *The Recurrent Shortage of Registered Nurses,* U.S. Department of Health and Human Services Publ. No. (HRA) 81-23. Bureau of Health Professions, 1981.

33. Aiken L: The impact of federal health policy on nurses, in Aiken L (ed): *Nursing in the 1980's: Crises, Opportunities, Challenges.* Philadelphia, Lippincott, 1982.

34. Fagin C, McClure M, Schlotfeldt R: Can we bring order out of the chaos of nursing education? *Am J Nurs* 1976; 76:98–107

35. *Resolution on Entry Into Professional Practice.* New York, New York Nurses Association, 1974.

36. Dolan A: The New York State Nurses Association 1985 Proposal: Who needs it? *J Health Politics, Policy, Law* 1979; 2:508–531.

37. *Physician Asisstants: Education, Accreditation, and Consumer Acceptance.* Chicago, American Medical Association, 1975.

38. *Report of GMENAC to the Secretary, DHHS: Vol 6: Nonphysician Health Care Provider Technical Panel,* Publ. No. (HRA) 81-656. U.S. Department of Health and Human Services, 1980.

39. Abdellah F: The nurse practitioner 17 years later: Present and emerging issues. *Inquiry* 1982; 19:105–116.

40. Kane R, Wilson W: The new health practitioner—the past as prologue. *West J Med* 1977; 127:254–261.

41. Record J, McCally M, Schweitzer S, et al: New Health professions after a decade and a half: Delegation, productivity and costs in primary care. *J Health Politics, Policy, Law* 1980; 5:470–497.

42. Lawrence D: The impact of physician assistants and nurse practitioners on health care access, costs, and quality. *Health Med Care Serv Rev* 1978; 1:1–12.

43. Kissam P: Physician's assistants and nurse practitioner laws: A study of health law reform. *Kansas Law Rev* 1975; 24:1–65.

44. Brooks E, Johnson S: Nurse Practitioner and Physician Assistant Satellite Health Centers—the pending demise of an organizational form. *Med Care* 1986; 24:881–889.

45. Ginzburg E: Investments in health manpower: A possible alternative, in MacLeod G, Redman R (eds): *Health Care Capital: Competition and Control.* Cambridge, MA, Ballinger, 1978.

46. Ginzberg E (ed): *The U.S. Health Care system—A look to the 1990's.* Totowa, NJ, Rowman & Allanheld, 1985.

CHAPTER 11

Financing
Health Services

Alma L. Koch

The system for financing health services in the United States reflects the general fragmentation of health care as a whole. One may say that it is not really a system at all; rather, that it is a patchwork of loosely connected financing mechanisms varying by provider type and reflective of the socioeconomic status of the specific patient groups being served. However, this type of observation only frustrates the study of the financing apparatus as it now exists. If one views the "system" in light of the role of tradition and the values of the American people, as well as the political philosophy of the times, the organization of health care financing in the United States comes into better focus.

This chapter examines the size and scope of the health care financing system in the United States. Where possible, comparisons are drawn between the United States and other countries, particularly those in the industrialized world. Particular attention is paid to differences and similarities in the public and private financing components of the system, reimbursement of various provider categories, and trends that we may expect to see by the end of the century. The role of health insurance as a financial conduit is explored, and monetary business objectives are contrasted with the altruistic goals of health care as a human service.

HEALTH EXPENDITURES

MAGNITUDE OF THE U.S. HEALTH CARE INDUSTRY

In dollar volume, the health care industry ranks second only to the automobile industry in the United States. In terms of U.S. general public expenditures, the health care industry ranks third following national defense and education. Furthermore, it is the largest service industry in the country (1). In 1985 Americans spent $425 billion on health care, constituting 10.7 percent of the gross national product (GNP), amounting to $1,721 per capita (2). The United States spends far more on health care than other industrialized democracies. For example, in 1983 the United Kingdom and Japan fell at the lower end of the spectrum, spending 6.2 and 6.7 of their respective gross domestic products on health care. Sweden and France came closest to U.S. figures, with 9.6 and 9.3 of their GDPs spent on health, while other comparable nations fell within the established range (3).

Growth in Health Expenditures

Since 1940, national health expenditures have grown at a rate substantially outpacing the GNP. Table 11-1 shows that prior to World War II, only 4.0 percent of the GNP was devoted to health care, both public and private. By 1985, the proportion of the GNP expended for health care increased by nearly 7 percent (2). Since the onset of Medicare and Medicaid in mid-1966, national health expenditures have grown particularly rapidly, from about 6.3 percent of the GNP to the present figure. In fact, 1984 was the first year since 1973 where the percentage of GNP devoted to health care actually showed a slight downturn of 0.1 percent from the previous year. One may speculate that recent changes in the Medicare reimbursement system, along with other cost control measures, accounted for this phenomenon.

Various factors have contributed to the disproportionate growth in health care spending relative to the growth in GNP. These include (1) rising expectations about the value of health care services, (2) rapid development and dissemination of medical technology which expanded the treatment of disease, (3) government financing of health care services, (4) the nature of third-party reimbursement, and (5) the lack of competitive forces in the health care system to increase efficiency and productivity in the delivery of health care services.

MONETARY FLOW

Payment Sources

Figure 11-1 contrasts the monetary inflow and outflow in the United States for total health spending in 1985. Private health insurance finances almost one-third of all

TABLE 11-1. Aggregate and Per Capita National Health Expenditures, United States, Selected Years

Year	Total (Billion $)	Per Capita[a]	GNP (Billion $)	Percent of GNP
1940	4.0	30	100	4.0
1950	12.7	82	287	4.4
1960	26.9	146	507	5.3
1970	75.0	350	1015	7.4
1980	247.5	1049	2632	9.4
1985	425.0	1721	3989	10.7

SOURCE: Adapted from Waldo DR, Levit KR, Lazenby H: National health expenditures, 1985. *Health Care Finan Rev* 1986; 8:1–21.

[a]Based on July 1 Social Security area population estimates.

health expenditures; direct patient payments finances another one-quarter. These payment sources, together with philanthropy, account for the 59 percent of all health expenditures that are privately financed in the United States. The other two-fifths is financed publicly by either federal or state and local governments. The largest single public program is Medicare, the federal Social Security health insurance plan for the elderly, the disabled, and other groups. Medicare, Medicaid (the federal/state welfare program for health care), and other government programs together account for 41 cents of each health care dollar (2).

Spending for Medicare and Medicaid has been increasing even more rapidly than total national health expenditures. In 1985 Medicare and Medicaid together constituted 26.8 percent of the total health care bill; in 1967 the two programs represented only 15 percent of the total health care bill. Out of approximately 238 million people in the United States in 1985, more than one in five (over 50 million people) were enrolled in either or both programs. Medicare's role was clearly most substantial for hospital care; Medicaid's role was most prominent for nursing home care, and the growth in these two services has indubitably been spurred on by the two public programs (4).

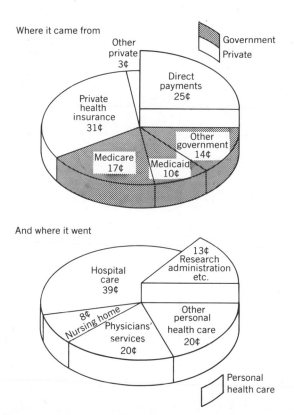

Figure 11-1. The nation's health care dollar, 1985. (SOURCE: Waldo DR, Leavit KR, Lazenby H: National health expenditures, 1985. *Health Care Finan Rev* 1986; 8:1–21.)

Outlays

In terms of outlays, almost half of the money spent for health in 1985 was used to purchase hospital and nursing home services. Hospital expenditures, $167 billion in 1985, grew less during the previous 2 years than at any other time in the previous two decades. Another 40 cents were evenly divided among physicians' services and other personal care items (i.e., dentists' services, drugs, eyeglasses and appliances, and other professional services). Research and construction, program administration, and public health activities made up the final 13 cents of the health care dollar for 1985 (2).

Personal Health Care

Figure 11-2 shows financing trends since 1950 for personal health care expenditures (total health expenditures minus program administration, public health activities, research, and construction) (2,5). Government and private insurance carriers, as funding sources for health care, have grown continuously in the postwar era, and out-of-pocket payments by patients have dropped commensurately. Compared to previous decades, the 1980s have thus far manifested considerable stability among payers.

Sources of funding for major providers of personal health care are depicted in Figure 11-3. Government funding dominates hospital reimbursement, with over 55 percent financed by Medicare, other government programs, and Medicaid, in that order. Another 35 percent of the national hospital bill is footed by private health insurance. Physician outlays are clearly dominated by the private sector. Private insurance and direct patient payments account for more than 70 percent of physician funding; Medicare picks up another 20 percent. Nursing home funding reflects the

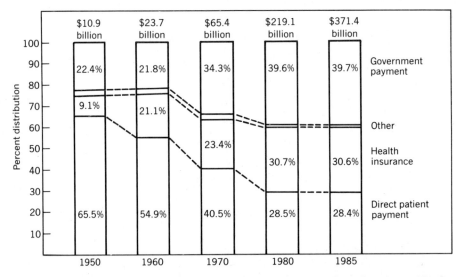

Figure 11-2. Percentage distribution of personal health care expenditures by source of funds, United States, selected years. (SOURCE: Adapted from Waldo DR, Leavit KR, Lazenby H: National health expenditures, 1985. *Health Care Finan Rev* 1986; 8:1–21.)

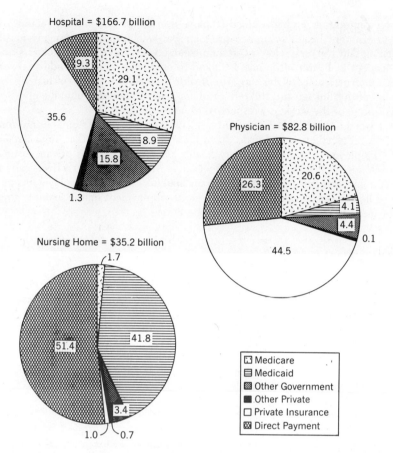

Hospital = $166.7 billion

Physician = $82.8 billion

Nursing Home = $35.2 billion

Medicare
Medicaid
Other Government
Other Private
Private Insurance
Direct Payment

Figure 11-3. Personal health care expenditures for total population, by type of service and source of funds, United States, 1985. (SOURCE: Adapted from Waldo DR, Leavit KR, Lazenby H: National Health Expenditures, 1985. *Health Care Finan Rev* 1986: 8:1–21.)

"rich man, poor man" dichotomy of the long-term care industry, wherein patients must "spend down" their assets in order to qualify for government assistance. Over 50 percent of nursing home revenues come directly from patients; another 42 percent come from Medicaid (2).

HEALTH INSURANCE

ORIGINS OF HEALTH INSURANCE

Health insurance originated in Europe in the early 1800s when mutual benefit societies arose to reduce the financial burden for those stricken with illness. The focus was on low-skilled, low-income workers who were industrially employed. (Providers in

Europe wanted to keep high-skilled employees in the private medical market.) The first government health insurance program was established in Germany in 1840, mandating that workers below a certain income level to belong to a "sickness fund." The concept of health insurance as linked to employment in the industrial sector persists internationally to this day. The health insurance networks of many nations grew out of this linkage and still reflect an emphasis on nonagricultural employment and coverage of the worker, irrespective of dependents (6,7).

Today in the United States, the framework of health insurance stems clearly from its European antecedents and breaks down into three categories that, in some sense, reflect employment status. Voluntary health insurance (VHI) is private insurance usually denoting current employment; social health insurance (SHI) reflects participation in a government entitlement program linked to previous employment; public welfare health care programs connote lack of employment or the inability to gain employment stemming from a disabling condition.

DISTRIBUTING RISK

Insurance is a way of pooling or distributing risk, the "risk" meaning the probability of incurring a loss. Risk stems from two kinds of occurrence: (1) unanticipated events such as fires, car accidents, or airplane crashes; and (2) anticipated events such as death, old age, and sickness. Health—or, more correctly, illness—is an anticipated event associated with old age and death. Thus, we know that illness is a likely event, but we don't know when it will strike, to whom it will happen, or how severe it will be. Therefore, health is uncertain for the individual but not for a group. Groups are actuarially (statistically) predictable.

Moral Hazard

In all insurance, it is assumed that risks are independent of each other: (1) what befalls one person does not affect another; and (2) for a single individual, risks are independent. Neither assumption applies in health insurance because one person's sickness may spread contagiously, and illness in one part of the body may weaken another part. These phenomena, together with the moral hazard inherent in medical care, make health insurance and health costs in general extremely volatile. Moral hazard means that, to the extent that the event insured against can be controlled, there exists a temptation to use the insurance. (The classic example of moral hazard is setting fire to a failing business in order to collect the insurance.) Health insurance usage is highly discretionary; physicians and patients can conspire (intentionally or not) to use the insurance. A common example is where the patient is kept in the hospital an extra day because it would be difficult or inconvenient for the family to receive the patient back home on the earliest possible discharge day. In this example, the insured's extra day in the hospital, at a cost of $500 or more to the carrier, is traded for a family member's day at work, and the expense is borne by purchasers of the policy, as reflected in the price of the premium.

Benefit Structure

Because of moral hazard, health insurance usually pays less than the total loss incurred by levying out-of-pocket or direct costs on the patient. In fee-for-service provider reimbursement, these take the form of deductibles and copayments. A *deductible* is a sum of money that must be paid, typically every year, before the insurance policy becomes active. Deductibles have long been criticized in health insurance for posing an impediment to first-contact care, discouraging the patient from seeking care until the condition becomes severe. Since higher costs may be incurred for more severe illness, deductibles have been postulated to contribute to health cost inflation rather than stimulate parsimonious consumer utilization. A *copayment* is paid as the beneficiary uses the insurance. For example, in a policy with an *indemnity benefit*, a fixed cash amount is paid to the beneficiary per procedure or per day in the hospital (e.g., $800 for a one-night stay in the hospital following a hernia repair). If the hospital charges $1100, the patient must pay a copayment of $300. Thus, the patient is liable for any amount in excess of the indemnity payment. An insurance plan with a *service benefit* reimburses on a percentage basis and the patient pays *coinsurance*. According to the preceding example, the insurance plan would pay 80 percent or $880 of the surgeon's charges, leaving only $220 in coinsurance to be paid by the patient. Thus, if the percentage rate is high, the reimbursement structure of service benefits usually works to the patient's advantage, in comparison to indemnity benefits.

Nowadays, to control health cost inflation, there is a growing trend toward hybrid benefit structures, combining both service and indemnity features. A plan may, for example, pay a percentage of charges up to a specified limit, beyond which point the patient becomes responsible for the balance. Preferred Provider Organizations (PPOs) utilize this technique, often in concert with low price ceilings, to reimburse nonparticipating providers. Again according to the preceding example, the PPO might pay 80 percent up to an $800 limit on charges for a nonparticipating hospital. The patient would thus incur a $460 copayment—a good incentive for the patient to utilize a participating provider in the PPO.

Premium Determination

Because of the financial implications of choosing one type of health insurance plan over another, and because the possibility of moral hazard is a real one in health care utilization, health insurance plans are particularly vulnerable to the phenomenon of *adverse selection*. Adverse selection may be at work when an insurance policy experiences a higher number of claims due to sickness than would be probable on a random basis. If an employee is offered an alternate choice of plans, for example, a "sicker" person or a potentially higher utilizer of health care services is likely to elect the plan with more generous provisions (i.e., lower deductible, copayments, and limitations, or fewer exclusions), even if the employee's share of the premium is higher. Therefore, more liberal plans may experience an adverse selection of sicker enrollees compared to a more restrictive fee-for-service plan or a Health Maintenance Organization (HMO). This may result in continuously spiraling claims for the plan as costlier patients join and as healthier individuals defect to the lower cost alternative plans.

Because of adverse selection, most health insurance plans today are *experience-rated*; the premiums are based on the demographic characteristics (e.g., age and sexual composition) of the employer group or on the actual experience of the group in that plan in prior years. *Community rating*, originated by Blue Cross and Blue Shield, bases premiums on the wider utilization of the defined geographic area (census tracts, city, county, etc.). Today, most fee-for-service plans are experience rated, as are the Blues, which must contend with stiff price competition from commercial carriers. Most

HMOs, on the other hand, use community ratings for their enrolled groups, but even this is fading as HMOs face price competition or enter the for-profit arena.

VOLUNTARY HEALTH INSURANCE

Voluntary or private health insurance in the United States can be subdivided into three distinct categories: (1) Blue Cross and Blue Shield, (2) private or commercial insurance company health insurance, and (3) HMOs. The respective sponsorship of these types of VHI are providers, third-parties or intermediaries, and patients or independent carriers.

Growth and Development

The year 1929 was a landmark year for VHI. In spite of active opposition from the American Medical Association (AMA) to any type of health insurance from 1920 onward, both Blue Cross and the HMO movement were launched in this last pre-Depression year. Blue Cross was initiated by Baylor University teachers in Dallas, Texas, who organized to provide hospital care for 3 cents a day. Michigan and New Jersey were next in the movement for hospital insurance. In 1934, the depths of the revenue depression for hospitals, the American Hospital Association (AHA) united these plans into the Blue Cross network. Today Blue Cross has broken away from its original AHA sponsorship, but the hospita-sponsored underpinnings remain strong in many locales (6,7).

In Oklahoma also in 1929, the Farmer's Union started their Cooperative Health Association, the first HMO. Independently, the same year in Los Angeles, two Canadian physicians founded the Ross-Loos group practice and sold the first physician-sponsored health insurance plan with prepayment to the Department of Water and Power and Los Angeles City workers.

As these and other plans grew during the 1930s, the AMA reversed its opposition to VHI in response to dwindling physician and hospital incomes, and, in 1939, the California Medical Society developed and sponsored a plan known as Blue Shield to pay physicians' bills in a hospitalized environment (6,7).

By 1946, private health insurance plans were experiencing astronomic growth as wage and price restrictions in the post–World War II period spurred the growth of fringe benefits, especially in unionized industries. Insurance companies, already having the inside track in sales and actuarial information in life insurance, went headlong into the health insurance business in competition with Blue Cross and Blue Shield.

Although voluntary health insurance plans were initiated by consumer cooperatives or employers and followed by provider-sponsored plans in the 1920s and 1930s, and supplemented by commercial insurance companies in the 1940s, the rate of growth in VHI programs has been in the reverse order. Most programs in the United States today are sponsored largely by insurance companies, followed by providers, with consumers lagging far behind. Blue Cross sponsors a network of 63 organizations extending its public service concept internationally. Similarly, Blue Shield administers 65 plans, 50 of which are administered jointly with Blue Cross. More than 1000 commercial insurance companies offer health insurance plans (6).

Population Coverage

More than two-thirds of all persons insured for health care in the United States rely on private insurance because most of the civilian population is not eligible for Medicare, Medicaid, or other public programs that finance health care. In addition, a majority of the elderly, who with few exceptions are covered by Medicare, purchase private coverage to supplement their Medicare benefits. Today, over 80 percent of the population under 65 have some form of VHI and about 80 percent of employees in the United States work for firms where they are eligible for health insurance. Firms that do not offer any health benefits at all tend to be small and nonunionized, hire seasonal workers, and employ relatively large numbers of low-wage employees. The industry groups supporting the highest rates of health insurance coverage are transporation, communication, utilities, manufacturing, and mining, which insure over 90 percent of the household heads employed. Construction, agriculture, and services (other than professional or financial) are the least insured groups, insuring about three-quarters of the household heads employed in those industries (8).

An unfortunate effect of employment-linked private health insurance is that people who are least able to pay for health care have the least insurance due to lack of employment (or full-time employment). The alternatives for these people are to purchase a nongroup or individual plan, usually a less generous and more expensive option in terms of out-of-pocket premiums, or to accept the risk of doing without any health insurance. Over 12 percent of the civilian noninstitutionalized population has no health insurance coverage at all, either public or private (9).

Benefits

Private health insurance coverage varies widely in terms of benefits provided, the extent of reimbursement for covered services, and exclusions or limitations. Figure 11-4 depicts the most commonly covered services for the privately insured. *Basic insurance* plans are designed to provide limited protection for the most expensive services and usually cover inpatient hospital and physician services and outpatient hospital services, including laboratory procedures. Limits may apply to a group of related services such as those provided during the course of a hospitalization. *Major medical insurance*, on the other hand, extends benefits to such services as physician office visits, outpatient mental health care, prescribed medicines, durable equipment and supplies, ambulance services, and the like. Thus, they are designed to protect against large medical bills as well as many expenses associated with routine types of medical care. The insurer typically pays a specified share of total covered expenses (e.g., 75–90 percent) in excess of a deductible (usually $100–$200 per year), with a high maximum allowance. The beneficiary pays the deductible and coinsurance, which constitute the share of the incremental expenses not covered by the plan, subject to a limited amount known as the "out-of-pocket limit" or "stop-loss provision." A limit of this kind may range from $1500 to $2500. Many major medical plans limit deductibles for family members to a specified amount (typically $300 per family) or waive the deductible for the rest of the family once two or three members have met their deductibles (8).

Comprehensive plans combine the features of both basic insurance and major medical plans. The deductible and other provisions apply to all expenses for all covered services. In contrast, "Medigap" plans are designed to reimburse only the deductibles

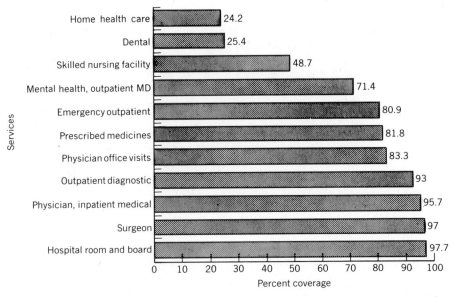

Figure 11-4. Coverage of the U.S. population: percent of privately insured persons under 65, by selected services. (SOURCE: Adapted from Farley PJ: *Private Health Insurance in the United States.* Data Preview 23, National Medical Care Expenditure Survey. DHHS Publication No. (PHS) 86-3406. National Center for Health Services Research and Health Care Technology Assessment, 1986, p 19.)

and coinsurance associated with Medicare covered services. About 70 percent of all Medicare beneficiaries privately purchase this type of limited benefit insurance (8).

Two other types of private insurance coverage are noteworthy: hospital indemnity plans and HMOs. Hospital indemnity plans offer specified cash payments (e.g., $100 per day) for each day of inpatient hospitalization, regardless of the expenses actually incurred. Thus, it is a type of disability insurance wherein the payment is not linked to the amount or type of medical services provided, but rather to length of the hospital stay, and the payment is not generous in relation to the actual hospital expenses. This type of coverage is held by less than 2 percent of the privately insured (8).

Prepaid Plans

HMOs and other similar plans provide fairly comprehensive coverage in return for a prepaid fee, usually without deductibles and coinsurance for most services, and therefore offer coverage against the risk of large health care financial losses. Prepaid health plans are a rapidly growing segment of the private health insurance market. Today, there are about 310 HMOs in the United States, compared to about 50 in 1973, prior to the passage of the HMO Act (1). This act requires employers with over 25 employees to offer a dual choice of health plans including one HMO, if one is available locally. It was anticiapted that the HMO concept would foster incentives toward prevention and cost-consciousness on the part of physicians who are encouraged to be frugal in the use of secondary services, particularly hospitalization. However, because the prepayment of premium does not necessarily translate into capitated provider reimbursement and tight prospective budgeting, cost-containment experience is mixed. In spite of legislative and economic incentives, only about 12.5 million Americans belonged to HMOs in 1983 (8).

SOCIAL HEALTH INSURANCE

The U.S. government sponsors two major mandatory social health insurance programs: (1) Worker's Compensation for the costs and pain of suffering job-related accidents and (2) Medicare for the elderly, disabled, and other special groups. Several states sponsor social insurance programs in the areas of temporary disability (California) or health insurance (Hawaii) (6).

Worker's Compensation

Worker's Compensation is offered in all 50 states to some extent. It is usually the first type of social insurance enacted in a nation, and, in 1975, 128 countries out of about 140 worldwide had industrial accident insurance. The first Worker's Compensation law in the United States was passed by New York State in 1914 in response to the tragic Triangle Shirt factory fire in which 146 women lost their lives. In 1950 Mississippi became the last state to enact Worker's Compensation. Today, about 80 percent of the U.S. workforce is covered to some extent by Worker's compensation, leaving about 21 million, many of whom are agricultural, casual, and domestic workers, without coverage. Unfortunately, it is often these same people who are not covered by any type of health insurance (6).

Worker's Compensation provides two basic benefits: (1) cash replacement of a portion of wages lost due to disability and (2) payment for all or part of the medical care necessary. Worker's Compensation may be underwritten by a private insurance company, a state government insurance fund, or a corporate contingency fund. Premiums are usually determined by experience rating. In 1985, Worker's Compensation paid out about $8.2 billion in disability claims.

Medicare

In 1935 national health insurance almost became a reality as part of the Social Security Act. Because of strong opposition from the AMA and conservative members of Congress, national health insurance was scrapped from the act by President Roosevelt, who did not want to risk passage by Congress. In 1939, and every 2 years for several Congresses thereafter, the Wagner, Murray, Dingell National Health Insurance Bill was proposed in Congress. This bill coincided with the growth curve of private health insurance enrollment, which precluded a pressing interest in national health insurance. However, private health insurance was largely sponsored by employers and thus did not serve the nonworking population, particularly the aged. Nonetheless, about 50 percent of the elderly enrolled in voluntary health insurance programs during the 1957–1964 pre-Medicare period (6).

In 1957 Representative Forand of Rhode Island introduced the bill that was the precursor of Medicare (Title XVIII of the Social Security Act). On July 30, 1965 Medicare became the first entry of the federal government into the provision of social health insurance rather than medical assistance (public welfare medicine) such as offered by the Kerr-Mills Act of 1960—"Medical Assistance for the Aged."

Strictly speaking, only Medicare Part A—Hospital Insurance (HI)—is social health insurance (Figure 11-5). Part B—Supplementary Medical Insurance (SMI)—is neither compulsory nor funded by a trust fund. Of the funds for SMI, 74 percent comes from the general treasury and the other 26 percent comes from Medicare Part A recipients who elect that Part B premiums be deducted from their monthly Social Security check (4).

Medicare utilizes an *indirect pattern* of finance and delivery, wherein the Health Care Financing Administration (HCFA), a branch of the U.S. Department of Health and Human Services, contracts with independent providers. Medicare recipients also access providers independently. HCFA sees to it that the provider is paid, but the providers are neither owned nor hired by the government, as in SHI systems utilizing the direct pattern of delivery. Generally speaking, if the private medical market is strong at the time when SHI is enacted, an indirect pattern of delivery emerges. If the market is weak, a direct financing route emerges.

WELFARE MEDICINE

Public assistance or welfare medicine is sponsored by a plethora of federal, state, and local government programs, but the most far-reaching program is Medicaid (Title XIX of the Social Security Act). Administered at the federal level by HCFA, Medicaid is financed by an average federal contribution from the general treasury of 55 percent and from state treasuries at an average contribution of 45 percent (Figure 11-5). Federal matching varies from 50.0 to 77.5 percent, depending on the income of the individual state (4). General treasury funds are generated from personal income tax, corporate income tax, and various excise taxes, and—to the extent that these taxes are borne by higher income individuals and organizations—Medicaid represents a type of transfer payment to the poor.

The distinction between welfare medicine and social health insurance, both of which are public programs, is an important one and rests on the philosophical difference between a transfer payment and entitlement. Medicaid is a transfer

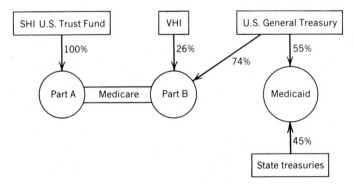

Figure 11-5. Flow of federal and state financing for Medicare and Medicaid.

payment "in kind," meaning that medical services are provided as a welfare benefit in lieu of cash. Welfare recipients also receive cash subsidies to cover their living expenses, but medical benefits are paid directly to the provider so that the recipients will not be tempted to spend the money on expense items other than health care. (Food stamps are another "in kind" benefit, providing vouchers solely for the purpose of purchasing food and groceries.) Thus, the transfer payment is a type of "relief" that government bestows on the poor; it is a form of charity.

Social health insurance is an *entitlement* program, not charity. It is a right earned by individuals in the course of their employment. The funds for SHI programs are contributed by a payroll tax, which in the case of Social Security is divided equally by the worker and the employer. Worker's Compensation is also financed, at least in part, by worker contributions. When the worker retires or suffers a temporary or sustaining injury related to employment, SHI becomes active for the worker and dependents. The fundamental aim of a compulsory, government-provided or government-supervised SHI program is social adequacy—to provide members of society with protection against hazards so widespread as to be considered risks that individuals cannot afford to deal with themselves. Eligibility in SHI is derived from contributions having been made in the program, and benefits are a statutory right not based on need. Recipients are thus entitled to the benefits of SHI. In 1975 71 countries had a SHI system for financing health care (6).

MEDICARE

Medicare, the principal SHI program in the United States, provides a variety of hospital, physician, and other medical services for (1) persons 65 and over, (2) disabled individuals who are entitled to Social Security benefits, and (3) end-stage renal disease victims. In 1985 Medicare financed $117.2 billion in health services, constituting 40.3 percent of all publicly financed health expenditures and 19.0 percent of personal health care expenditures. Medicare reimbursed 29.1 percent of all hospital expenditures and 20.6 percent of all physician expenditures in 1985 (2).

HOSPITAL INSURANCE

Ninety-five percent of the aged population of the United States is enrolled in Part A of Medicare, Hospital Insurance (HI). Part A finances four basic benefits for the covered population:

1. Ninety days of inpatient care in a "benefit period." (A benefit period is a spell of illness beginning with hospitalization and ending when a beneficiary has not been an inpatient in a hospital or skilled nursing facility for 60 continuous days. There is no limit to the number of benefit periods a beneficiary can use.)
2. A lifetime reserve of 60 days of inpatient care, once the 90 days are exhausted.
3. One hundred days of posthospitalization care in a skilled nursing facility.
4. Home health agency visits.

Since the inception of the Medicare program, Hospital Insurance has required the beneficiary to participate in cost sharing. The patient is required to pay an inpatient hospital deductible in each benefit period which approximates the cost of one day of hospital care ($520 in 1987). Coinsurance based on the inpatient hospital deductible is required for the 61st to 90th day of inpatient hospitalization and is always equal to one-fourth of the deductible ($130 in 1987). For the 21st to 100th day of SNF care, the coinsurance equals one-eighth of the deductible, and for the 60 lifetime reserve days, the patient pays one-half of the deductible for each day of inpatient hospitalization. The patient is also liable for the cost or replacement of the first three pints of blood. Nearly 70 percent of Medicare enrollees have private Medigap policies, which primarily cover some or all of the deductibles and coinsurance under Medicare. About 15 percent of the aged and 21 percent of the disabled have Medicaid coverage also (a group known as "crossovers"), and Medicaid usually assumes responsibility for the cost sharing under Medicare (4).

While hospital expenditures have grown at a rapid rate since the inception of Medicare, skilled nursing facility, home health agency, and outpatient benefits have all shifted significantly as a percent of total Medicare benefit payments. Skilled nursing facility payments dropped sharply from 6.5 percent in 1967 to only 0.8 percent in 1983. Home health agency payments rose from 1.0 to 2.6 percent, and outpatient outlays, the fastest growing component in Medicare, climbed dramatically from 0.9 percent to 6.4 percent over the same period (4).

SUPPLEMENTARY MEDICAL INSURANCE

Ninety-seven percent of Part A beneficiaries are enrolled in Part B—Supplementary Medical Insurance (SMI). Part B is the third largest federal domestic program, exceeded only by the Social Security cash benefit program and Medicare's Part A program. SMI requires a monthly premium and was designed to complement the HI program. It provides payments for physicians, physician-ordered supplies and services, outpatient hospital services, rural health clinic visits, and home health visits for persons without Part A coverage. Under "buy-in" agreements, most state Medicaid programs pay the premiums for Medicaid enrollees who qualify to participate in SMI (4).

Drugs on an outpatient basis, dental care, routine eye examinations and eyeglasses, preventive services, and long-term institutional services are not covered by either Part A or Part B of Medicare. Hospice benefits, however, became available for persons who are terminally ill in 1983. Enrollees in Medicare can elect the hospice benefit for two 90-day periods and one 30-day period.

From 1967 to 1984, Part B of Medicare has grown faster than Part A—a compound rate of growth, corrected for inflation, of 10.3 percent as compared to 8.6 percent. Therefore, although Part B represents only about 31 percent of Medicare expenditures, Part B has grown by 5 percent since 1967, and Part A has shrunk commensurately (4).

Under SMI, in addition to paying a monthly premium ($17.90 in 1987), the beneficiary must meet a deductible (currently $75) each year. On each claim for payment, physicians can accept or reject assignment. Acceptance means that the physician agrees to accept as payment in full the amount Medicare designates for the service. On assigned claims, the program reimburses 80 percent of allowed charges directly to the physician. Beneficiaries are liable for the remaining 20 percent coinsurance. On unassigned claims the beneficiary is also liable for the difference between the physician's charge and the allowed charge; Medigap policies generally do not cover charges above Medicare's allowed charge.

During the first 20 years of the Medicare program, the annualized rate of growth of Medicare reimbursements for physicians' services has been nearly equal to the rate of growth of reimbursement for inpatient hospital care: 16.3 percent as compared to 17.4 percent (4). To constrain SMI inflation, the Deficit Reduction Act of 1984 imposed a freeze on Medicare maximum payment levels (originally slated for 15 months beginning July 1, 1984, but continuing to date with a one percent across-the-board increase on January 1, 1987) and introduced the concept of "participating physicians," who are those who accept assignment for all services. Incentives to participate were introduced and resulted in substantial increases to assignment.

PROVIDER REIMBURSEMENT

Medicare has operated primarily on a fee-for-service basis for physicians and related services and, until 1983, on a cost-based retrospective basis for hospital services. Hospitals were reimbursed for any reasonable costs incurred in the provision of covered care to Medicare patients. Commencing October 1, 1983, payment rates were prospectively determined on a case basis. The Medicare hospital prospective payment system (PPS) uses diagnosis-related groups (DRGs) to classify cases for payment.

Claims are processed by intermediaries or fiscal agents, such as Blue Cross or a commercial insurance company, contracted for by the Medicare program to review and pay the bills. Enrollees can also join HMOs and similar forms of prepaid health care and special reimbursement provisions apply to these organizations. The Tax Equity and Fiscal Responsibility Act of 1982 (TEFRA) included major revisions to the Medicare law to encourage growth in the number of HMOs and other comprehensive medical plans enrolling Medicare beneficiaries. TEFRA also set limits on Medicare reimbursements for hospital costs at the per-case level and also placed a limit on the annual rate of increase for Medicare's reasonable costs per discharge.

The average-aged Medicare enrollee spent $1724 in 1983. As in any insurance program, however, utilization is uneven. Over two-thirds of the enrolled population had small claims of $500 or less or none at all. The highest 9.6 percent of users had reimbursements of $5000 or more, and these enrollees consumed 72.2 percent of program payments (4). Several studies have demonstrated that high Medicare reimbursements are related to terminal illness. Lubitz and Prihoda (10) found that reimbursements for decedents averaged $4527 for the last year of life, whereas reimbursements averaged $729 for a comparison group who survived the period under study. Fuchs (11) showed that the greatest proportion of medical care costs are incurred in the year prior to death, regardless of the age of natural death. For Medicare enrollees in 1976, the average reimbursement for those in their last year of life was 6.6 times as large as for those who survived for at least 2 years. Thus, one may surmise that the principal reason why health expenditures rise with age is that the proportion of persons near death increases with age. Other studies have revealed a great deal of consistency over time in the utilization of health expenditures by the highest users, the top 1 percent accounting for 20 or more percent of health care dollars (4).

MEDICAID

PROGRAM STRUCTURE

Medicaid was enacted into law on July 30, 1965 as Title XIX of the Social Security Act and became part of the existing federal-state welfare structure to assist the poor. Until 1956, there had been no federal participation in health care for the poor. This public obligation was delegated to the states as part of their police powers. Prior to Medicaid, many physicians donated their services or used a sliding scale of fees in treating the poor and, as a rule, hospitals admitted charity cases. However, under the purview of the states, health care for the poor varied widely from state to state and manifested all the forms of discrimination tolerated in each locale. The Kerr-Mills Act of 1960—Medical Assistance for the Aged—was the forerunner of the Medicaid model and was later subsumed under Title XIX.

Eligibility

Supported by federal grants and administered by the states, Medicaid is limited to specific groups of low-income individuals and families. Medicaid is welfare medicine and thus has no entitlement features. Recipients must prove their eligibility according to their income, and, prior to 1976, states were permitted to put a lien on a recipient's home or other personal property.

The program was designed to cover those groups who are eligible to receive cash payments under one of the two existing welfare programs established under Social Security—Aid to Families with Dependent Children (AFDC) and Supplemental Security Income (SSI). The four "categorical" assistance groups covered by Medicaid are (1) children of AFDC families; and those covered by SSI including (2) the aged, (3) the blind, and (4) the permanently and totally disabled. In most instances, receipt of a welfare payment under one of these programs means automatic eligibility for Medicaid. Figure 11-6 compares the distribution of Medicaid recipients to that of expenditures by eligibility category. AFDC families were the largest group of recipients (67.8 percent) in 1984, but accounted for a relatively small part of the Medicaid budget (25.2 percent), reflecting the relatively good health of most Medicaid children. Largely because of high utilization of nursing home services, 37.3 percent of total Medicaid outlays was attributable to aged SSI recipients, who comprise only 14.8 percent of the Medicaid population. Similarly, outlays for the disabled totaled 34.3 percent of Medicaid expenditures, as compared to 13.4 percent of recipients, reflecting in part the high rate of expenditures for the 139,000 persons in intermediate-care facilities for the mentally retarded (4).

In addition to the categorical groups, states may provide Medicaid to two optional "medically needy" groups of people who are not recipients of cash assistance. The first group is the "categorically related medically needy," people who fit into one of the four categories covered by the cash assistance programs and whose income and assets fall within the medically needy standards (i.e., 1.33 times the "poor" level). The second optional group is the "medically needy only," the near poor who spend down their income and wealth, due to medical bills, to the medically needy standard. Under federal guidelines, states set income and asset levels for cash assistance and medical eligibility. Because there is considerable variation in the coverage of optional groups by

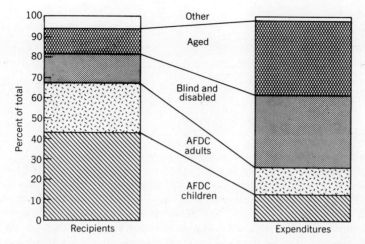

Figure 11-6. Distribution of Medicaid recipients and expenditures, by eligibility category: United States, 1984 (AFDC, Aid to Families with Dependent Children). (SOURCE: Gornick M, Greenberg JN, Eggers PW, et al: Twenty years of Medicare and Medicaid: Covered populations, use of benefits, and program expenditures. *Health Care Finan Rev* 1985; (Ann Suppl):13-59.

the states and in income standards across Medicaid jurisdictions, the degree to which programs cover more than the poverty population varies considerably.

BENEFITS PROVIDED

Services

Title XIX of the Social Security Act mandates that every state Medicaid program provide specific basic health services:

- Hospital inpatient care
- Hospital outpatient services
- Laboratory and x-ray services
- Skilled nursing facility (SNF) services for those aged 21 and older
- Home health services for those eligible for SNF services
- Physicians' services
- Family planning
- Rural health clinic services
- Early and periodic screening, diagnosis, and treatment for children under 21 years of age

States may determine the scope of services offered (e.g., limit the days of hospital care or the number of physician visits covered) and provide a number of other elective services including:

- Drugs
- Eyeglasses
- Intermediate care facility services
- Inpatient psychiatric care for the aged and persons under 21 years of age
- Physical therapy
- Dental care

Administration

Medicaid operates primarily as a vendor payment program. Payments are made directly to providers of service for care rendered to eligible individuals. Methods for reimbursing physicians and hospitals vary widely among the states, but providers must accept the Medicaid reimbursement level as payment in full. Medicaid physician reimbursement rates are usually less generous than Medicare. In long-term care facilities, individuals are required to turn over income in excess of their personal needs and maintenance needs of their spouses (the monetary level being determined by the state) to help pay for their care. States may require cost sharing by Medicaid recipients, but they may not require the categorically eligible to share costs for mandatory services. As noted previously, most state Medicaid programs have buy-in agreements with Medicare in which Medicaid assumes the responsibility for the Medicare cost-sharing for persons covered under both programs. About 12 percent of the aged and disabled Medicare enrollees are also covered by state Medicaid programs (4).

States participate in the Medicaid program at their option. All states except Arizona (which has a demonstration project of capitated health delivery that excludes long-term care services) currently have Medicaid programs. The District of Columbia, Puerto Rico, Guam, The Northern Marianas, and the Virgin Islands also provide Medicaid coverage.

The states administer their Medicaid programs within broad federal requirements and guidelines. These requirements allow states considerable discretion in determining not only eligibility but also covered benefits and provider payment mechanisms. Some states also include in the Medicaid program persons known as "state-only" enrollees, who do not meet federal requirements and hence do not qualify for federal matching funds. As a result of state options and policy decisions, the characteristics of Medicaid programs vary considerably from state to state. In the Omnibus Budget Reconciliation Act of 1981, the states were given even more flexibility in the administration of their programs as well as additional options, including the introduction of home- and community-based service programs as alternatives to institutionalization.

Medicaid expenditures vary widely across the states. In 1984 four states had per capita Medicaid expenditures of less than $70, whereas four states had more than $190. Similarly, seven states had Medicaid expenditures per person in poverty of less than $500, and eight states had expenditures of $1500 or more (4).

GROWTH OF MEDICAID

Providers

Although Medicaid expenditures have grown by 195 percent from 1975 to 1985, the rate of growth is far less than that of Medicare, which has grown by 352 percent over the same period. Inpatient hospital care, which has experienced the greatest amount of inflation in 20 years following passage of Medicare and Medicaid, accounts for a much smaller proportion of Medicaid program dollars (26 percent in 1984) compared with Medicare program dollars (64 percent in 1983). Nursing home care, including skilled nursing facilities (SNF), intermediate care facilities (ICF), and intermediate care facilities for the mentally retarded (ICF/MR), is the largest component of the Medicaid budget. Although growth in spending for SNFs and ICFs has slowed considerably in recent years, ICF/MRs have expanded so rapidly since their inclusion as a benefit in 1972 that the overall growth in the proportion of Medicaid spending for nursing home care can be attributed solely to them. In 1975, 38 percent of total Medicaid outlays went for nursing home care; in 1984, 43 percent went for this service. During the same period, ICF/MR expenditures rose from 3 to 12 percent of the Medicaid budget, covering 139,000 mentally retarded beneficiaries. (The share of nursing home care financed by all public programs has also declined since 1979, from 56 to 48 percent in 1983). Compared with other services that Medicaid provides, Medicaid payments for long-term care are also the most costly per user. In 1984 the average Medicaid payment for SNF services was $8594: for ICF services, the payment was $7377; and for ICF/MR, the payment averaged $29,995 (4).

Budgetary

Medicaid is the fastest growing component of aggregate state spending, increasing at a compound rate of 16.9 percent as compared to an 11.4 percent growth rate for state revenues. Between 1965 and 1981, state Medicaid expenditures have increased from 2 percent of total state spending to 7.7 percent, a relative increase of 285 percent. During that same period of time, Medicaid payments have risen from 23.8 percent of state welfare expenditures to 60.2 percent, reflecting in part the fact that cash assistance payments have risen very slowly compared with the rise in the cost of health care services (4).

PHYSICIAN REIMBURSEMENT

Paying the physician traditionally calls on one of three reimbursement mechanisms: fee-for-service, prepayment, or salary. Health insurance plans, either public or private, may utilize any or all of the three reimbursement types; there is no optimal system. Today, private insurance covers over 80 percent of the U.S. population under 65 years of age for physician office visits, over 95 percent for physician inpatient medical care and surgeons' fees, and over 70 percent for outpatient mental health care (8).

FEE-FOR-SERVICE

Fee-for-service is widely used throughout the world for paying the physician and is typically the physician's preferred mode of payment. In fee-for-service, the unit of remuneration is the medical act, either a service or a procedure. In the days before health insurance for physician reimbursement was widespread, most physicians had a sliding fee scale wherein the poor paid lower fees than wealthier patients. With the advent of health insurance in both the public and private sectors, physician payment became more regulated, and today most physicians have one schedule of charges used for all payers, whether they are individuals or third parties.

Indemnity

Insurance policies that reimburse on a fee-for-service basis offer payment either by indemnity or service benefits or by fixed fees. *Indemnity payment* stipulates a certain dollar value per procedure, usually according to a "Table of Allowances." The provider can charge anything above the stipulated amount and collect the remainder directly from the patient. Often, the Table of Allowances is based on a "Relative Value Scale," in which each procedure is rated according to a point system that reflects the relative technical difficulty and time cost of the procedure, and each point is worth so many dollars. This type of system is easy to administer and update for inflation and changing practice patterns, but no provision is made by the insurer to protect the patient from outlandish charges.

Service Benefits

Service benefits pay a percentage per procedure, usually 75 or 80 percent of "usual, customary, and reasonable" (UCR) fees. In this scheme, the UCR fee schedule protects the carrier from unlimited liability in the wake of high charges and also may give the patient information about reasonable fee norms. UCR means that the fee is "usual" in that physician's practice, "customary" in that community, and "reasonable" in terms of the distribution of all physician charges for that service in the community. The latter is commonly expressed as a percentile (e.g., the policy will pay up to the 75th percentile). Medicare Part B currently uses a similar standard, "CPR," which stands for customary, prevailing, and reasonable fees. In this nomenclature, the "customary" charge is determined through development of a fee profile for each individual physician and a median figure is determined for each procedure. "Prevailing" denotes the community standard and is figured by arraying the customary charges for all physicians in the community. A "reasonable" fee is one that is justifiable in the opinion of a duly constituted professional review panel or Peer Review Organization (PRO). Under the Deficit Reduction Act of 1984, Medicare pays physicians at the lowest of their actual charge, their customary charge, or the prevailing charge for the community. The enactment of this legislation has frozen reimbursement levels for physicians' services at specified levels, with only a 1.0 percent increase to date (12).

Physicians may elect one of two reimbursement strategies under Medicare Part B. They may accept the Medicare fee determination as payment in full, billing Medicare directly and receiving payment from the Medicare intermediary (a practice called "accepting the assignment"). The second strategy is to bill charges to the patient, who, in turn, receives the CPR reimbursement from Medicare, leaving it up to the physician to collect the fee from the patient. The Deficit Reduction Act of 1984 also created two classes of physician: "participating" and "nonparticipating." A participating physician must accept assignment for all claims for all Medicare patients. Several incentives of a pecuniary and marketing nature have been employed by Medicare to entice physicians to participate. A nonparticipating physician can continue to treat Medicare patients, accepting assignments or not on a claim-by-claim basis, subject to the freeze-period prohibition on increasing their actual charges to Medicare beneficiaries (12).

Fixed Fees

In some reimbursement plans, physicians can only charge, and will only be paid, according to fixed fees. A provider who accepts the plan must accept the fee schedule. This arrangement exists in Medicaid, and many private plans also stipulate fixed fees in order to protect the patient and contain costs.

One advantage to fee-for-service reimbursement is that the remuneration adjusts automatically for case complexity, linking the provider's reward closely to the output of services. The billing system, in turn, provides a great deal of "transparency" of the physician's profile of practice. The ease with which patients may change physicians in a fee-for-service system enables them to directly exercise considerable economic clout over practitioners (13).

PREPAYMENT

In prepayment or capitation, the person served, rather than the medical act, is the unit of remuneration. The capitation payment takes care of reimbursement for a stipulated length of line, usually a year. Using capitation as a reimbursement methodology, physicians have formed contracted networks known as Independent Practice Associations (IPAs), usually organized around an HMO. In recent years, IPAs have been gaining in popularity for physicians and consumers along with the HMO movement. Advantages to prepayment are that it is administratively simple, facilitates advance global budgeting, and gives physicians incentive to control the cost of medical treatments. If patients can switch physicians from time to time, they still retain some economic clout over physicians (13).

SALARY

Salary is payment to the physician for that physician's time, irrespective of the units of service or the number of patients. On a large scale, salaried practice almost always takes place in a highly organized network such as the National Health Service in Great Britain. On a smaller scale in the United States, urban public hospitals that serve indigent populations often have large attending staffs who are salaried. Countries in which salaried practices are common rarely include specialists in this payment mechanism. Instead, general practitioners or primary care providers have a "panel" of patients in the community. Advantages to salaried reimbursement for physicians are that it is administratively simple, the medical treatments selected are not influenced by relative profitability, and it encourages cooperation among physicians. Furthermore, salaries facilitate budgeting for health expenditures ex ante (13).

MONITORING

All payment mechanisms have faults, and each must be monitored for abuses. In fee-for-service, the incentives are for overwork by the physician and overutilization by the patients. Fee-for-service fosters unnecessary or duplicative service to the point where the high volume of services may actually affect the quality of care adversely.

Unfortunately, in the United States, malpractice suits have encouraged defensive medicine, wherein overutilization and extra fees are simply passed on to the consumer in higher insurance rates. Also, if fees for all procedures do not stand in constant proportion to costs incurred, the choice of treatment may favor more profitable procedures. For these and other reasons that foster inflation, fee-for-service reimbursement is very difficult to budget for in advance (13).

In prepayment, on the other hand, underutilization must be monitored because the incentives are to decrease costs and services provided vis-à-vis the capitation payment. In many prepayment schemes, any cost savings realized are distributed to the participating physicians, which may be an inducement to cut costs too far. In HMOs where only the primary care physicians are capitated, for example, there also exists the incentive to excessively refer patients to specialists. Likewise, capitation gives physicians incentives for "dumping" patients with complex, costly conditions onto other providers. Finally, the administrative system for prepayment yields little insight as to the physician's practice profile (13).

In salaried practice, incentives favor underwork or seeing too few patients. Physicians literally "get paid by the hour," resulting in no inducement toward higher volume. According to Reinhardt, unless the salary is linked to output and patient satisfaction, patients lose economic clout over the physician—who, in turn, may render care as an act of noblesse oblige. Like capitation, salaried practice gives little transparency as to the physician's practice profile (13).

RECENT INITIATIVES IN HEALTH CARE FINANCE

FACTORS IN HEALTH CARE COST INFLATION

The implementation of Medicare and Medicaid in 1966 heralded a 20-year era of unprecedented health care cost inflation. Gornick et al. succinctly list the multiplicity of factors feeding the inflationary process (4:16):

> Several different factors in the health care system have been identified with the continuing increase in costs: the rise in wages and price levels in the health care industry; increases in the number of certain customary services, such as laboratory tests; the development of new and costly medical technologies, such as open-heart surgery; changes in the organization of care, such as the growth of intensive care units in hospitals and increases in personnel; and the growth of institutions for long-term care.
>
> Factors often cited as giving impetus to these changes include: the increase in demand for more costly health care services, as a result of Medicare, Medicaid, and other third-party payment that removed the individual from direct consequences of the cost of services; the response of health care providers to reimbursement methods that offered financial incentives to increase medical care spending; and the rising expectations in the nation with regard to health care services.

Cost-Containment Measures

In the 1970s the federal government experimented with a number of programs and reimbursement methods to contain health care costs. Major programs included (1) the establishment of reasonable cost limits for hospitals, (2) the initiation of state and local networks of health planning agencies along with the certificate-of-need (CON) procedure for augmenting capital plant and equipment, (3) the establishment of the Professional Standards Review Organization (PSRO) program to review care and eliminate unnecessary hospital days for federally funded patients, and (4) encouragement of the growth of HMOs to promote the use of preventive services and decrease the utilization of hospital inpatient care.

It can be safely said that the programs of the 1970s were unsuccessful in containing health care costs. Early in the Reagan Administration, legislative efforts to change the monetary incentive system in health care began in earnest. Today, the seeds of deceleration in health costs are manifesting themselves, but not without painful consequences for many groups of people. The balance between reasonable costs and equitable access has not yet been struck, but what is clear is that the traditional health care market, based on cost reimbursement, has no apparatus to reflect social or economic rationing decisions regarding the provision of health care that might help to stem inflation. The cost-based reimbursement market holds no incentives for efficiency, productivity, and management coordination; yet, even in this market of seemingly never-ending growth, universal realized access to health services remains illusive.

Procompetition

Early in this decade, Enthoven (14–16) and other health economists exposited strategies of "procompetition" that were meant to stem health care costs by creating competitive market conditions by means of direct incentives both for consumers and for employers who purchase group health insurance policies. These strategies included the imposition of a "tax cap" on employer income tax deductions for health insurance expenses, raising the threshold for individual income tax deductions, and offering multiple choices by employers in health insurance plans. While the threshold for personal income tax deductions for medical out-of-pocket expense has been raised in the past few years to 7.5 percent of adjusted gross income, the other strategies, while not enacted, had a profound effect on the thinking of health policymakers. The programs described below reflect this "neoconservative" philosophy, and, in most cases, the scorecards on their success are not in. Nevertheless, these programs point in likely future directions for health finance.

TEFRA

The Tax Equity and Fiscal Responsibility Act (TEFRA), signed into law in September 1982, set limits on Medicare reimbursements on a per-case basis for hospital costs and also placed a limit on the annual rate of increase for Medicare's reasonable costs per discharge. TEFRA was expected to reduce Medicare reimbursement by 4.5 percent in real dollars over the ensuing 3 years, during which time reimbursement increases, based on projected inflation rates, would be in effect. Considering the rapid enactment of the Prospective Payment System 1 year later, it is difficult to evaluate the impact of the act. However, TEFRA was the harbinger of prospective payment, and a number of features of the latter program were borrowed from it. These features were part of the Section 223 limits on hospital costs. They included (1) grouping hospitals by bed size and size of locale, (2) wage adjustments by locality, (3) an adjustment for teaching hospitals, and (4) an adjustment for case-mix index.

The Section 223 limits were calculated according to a complicated formula whereby the labor-related component for the hospital region, adjusted by a geographic wage index, was added to a regional nonlabor component (Table 11-2). The product was then multiplied by a case-mix index, specific to each hospital. Finally, the result was multiplied by a cost reporting year adjustment factor so that the hospital's fiscal year coincided with the federal fiscal year, which starts each October 1. (These figures were all specified by HCFA and published in the *Federal Register* on September 30, 1982, the day prior to enactment of the legislation.) The formula used to calculate the Section 223 limits was substantially retained for figuring the hospital-specific portion of the rates "blended" with a federal portion in the Prospective Payment System, enacted October 1, 1983. HCFA developed institutional-specific case-mix indexes based on a

TABLE 11-2. Computation of Allowable Cost per Discharge with the Actual Cost and Target Rate above the Section 223 Limit

Hospital A is a 425-bed general acute-care hospital located in Columbus, Ohio. The hospital operates on a March 31 fiscal year; therefore, the first year in which the hospital is subject to the provisions of Section 101 of the act is the year ending March 31, 1984. The following facts apply to this situation:

Section 223 information published in the September 30, 1982, *Federal Register:*

Per discharge labor-related component	$2,897.76
Per discharge non-labor-related component	$ 765.57
Geographic wage index	1.0803
Cost reporting year adjustment factor	1.04125
Case-mix adjustment factor	1.0067
Nonteaching hospital, thus no education adjustment	

Other information:

Actual base period (3/31/83) cost per Medicare discharge	$3,900.00
Actual target period (3/31/84) cost per Medicare discharge	$4,200.00
Market basket index, plus 1%	8.075%
Index for calendar 1984—7.9%	
Index for calendar 1984—8.6%	
Weighted —8.075%	

Hospital A's Section 223 limit for the year ended March 30, 1984, is computed as follows:

Labor-related component	$2,897.76
Geographic wage index	1.0803
Adjusted labor component	$3,130.45
Nonlabor component	765.57
Labor adjusted limit	$3,896.02
Case-mix index	1.0067
Case-mix adjusted limit	$3,922.12
Cost reporting year adjustment factor	1.04125
Section 223 limit per discharge	$4,083.91

SOURCE: Deloitte Haskins & Sells: *Tax Equity and Fiscal Responsibility Act of 1982: Management Strategies for Health Care Providers.* New York, Deloitte Haskins & Sells, 1982.

diagnosis-related group (DRG) system designed at Yale University. The DRG classification system sorts patients into uniform, clinically compatible groups that have been categorized on the basis of traditional resource use by patients with similar diagnoses. The original Yale DRGs were modified to reflect variation only in Medicare cases. For each hospital, HCFA used a 20 percent sample of the Medicare billing forms submitted for calendar year 1980. Using the 10,167 ICD-9-CM diagnosis codes from these claims and each hospital's Medicare cost report, HCFA developed the case-mix index (Table 11-3). In essence, this case-mix index is intended to compare a particular hospital's case mix with that of all other hospitals in the nation (17).

Target Rates

Another ceiling established by HCFA, also published in the *Federal Register* on September 30, 1982, was the *target rate ceiling*. The regulations establishing the target rate ceiling limited the allowable amount of growth in Medicare reimbursable inpatient operating costs and were, at the time, expected to be substantially more severe in terms of impact than that of the Section 223 limits. The target cost per Medicare discharge was computed by using 1980 base period allowable Medicare operating costs per discharge, increased by an inflation factor. This factor was based on a market basket index, plus one percentage point (and were the same as those used to calculate the cost reporting adjustment factor used in the Section 223 limits). Medicare operating costs were defined as routine operating costs, ancillary service costs, and special care unit costs, excluding capital-related costs, medical education program costs, and medical insurance costs.

The TEFRA regulations gave bonuses to hospitals whose inpatient operating costs per discharge were less than the target rate, provided the target rate was below the Section 223 limit. If a hospital's per-discharge costs fell below the target rate, the hospital would be given 50 percent of the difference. On the other hand, if a hospital's per-discharge costs were above the target, the hospital would be reimbursed only at the target rate plus 25 percent of the costs in excess of it, so long as the reimbursement rate was below the limit. If the limit was below the target rate, the limit became the rate of reimbursement regardless of actual costs (17). In this way, TEFRA provided the first incentive system for hospitals to lower their costs on Medicare discharges rather than to contribute to the cost spiral induced by the cost-based reimbursement system. Incidentally, the TEFRA system more closely resembled the economic theory of prospective payment than the subsequent reimbursement system that came to be known as the Prospective Payment System.

THE PROSPECTIVE PAYMENT SYSTEM

The Prospective Payment System (PPS) was enacted on October 1, 1983, 2 years ahead of schedule. The Social Security Amendments of 1983 (PL 98-21) initiated the Medicare prospective payment system and contained provisions to base payment for hospital inpatient services on predetermined rates per discharge for 468 DRGs. Under PPS, the majority of hospitals in the United States would no longer be reimbursed for inpatient services on the basis of reasonable costs. The legislation excluded psychiatric, rehabilitation, and children's hospitals and long-term care facilities from prospective payment; these facilities remained on TEFRA regulations. Hospitals with distinct part

TABLE 11-3. Calculation of Medicare Case-Mix Index[a]

Hospital	DRG 1	DRG 2	DRG 3	DRG 4	DRG 5	Total (Percent)	DRG Weighted Expected Cost Per Case ($)[b]	Case-Mix Index[c]
A	2.5	27.3	10.5	41.5	18.2	100	1660.40	0.8900
B	21.0	.9	30.1	2.0	46.0	100	2401.30	1.2872
C	40.6	5.0	2.3	47.2	4.9	100	1346.30	0.7227
D	5.1	18.4	62.5	10.0	4.0	100	2990.70	1.6031
E	30.4	65.0	1.0	1.6	2.0	100	929.00	0.4980
Average proportion for all hospitals	19.92	23.32	21.28	20.46	15.02	100	1865.54	—
DRG cost weight	$1000	$800	$4100	$1500	$2000	—	—	—

SOURCE: Deloitte Haskins & Sells: *Tax Equity and Fiscal Responsibility Act of 1982: Management Strategies for Health Care Providers*. New York, Deloitte Haskins & Sells, 1982.

[a]Adjusted to make these 5 DRGs hypothetically represent all 356 Medicare DRGs.

[b]For hospital A, calculated as follows:

$$0.025 \ (1000) + 0.273 \ (800) + 0.105 \ (4100) + 0.415 \ (1500) + 0.182 \ (2000) = \$1660.40$$

[c]For hospital A, calculated as $1660.40 divided by $1865.54 = 0.8900.

psychiatric and rehabilitation units, sole community hospitals, cancer hospitals, and referral centers had the option to elect prospective payment for Medicare cases (18). By the end of the first year of PPS, a total of 5405 hospitals, which constituted 81 percent of all Medicare participating hospitals, were operating under PPS. This figure represents virtually all the short-stay acute-care hospitals participating in the Medicare system (19).

PPS is a major departure from cost-based reimbursement in that payment has no direct relationship to length of stay, services rendered, or current costs of care. Certain costs, such as capital depreciation and direct medical education costs, are exempt from the PPS provisions and continue to be reimbursed on a reasonable cost basis. Payment for physician services (e.g., radiology, anesthesiology) previously reimbursed on the basis of reasonable costs under Medicare Part A are included in the hospital's PPS rate. Hospitals with costs below their predetermined rates are permitted to keep the difference in payment. If costs exceed the payment levels, however, hospitals are required to absorb the loss.

Blending Rates

Originally slated for a 3-year phase-in period beginning with cost reporting periods starting on or after October 1, 1983, the movement to a purely national rate schedule has been extended by "blending" hospital-specific DRG rates, based on the hospital's 1981 calendar year costs and regionally established DRG rates, with national DRG rates. After the phase-in period, the payment rates will be established by HCFA on a national basis, without regard to a hospital's specific costs. For fiscal year 1987, the blending consisted of 25 percent hospital-specific and 75 percent federal rates, except for Oregon, which assumed the 100 percent federal rate. The rate, whether blended or national, is multiplied by the DRG weight specific to each Medicare discharge to arrive at total reimbursement for the case.

The hospital-specific portion of the blending, computed by a case-mix index derived from 1981 cost and billing information, differs from the index used under TEFRA. To figure the hospital-specific portion of the rate, the Medicare cost per discharge for the base year (the hospital's 1982 fiscal year) is divided by the case-mix index, and then adjusted for outliers and inflation. Reimbursement rates to individual hospitals also increase with the number of full-time equivalent interns and residents per bed (i.e., the indirect medical education adjustment) (18).

It should be noted that in the hospital-specific portion of the blending, costs are divided by the case-mix index. Therefore, the higher the costs incurred relative to the case-mix index, the higher the hospital-specific portion will be, which may be interpreted as rewarding less efficient hospitals. This phenomenon had a large effect on reimbursement rates early in the PPS phase-in when blending was 75 percent hospital-specific and 25 percent federal. By 1987, however, with 25/75 blending, the influence of this phenomenon was dissipating.

DRG Weights

The DRG weight classifications used in TEFRA were updated for use in PPS by using a stratified sample of 400,000 medical records drawn from patient discharges in 332 hospitals during the latter half of 1979. Ultimately 468 DRGs wre developed, 467 representing principal diagnoses and 1 for "other" procedures. A contracted fiscal intermediary, such as Blue Cross or a commercial insurer, assigns a DRG from a bill submitted by the hospital for each case. Using classifications and terminology consistent with the ICD-9-CM and the Uniform Hospital Discharge Data Set (UHDDS), the intermediary assigns the DRG using the Grouper Program (an automated classification algorithm), which compares information contained in the bill with appropriate DRG criteria. Criteria include the patient's age, sex, principal and secondary diagnoses, procedures performed, and discharge status (20). (Figure 11-7 presents a schematic diagram of the Grouper Program.) If the discharge is classified under DRGs 1 to 467, the intermediary determines the payment amount and pays the hospital; if the case falls into DRG 468, the intermediary returns the claim to the hospital for clarification before the payment amount is determined.

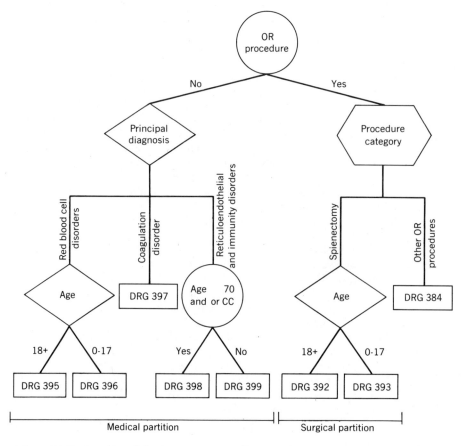

Figure 11-7. Flowchart of the Grouper Program for major diagnostic category 16: Disease and Disorders of the Blood and Blood-Forming Organs and Immunological Disorders. (OR, operating room; CC, comorbidity and/or complication.) (SOURCE: American Medical Association: *Diagnosis-Related Groups (DRGs) and the Prospective Payment System.* Chicago, American Medical Association, 1984.)

Outliers

Bills for "outliers" require special consideration. Length-of-stay or day outliers are identified by the intermediary, and, after appropriate review, payment is made to the hospital. Cost outliers, however, are not identified by the intermediary. The hospital must identify cost outliers and request payment. (It is important to note that the classification of DRGs depends largely on the principal diagnosis, which may not be the diagnosis consuming the most resources.) The original DRG rates were reduced by 5.7 percent to accommodate the expected outlays for outliers. HCFA estimated that 6 percent of all cases would be outliers. However, in the first year of PPS, outliers accounted for only 1.6 percent of all cases submitted for payment. This phenomenon may be related to actual hospital cost savings or length-of-stay reductions stimulated by PPS (thus precluding outliers) or may reflect cut-rate care induced by the stringent rates of reimbursement for outliers. Whatever the reason, HCFA has not adjusted the 5.7 percent reduction in DRG rates to accomodate the overestimation in outliers.

Incentives in PPS

A clear incentive in the PPS system is for hospitals to expand services still qualifying for cost-based reimbursement. Opportunities for marketing new services include specific ambulatory programs, satellite clinics, health-related services such as family planning, chemical dependency treatment, and laboratory or other ancillary services used by physicians. Hospital-sponsored skilled nursing, rehabilitation, home health services, and other services that may facilitate earlier discharge of patients and provide additional sources of revenue for hospitals have experienced marked growth since the inception of PPS. Many of these programs may be accomplished by conversion of acute-care beds, replacing services eliminated by PPS-induced financial considerations or making use of excess capacity (18).

The major deleterious incentives anticipated in the enactment of PPS are (1) multiple, unnecessary admissions of the same patient for a set of related procedures, resulting in more discreet DRG payments, a practice known as "churning"; (2) "skimming" more profitable, less severely ill patients in each DRG, or "dumping" high-cost patients; and (3) reducing length of stay, tests, and procedures per admission to dangerously low levels. Data for the first and second years of the program reveal no conclusive evidence that these phenomena are occurring (19,21,22). Indeed, some of the empirical findings are counterintuitive. Hospital admissions have been falling for all payers for several years, and since PPS was enacted, Medicare admissions are down as well. The figures for the fiscal year 1984 indicate a decrease in admissions per 1000 enrollees of 3.5 percent, which is contrary to the steady rise in Medicare admissions during the 1978–1984 period (19). While isolated examples of skimming and dumping do surface, widespread usage of these practices by hospitals has been documented largely for the uninsured and, in some states in particular, for Medicaid patients. Length of stay has been falling for Medicare since the inception of TEFRA. In 1967, the average length of stay was 13.8 days per Medicare patient; in 1985, it was 8.4 days. However, length of stay has dropped dramatically since PPS—0.9 days in 1984 and 0.6 days in 1985, compared to an average drop of 0.2 days per year from 1967 to 1983 (4,19,21). Conclusive data are not yet available for tests and procedures, but it is safe to say that anecdotal evidence points to significant reductions. Whether these cuts were taken from the "fat" in the system or whether they impinge on the quality of care is unknown. Mortality and morbidity rates, figured in a variety of ways, are thus far inconclusive (23).

Preliminary research indicates a tendency under PPS to increase the care provided to patients in other than inpatient settings (19). A survey of 200 physicians in five states shows that under prospective payment, hospitals encourage physicians to reduce ancillary services, shorten hospital stays, and increase outpatient testing. Data on SNF admissions show a slight acceleration in actual admissions as compared to projected rates for 1984. In general, there is no systematic evidence that access to needed care has been thus far hampered by PPS (22).

Criticisms of PPS

A number of criticisms have been levied against the incentives inherent in the DRG system. First, there is speculation that DRGs may not be "economically neutral" in that a hospital may be rewarded or penalized for performing a particular activity. To the extent that DRGs reflect procedures performed (i.e., types of surgery) as well as diagnosis, the choice of treatment may vary according to the "profitability" of that DRG, and treatment decisions may not be made on purely clinical grounds. In a similar vein, physicians, in their clinical notes, and medical records administrators, in abstracting data for the DRG grouper program, might employ "gaming" strategies to assure "DRG creep" to higher-level, more revenue enhancing diagnoses (24). Other criticisms involve the structure and mathematical integrity of DRGs. Several methods for changing PPS to a severity-based, rather than diagnosis-based, case-mix system have been postulated along with schemes for refining DRG coding to reflect the severity of the condition (24–27). Lave has shown that the mathematical constructs of the DRGs lend themselves to "compression" in DRG prices; the prices of the truly high cost DRGs are set low relative to their actual costs, whereas the prices of truly low cost DRGs are set high relative to their costs (28). This could create a situation in which hospitals may want to discriminate against providing service to patients in the high-cost DRGs or, on the bright side, could encourage a few hospitals in competitive markets to specialize in efficiently providing "high-cost" services, such as coronary bypass surgery, at more profitable rates.

Performance

How are hospitals faring financially under PPS? Across the board, hospitals are showing large operating margins, with large urban hospitals and major teaching facilities leading the pack. On the other hand, rural hospitals and proprietaries are not doing as well (29,30). The spate of hospital bankruptcies that were forecast at the inception of PPS has not taken place, but acquisitions and mergers are rampant in the health care industry (as they are in many American industries in the 1980s).

While a final verdict on PPS would be premature at this point in time, evidence on the "bottom line" is encouraging. From fiscal year 1974 (which marked the end of wage and price control under the Nixon Administration) through fiscal year 1982 (the last year prior to the enactment of TEFRA), Medicare inpatient hospital benefit payments increased at an annual rate of 19.9 percent (10 percent in real terms). Under TEFRA, this rate of increase dropped to 10.2 percent (6.8 percent in real terms), which was more than four percentage points lower than any time in the previous 10 years. Furthermore, the estimated rate of increase under PPS, for fiscal year 1984, was 8.2

percent (3.8 percent in real terms), which is among the smallest percent increases in Medicare's history (19). This deceleration in the costs of Medicare, along with numerous other findings, underlines the responsiveness of provider behavior to changing the economic incentive system in health care; economic control may well be shifting from the providers to the purchasers of health care.

SELECTIVE CONTRACTING

In 1982 the California legislature cleared the way for the state Medicaid program (Medi-Cal) and private insurers to enable payers to draw up contracts for the delivery of health services to their beneficiaries, selecting only hospitals and physicians who agreed to accept a negotiated price for their services. This practice of "selective contracting" was first embraced by the Medi-Cal program to contract hospitals at low per diem rates. The selection rule was uncomplicated; if the price (and other specified conditions) was right, a contract would be secured. Not all hospitals competing for contracts, including large traditional Medi-Cal providers, gained them, and, as a result of these shocks in the health care marketplace, the contracting process was enormously successful, with 67 percent of California hospitals, accounting for 72 percent of the Medi-Cal patients, awarded contracts by the end of the first year of negotiations. Furthermore, for the first 2 years of selective contracting, there was no evidence of reduced access to health resources for Medi-Cal patients or any change in the quality of care they received. Savings to the state were estimated at $165 million for the first year of the program and $235 million for the second year. Cost cutting on an unprecedented scale was reported by hospitals receiving Medi-Cal contracts (31,32).

Preferred Provider Organizations

The entry of private insurers and firms into selective contracting began in earnest in 1984 and quickly became known as "Preferred Provider Organizations" (PPOs). A PPO is an arrangement or contract between a panel of health care providers, usually hospitals and physicians, and purchasers of health care services, wherein the providers agree to supply services to a defined group of patients on a discounted fee-for-service basis. Purchasers are usually insurance companies or self-insured employers (33). PPOs generally have five key elements: (1) a limited number of physicians and hospitals, (2) negotiated fee schedules, (3) utilization review, (4) consumer choice of provider with incentives to use PPO participating providers, and (5) expedient settlement of claims (34).

PPOs have become a rapid growth area in health insurance. By February 1986, enrollment in PPOs had increased to 6.2 million people with 28 percent of the nation's patient care physicians contracting with a PPO. With California leading the pack in selective contracting, 5 out of the 10 nation's largest PPOs are in that state. Utilization review is the principal mechanism for controlling costs by reducing inappropriate use of services. Other mechanisms utilized by PPOs for cost control are contracting with low-cost providers and establishing a reimbursement system that realizes savings through discounted provider charges or incentives for reduced utilization. Discounts are generally in a range of 10–13 percent below usual charges and insurers are reporting premiums at 10–20 percent below standard indemnity plans (33). While many believe that PPOs have the potential to increase competition in the health care sector, there is little empirical evidence to substantiate this supposition (32).

FUTURE POSSIBILITIES

PHYSICIAN PAYMENT REFORM

From 1975 to 1982, Medicare's total payments for physician services grew at a faster rate than payments for hospital services. By 1985, physician services reached 23.6 percent of total Medicare spending, up from 21.4 percent in 1975. Over the same period, hospital care dropped as a percentage of total Medicare expenditures from 74.4 to 67.1 percent. Although the Reagan Administration had intended to reform physician reimbursement for Medicare, these plans have been postponed indefinitely as a result of pressures from opponents of government regulation in the private sector. Nonetheless, there is general agreement that physician payment under Medicare needs to be revised (4,35).

Congress directed the Reagan Administration to study physician payment reform when it established Medicare's DRG-based prospective payment system for hospital care. One of the favored options was to develop a national fee schedule that would set a price for each type of service with adjustments for local wage costs. Another possible reform alternative was to establish physician DRGs. Research into this option, however, disclosed thorny problems in (1) applying DRGs to outpatient care, which is typified by a large number of encounters at a relatively small price per visit; (2) dividing the DRG payment among a number of physicians who may be involved in one illness episode; (3) marked geographic variations in practice patterns; and (4) cost variability in DRGs used to reimburse the medical versus the surgical specialties, the latter of which are more homogeneous and lend themselves better to DRG-based payment (36,37).

These approaches to physician payment have been viewed by HCFA as impediments to the overall objectives of Medicare reform, which is more likely to be based on more competitive strategies using capitation as the basic payment mechanism. Under this alternative, the objective is to have a single capitated payment for physician, hospital, and other Medicare-covered services. Demonstrations of various capitated approaches to consider quality, beneficiary access, out-of-pocket liability, and cost-effectiveness of service provision are currently being developed. In 1985 the number of Medicare beneficiaries enrolled in HMO-type prepayment organizations reached 1,117,000 or 3.7 percent of Medicare enrollees (up from about 2 percent in 1981) (4).

NATIONAL HEALTH INSURANCE

National health insurance (NHI) is a concept espoused by many for over 50 years for containing health care costs and for providing universal access for the population. This concept should not be given short shrift, however, just because it is out of fashion politically at this time. As mentioned previously, NHI came close to becoming part of the Social Security Act of 1935 and numerous bills, representing a spectrum of schemes, have been introduced and seriously debated in every Congressional session since then. In the mid-1970s the issue of NHI became so heated that both political parties introduced some bills that were strikingly similar. NHI bills ran the gamut from expanding Medicare to new population groups (e.g., children under 5 years of age) to a national health service (NHS) concept such as that in Sweden or Great Britain, where the government owns the hospitals and physicians are paid on the basis of capitation or salary by the NHS. When Jimmy Carter was elected to the presidency in 1976, many in the health arena assumed the NHI would be an eventuality in a Democratic administration, but early on Carter took little interest in health issues. Later in his tenure, the energy crisis and the Iranian hostage situation overshadowed NHI and other health finance agendas.

Before one discards the idea of NHI as politically infeasible in the United States, two points should be borne in mind. First, the new competitive financing programs outlined above hold the potential for social disaster. PPS, for example, may contain health care costs at the expense of high-quality care for the elderly and other groups. To the extent that quality of health services is related to quantity (and surely there is some relationship), the incentives favor a reduction in services rendered. The same holds true for the HMO movement and Medicaid services in states that reimburse providers below marginal costs. In fact, it may be cost-based reimbursement in the private sector, as a competing strategy, that holds cost-cutting systems in check. In other words, so long as a discernible proportion of patients still have access to full utilization of services, with little or no incentive to cut back, there exists a high standard of service in the minds of patients and physicians. Should this standard be breeched for large groups of people, such as the elderly, the public outcry might result in NHI, particularly if the pendulum swings back to more liberal philosophies. Second, national health services have existed as a movement in Europe. Abel-Smith (38) has shown that among 12 European nations (10 European Community members plus Spain and Portugal), 6 now have a NHS model: the United Kingdom, Denmark, Spain, Italy, Greece, and Portugal. France, West Germany, Belgium, Luxembourg, Ireland, and the Netherlands remain without a NHS. He also notes that increasing regulation of health care is notable in western Europe. Many would hold that in social services, European countries portend U.S. trends to a large extent. This does not necessarily point the United States in the direction of a NHS model per se, but movement in the direction of some type of NHI plan, such as government-mandated universal health coverage of employees, should not be precluded from consideration.

Financing health services in the United States includes a plethora of institutions and activities. The growth of employer-based private health insurance has stimulated unprecedented growth in health expenditures and biomedical advancement for the nation in the postwar era. The advent of Medicare and Medicaid in 1966 heralded a period of even more rapid growth, along with unbridled inflation, in the health care sector for the ensuing period. Only recently is there evidence that the health care industry may be slowing down in terms of expansion.

Inequities in access to health care, thought to be alleviated by Medicare and Medicaid, along with extensive provision of voluntary health insurance for employed groups, have not been resolved. Universal health coverage has not been realized, and about 12 percent of the population in the United States are uninsured. The Medicare PPS, with its emphasis on cost controls, holds incentives for creating new groups of severely ill, medically underserved patients. State revenues have grown at rates slower than health care costs, inducing across-the-board reductions and more restrictive eligibility requirements for state Medicaid programs.

The PPS, selective contracting, and prepaid plans hold potential for ameliorating uncontrolled inflation in health care spending. However, effective means for identifying and monitoring the adequateness and appropriateness of health care, in an environment of either over- or underutilization, have not been developed. Perhaps the savior of the American system of health care finance will lie in payment source pluralism, making it virtually impossible for most providers and patients to make decisions based on any criterion other than clinical prudence.

REFERENCES

1. U.S. Bureau of the Census: *Statistical Abstract of the United States: 1986* (106th edition). Washington, DC, U.S. Government Printing Office, 1985.

2. Waldo DR, Levit KR, Lazenby H: National Health expenditures, 1985. *Health Care Finan Rev* 1986; 8:1–21.

3. Organization for Economic Cooperation and Development. *Measuring Health Care, 1960–1983.* Paris, Organization for Economic Cooperation and Development, 1985.

4. Gornick M, Greenberg JN, Eggers PW, et al: Twenty years of Medicare and Medicaid: Covered populations, use of benefits, and program expenditures. *Health Care Finan Rev* 1985; (Ann Suppl):13–59.

5. Gibson, RM: National health expenditures, 1979. *Health Care Finan Rev* 1980; 2:1–36.

6. Roemer MI: *Social Medicine: The Advance of Organized Health Services in America.* New York, Springer, 1978.

7. Roemer MI: *Comparative National Policies on Health Care.* New York, Marcel Dekker, 1977.

8. Farley PJ: *Private Health Insurance in the United States.* Data Preview 23, National Medical Care Expenditure Survey. DHHS Publ. No. (PHS) 86-3406. National Center for Health Services Research and Health Care Technology Assessment, 1986, pp 1–106.

9. Walden DC, Wilensky GR, Kasper JA: *Changes in Health Insurance Status: Full-Year and Part-Year Coverage.* Data Preview 21, National Health Care Expenditures Study. DHHS Publ. No. (PHS) 85-3377. National Center for Health Services Research and Health Care Technology Assessment, 1985, pp 1–15.

10. Lubitz J, Prihoda R: Use and costs of Medicare services in the last two years of life. *Health Care Finan Rev* 1984; 5:117–131.

11. Fuchs VR: "Though much is taken": Reflections on aging, health, and medical care. *Milbank Mem Fund Quart* 1984; 62:143–166.

12. American Medical Association, Department of Federal Legislation, Division of Legislative Activities: *Q & A: New Provisions for Physician Reimbursement under Medicare.* Chicago, American Medical Association, July 30, 1984, pp 1–7.

13. Reinhardt UE: The compensation of physicians: Approaches used in foreign countries. *Quality Rev Bull* 1985; 11:366–377.

14. Enthoven AC: Consumer-choice health plan. Inflation and inequity in health care today: Alternatives for cost control and analysis of proposals for national health insurance. *New Engl J Med* 1978; 298:650–658.

15. Enthoven AC: Consumer-choice health plan. A national-health-insurance proposal based on regulated competition in the private sector. *New Engl J Med* 1978; 298:709–720.

16. Enthoven A: The competition strategy; status and prospects. *New Engl J Med* 1981; 304:109–112.

17. Deloitte Haskins & Sells: *Tax Equity and Fiscal Responsibility Act of 1982: Management Strategies for Health Care Providers.* New York, Deloitte Haskins & Sells, 1982.

18. Deloitte Haskins & Sells: *Medicare Prospective Payment System—1983: Strategies for Health Care Providers.* New York, Deloitte Haskins & Sells, 1982.

19. Guterman S, Dobson, A: Impact of the Medicare prospective payment system for hospitals. *Health Care Finan Rev* 1986; 7:97–114.

20. American Medical Association: *Diagnosis-Related Groups (DRGs) and the Prospective Payment System.* Chicago, American Medical Association, 1984.

21. Guerman S, Dobson A: The Impact of PPS: Evidence from the second year. *The Official Program of the 114th Annual Meeting of the American Public Health Association,* Session 1082. Las Vegas, NE, American Public Health Association, 1986, p 43.

22. DesHarnais S, Kobrinski E, Chesney J, et al: The early effects of the Prospective Payment System on inpatient utilization and the quality of care. *Inquiry* 1987; 24:7–16.

23. Eggers P, Riley G: Beneficiary impact of the Medicare Prospective Payment System for Hospitals. *The Official Program of the 114th Annual Meeting of the American Public Health Association,* Session 1082. Las Vegas, NE, American Public Health Association, 1986, p 43.

24. Jencks SF, Dobson A, Willis P, et al: Evaluating and improving the measurement of hospital case mix. *Health Care Finan Rev* 1984 (Ann Suppl):1–11.

25. Conklin, JE, Lieberman JV, Barnes, CA et al: Disease staging: Implications for hospital reimbursement and management. *Health Care Finan Rev* 1984 (Ann Suppl):13–22.

26. Smits HL, Fetter RB, McMahon LF Jr: Variation in resource use within diagnosis-related groups: The severity issue. *Health Care Finan Rev* 1984 (Ann Suppl):71–78.

27. Horn SD, Horn RA: Reliability and validity of the Severity of Illness Index. *Med Care* 1986; 24:159–178.

28. Lave, JR: Is compression occurring in DRG prices? *Inquiry* 1985; 22:142–147.

29. Kidder D, Coelan C: Prospective payment and hospital finance. *The Official Program of the 114th Annual Meeting of the American Public Health Association,* Session 1082. Las Vegas, NE, American Public Health Association, 1986, p 43.

30. Feder J, Hadley J, Zuckerman, S: Hospitals' Behavioral responses to the PPS. *The Official Program of the 114th Annual Meeting of the American Public Health Association,* Session 1082. Las Vegas, NE, American Public Health Association, 1986, p 43.

31. Johns L, Derzon RA, Anderson MD: Selective contracting in California: Early effects and policy implications. *Inquiry* 1985; 22:24–32.

32. Johns L, Anderson MD, Derzon RA: Selective contracting in California: Experience in the second year. *Inquiry* 1985; 22:335–347.

33. Gabel J, Ermann D, Rice T et al: The emergence and future of PPOs. *J Health Politics, Policy, Law* 1986; 11:305–322.

34. de Lissovoy G, Rice T, Ermann D et al: Preferred provider organizations: Today's models and tomorrow's prospects. *Inquiry* 1986; 23:7–15.

35. Hadley J: How should Medicare pay physicians? *Milbank Mem Fund Quart* 1984; 62:279–299.

36. Mitchell JB: Physician DRGs. *New Engl J Med* 1985; 313:670–675.

37. Culler S, Ehrenfried D: On the feasibility and usefulness of physician DRGs. *Inquiry* 1986; 23:40–55.

38. Abel-Smith, B: Who is the odd man out?: The experience of western Europe in containing the costs of health care. *Milbank Mem Fund Quart* 1985; 63:1–17.

PART FIVE

Assessing and Regulating System Performance

CHAPTER 12

Health Services Planning and Regulation

Thomas W. Bice

In the wake of World War II, modern nations of all political and economic coloration turned to planning and regulation to guide economic and social development (1). Expanding conceptions of the welfare state, imperatives of technological change, and unwanted consequences of industrialization and urbanization gave rise to forms of public controls that were extended over enlarging segments of economic and social life. Nowhere is this trend more evident than in modern nations' health services industries. While the basic forms of their organization and financing vary considerably among countries, all are being subjected to direction by mixtures of market forces and state planning and regulation (2).

This chapter reviews these trends as they materialized in the United States. We begin by defining planning and regulation and explicating rationales for their use. Following this, we identify major milestones in the development of planning and regulation aimed at improving the health industry's performance and review evidence pertaining to the effectiveness of the most prominent programs. In the concluding section, we speculate about the future of health planning and regulation in the United States.

PLANNING AND REGULATION

DEFINITIONS

Rational action involves four fundamental steps: (1) delineation of problems and objectives, (2) formulation and valuation of alternative means of attaining objectives, (3) implementation of chosen means, and (4) evaluation of processes and outcomes (3). When performed by individuals, these steps constitute rational behavior; when performed by groups, the entire process is ordinarily considered planning.

This chapter makes a somewhat arbitrary distinction between the steps involving decision making about problems, objectives, means, and program effectiveness, which we consider planning, and the implementation stage, which in many instances involves regulation. Accordingly, "planning" is viewed as an essentially symbolic process, the results of which are statements of alternative ends and means and choices among them. "Regulation," by contrast, refers to a diverse set of means by which individuals or organizations are either induced or compelled to behave in specified ways. More specifically, regulation entails government's intervention in private markets for the purpose of promoting some desired public objective that otherwise could not be realized.

RATIONALES FOR HEALTH CARE PLANNING AND REGULATION

Planning

The need for planning arises from the growing complexity and interdependence among specialized institutions and the rapidity of social and economic change. In the modern era decisions made today affect actions and outcomes in the near- and long-term futures, both of which may differ drastically from existing situations. In consequence, firms and governments engage in planning: they anticipate the future and decide today how they will shape their destinies or respond to scenarios of alternative futures.

Markets and government planning are alternative means to accomplish the necessary coordination among social and economic activities (4). Differences among nations' public philosophies and administrative traditions dictate the predominant locus of planning activities and their extensiveness. In socialist countries, where virtually all social and economic institutions are owned and operated by the state, planning is either centralized in national governments or decentralized among lower units of government and is comprehensive, encompassing virtually all social and economic activities. Liberal democratic welfare states have removed particular sectors of their economies from markets by bringing them under the control of the state. In those countries, sectoral public planning is exercised, typically encompassing the totality of economic decisions and activities within those particular sectors. In capitalist nations, especially the United States, public philosophies and traditions place the principal responsibilities for planning in the private sector. Corporations and private associations accomplish the bulk of societies' coordinative and planning activities through mutual accommodation, contractual agreements, and other private means. Governments confine their planning to such public functions as the implementation of fiscal and monetary policies, the provision of public goods, and the management of public services.

Because capitalist nations presume that private markets and associations will carry out most of societies' planning, positive rationales and political strategies must be developed to support government intrusion into private arrangements. Government planning typically receives widespread support only during periods of national peril, which, for example, permitted presidents to extend national coordination over basic industries during the depression of the 1930s and during World War II. Correspondingly, because extensive public planning is viewed as an exceptional, temporary expedient, its political support terminates with the close of the crisis that occasioned it

(5). Government planning in the absence of enduring crisis is therefore marked by cycles of fitful starts and endings, always lacking secure institutional bases and forever subject to partisan assaults.

Regulation

Government regulation occurs in nations where major sectors of their economies are organized by markets, for the very definition of regulation presumes the existence of private markets. Where significant, officially endorsed private markets have never existed (as in the postrevolutionary Union of Soviet Socialist Republics) or where they have been preempted in particular sectors by state control (as in the National Health Service of the United Kingdom), comprehensive or sectoral state planning is merely one ingredient of public *management* of state-owned and state-operated industries. In such circumstances, government does not regulate affected industries; rather, its authority to control them flows from the statutory function of delivering public services.

In capitalist nations, regulation, like state planning, conventionally is viewed as an exceptional governmental intrusion, an avenue to be pursued only when all else fails. Success in attempts to promulgate regulatory solutions therefore requires proponents of regulatory solutions to develop politically persuasive arguments and to marshal effective political support. Only then will they prevail over strongly entrenched ideologies that favor markets and market reforms and, as well, overcome the presumptions in American law that favor private sector solutions.

Ordinarily, arguments favoring regulation begin by identifying "market failures," that is, imperfections in behaviors of markets that are so severe as to demonstrably compromise the attainment of important public objectives. Moreover, rationales for regulation must withstand an additional test: the proposed regulatory intervention must be capable of achieving results that are verifiably superior to those that could be realized by market reforms (6).

The theoretical expectation that freely operating markets will produce the socially optimal allocation of resources rests on assumptions about the nature of markets. When any of these is untenable, some degree of market failure occurs. The principal assumptions of well-functioning markets are that (1) individuals know what they want and are able to make informed choices among alternative products, (2) one's consumption decisions affect only oneself, (3) people can select from products offered by a large number of independent suppliers who are able to freely enter and leave markets, and (4) suppliers bear the full costs of producing their products.

In their aggregate, these assumptions place heavy reliance on rationality, self-sufficiency, and fairness. People and firms are assumed to be aware of the personal values that they seek to optimize and to command the resources required to satisfactorily attain them. Moreover, the expectation that markets will be self-regulating presumes open and fair competition among suppliers.

From their original formulations, however, conceptions of markets have recognized inevitable exceptions that require remedial actions by collectivities, either voluntary groups or governments. Exceptions to the first two assumptions, which apply to consumers, arise from the limits of rationality, the interrelatedness of individuals' decisions and behaviors, and differences in individuals' personal resources. Such individuals as children and the mentally ill, who cannot be assumed capable of exercising judgment, require assistance and protection. Free rein of individual rationality fails to provide sufficient quantities of so-called public goods and resources such as military security, whose enjoyment by one person does not diminish their availability to others (7). The task of providing such goods falls to governments. Interdependence of individuals' so-called utility functions also invites collective action. The assumption that one person's consumption affects no other's is violated, for example, by those who operate air-polluting automobiles. Hence, governments intervene by requiring consumers to purchase emission control devices. Finally, societies recognize that some people, lacking either the means or the will to compete in labor markets, are incapable of securing even basic necessities of life. The poor, the infirm, and others so afflicted are thus accorded charity and public assistance.

Inevitable departures from the second pair of assumptions pertaining to market structures and externalities of production also invite intervention into markets. Theories of markets assume that industries represent large numbers of competitive suppliers who freely enter and leave markets and who independently decide what to produce and what to charge for their products. The several circumstances that violate these assumptions often call for regulation. In markets where it is economically efficient for particular goods or services to be supplied by a single producer (e.g., natural monopolies), government applies public utility regulation to protect the public against monopolistic practices. Where publicly owned facilities required for the conduct of businesses are limited, governments allocate those facilities by regulation, as, for example, in the licensing of taxi cabs and television stations. Finally, as in the case of the polluting driver, collective intervention is evoked by producers who externalize costs to the public through such means as discharging harmful waste products into public water supplies.

As the public benefits of competition accrue only when economic behaviors of both consumers and suppliers are fair and open, governments inevitably must intervene to ensure that transactions are conducted in accordance with general rules. Such rules are encoded in laws that seek primarily to ensure that the various assumptions noted above are not willfully violated. These include such regulations, for instance, as those that prohibit the making of untruthful claims by advertisers and insider trading among stockbrokers.

The diverse means employed by government to regulate markets comprise the following six general types: (1) subsidies, (2) entry controls, (3) rate or price setting, (4) quality controls, (5) social regulation, and (6) market-preserving controls. The first and sixth types generally are relatively benign forms of regulation: subsidies aim to induce particular economic activities by offering positive incentives; market-preserving controls punish willful violators of general rules. By contrast, the second through the fifth forms of regulation generally intrude more directly into the daily functioning of industries, imposing some degree of management by public bureaus. The greater intrusiveness of entry controls, price and rate setting, and quality controls is recognized by their being regarded as "command-control regulation" (8). The class of so-called social regulation differs from the others—"economic regulation"—in that it aims not to attain particular economic consequences through regulation. Rather, social regulation attempts to realize such socially desired ends as fair employment practices and safety in the workplace (9).

Subsidies. Subsidies are intended to alter demand for or supplies of particular goods and services and to guarantee citizens access to basic necessities of life. Public transfers to the poor, for instance, attempt to provide necessities that otherwise could not be secured. The United States typically has followed the categorical policy of restricting subsidies to specific groups, while more advanced welfare states have conferred universal entitlement to subsidies through enactments of resource-using rights (10).

Supply-side subsidies aim to increase supplies of particular goods and services that markets undersupply. Subsidies to medical schools, for instance, historically have been justified on the grounds that private markets produce too few physicians and invest insufficiently in the pursuit of biomedical knowledge. Similarly, rationales for public subsidies for the construction of voluntary hospitals recognized that capital markets would not support the development of such institutions in sparsely populated, low-income regions of the nation.

Entry Controls. Entry controls limit potential suppliers' access to markets. Such controls include licensing professionals to ensure that they meet at least minimal standards of competence and to such institutions as hospitals to protect public safety. A second form of entry control arises from the recognition that such limited public resources as air waves and streets can be used efficiently by only relatively few suppliers who use such resources. Hence, as noted above, government allocates access to them via the issuance of certificates of public necessity and convenience to, for example, taxi cabs and television stations.

Rate or Price Controls. Rate or price setting authorities impose limits on prices suppliers can charge for their products. In the classic circumstance for their use, that of public utility regulation, controls are invoked by governments as a quid pro quo for protection afforded producers subject to mandated entry restrictions. This rationale is applied most purely in such so-called natural monopolies as found in the production and distribution of electrical power and local telephone services. In these and similar situations, where a sole producer is presumably optimally efficient, governments protect monopolies from competition by restricting entry and, in turn, protect the public from the monopolies by controlling their rates and the quality of their products.

In other situations, rate or price setting is invoked to guarantee citizens access to necessities of life. This accounts for the adoption of rent controls by several municipalities and underlies the imposition of rate regulation on hospitals in several states.

Quality Controls. Quality controls aim to ensure the safety and efficacy of products. Such regulations usually are justified on the grounds that consumers lack knowledge sufficiently to evaluate some products and, more importantly, that gaining such knowledge by experimentation could be injurious or even lethal. This accounts for the imposition of, for example, regulation of pharmaceutical products by the Food and Drug Administration (FDA).

Social Regulation. The broad class of social regulation includes controls that aim variously to reduce health and safety risks to consumers and workers in workplaces, to eliminate socially undesirable practices associated with the production or consumption of goods and services, and to reduce negative externalities of production. This class of controls subsumes, for instance, fire and safety codes, fair employment practices, and environmental protection laws. Unlike economic regulations, which are imposed on particular industries and aimed at attaining economic objectives, social regulations typically apply to all producers, and, while they have secondary economic effects, their principal objectives are "noneconomic."

Market-Preserving Controls. As the notion of pure competition does not recognize such human failings as greed and miscalculation, even the most minimal notion of government calls for public involvement in establishing and enforcing rules of private conduct. Where private markets are highly valued, such rules are elaborated extensively in laws, the most prominent of which enforce contracts and punish antitrust violations. Antitrust laws are especially crucial, for they attempt to maintain conditions that correspond to the market assumptions described above (11). While antitrust and other market-preserving laws are, technically speaking, regulatory devices, they are essentially passive, being invoked only when violated. By contrast, direct, command-control regulation, such as public utility regulation, requires ongoing policing and some degree of publicly sponsored management of regulated firms. The limited intrusiveness of market-preserving instruments thereby appeals to those who identify market failures but eschew direct, command-control regulatory solutions.

Planning cum Regulation

While we have distinguished conceptually between planning and regulation, in theory they are symbiotic processes. Planning in the absence of means for intervention breeds futility; regulation devoid of planning conduces caprice. Indeed, theories of planning and regulatory process join these functions, and laws establishing planning and regulatory bodies typically make at least passing reference to each function. The symbiosis is particularly crucial for regulatory agencies, for administrative law requires them to establish general rules to guide decision making in particular instances (12). Also, because many modern regulatory agencies pursue statutory mandates to guide the development of entire industries, planning is in principle a vital part of regulation (12,13). In general, needs for planning expand with the extensiveness and intrusiveness of regulatory authority.

Planning in complex, volatile industries entails high levels of technical acumen. Such techniques as forecasting and modeling are essential. *Public* planning and regulation require these but must satisfy canons of public accountability as well. Public planning and regulation, therefore, are political processes intermingled with technocratic functions. As such, evaluation of planning and regulatory programs requires attention to their means and processes as well as to their outcomes.

Political assumptions underlying much of the public planning and regulation that emerged in the 1960s, including health planning, fundamentally affected the nature of public interventions, vastly complicated their processes, and significantly affected their abilities to attain prescribed objectives. The outpouring of federal programs during the Johnson Administration greatly extended the reach of public planning and regulation and established new mechanisms of public accountability. Breaking with traditional conceptions of federalism, programs launched over the War on Poverty and many planning and regulatory programs were established outside the orbits of state and local government (14).

As traditional mechanisms of public accountability—election and executive appointment—had been circumvented, new forms of accountability were required. Political and consumer movements of the times dictated the choice of "maximum feasible participation" as the preferred mode (15). Accountability came to imply two ingredients: (1) broadly based representation of statutorily identified categories of people on governing boards of planning and regulatory agencies and (2) the extension of standing before regulatory bodies to virtually all citizens (16).

The health services industry embodies several features that historically have invited planning and regulation. It is a complex industry whose aggregate success requires the orchestration of multiple and diverse resources. Health care is also undeniably cloaked in the public interest, being considered among the necessities of life. The relentless upward spiraling of expenditures for health services is thus a public issue, for it threatens families' abilities to secure adequate care while depleting the public treasuries.

Inspection of the organization and innerworkings of the health care industry as of the late 1960s also revealed numerous departures from market assumptions. Ignorance of the complexities of medical care was assumed to preclude consumers from making informed choices among providers and treatment modalities, while ethical prohibitions prevented providers from advertising. Widespread insurance coverage blunted consumers' interest in seeking lower-priced services and relieved providers of the need to control costs, the sine qua non of efficient markets. Price competition was thwarted as well by its prohibition in providers' codes of ethics and by the freedom dominant providers exercised to boycott colleagues who would offer lower-priced alternatives (17). Private health insurers, who in most insurance markets act as prudent buyers, exercised little leverage over either insurees or providers, and employers, the principal purchasers of insurance, paid scant attention to mounting insurance premiums (18).

Despite these egregious and widespread market failures, the health care industry was virtually free of public control. Whatever planning and regulation occurred was sponsored and conducted by groups of health care providers that were essentially closed to the public at large.

By the mid-1960s, the mounting costs of health care had transformed the industry's market failures and lack of accountability into major public issues, undeniably demanding public reform. Opinions differed, however, as to the means to be employed and whether the responsibility for action lay primarily with the federal or state governments. Few public officials supported the idea of socializing the industry as had been done by welfare states, and the market reform strategy had yet to be articulated. Hence, the public planning and command-control regulation were adopted as the compromise strategy. Some forms were initiated primarily by the federal government, others primarily by states. As a result, considerable variability existed among states in the nature and vigor of public control over their industries, and, even where the political will to plan and regulate was relatively strong, public control was fragmented among several programs.

ORIGINS, DEVELOPMENT, AND DECLINE OF HEALTH SERVICES PLANNING

The history of health services planning in the United States can be divided into three rather distinct periods based on (1) the locus of sponsorship of planning and (2) its degree of comprehensiveness. The first period began in the 1930s and extended through World War II. Planning was conducted by voluntary organizations and was relatively narrowly concentrated on developing services for the poor and on coordinating fund-raising efforts among voluntary hospitals. The second period began following the war with the appearance of federally sponsored, communitywide planning aimed primarily at determining appropriate numbers and locations of hospitals. The third period opened with the extension of federally sponsored planning to *comprehensive*, communitywide planning that embraced the totality of personal and environmental health services. The final period of public planning as of the late 1980s began with the election of the Reagan Administration in 1980. At that point the federal government began withdrawing its support of health planning, leaving states to determine the nature and extent of public planning that they were willing to sponsor. This period also witnessed the return to privately sponsored planning, conducted sporadically by coalitions of major employers.

Since the beginning of the federal government's involvement in the 1940s, the objectives, scope, and organization of planning have been determined largely by federal policy as expressed in the following five programs: (1) the Hill-Burton Program (the Hospital Survey and Construction Act of 1946 [PL 79-725]), (2) the Regional Medical Programs (the Heart Disease, Cancer, and Stroke Act of 1965 [PL 89-239]), (3) the Comprehensive Health Planning Program (the Partnership for Health Act of 1967 [PL 90-174]), (4) the Experimental Health Services Delivery Program, and (5) the National Health Planning and Resources Development Act of 1974 (PL 93-641). The processes and organizational structures established under these programs are milestones in the transformation of health planning from its origins in elite-dominated, categorical planning to the more recent participatory, comprehensive planning, and from planning in the absence of regulation to the partial joining of these functions.

ORIGINS OF HEALTH PLANNING

Health services planning emerged in the United States in the 1930s, joining two elements that shaped the organization and objectives of planning until its decline in the early 1980s. One established the organizational foundations of health planning in local voluntaristic groups. The other developed the idea of a regionalized health services system that remains the ideal to which comprehensive health planning is dedicated.

Prior to the 1940s, health planning was limited to localized efforts aimed primarily at coordinating activities of municipal public health and welfare departments and hospitals. The attention of the health and welfare councils established to accomplish these ends focused on problems of providing services for the indigent rather than on fundamental reforms of the health services industry (19). The first organized attempt to deal specifically with such matters was initiated in the 1930s in New York City with the founding of the Hospital Council of Greater New York (20). The economic depression had produced severe overcrowding of municipal facilities that provided free services and had depleted patient censuses in the voluntary hospitals. These and other conditions were documented in an extensive survey of hospitals, leading the group of prominent citizens that sponsored the study to recommend the establishment of a permanent planning body. A few other cities followed New York's example, urged by philanthropists interested in seeing that their contributions to hospitals were being wisely used (21).

Supported largely by philanthropic donations, these early planning agencies functioned outside the ambit of government. Their governing boards typically comprised influential citizens who oversaw the activities of their small staffs. Initially, planning concentrated almost exclusively on estimating the numbers of hospital beds needed in communities.

The concept of health services planning achieved national prominence in the early 1930s with the publication of findings and recommendations of the prestigious Committee on the Costs of Medical Care. The Committee had been established in 1927 following a national conference on health care attended by leading physicians, social scientists, public health practitioners, and the lay public (22). With funds provided by several philanthropic foundations, the Committee undertook extensive studies of the use, organization, and financing of health services that culminated in 28 published reports and numerous staff papers. Among the Committee's principal conclusions was a recommendation calling for the establishment of local and state agencies for the purposes of conducting research and devising plans for coordinating health services. Further, the Committee presented a plan for organizing health services institutions and personnel in accordance with the principles of regionalization detailed in the Dawson Report issued 12 years earlier in the United Kingdom (23).

The notion of regionalization outlined in the Dawson Report and in the recommendations of the Committee on the Costs of Medical Care envisioned a division of functions among hospitals, clinics, and medical personnel based on vertically integrated levels of specialization and intensity of services. Choices of sites of care and the placement of patients would be dictated by the levels of services required. The beginnings of such arrangements were already recognizable in Sweden and Denmark by the opening of this century, and the idea has been adopted as a guiding principle for health planning in the United Kingdom and elsewhere.

The rationales offered for health services planning in the 1930s and early 1940s combined several notions that appealed to deeply rooted social values. As practiced in New York City and later in Rochester (New York), Detroit, and Pittsburgh, planning was a voluntary endeavor in which leading citizens and health care providers applied the tools of business management to attain greater efficiency and improved health care. Moreover, the concept of regionalization embodied ultimate designs of rationality and offered possibilities for resolving the then pressing problem of providing health services to the nation's small towns and rural areas.

THE HILL-BURTON PROGRAM

World War II and its aftermath placed health services planning on the public agenda as the Great Depression had done the decade before. Concerns about the educational and physical fitness of the population raised in findings from examinations of military inductees led to a Senate inquiry into the adequacy of the nation's health services and their bearing on the health of the population. Pursuant to its charge, the Subcommittee on Wartime Health and Education conducted hearings at which the then Surgeon General of the U.S. Public Health Service proposed establishing planning agencies throughout the country to guide the development of "coordinated hospital systems" (24). His testimony and subsequent discussions with members of the Subcommittee clearly evidenced the influence of the Dawson Report, and, although the label attached to his proposal referred specifically to "coordinated hospitals," the plan itself extended to virtually all aspects of contemporary comprehensive health planning.

Following World War II the conditions of hospitals prompted the federal government to establish the nation's first major health services planning and construction subsidy program. Having suffered two decades of neglect imposed first by the Depression and then by the war, the country's stock of hospital facilities was obsolete and unevenly distributed; and wartime migrations of people from rural areas to cities, rapid population growth, and rising construction costs strained the private sector's ability to make needed improvements. In response, Congress enacted the Hospital Survey and Construction Act of 1946, discussed in Chapter 5, a two-part law that provided funds for states to

1. Inventory their existing hospitals, to survey the need for construction of hospitals, and to develop programs for construction of such public and other non-profit hospitals as will, in conjunction with existing facilities, afford the necessary physical facilities for furnishing adequate hospitals, clinics, and similar services to all people.
2. Construct public and other nonprofit hospitals in accordance with such programs (25).

The avowed purpose of the program was to eliminate shortages of hospitals, particularly in the nation's rural and economically depressed regions. This objective was incorporated in the formula devised to allocate funds among the states and, within the states, in the fixed bed:population ratios used to identify underserved areas. Over its more than 20 years of operation, the program was successful in distributing construction funds to hospitals. As the shortage of hospital beds diminished, the act was repeatedly amended to extend its benefits to hospital modernization and replacement, and later to neighborhood health centers and emergency rooms. Additionally, the thought that increasing the numbers of hospitals in rural areas would entice physicians to locate in them appears in retrospect to have had at lease some validity (26).

The record of Hill-Burton in planning and inducing coordination among hospitals is less favorable, however. The program was administered in each state by an agency of state government assisted by an advisory Hospital Planning Council typically comprising hospital administrators and representatives of trade associations and local government agencies. These councils reviewed applications for grants and provided other assistance. In view of their members' ties to the industry, one would not have expected them to be vigorous proponents of major changes, and, even if they had been so, Hill-Burton agencies faced other problems that limited their abilities to plan and coordinate. Initially, they were provided few resources with which to plan. Consequently, their decisions on whether to award grants to particular applicant hospitals were often made without the benefit of well-formulated guidelines (27). Furthermore, agencies' purviews encompassed only a minority of the nations's hospitals, and their authorities to enforce compliance with plans were strictly circumscribed. Applicants who were denied assistance were free to engage in construction projects using funds from other sources, and those who were either ineligible for subsidies or chose not to apply for them were outside the agency's control altogether.

Despite these limitations, the program provided states with at least some experience in planning hospital facilities and in dealing with the difficult problems of defining and estimating populations' needs for hospital beds. The replacement of the bed:population formula by a more sensitive indicator of need represented an important advancement in the techniques of planning, and the grants for research and demonstration programs authorized in 1964 stimulated investigation into a variety of issues pertaining to the structure and dynamics of hospitals.

By the early 1970s, however, history had reversed itself: the problem of shortages of hospital beds had been eclipsed by concerns about their oversupply. Hence, Hill-Burton's raison d'etre evaporated. The program's planning functions had already been allocated elsewhere with the enactment of the Regional Medical Programs and Comprehensive Health Planning Programs in the mid-1960s. In 1974, the Hill-Burton authority was allowed to expire, and its few remaining functions were blended into the National Health Planning and Resources Development Act.

REGIONAL MEDICAL PROGRAMS

Among the enduring problems of the American health services industry has been the variance in the quality of health services rendered in the nation's medical research and teaching centers versus that provided by community-based practitioners. Once licensed on completion of their training, physicians find it difficult and have few incentives to stay abreast of new discoveries and improved techniques. Medical schools, in turn, have had little contact with community-based providers. Throughout this century the lacuna has widened, as specialization has accelerated the growth of medical knowledge.

To remedy this situation, in 1965 Congress enacted an amendment to the Public Health Service Act intended, among other purposes, "to encourage and assist in the establishment of regional cooperative arrangements among medical schools, research institutions, and hospitals, for research and training (including continuing education) and related demonstrations of patient care" (28). The law was an outgrowth of a report by the President's Commission on Heart Disease, Cancer, and Stroke, which had been empanelled to make recommendations regarding the control and treatment of these three dreaded diseases (29). On completion of its task, the Commission envisioned the establishment of regional centers through which advanced technology would be channeled to communities from research and training institutions, and where services would be delivered and community-based physicians informed of new techniques through continuing education.

The amendment, however, authorized considerably less than the Commission had recommended. The program was essentially stripped of its services providing authorities and, thereby, was transformed primarily into a grants-in-aid program (30). Powerful interest groups, particularly the American Medical Association (AMA), opposed the federal government's sponsoring centers that would compete with local practitioners in the practice of medicine. Hence, the compromises required to attain passage led to a program that was to coordinate services without interfering with existing patterns of health services delivery.

The Regional Medical Programs Act was implemented by Regional Advisory Groups (RAGs) constituted in 56 regions. Comprised of representatives of medical schools, teaching hospitals, state and local health departments, private practitioners, and the general public, RAGs were charged with devising plans and authorizing expenditures of federal grant monies for innovative programs. The Regional Medical Programs thereby were designed to enhance coordination and integration of health services through a voluntary, pluralistic mechanism that decentralized decision making directly from the federal government to the 56 RAGS, which were dominated by the interests of providers, particularly by those of the medical schools and teaching hospitals. State governments were given no role in the program's implementation or funding.

As the substance of Regional Medical Programs was left within broad limits to local determination, considerable variation occurred in both their structures and activities. In consequence, it became increasingly difficult to characterize the program's national purposes (31,32). The RAGs stimulated federally funded demonstrations of a variety of innovations, including continuing education for physicians and training for ancillary personnel. However, no overarching plans appeared in any of the 56 regions. When other local planning agencies began to be established pursuant to the Partnership for Health Amendments of 1967, the Regional Medical Programs' stated goals shifted from concern with specific diseases to the promotion of comprehensive health services. Federal monies were then made available through the programs for several types of system-oriented demonstration, most prominently efforts to develop and improve emergency medical services (33). In Glaser's words, "the Regional Medical Programs became an effort to obtain federal money for worthy projects rather than a disciplined system for framing and implementing plans" (34).

Because the Regional Medical Programs Act was popular among the nation's medical schools and teaching hospitals, it was able to withstand the Nixon Administration's attempts to abolish it. However, in 1974 the program was swept with Hill-Burton and other planning efforts under the umbrella National Health Planning and Resources Development Act, and shortly thereafter the Regional Medical Programs became extinct.

THE COMPREHENSIVE HEALTH PLANNING PROGRAM

Although the federal government attempted to promote planning and coordination of health services through Hill-Burton and the Regional Medical Programs, it had done so following categorical approaches. Hill-Burton dealt only with construction of and planning for facilities; the Regional Medical Programs ostensibly concentrated, at least at the outset, on particular diseases. No agency had responsibility for overall, comprehensive health planning. Only 1 year after enactment of the Regional Medical Programs' legislation, Congress moved to fill this void. The instrument was to be a network of voluntary, comprehensive health planning agencies with mandates to develop long-range, statewide, and local plans for environmental as well as personal health services.

As with the Regional Medical Programs, Comprehensive Health Planning legislation was preceded by a report of a national commission that called for more sweeping roles and authorities than were ultimately incorporated in the authorizing structure (35). "Planning" was defined as an "action process" in which councils would not only devise blueprints but would also take steps to implement their plans. On the basis of careful and extensive study of health service needs and through exercise of their pluralistic influence, councils were to effect major and permanent changes in health services delivery (36).

However, legislation authorizing the program, such as the Regional Medical Programs before it, specified that planning was to be accomplished without interfering with the prevailing patterns of medical practice. This constraint and the absence of any regulatory authority over health services institutions left Comprehensive Health Planning agencies created under the act devoid of official powers to pursue "active planning" as defined by the National Commission. In effect, these agencies were given the mandate to develop plans but were prevented from implementing them.

Comprehensive Health Planning (CHP) was organized in two layers. Each participating state established a statewide [CHP(a)] agency to oversee planning throughout the state. At the local level, areawide [CHP(b)] agencies were responsible for planning within designated regions. Plans developed by these so-called "b" agencies were to be reviewed by the umbrella "a" agency and incorporated in its statewide plan.

Unlike the Regional Medical Programs, CHP was structured as a cooperative effort among the federal and state governments and local areas rather than as a direct federal-to-local decentralization. Moreover, the Partnership for Health Amendments reflected the policy of encouraging maximum feasible participation that was incorporated in much of the social legislation of the 1960s. CHP(a) agencies were to be advised by councils made up of not less than 51 percent of consumer members. CHP(b) agencies were to be voluntary corporations with equivalently constituted boards. To preserve local autonomy, CHP agencies were funded by formula grants in which federal monies were to be augmented by roughly equal contributions from state and local sources (37).

It is generally agreed that CHP agencies were unable to accomplish all of their intended aims. Empirical data on improvements in health levels, health care costs, and the like attributable to CHP planning are virtually nonexistent (38). However, observations accumulated since 1967 on the organization and process of planning in various sites suggest that CHP was structurally, fiscally, and politically unable to bring about the changes required to significantly affect major trends in the costs, quality, and accessibility of health services (39). Few statewide or areawide agencies were able to develop long-range plans, most lacked the resources needed to gather information to develop them, and none had the power to enforce compliance with their recommendations. As a result, CHP agencies existed on the fringes of the major forces that shape the nation's health services industry. They attempted to plan in a turbulent and recalcitrant environment, while the power to act remained in the hands of institutions and associations that represented their memberships and provided local funds.

During the late 1960s and early 1970s, CHP agencies began to acquire advisory roles in federal and state regulatory processes. In keeping with its New Federalism policy, the Nixon Administration delegated to CHP agencies the function of reviewing and commenting on requests for federal Public Health Service grants by institutions within their jurisdictions. Also, several states assigned advisory roles to CHP agencies in their implementation of certificate-of-need (CON) controls. For the most part, however, CHP agencies continued to practice "consensus planning," lacking the "teeth" to move forcefully to the implementation stage. Moreover, by the early 1970s, it had become apparent to officials in the Nixon Administration that federal agencies engaged in planning had become as ill-coordinated as the health services industry itself. On that point, the then Secretary of the Department of Health, Education, and Welfare remarked that:

Six years ago, the federal government attempted to systematize and bolster planning efforts by creating and funding state and local comprehensive health agencies (sic). Today, all states and territories have comprehensive health planning agencies. And more than 170 local and areawide agencies now serve about 70 percent of the nation's population.

From their inception, however, these agencies have been underfunded and under-staffed. Even more pertinent, they haven't had any real authority to coordinate planning. They have served principally as advisory groups, and, while some can claim successes here and there, their advice has been largely ignored.

We thus see a planning system in which, as with its operational counterpart, interrelationships among functions are very poorly thought out—if any real thought has ever been given to the possibility of interrelationships—and that is thus hopelessly confusing and sometimes duplicative and overlapping.

It is, again, a "nonsystem" incapable of either rationally identifying shortfalls or gaps in performance or of rationally addressing needs (40).

Dedicated to the elimination of programs that "don't work" and to streamlining the federal bureaucracy (41), the Nixon Administration had sought to combine the Regional Medical Programs and the Comprehensive Health Planning Program under a single authority. Its proposal, submitted to Congress as the "National Health Care Improvement Act of 1970," had failed, leaving these programs intact as separate entities. The consolidation was ultimately accomplished with the enactment of the National Health Planning and Resources Development Act of 1974, following which Comprehensive Health Planning gave way to a more vigorous form of planning linked to regulatory controls.

THE EXPERIMENTAL HEALTH SERVICES DELIVERY PROGRAM

The federally sponsored health services planning programs described to this point shared an important feature: the principal impetus behind each was the federal government's recognition of deficiencies *within* the health services industry. By the late 1960s, however, other elements were begining to concern the federal government, namely, the "bureaucracy problem" (42) and rapidly escalating health care costs stemming from the Medicare and Medicaid programs. Several problems within the health services industry were increasingly being attributed to the federal government's involvements. Such recognitions gave rise to yet another health planning effort, the Experimental Health Services Delivery System (EHSDS) program.

The EHSDS program grew out of attempts to reorganize the internal affairs of the federal bureaucracy and its dealings with local communities. Beginning with the Johnson Administration's War on Poverty in the early 1960s and continuing throughout the decade, Congress enacted a landslide of health legislation that vastly increased the federal government's administrative responsibilities (43). Characteristically, program funding and authority bypassed the states, going directly to "targeted" areas in which local groups dealt directly with federal agencies (44,45). A variety of demonstration authorities had established health centers for the impoverished—first under the Office of Economic Opportunity and later others under the Partnership for Health Programs—migrant workers' health centers, maternal and infant care centers, mental health centers, and Model Cities health clinics. All were supported with federal funds administered by newly created or expanded federal agencies (46).

Several of these agencies were brought together in 1968 under the newly created Health Services and Mental Health Administration (HSMHA). Established as part of a general reorganization of the health activities of the Department of Health, Education, and Welfare (41), HSMHA's nine agencies and Fiscal Year 1970 budget of $1.3 billion made it one of the three largest federal organizations concerned exclusively with health and health services (47–49).

Impressive as the scope of activities subsumed under HSMHA was, the creation of the agency by no means brought effective coordination among the federal government's health programs. Most of the government's health effort, as measured by budgets, remained with other agencies, (e.g., Medicare and Medicaid), and each of HSMHA's programs operated under Congressional authorizations that defined at least in general terms how their appropriations were to be allocated. HSMHA was not an integrated agency with a set of well-ordered priorities or abilities to combine budgets and personnel of its member programs. It was, rather, a confederation of programs, each with its own purposes, procedures, constituencies, and interests.

The need for bringing coherence to HSMHA's disparate functions and programs gave rise to ideas that ultimately led to the EHSDS program. A solution that emerged was the notion of "conjoint funding": HSMHA programs were to increase their efficiency by working together and, more importantly, pooling their resources and delegating allocative decisions to local community groups.

Within HSMHA, the National Center for Health Services Research and Development (NCHSR&D) was designated as the "lead agency" to develop the EHSDS program. NCHSR&D was a newly established agency whose principal mission was to provide grants and contracts for research into and development of health services (50). The agency came to view ESHDS as the ultimate embodiment of rationality and as a mechanism for concerting various innovations being developed and tested under its grants and contracts (51). The EHSDS plan called for systemwide planning based on research and development combined with the rational allocation of funds by local management agencies, known as "ESHDS corporations." These funds were to be channeled from various federal agencies directly to the management corporations, thus eliminating federal agencies' direct administrative involvement in determining the uses of federal monies in local communities.

To accomplish these aims, in 1971 NCHSR&D established 12 EHSDS corporations scattered throughout the United States, and six others were added in the following year. Like Comprehensive Health Planning "b" agencies, ESHDS corporations were voluntary, nonprofit corporations. Unlike the "b" agencies, however, boards of ESHDS corporations were mandated to include representatives of four interest groups (the "4 Ps")—public, providers, payers (i.e., insurance companies and government agencies), and politicians—in proportions such that no group constituted a majority.

While ESHDS members could also participate on Comprehensive Health Planning and Regional Medical Program boards, the EHSDS corporations were to remain corporately distinct from these and other agencies. NCHSR&D developed a triangular model of the division of labor among Regional Medical Programs, Comprehensive Health Planning, and EHSDS bodies. Regional Medical Programs were seen as instruments of providers to develop and test innovations in the delivery of health services. Comprehensive Health Planning agencies would, in turn, incorporate these ideas into their long-range plans and communicate to the Regional Medical Programs the issues that planners deemed important for research and development. EHSDS bodies would then incorporate these priorities in their shorter-term investment decisions. In sum, NCHSR&D envisioned a network of cooperative and mutually facilitating exchanges among the three planning and coordinating bodies.

As the EHSDS experiment proceeded, none of the prerequisites required for its full implementation materialized. Each ESHDS site was given 2 years to charter a conforming corporate body and conduct community surveys and other studies with which to establish priorities. Meanwhile, NCHSR&D and HSMHA endeavored to conjoin funds of HSMHA and other federal agencies and to deliver these to EHSDS corporations. No such conjoining occurred, however. As might have been expected, other HSMHA agencies resisted NCHSR&D's urgings to delegate funding decisions to EHSDS bodies and declined even to give EHSDS communities priority claims on their funds. In consequence, the principal functions of the EHSDS corporations were vitiated, and their activities became increasingly indistinguishable locally from those of Comprehensive Health Planning and Regional Medical Programs. Instead of mutual cooperation and coordination, conflict and duplication characterized the triangle of agencies. On this point, a federal official observed in 1974 that the EHSDS experiment demonstrated that communities will accept federal funds when they are offered and will engage in conflict when competing programs are established (52).

While the EHSDS experiment failed to attain its principal objectives, it introduced a new element into the evolving debate about health planning that had reemerged in the early 1970s, and it contributed valuable experience to the body of planning methods. The experiment's focus on implementation and systemwide management of conjoined federal funds—although none were forthcoming—was in marked contrast to the long-range perspective of Comprehensive Health Planning and the narrower, categorical interests of the Regional Medical Programs. Also, EHSDS' emphasis on linking decisions to thorough empirical research on communities' needs for and use of health services and their flows of health services monies was notably different from the paucity of such information in most Comprehensive Health Planning agencies. Indeed, the vision of regional health authorities, not unlike those in the United Kingdom, that underlay the EHSDS ideology, anticipated by several years contemporary debate about the roles of planning agencies in gathering and analyzing data and in implementing regulatory controls.

The experiment never gained the support of officials in the Nixon Administration, who in 1973 ordered its orderly termination. Lacking explicit legislative authorization, the EHSDS program thus died within the bureaucracy, causing little comment. With Hill-Burton and the two other sides of the planning–innovation–management triangle, EHSDS corporations closed their doors shortly after the enactment of PL 93-641.

THE NATIONAL HEALTH PLANNING AND RESOURCES DEVELOPMENT ACT OF 1974

The National Health Planning and Resources Development Act of 1974 (PL 93-641) existed for more than a decade as the nation's principal federal health planning legislation. Although the program's federal authorities were allowed to expire in the mid-1980s, the planning and regulatory processes and organizational structures it established were maintained by many states. It remains, therefore, into the late 1980s, the principal vehicle for public planning and regulation in the health services industry.

Public Law 93-641 embodied several features that built on experience of its predecessors and others that sought improvements (53). The organizational entities it established further democratized community planning by preserving requirements for consumer majorities on governing boards and by adding to these explicit requirements for representation of racial, ethnic, linguistic, and low-income persons in proportion to their numbers in local communities (54). At the same time, however, the statute sought to give state and local governments greater roles and authorities than had been conferred on them by previous efforts. Local planning agencies, known as Health Systems Agencies (HSAs), were to be free-standing corporations. However, the law permitted HSAs to be created by groups of local governments, not unlike Councils of Governments. To give state governors greater roles than previous programs had provided, the statute called for two statewide organizations and awarded them explicit functions and authorities. State Health Planning and Development Agencies (SHPDAs) housed in state agencies were to oversee planning among HSAs and issue regulatory decisions. A new element, the State Health Coordinating Council (SHCC), was to comprise representatives of the state's HSAs and other members appointed by the governor. SHCCs were to advise governors and set overall policy pertaining to the programs' planning and regulatory missions. Finally, PL 93-641 awarded explicit functions and authorities to the federal government and established a National Health Planning Council charged with advising the Secretary of the Department of Health and Human Services on the national health planning goals and standards that that person was directed to formulate and disseminate.

The planning processes established by PL 93-641 also attempted to remedy weaknesses that inhered in the CHP program. The law required HSAs and SHPDAs to develop both long- and short-term plans, base them on reliable information, and deal explicitly with specific performance measures (viz., the accessibility, availability, acceptability, quality, and costs of health services). HSAs and SHPDAs were to devise long-range, comprehensive plans (known as *Health Systems Plans*). In addition, they were to develop long-range Health Facilities Plans concentrating on personal health services institutions and Annual Implementation Plans focusing on short-range, action-oriented strategies to be employed in effecting change. To guarantee that the various plans complied with federally defined standards, a series of reviews was established: SHPDAs reviewed HSAs' plans, and federal regional offices reviewed SHPDAs' plans.

The basic program was funded on a formula basis entirely with federal revenues, with allowances for additional federal matching of contributions by state and local governments and other permissible donors. The latter excluded named groups and organizations whose contributions might be construed as constituting conflicts of interest (e.g., individual hospitals).

The most important difference between PL 93-641 and its predecessor planning programs was the incorporation in the new program of explicit regulatory functions and other authorities. To qualify for federal grants-in-aid, states were required to enact CON laws (discussed below) that conformed to federal guidelines. Furthermore, states were directed to authorize their SHPDAs to review and approve proposals from designated health care institutions for grants-in-aid made available by Title XVI of the act.

Although the framers of PL 93-641 had attempted to redress the weaknesses of predecessor programs, many of their reforms created conflict at each stage of the program's implementation. Had the new program only bestowed subsidies, as had Hill-Burton, or had it been denuded of authorities to act, as had RMP, CHP, and EHSDS, PL 93-641 probably would have attracted little attention. However, the joining of planning with command-control regulation and other potentially penalizing authorities evoked considerable interest in and debate about where ultimate control over the structure rested. Clearly, much more control than before lay with the federal government: the Secretary of Health and Human Services was awarded authority to approve states' designations of planning regions, the structures of planning agencies and the compositions of their governing boards, the formats and contents of areawide and state plans, and the provisions of states' CON laws (55).

Complaints were voiced at all levels. Powers conferred on the Secretary of Health and Human Services offended many state governors, who preferred to retain such authorities for themselves. Associations representing health care providers generally opposed the regulatory programs and other authorities altogether and held strongly to the view that, if they were to be joined with planning, the joining should occur at the local level in HSAs. Perhaps unexpectedly, representatives of citizens' groups and professional health planners were also divided in terms of support of PL 93-641. Some feared that the wedding of planning and regulation would breed litigiousness and thereby undermine the voluntarism and cooperative spirit so vital to consensus-oriented planning, and many joined provider groups in decrying the upward drift of authority away from the grass roots into the hands of governors and federal officials.

These conflicting views, apparent in the hearings preceding enactment of PL 93-641, gave rise to numerous lawsuits challenging various features of the program. Several state governors who found portions of their states being joined in HSAs with portions of other states challenged the Department's designations of Health Services Areas. Some entered with the AMA and other parties into suits alleging that the law's CON provisions violated constitutional guarantees of states' rights by coercing (through the threat of terminating particular federal health subsidies) states to enact such regulatory programs. Still others challenged the compositional requirements of HSAs and SHCCs (56). Later, the issuance of the first set of planning guidelines detailing quantitative criteria for hospital beds and other health services per population (57) evoked a veritable flood of dissenting comments.

Despite its stormy beginnings, the new program was implemented in most states with little apparent difficulty. HSAs were created largely from people who had staffed and governed CHP(b) agencies, and CHP(a) agencies became SHPDAs. Most states enacted CON laws that satisfied federal guidelines. HSAs and SHPDAs began preparing their various plans.

The relative calm of the new program's development did not imply, however, that the program was accomplishing the expansive ends to which PL 93-461 had committed it. The new effort, while differing in many important respects from predecessors, suffered three enduring problems. First, funding was severely limited in view of the extensive planning and planning products mandated by the law. Second, commitment to comprehensive public planning was lacking among most state and local officials and provider groups (58). Finally, the ambitions of comprehensive planning in so complex and turbulent an environment as that of the health services industry far outstripped the theories and techniques available to health care planners. Planning in most states went along, as before, largely unheeded by public officials and providers, producing plans lacking useful or reliable details and having little consequence.

No one has determined whether planning per se has materially attained its expansive ends. Given the logic of PL 93-641, the question is largely moot. The program's regulatory authorities, not its planning activities, were expected to effect the desired changes. In the few states where regulatory authorities were being vigorously applied, planning under PL 93-641 played the subsidiary role of establishing the record required to justify regulatory decisions. Elsewhere, planning proceeded as it had under CHP, directed largely by vague purposes with only slight and sporadic effect.

While the program created by PL 93-641 was being put into place, public debate about national health insurance was under way in Congress, where newly voiced alternatives to public planning and command-control regulation were being heard. While cost containment loomed as the principal public issue, the enduring goal of securing universal, publicly sponsored health insurance moved Senator Edward Kennedy and a few other members of Congress to propose schemes that would join universal insurance coverage with elaborate regulation of the health services industry.

The prospect of extensive and permanent public planning and regulation, however, gave impetus to a counter view, one that stressed remediation through reform of the market. That view, embodied in the Carter Administration's "Consumer Choice Health Plan" (59), expressed no confidence in public planning and command-control regulation and, indeed, held that they militate against both the realization of more equitable access to care and the moderation of cost increases. It preferred to employ market-preserving regulation alongside rollbacks of market-distorting subsidies to remedy market failures, thereby obviating the need for command-control regulation.

Although prospects for enactment of a national health insurance soon dissipated, debate about command-control regulatory strategies versus market-reform strategies broadened. The latter, having been bolstered by landmark court decisions that had opened hospitals to liability claims and all health care providers to antitrust litigation, was given great encouragement by the 1980 elections. The Reagan Administration brought to the federal government a strongly held ideology opposing command-control regulation and a consonant legislative agenda calling for the repeal of federal efforts that imposed them. Among the programs slated for extinction was that created by PL 93-641.

Outright repeal of PL 93-641 proved impossible owing to the strong support for planning and regulation among a few powerful members of Congress. The Reagan Administration countered by starving the program of funds in its annual budget proposals. By middecade the program had become so severely depleted and correspondingly unable to perform that Congress allowed its authorities to expire. Many states, in turn, dismantled their agencies and repealed their CON laws. Others, principally those that had supported planning and regulation before enactment of PL 93-641, reassumed responsibilities for continuing their efforts.

Bolstered by decisions of the court that had removed hospitals' protections from liability suit and that had opened health care providers to antitrust prosecution, proponents of market reform offered a new avenue of debate. Market-preserving devices, especially those available in antitrust laws, were to be employed to rid the health services industry of anticompetitive practices. At the same time, various public subsidies that had, in their view, distorted health care markets were to be abolished. Chief among these were tax subsidies that encouraged the purchase of too much shallow insurance and, correspondingly, fostered the economically devastating disregard for costs among providers and consumers alike (60).

ORIGINS AND DEVELOPMENT OF HEALTH SERVICES REGULATION

It was noted at the outset of this chapter that regulation subsumes a variety of instruments by which government induces or compels persons to engage in (or refrain from) behaviors that promote (or are injurious to) the public interest or general welfare. The objectives pursued through regulation embrace a large set of socially desirable ends, including directing the development of entire industries and sectors of the economy, and protecting individuals from a host of hazards accompanying modern life. The means available to government to pursue such ends are nearly limitless. They range from subsidies provided either indirectly through tax policies or directly through cash transfers to direct command-control mechanisms enforced by varieties of legal and economic sanctions (61). Further, the types of agency involved in the implementation of regulatory programs defy simple enumeration. All branches of government—legislative, executive, and judicial—participate, and in many instances private bodies are enlisted into governments' regulatory efforts.

In view of this complexity, one cannot hope to comprehend either the entirety of regulation within the United States or even its totality within a single sector of the nation's economy. Accordingly, the discussion that follows is selective and highlights the general features of, and trends in, regulation rather than attempting comprehensively to deal with details of the highly fluid and uncertain regulatory environment surrounding the health services industry.

Specifically, we examine the origins and development of three types of command-control regulation that have been applied the health services industry: (1) capital expenditures and services (CES) controls, (2) utilization review as practiced by the Professional Standards Review Organizations (PSROs), and (3) prospective rate setting. Each of these programs was intended inter alia, to contain health care cost inflation, and each has contributed to a regimen of external control that through the 1970s approximated public utility regulation. Additionally, we briefly discuss the main features of antitrust regulation, the principal market-preserving instrument recommended by those who prefer market reform strategies to those that rely on public planning and command-control regulation.

THE BASES OF CONTROLS ON HOSPITALS

Hospitals have been the principal targets of regulatory programs aimed at controlling health care cost inflation. This may be due to the hospital industry's large and growing share of the nation's health care expenditures. It accounts for about 40 percent of the total and has been increasing annually at rates that greatly exceed growth in the general economy. The concentration on hospitals may also reflect tradition and political forces. As discussed previously, hospitals have been the major focus of the health planning movement from its inception. Since the regulatory movement that began in the 1960s built on that tradition, it follows that controls on hospitals would be the first to appear. It is also the case, as noted in Chapter 6, that hospitals have historically been a less potent political force than physicians and, therefore, are correspondingly more vulnerable to government intervention. Alternatively, if one takes the view that regulatory controls—particularly entry restrictions—are sought by industries to thwart competition (62), it might be argued that physicians' greater power was exercised earlier in this century in the establishment of their cartel and that hospitals have only recently been able to accomplish this feat. Regardless of one's conception of the origins of regulation, the fact remains that the newest forms of regulation have concentrated on hospitals.

The principal problem that stimulated regulation of hospitals is cost inflation attributable to long-standing inefficiencies in the industry. While sweeping changes in the hospitals' financing and market structures began to emerge in the early 1980s, until that time the case for regulating hospitals was compelling. Two related but conflicting arguments were advanced: (1) that hospitals "overinvest" in sophisticated and expensive services and (2) that such services are "overutilized" by the population (63). The overinvestment and overutilization, in turn, result in "unnecessary" expenditures for health services that contribute wastefully to cost inflation (64).

Recalling the earlier comments on the structure and financing of the health services industry, the inpatient hospital services market appeared to warrant regulation.

Specifically, assuming consumer ignorance, four features have combined to justify regulation: (1) the nonprofit status of most hospitals, (2) the relationships between these hospitals and community-based physicians, (3) the so-called Roemer Law (more generally, the availability effect), and (4) insurance (65).

Throughout the first three-quarters of this century the hospital industry has been dominated by multiproduct, nonprofit firms whose investment and output decisions have been amalgams of interests of their communities, lay boards of trustees, management, and medical staffs. Because hospitals have had to be responsive to the demands of these various constituencies, their investment decisions have reflected considerations other than profit maximization. Among the various objectives attributed to hospitals by economists are prestige and status (66), the quality and quantity of services produced (67), and social welfare (68). While all such specifications are conceived as being subject to the constraint that revenues must cover costs, all imply that investment and output decisions of nonprofit hospitals have not conformed to the model of a pure profit maximizer.

Related to these observations is the argument that hospitals' investment and output decisions have been strongly influenced by physicians' preferences (69). Because physicians select both the hospitals into which their patients are admitted and the mixes of services patients receive, physicians have exerted pressures on hospitals to provide the types and amounts of facilities, services, and support personnel that they desired. These pressures have joined with competition among hospitals for prestige to encourage investment in expansion and, more importantly, in upgrading styles of care (70). As physicians' incomes are enhanced by their use of hospital services, whose costs were being paid by insurers, one would expect physicians to have given little attention to hospital cost inflation.

The availability effect observed in the hospital industry protects the hospital from losses due to investment in facilities and services for which demand is low (71). This phenomenon implies, in effect, that the availability of health services stimulates their use. To the extent that this has occurred in markets for inpatient services, hospitals have been free to expand capacity and services with the assurance that additional beds would be filled and services used.

Insurance for hospital services has affected hospital investment in two ways. First, the typically more extensive coverage of inpatient services versus those rendered in ambulatory care settings has shifted patients into hospitals, where, because of low deductibles and coinsurance rates, patients have paid out-of-pocket only a small portion of their charges. Patients therefore have been relatively indifferent to costs incurred at the time of treatment. Second, retrospective cost-based reimbursement schemes have protected hospitals from losses caused by poor investment decisions. Together, the assurances of high cash flows due to the availability effect and insurance and the guaranteed retroactive payment of costs (including debt service) placed hospitals in favored positions in the capital market (72–74). This, in turn, facilitated more investment. The three types of regulation discussed next were intended to rectify the consequences of these structural and financial characteristics.

CAPITAL EXPENDITURES AND SERVICES CONTROLS

CES controls attempt to eliminate unnecessary investment in expansion of capacity and to halt offerings of new services that are deemed to duplicate existing ones (75). To the extent that this occurs, needless expenditures for health services will be averted by preventing initial outlays for construction, renovation, and new equipment and avoiding future operating costs. Proponents of CES regulation point to two indicators of unnecessary expenditures: excess capacity and inappropriate utilization. Excess capacity, as evidenced by empty hospital beds and idle equipment and services, is taken to be an obvious sign of overinvestment and a portion of their fixed costs as an indication of unnecessary expenditures. Also, expenditures for inpatient services are considered unnecessarily high in instances where patients' problems are viewed as amenable to treatment in less expensive ambulatory care settings and, for patients who require hospitalization, where less expensive combinations of diagnostic and therapeutic services could be substituted for more costly ones.

CES controls on hospitals first appeared in the mid-1960s when the State of New York enacted its CON, and, by 1972, about half the states had imposed such regulation. That year brought the federally sponsored Section 1122 program, and, in 1974, the National Health Planning and Resources Development Act mandated all states to enact CON statutes. By the close of the 1970s, all states imposed CES controls on their hospitals, either CON or Section 1122 regulation, or both. As noted earlier, many states adopted CON programs only to satisfy requirements of PL 93-641 and, with the removal of that requirement abandoned them. As of the late 1980s, about half the states continued to apply some form of CON to hospitals and other designated health care institutions.

CES controls attempt to attain equilibria between supplies of and needs for services by requiring hospitals' plans for major capital investments and offerings of new services to be certified by regulatory agencies as needed in their communities. State CON statutes typically levy legal sanctions against institutions that either fail to seek certificates or proceed with their plans after certificates have been denied. The Section 1122 program employs only financial sanctions: institutions that implement plans that have not received prior authorization are denied reimbursement for costs associated with their investments (e.g., interest payments) by the Medicare, Medicaid, and Maternal and Infant Care programs.

CES programs are administered by state agencies, in most cases those that were initially established under PL 93-641. The review process typically is initiated when a hospital submits a proposal for a major capital investment or a significant change in its services to the regulatory agency. The agency determines whether the application justifies the need for the proposed project and either issues or denies a CON. Failure to do so prohibits the applicant from pursuing the proposed project, and sanctions are applied to those that proceed without certification.

Since the early 1970s, several evaluations of the effectiveness of CES regulation have been carried out, focusing primarily on CON programs. Without exception, studies have revealed that such controls have had no appreciable effects on either amounts or patterns of capital investment by hospitals or growth in aggregate expenditures for hospital services (76). On the basis of these findings, most observers conclude that CES regulation as practiced from the late 1960s and throughout the 1970s were generally ineffective as cost-control devices.

PROFESSIONAL STANDARDS REVIEW ORGANIZATIONS

The soaring costs of Medicare and Medicaid prompted Congress to enact in 1972 sweeping reforms in these programs' reimbursement procedures. Among the amendments attached to the Social Security Act by PL 92-603 were provisions establishing

Professional Standards Review Organizations (PSROs), discussed also in Chapter 13. These organizations were (77)

> To promote the effective, efficient, and economical delivery of health care services of proper quality for which payment may be made (in whole or in part) under this Act and in recognition of the interests of patients, the public, practitioners, and providers in improved health care services, it is the purpose of this part to assure, through the application of suitable procedures of professional standards review, that the Social Security Act will conform to appropriate professional standards for the provision of health care.

The clear intent of the statute was to curtail overutilization and excessive costs of inpatient hospital services by subjecting physicians' admitting and treatment decisions to review by colleagues. To accomplish this, PSROs comprised of local physicians were created throughout the nation. These bodies were to establish standards of medical care for categories of health problems, develop profiles of individual physicians' practices, and monitor the inpatient services they provide or order for beneficiaries of the Medicare, Medicaid, and Maternal and Infant Care programs (78). Failing this test, the federal government was to withhold payment to the offending physician for the unnecessary services and to levy more severe financial penalties on repeating and fraudulent offenders.

At the federal level, a National PSRO Council was empaneled, inter alia, to review local PSRO's standards and to advise the Secretary of Health, Education, and Welfare on the program's structure and operation.

From its inception the PSRO program was beset by controversy. During the legislative process, the AMA mounted a ferocious, albeit belated and unsuccessful, campaign to defeat the bill. While the AMA endorsed the bill's delegations of responsibilities and authorities to its members, it was appalled by what it regarded as an unwarranted and ominous gambit that allowed the federal government to intrude directly in individual physicians' practices. Associations representing other health professions viewed the program as a government endorsement of the dominance of physicians, and spokespeople for consumers' interests saw it as a sellout akin to appointing the fox to guard the henhouse (79). Moreover, as the program developed, its principal mission become clouded. Physicians were inclined to view it primarily as aimed at improving the quality of health services, while advocates of PSRO in Congress and the federal bureaucracy saw it as a cost-containment effort (80).

As a result of lingering opposition from most of the nation's physicians, the program was implemented in a desultory manner. Perhaps because of this, evaluations of PSRO have found few indications of effectiveness. Studies revealed that, as of 1976, the program had had no profound impacts on the use of inpatient hospital services on their costs and had produced no measurable improvements in the quality of care (81). While some savings were identified in some areas of the nation and for selected types of expenditure (82,83), informed opinion held that PSRO did not materially lower hospital cost inflation.

With the election of the Reagan Administration, the PSRO program joined PL 93-641 in being slated for repeal, and by the mid-1980s this had been accomplished. PSROs were replaced, however, by private Professional Review Organizations (PROs), which contract with the federal government and private insurers to conduct review of care rendered to hospitalized patients. Backed by the authority of the federal government and its avowed objective of controlling costs, PRO reviews are considerably more focused and vigorous than those of the predecessor PSRO program.

PROSPECTIVE RATE SETTING

By the late 1960s, the brunt of health care cost inflation from the Medicaid program was being felt in state legislatures. Among the several factors identified as causing the problem was the prevailing mode of paying hospitals for their services. The reimbursement scheme for the Medicare and Medicaid programs had initially been modeled after the Blue Cross procedure of retroactively paying hospitals their costs plus a fixed percentage. As noted earlier, this approach to financing in combination with other features of the hospital industry reinforced its tendencies toward inefficiency.

To remedy this, in the early 1970s several states established rate-setting programs by which hospitals' budgets are set prospectively (84). Although the several programs currently in operation employ various means to establish budgets, all are based on the assumption that the strategy will impel hospitals toward more cost conscious behavior and greater overall efficiency (85,86). In effect, hospitals' revenues are set at the outset of a budget period. Those whose actual costs are lower than the budgeted amount may retain the net revenues; those who overspend must cover costs with monies from other sources.

By 1978, some form of prospective rate setting was in force in at least portions of 28 states (87). About half of these programs were voluntary efforts involving Blue Cross plans and/or bodies established by state hospital associations. In six other states rate setting was mandated by state laws implemented by commissions. During the 1970s, the Health Care Financing Administration of the U.S. Department of Health and Human Services promoted rate setting, providing grants-in-aid to states that would establish experimental programs, and the Carter Administration included a federally sponsored program in its legislative proposals for a national strategy to contain the costs of health services (88). Having been defeated in Congress, the federal program never materialized, leaving mandatory rate setting to the few states that chose to impose it.

Several studies have shown that hospital rate-setting programs have been somewhat successful in controlling the growth of expenditures for hospital services. Evidence suggests that, where rate setting has been pursued vigorously (e.g., in New York State), rates of increase have been lowered in both average daily hospital costs and per capita spending for hospital services (89,90). Studies find that stringent rate setting may have lowered the rate of increase in per diem costs by as much as ten percent (91).

While rate setting appears to have achieved at least some success in dampening cost increases in hospital care, concern exists about how this has occurred and regarding the potential negative side effects of stringent regulation. As noted earlier, the aim of rate setting is to effect economies by fostering greater efficiency. Hospitals have several ways of lowering their costs, however, and some of those strategies would result in undesirable outcomes. One concern is that strict rate setting has prompted hospitals to forego needed capital improvements and saving (92). Were this so, the industry may lack sufficient capital to finance necessary expansion and renovation. Another holds that hospitals subject to rate setting will concentrate on providing the most profitable services and cease to offer such unprofitable services as ambulatory care, home care, and social services (93). Finally, some observers fear that stringent controls on revenues will bring about poorer quality of care by, for instance, leading to cutbacks in nursing services. Evidence pertaining to these matters remains sketchy. With the advent of Medicare's diagnosis-related groups (DRGs) mode of paying hospitals, however, considerable attention is being devoted to the potential deleterious consequences of restricting hospital rates and prices.

The underlying logic of hospital rate setting and its seemingly favorable outcomes have protected it somewhat from the deregulatory mood of the 1980s. Rate setting is a more flexible means of regulation than the others discussed above. Rate setting controls revenues, leaving hospitals to determine how they will use their available funds. The possibility of realizing higher net revenues by exercising cost-consciousness presumably moves hospitals to seek innovative efficiencies.

While these features recommend rate setting over other more intrusive forms of command-control regulation, debate has surfaced about the need for controlling hospitals revenues through direct regulation. The 1980s witnessed the beginnings of profound changes in health care markets that some believe have so dramatically altered incentives as to render external rate setting unnecessary. As of the late 1980s, it would appear that rate setting will continue to be practiced in a few states, but neither the federal government nor most other states are inclined to adopt such regulation.

ANTITRUST REGULATION

As noted earlier, antitrust regulation differs markedly from command-control regulation in both its underlying rationale and its modus operandi. Command-control regulation, presuming that markets will not function properly, substitutes some degree of external bureaucratic control over regulated firms. It exercises direct and usually enduring influence on decisions made by firms in industries singled out for regulation. By contrast, antitrust regulation presumes that markets do (or can be made to) function properly when market assumptions are met. Antitrust enforcement aims to ensure that such circumstances prevail by establishing general rules of conduct to which all commercial enterprises are subject and levying sanctions against those who willfully violate them (94).

Although the enforcement of antitrust laws is often complex, the basic rules of antitrust are straightforward. They aim to identify and punish compacts and conspiracies among businesses that either thwart or aim to thwart competition. Two general types of evidence are employed in identifying antitrust violations. Some behaviors are so unarguably anticompetitive that their mere existence suffices to evoke punishment. These so-called per se violations include such offenses as boycotts organized against competitors and price fixing among presumed competitors. Other offenses are identified by the rule of reason, which, in effect, seeks to determine whether particular behaviors could reasonably have been expected by those engaging (or conspiring to engage) in them to have the effect of thwarting competition. When activities are judged in the affirmative in this respect, they are deemed to be antitrust violations.

Antitrust laws apply to all commercial enterprises that are not explicitly exempted. Common law traditions, however, historically have conferred exemption on various classes of business, including such professional groups as lawyers, engineers, and physicians. Legal tradition presumed that codes of ethics governing behaviors of professionals evoke sufficient public-spirited service as to justify their being granted immunity from antitrust regulation.

Removed from the reach of antitrust laws, physicians and other professionals historically were free to engage in activities with impunity that, by today's standards, would be considered egregious instances of restraint of trade. These include, for example, price fixing, boycotting Health Maintenance Organizations (HMOs) (95), and insurance companies (96), and prohibiting advertising among their colleagues.

Committed under the guise of being enforcements of professional ethics, however, most such practices escaped antitrust prosecution.

By the 1970s, critics of command-control regulation had begun to espouse the view that many of the market failures to which regulation was being addressed had arisen from and were being perpetuated by physicians' and other health care providers' privileged status under the antitrust laws (97). Moreover, they regarded many of the organized practices of providers to be blatantly self-serving and at the expense of the public at large. They called, therefore, for more extensive use of antitrust regulation in the health services industry. By the late 1970s, several landmark court decisions had swept aside professional groups' blanket immunities, first in cases involving price fixing among lawyers and later in cases involving competitive bidding among engineers. These created the possibility of removing long-standing privileges of physicians, hospitals, and other health care providers that had militated against the reign of market forces within the health care industry.

In the environment of the 1970s, with its heightened consumerism and consumer advocacy, agencies of government charged with implementing antitrust regulation initiated numerous proceedings against health care providers. The Federal Trade Commission, the U.S. Department of Justice, and many state attorneys-general launched investigations and filed suits that established legal precedents and, perhaps as importantly, sent the unambiguous message to health care providers that they no longer enjoyed the privilege to exercise professional power for the purpose of obstructing market forces (98).

The rush of official actions against such fundamental violations as restraining advertising had subsided by the mid-1980s. Those charged with enforcing antitrust violations, however, keep watch over the industry, and new generations of health care providers and administrators are unlikely even to consider engaging in the standard anticompetitive practices of the preantitrust era.

Proponents of market-reform strategies never expected that antitrust enforcement alone would rid the health care industry of all its market failures. Rather, it was viewed as an important element that at least cleared the way for latent market forces to begin to operate. They sought increased cost-consciousness among providers and consumers by advocating changes in the nature and extent of health insurance coverage and promoting such alternatives to fee-for-service medicine as HMOs (99). In our concluding section, we will comment on trends of the 1980s that have given substance to those hopes.

By the late 1980s, the antiregulatory mood that had begun to surface in the mid-1970s had taken firm hold. The federal government and most states had withdrawn their support of community wide comprehensive health planning and command-control regulation. Federally sponsored regulation was confined largely to utilization review associated with the Medicare program. Responsibility for controlling the industry had been returned largely to the private sector. That did not imply, however, a return to the form of industry-dominated control that had prevailed before the 1960s. Antitrust laws now prohibited such cartel arrangements. More importantly, however, the 1980s witnessed the rise of new forms of control approximating those desired by proponents of market reform.

Impetus for change gathered from several sources. In 1981 Congress enacted laws that permitted states greater freedom in the administration of their Medicaid laws (100). Several responded by establishing preferred provider schemes in which providers competed for Medicaid contracts (101). The business community also added a new element. Business coalitions representing major employers began to pressure insurers for less costly premiums and to extend to their employees options of joining HMOs. Insurers responded, in turn, by offering benefit plans including more extensive cost sharing and provisions for utilization review (102) and themselves began to promote preferred provider arrangements and HMOs (103).

As of the late 1980s, these dramatic changes in the health services industry have yet to run their course. They portend, however, an industry very different from that of the past, one in which market controls stimulate greater competition to attain results previously sought through externally imposed command-control regulation. Whether such changes will effect the efficiencies and controls over increasing expenditures to which regulation has been directed remains to be seen.

It would appear, however, that the newly unleashed market forces will not remedy the problem of the limited access to health care that many citizens continue to suffer (104). As this issue regains the center of public attention, as it inevitably will, the federal and state governments may find themselves with a compelling purpose to extend public subsidies to larger segments of society. Were this to occur, renewed public interest in the performance (not only its costs) of the health services industry would surely follow. Whether that interest would reenliven public planning and new forms of regulation also remains to be seen.

Were public planning and regulation again to become an important instrument of public policy, the principal lessons drawn from the experiences recounted in this chapter would require close attention. Public planning and regulation cannot serve the public interest when objectives set for them are vaguely and expansively defined and when sustained political commitment is lacking.

REFERENCES AND NOTES

1. Lindblom CE: *Politics and Markets: The World's Political-Economic Systems.* New York, Basic Books, 1977.

2. Roemer MI: *National Strategies for Health Care Organization: A World Overview.* Ann Arbor, MI, Health Administration Press, 1985.

3. Dahl RA, Lindblom CE: *Politics, Economics, and Welfare.* New York, Harper, 1953.

4. Lindblom, op cit (Ref 1).

5. Wilson JQ (ed): *The Politics of Regulation.* New York, Basic Books, 1980.

6. Breyer S: Analyzing regulatory failure: Mismatches, less restrictive alternatives, and reforms. *Harv Law Rev* 1979; 92:549–609.

7. Schelling TC: *Micromotives and Macrobehavior.* New York, Norton, 1978.

8. Schultze CL: *The Public Use of Private Interest.* Washington, DC, The Brookings Institution, 1977.

9. Weidenbaum ML: *Business, Government, and the Public.* Englewood Cliffs, NJ, Prentice-Hall, 1977.

10. Okun AM: *Equality and Efficiency: The Big Tradeoff.* Washington, DC, The Brookings Institution, 1975.

11. Posner RA: *Antitrust Law: An Economic Perspective.* Chicago, University of Chicago Press, 1976; Posner RA: *Economic Analysis of Law,* 2nd ed., Boston, Little Brown, 1977, pp 211–237.

12. Stewart RB: The reformation of American administrative law, *Harv Law Rev* 1975; 88:1667–1814.

13. Lowi TJ: *The End of Liberalism,* 2nd ed. New York, Norton, 1979, pp 92–126.

14. Sundquist JL, Davis DW: *Making Federalism Work.* Washington, DC, The Brookings Institution, 1969.

15. Moynihan DP: *Maximum Feasible Misunderstanding: Community Action in the War on Poverty,* New York, The Free Press, 1969.

16. Stewart RB, op cit (Ref 12).

17. Goldberg LG, Greenberg W: The effect of physician-controlled health insurance: U.S. v. Oregon State Medical Society. J Health Politics, Policy, Law 1977; 2:48–78; Kessel RA: Price discrimination in medicine, *J Law Econ* 1958; 1:20–53.

18. Havighurst CC, Hackbarth GM: Private cost containment. *New Engl J Med* 1979; 300:1298–1305.

19. Palmiere D: Community health planning, in Corey L, Saltman SE, Epstein MF (eds): *Medicine in a Changing Society.* St. Louis, Mosby, 1972, pp 59–82.

20. Klarman HE: Planning for facilities, in Ginzberg E (ed): *Regionalization and Health Policy.* Washington, DC, U.S. Government Printing Office, 1977, pp 25–36.

21. Thompson P: Voluntary regional planning, in Ginzberg E (ed): *Regionalization and Health Policy.* Washington, DC, U.S. Government Printing Office, 1977, pp 123–128.

22. Pearson DA: The concept of regionalized personal health services in the United States, 1920–1975, in Saward EW (ed): *The Regionalization of Personal Health Services.* New York, Prodist, 1976, pp 10–14.

23. Ibid, pp 5–10.

24. Ibid, pp 14–19.

25. Cited from May JJ: *Health Planning: Its Past and Potential.* Chicago, Center for Health Administration Studies, Perspectives No. A5, University of Chicago, 1967, p 25.

26. Lave JR, Lave LB: *The Hospital Construction Act: An Evaluation of the Hill-Burton Program.* Washington, DC, The American Enterprise Institute for Public Policy Research, 1974, pp 41–43.

27. Gottlieb SR: A brief history of health planning in the United States, in Havighurst CC (ed): *Regulating Health Facilities Construction.* Washington, DC, The American Enterprise Institute for Public Policy Research, 1974, pp 7–26.

28. Cited from Hilleboe HE, Barkhuus A: Health planning in the United States: Some categorical and general approaches. *Internatl J Health Serv* 1971; 1:137.

29. President's Commission on Heart Disease, Cancer and Stroke: *A National Program to Conquer Heart Disease, Cancer, and Stroke.* Vol I, Washington, DC, U.S. Government Printing Office, 1964.

30. For a comparison of the Commission's recommendations and the actual provisions of the amendment, see Pollack J: Health services and the role of medical school, *Milbank Mem Fund Quart* 1968; 46:151–152, Part 2.

31. Glaser, WA: Experiences in health planning in the United States (mimeograph). Paper prepared for the Conference on Health Planning in the United States: Past Experiences and Future Imperatives, New York, Columbia University, June 1973.

32. Bodenheimer TS: Regional medical programs: No road to regionalization. *Med Care Rev* 1969; 26:1125–1166.

33. Regional Medical Programs Service: *Selected Vignettes on Activities of Regional Medical Programs,* Washington, DC, Health Services and Mental Health Administration, U.S. Department of Health, Education, and Welfare, 1971.

34. Glaser WA, op cit (Ref 31), p 16.

35. National Commission on Community Health Services: *Health is a Community Affair.* Cambridge, MA, Harvard University Press, 1966.

36. Ibid, p 131.

37. Comptroller General of the United States: *Comprehensive Health Planning As Carried Out by State and Areawide Agencies in Three States.* Washington, DC, U.S. General Accounting Office, Congress of the United States, April 1974, p 8.

38. May's studies are a notable exception; see May JJ, op cit (Ref 25), pp 25–36.

39. Havighurst CC: Regulation of health facilities and services by "certificate of need." *Virginia Law Rev* 1973; 59:1143–1232.

40. Richardson EL: Address before the Institute of Medicine. Washington, DC, National Academy of Sciences, May 10, 1972.

41. Iglehart JK, Lilley III W, Clark TB: New federalism report/HEW department advances sweeping proposal to overhaul its programs. *Natl J* 1973; Jan. 6:1.

42. Wilson JQ: The bureaucracy problem. *The Public Interest* 3–9 (Winter), 1967.

43. U.S. Congress, Senate Committee on Government Operations, Subcommittee on Executive Reorganization and Government Research: *Federal Role in Health: Report Pursuant to S. Res. 390. 91st Congress.* 2nd Session, S. Report 91-801, 1970.

44. Sundquist JL, Davis DW, op cit (Ref 14).

45. Liebman L: Social intervention in a democracy. *The Public Interest* 1974; 14–29.

46. Stevens R: *American Medicine and the Public Interest.* New Haven, CT, Yale University Press, 1971, pp 496–527.

47. U.S. Congress, House of Representatives: *Hearings Before the Subcommittee on Labor and Health, Education, and Welfare and Related Agencies of the Committee on Appropriations,* 91st Congress, 1st Session, 1969, pp 426–431.

48. English JT: Mission of the Health Services and Mental Health Administration. *Public Health Rep* 1970; 85:95–99.

49. U.S. Congress, op cit (Ref 43).

50. The National Center for Health Services Research and Development is now the National Center for Health Services Research and Technology Assessment. For a description of this agency's history, see The Institute of Medicine: *Health Services Research.* Washington, DC, Institute of Medicine, National Academy of Sciences, 1979, Chapter 5.

51. Sanazaro PJ: Federal Health Services Research and R and D Under the Auspices of the National Center for Health Services Research and Development, in Flook

EE, Sanazaro PJ (eds): *Health Services and R and D in Perspective.* Ann Arbor, Health Administration Press, 1973, pp 150–183.

52. Rubel EJ: Testimony before the U.S. Congress, House of Representatives, Committee on Interstate and Foreign Commerce, Subcommittee on Public Health and Environment. *Hearings on the National Health Policy and Health Resources Development Bill and Related Bills.* 93rd Congress, 2nd Session, March 15; April 30; May 1, 6–9, and 14, 1974, p 408.

53. Klarman HE: Health planning: Progress, prospects, and issues. *Milbank Mem Fund Quart Health Society* 1978; 56:78–112.

54. Checkoway B: Consumerism in health planning agencies, in *Health Planning in the United States: Selected Policy Issues.* Institute of Medicine, National Academy of Sciences, 1981, pp 143–166; Marmor TR, Morone JA: Representing consumer interests: Imbalanced markets, health planning, and the HSAs. *Milbank Mem Fund Quart Health Soc* 1980; 58:125–165; Vladeck BC: Interest-group representation and the HSAs: Health planning and political theory. *Am J Public Health* 1977; 67:23–29.

55. Vladeck BC: The design of failure: health policy and the structure of federalism. *J Health Politics, Policy, Law* 1979; 4:522–535; Brown LD: Some structural issues in the health planning process, in *Health Planning in the United States: Selected Policy Issues.* Institute of Medicine, National Academy of Sciences, 1981, pp 1–45; Rabb GG: National/state/local relationships in health planning: Interest group reaction and lobbying, in *Health Planning in the United States,* ibid, pp 105–130.

56. Public Health Service, U.S. Department of Health, Education, and Welfare: National guidelines for health planning. *Fed Reg* March 28, 1978; 43:12,040–12,050.

57. Glantz, LH: Legal Aspects of health facilities regulation, in Hyman HH (ed): *Health Regulation: Certificate of Need and Section 1122.* Germantown, MD, Aspen Systems Corp. 1977, pp 75–104.

58. Cohodes DR: Interstate variation in certificate of need programs—a review and prospectus, in *Health Planning in the United States: Selected Policy Issues.* Institute of Medicine, National Academy of Sciences, 1981, pp 47–80.

59. Enthoven AC: Consumer choice health plan (first of two parts). Inflation and inequity in health care today: Alternatives for cost control and an analysis of proposals for national health insurance. *New Engl J Med* 1978; 298:650–658; Enthoven AC: Consumer choice health plan (second of two parts). A national-health-insurance proposal based on regulated competition in the private sector. *New Engl J Med* 1978; 298:709–720.

60. Taylor AK, Wilensky GR: The effect of tax policies on expenditures for private health insurance, in Meyer JA (ed): *Market Reforms in Health Care: Current Issues, New Directions, Strategic Decisions,* Washington, DC, The American Enterprise Institute for Public Policy Research, 1983, pp 163–184; Ginsburg PB: Altering the tax treatment of employment-based health plans. *Milbank Mem Fund Quart Health Society* 1981; 59:224–255.

61. Breyer S, op cit (Ref 6).

62. Stigler GJ: The theory of economic regulation. *Bell Econ Manage Sci* 1971; 2:3–21.

63. Salkever DS, Bice TW: *Hospital Certificate of Need Controls: Impact on Investment, Costs, and Use*. Washington, DC, American Enterprise Institute for Public Policy Research, 1979.

64. For essays on the health care industry of this period, see Zubkoff M (ed): *Health: A Victim or Cause of Inflation*. New York, Prodist, 1976; Havighurst, op cit (Ref 39).

65. Such terms as "need," "overinvest," "unnecessary costs," and the like are elusive concepts. For a critique of the practice of basing health planning on notions of needs, see Klarman HE, op cit (Ref. 20). For a more general critique of the language of health planners, see Kessel R: Commentary on the papers, in Havighurst CC (ed), op cit (Ref. 27), pp 33–35; Posner RA: Certificates of need for health care facilities: A dissenting view, in Havighurst CC (ed), op cit (Ref 27), pp 113–118.

66. Lee ML: A conspicuous production theory of hospital behavior. South Econ J 1971; 38:45–58.

67. Newhouse JP: Toward a theory of nonprofit institutions: An economic model of a hospital. *Am Econ Rev* 1970; 60:64–74.

68. Feldstein PJ: *An Empirical Investigation of the Marginal Cost of Hospital Services*. Chicago, Graduate Program in Hospital Administration, University of Chicago, 1961.

69. Redisch MA: Physician involvement in hospital decision making, in Zubkoff M, Raskin IE, Hanft RS (ed): *Hospital Cost Containment*. New York, Prodist, 1978.

70. Feldstein MS: Hospital cost inflation: A study of nonprofit price dynamics. *Am Econ Rev* 1970; 60:853–872; Pauly MV, Redisch M: The not-for-profit hospital as a physicians' cooperative: *Am Econ Rev* 1983; 63:87–99.

71. Feldstein MS, op cit (Ref 70), pp 871–872.

72. Clapp DC, Spector AB: A study of the American capital market and its relationship to the capital needs of the health care field, in MacLeod GK, Perlman M (eds): *Health Care Capital: Competition and Control*. Cambridge, MA, Ballinger, 1978, pp 275–304.

73. Kelling RS Jr, Williams PC: The projected response of the capital markets to health facilities expenditures, in MacLeod GK, Perlman M (eds): *Health Care Capital: Competition and Control*. Cambridge, MA, Ballinger, 1978, pp 319–348.

74. Cohodes DR, Kinkead BM: *Hospital Capital Formation in the 1980s*. Baltimore, The Johns Hopkins University Press, 1984.

75. Salkever DS, Bice TW, op cit (Ref 63).

76. Steinwald B, Sloan FA: Regulatory approaches to hospital cost containment: A synthesis of the empirical evidence, in Olson M (ed): *A New Approach to the Economics of Health Care*. Washington, DC, The American Enterprise Institute for Public Policy Research, 1981, pp 273–317; Sloan FA, Steinwald B: Regulation and the rising cost of hospital care. *Rev Econ Stat* 1981; 3:4790–487.

77. 42 United States Code 1301, Section 1151.

78. Blumstein JF: The role of PSROs in hospital cost containment, in Zubkoff M, Raskin IE, Hanft RS (eds), op cit (Ref 69) pp 461–488.

79. Bellin LE: PSRO: Quality control? Or gimmickry? *Med Care* 12:1974; 1012–1018.

80. Havighurst CC, Blumstein JF: Coping with quality/cost tradeoffs in medical care: PSROs. *Northwest Law Rev* 1975; 70:6–68.

81. Office of Planning, Evaluation, and Legislation, Health Services Administration, U.S. Department of Health, Education, and Welfare: *Professional Standards Review Organizations: Program Evaluation, Vol I.* Washington, DC, U.S. Department of Health, Education, and Welfare, 1978.

82. Ibid pp 22–29.

83. Brook RH, Williams KN, Rolph JE: *Controlling the Use and Cost of Medical Services: The New Mexico Experimental Medical Care Review Organization-A Four-Year Case Study.* Santa Monica, CA, The Rand Corporation, November 1978.

84. Bauer KG: Hospital rate setting—this way to salvation?, in Zubkoff M, Paskin IE, Hanft RS (eds), op cit (Ref 69), pp 324–369.

85. Dowling WL: Prospective reimbursement of hospitals. *Inquiry* 1974; 11:163–180.

86. Esposito A, Hupfer M, Mason C, et al: Abstracts of stated legislated hospital cost-containment programs. *Health Care Financ Rev* 1982; 4:129–158.

87. Status of state regulation programs. *Federat Am Hosp Rev* 1978; 11:12–13.

88. Dunn WL, Lefkowitz B: The Hospital Cost Containment Act of 1977: An analysis of the Administration's proposal, in Zubkoff M, Raskin IE, Hanft RS (eds), op cit (Ref 69), pp 166–216.

89. Sloan FA: Rate regulation as a strategy for hospital cost control: Evidence for the last decade. *Milbank Mem Fund Quart Health Society* 1983; 61:195–221; Eby CL, Cohodes DR: What do we know about rate-setting? *J Health Politics, Policy, Law* 1985; 10:299–323.

90. Coelen C, Sullivan D: An analysis of the effects of prospective reimbursement on hospital expenditures. *Health Care Finan Rev* 1981; 2:1–40; Cromwell J, Kanak JR: The effects of prospective reimbursement programs on hospital adoption and service sharing. *Health Care Finan Rev* 1982; 4:67–88; Kidder D, Sullivan D: Hospital payroll costs, productivity, and employment under prospective reimbursement. *Health Care Finan Rev* 1982; 4:89–100.

91. Eby CL, Cohodes DR, op cit (Ref 89).

92. Ting HM, Valiante JD: Future capital needs of community hospitals. *Health Affairs* 1982; 1:14–27; Cohodes DR: Which will survive? The $150 billion capital question. *Inquiry* 1983; 20:5–11.

93. Conrad D, Morrissey M, Shortell S, et al: All-payer rate regulations: An analysis of hospital response, in Lewin ME (ed): *The Health Policy Agenda: Some Critical Questions.* Washington, DC, The American Enterprise Institute for Public Policy Research, 1985, pp 65–84.

94. For overviews of antitrust regulation, see Posner, RA, op cit (Ref 11, both Posner works); Bork RH: *The Antitrust Parados: A Policy at War with Itself.* New York, Basic Books, 1978; Letwin W: *Law and Economic Policy in America.* Chicago, University of Chicago Press, 1965; Gellhorn E: *Antitrust Law and Economics in a nutshell.* St. Paul, MN, West Publishing, 1976.

95. Kessel RA, op cit (Ref 17).

96. Goldberg LG, Greenberg W, op cit (Ref 17).

97. Havighurst CC: Professional restraints on innovation in health care financing. *Duke Law J* 1978; 19:321–326.

98. Havighurst CC: Antitrust enforcement in the medical services industry: What does it all mean? *Milbank Mem Fund Quart Health Society* 1980; 58:89–123.

99. Enthoven AC: *Health Plan*, Menlo Park, CA, Addison-Wesley, 1980.

100. Gibson R: Quiet revolutions in Medicaid, in Meyer JA (ed): *Market Reforms in Health Care: Current Issues, New Directions, Strategic Decisions*, Washington, DC, The American Enterprise Institute for Public Policy Research, 1983, pp 75–102.

101. Gabel J, Ermann D: Preferred provider organizations: Performance, problems, and promise. *Health Affairs* 1985; 4:24–40.

102. Goldsmith JC: Employers' self-funding surge adds a new dimension to competition in health insurance. *Federat Am Hosp Rev* 1985; 18:28–30; Goldsmith JC: Death of a paradigm: The challenge of competition. *Health Affairs* 1984; 3:5–19.

103. Tarlov AR: HMO enrollment growth and physicians: The third compartment. *Health Affairs* 1986; 5:22–35.

104. Feder J, Hadley J, Mullner R: Poor people and poor hospitals: Implications for public policy. *Milbank Mem Fund Quart Health Society* 1984; 62:544–566; Wilensky GR: Solving uncompensated care. *Health Affairs* 1984; 3:50–62.

CHAPTER 13

The Quality
of Health Care

James P. LoGerfo
Robert H. Brook

The purpose of this chapter is to create an understanding of major issues relevant to the assessment of the quality of health care and to provide an overview of existing mechanisms that have been established to ensure that patients receive good personal medical care. The first portion of the chapter will discuss the relationship between health and medical care; potential sources and selection of data on provider performance; issues of measurement including reliability of data, sensitivity, and specificity concerning judgments about the quality of care; specific methods of measuring quality of care and each method's strengths and limitations; and the implications of imperfect knowledge concerning the true effectiveness of many medical services. Illustrative studies of the quality of care are presented. The last portion of the chapter deals with those mechanisms and programs that have been established to assure that medical care is of appropriate quality. While the chapter addresses most of the major issues in the above areas, it is not an exhaustive review; the reader may wish to consult other reviews and bibliographies on the assessment and assurance of the quality of medical care (1–5).

Assessment of the quality of care is inextricably intertwined with societal, professional, and patient expectations concerning the role of health care in society. Quality—the degree of excellence or confirmation to standards—cannot be definitively assessed without a clear understanding about the expected standards of excellence. Unfortunately, many of society's expectations concerning health and medical care have not been explicitly delineated. However, improvement in the health of society at large, or of some persons within that society, is an expectation of the medical care system. With this fact in mind, the quality of health care could be assessed by the extent to which the society's or the person's health is improved by a specified level of resources, provided in a manner that is most consonant with the cultural and social mores of the society. If there are good methods for measuring health, the quality of a system could be measured by the relationship between actual health and the expected level for the amount of resources used. Unfortunately the relationship between medical care and the improvement of health is not as well defined as one would like,

406

and this ambiguity raises significant problems for the assessment of the quality of medical care. The following section deals with some of these important implications.

THE RELATIONSHIP BETWEEN HEALTH AND MEDICAL CARE

The improvement and maintenance of health are nearly universally accepted as objectives of medical care. These objectives would ideally be achieved by the sequence of events, represented in Figure 13-1 and discussed in more detail in other chapters of this book. As has been known for more than 20 centuries, however, many factors other than medical care have a profound effect on health, including personal behavior, environmental factors, and genetic endowment. In addition, as reflected in various ancient codes of law dealing with the adverse outcomes of care, such as removing the hand of a surgeon for a poor-quality operation, not all care is efficacious; that is, not all care contributes to a positive outcome. Indeed, some care has the potential to be harmful, leading to iatrogenic illness caused by the care itself (e.g., infections after surgery). Accordingly, a more extensive model is presented in Figure 13-2.

The final outcome of care for any patient is a function of the likelihood that the patient actually needs care, that a correct diagnosis is made, that the correct treatment is given, that the treatment is efficacious, and that the treatment was adhered to by the patient. The probability of all of these events occurring represents the positive contribution of medical care to health. Most of these probabilities are not precisely known. Even if the probabilities are known for specific medical care interventions, it is critical to recognize the contributions of the nonmedical factors (such as environment) to the production of health. This recognition is important because lack of an understanding of the multifactorial determinants of outcomes of disease process can lead to major errors in evaluation of health services. For example, critics of the U.S. health care system often cite this country's higher infant death rate and lower life expectancy compared to those of selected European nations as evidence that the health care system in this country is inferior. Infant death rates, however, are influenced by demographic and social factors that are difficult to adjust for when performing these comparisons. Similarly, life expectancy is influenced by personal

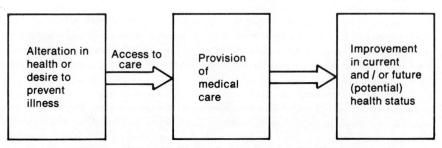

Figure 13-1. Idealized model of an episode of medical care.

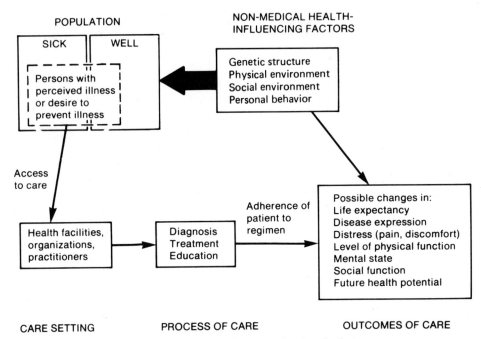

POPULATION

NON-MEDICAL HEALTH-
INFLUENCING FACTORS

SICK   WELL

Persons with
perceived illness
or desire to
prevent illness

Genetic structure
Physical environment
Social environment
Personal behavior

Access
to care

Health facilities,
organizations,
practitioners

Diagnosis
Treatment
Education

Adherence of
patient to
regimen

Possible changes in:
Life expectancy
Disease expression
Distress (pain, discomfort)
Level of physical function
Mental state
Social function
Future health potential

CARE SETTING   PROCESS OF CARE   OUTCOMES OF CARE

Figure 13-2. Model of a single episode of medical care.

behaviors such as smoking, drinking, and involvement in violence. Thus, criticism of a health care system based on mortality statistics is less a condemnation of that system than might be thought at first glance. This statement is not meant to imply that medical care has no influence on health as measured by mortality rates, but rather that the rates are imperfect measures for the evaluation of medical care. Accordingly, planners, policymakers, and providers should be cautious in the use of such global measures as the sole basis for criticizing a health care system or recommending changes in it. This argument also applies to other measures of health that are affected by nonmedical factors.

While the above discussion sounds a cautionary note about the use of broad measures of health in assessing medical care, it is also important to note that a focus on very narrow, professionally defined technical measures of health might also cause distortion if they are used as the sole basis of evaluation. For example, triumphs in the treatment of congenital heart disease by surgery and the prevention of strokes through the treatment of high blood pressure are often cited as unequivocal examples of effective medical care. Even in these two areas of undisputed efficacy, however, there could be harmful effects if, for instance, people who do not have the disease were erroneously labeled.

The negative effect of medical care on the health of nondiseased persons was demonstrated in a study of 93 junior high school children in Seattle, Washington, who had notations in school records indicating the presence of a heart condition (6). On detailed examination of these students, only 18 had evidence of heart disease; the other 75 were probably misdiagnosed. In the latter group, 30 were significantly restricted either psychologically or physically. The result was that screening for cardiac disease that is potentially curable by surgery may have produced more disability among those with no disease than it cured in those with heart disease.

In another study, the effects of labeling were noted in a hypertensive screening program. Absenteeism significantly increased when persons were identified as hypertensive even though many had had documented but unlabeled elevated blood pressure before screening (7). If the program had used narrowly defined measures of program outcome, such as number of cases identified, this important effect would have been missed. After the demonstration of the labeling effect, another study has shown that special attention can partially offset the effect of labeling. These examples illustrate the importance of knowing the effects of medical care on the health of populations and being careful to select appropriate measures to assess health programs.

USE OF POPULATION-BASED RATES FOR ASSESSING QUALITY

An important and often neglected concern in assessing the quality of care by a system or institution is the use of measures that are directed at the entire population at risk rather than simply the users of services. The latter approach commonly implies assessment of care only for patients definitively diagnosed as having a specific disease (case rate analysis). The importance of using population-based rates (occurrence of diseases in populations) rather than case rates has always been accepted by epidemiologists concerned with "denominators." The point is vividly illustrated in assessing the effect of various organizations or hospitals on the disease appendicitis, which is frequently included in evaluations of care.

In cases of appendicitis, the dilemma confronting physicians is a choice between operating on patients who have abdominal pain at a time when the signs and symptoms are such that some of the patients may have a less serious, nonsurgical illness mimicking appendicitis versus waiting until the signs and symptoms are more definite and clearly indicate that an inflamed appendix is the cause of the pain. Unfortunately, if one waits too long, the inflamed appendix may perforate and produce peritonitis (a general inflammation and infection of the abdomen). The choice is between operating too early on some people with abdominal pain and removing some normal appendices versus operating too late and having a few patients with appendicitis progress to peritonitis. Recognition of this trade-off has led to acceptance of the fact that even the best surgeons will sometimes operate at a time when the diagnosis is not certain so as to decrease the number of perforations. This means that some people who have undergone surgery will be found to have a normal appendix. The optimum rate of such removals per 100 cases of true appendicitis has not been rigorously defined, but the implications of the trade-off have been discussed in detail (8).

In view of these considerations, the logical inference is that the evaluator could assess the results described in the operative and pathology reports to classify the proportion of a facility's cases that are either normal (unnecessary), or abnormal but not perforated (best result), or perforated—possibly reflecting unnecessary delay before surgery. The case rate for these outcomes has been used to judge the extent to which a hospital or provider organization acts to reduce unnecessary surgery without significantly increasing the risk of perforation. Interestingly, the natural course of appendicitis is such that not all abnormal appendices will perforate; rather, some will improve without specific therapy or surgical intervention. The possible fate of patients who have abdominal pain are represented in Figure 13-3. Surgical intervention is beneficial

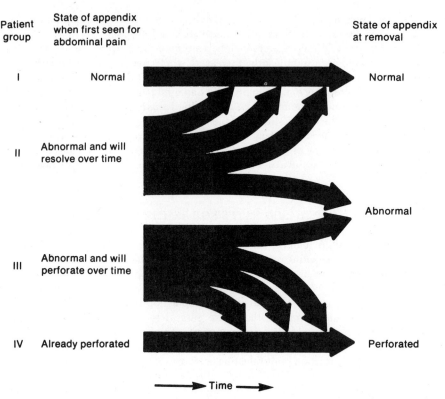

Figure 13-3. Changes in the condition of the appendix in patients with abdominal pain.

only to groups III and IV, in the former case to prevent perforation and in the latter to prevent continued leakage of bacteria into the abdomen by removing the source of the bacteria and draining any abscess that might be present. Note that in an absolutely biologic sense, all operations on patients in groups I and II are unnecessary. In assessing the performance of a provider, a crucial question is the extent to which physicians can differentiate between groups II and III. If they can, and if case rates are used, the relative sizes of those groups in any population will have a dramatic impact on the results of an assessment of care (Fig. 13-4).

Assume that two different medical organizations provide care to biologically similar populations of 100,000 people each. The staff in organization A cannot distinguish patients with abdominal pain who have abnormal appendices that are likely to perforate, either initially or after careful observation, from those patients whose abnormal appendices are not likely to perforate. Thus, they admit all such patients to the hospital and operate on them. The physicians in organization B can make this distinction and do not admit or operate on patients in group II. In addition, they are able to distinguish correctly all patients with normal appendices from those with abnormal ones and thus do not hospitalize or operate on anyone in group I. Analysis of operative case rates using only hospitalized patients would suggest that organization B is trading off lives (more than 50 percent higher death rate) for efficiency. On a population basis, however, organization B has exactly the same number of deaths as

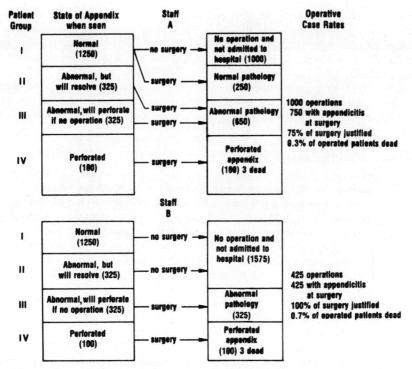

Figure 13-4. Hypothetical outcomes of care for two cohorts of 2000 patients each with abdominal pain managed under two different systems of care.

organization A and, in addition, performed less than one-half as many operations. A practical demonstration of this problem in evaluating health care has been described (9).

This illustration has implications for both quality assurance and cost-containment programs that are aimed at hospitals. For example, a hospital might respond to a cost-containment program by reducing admissions. An evaluation of the effect of that program on the quality of care may require a population-based assessment. Unfortunately, the identification of a hospital's denominator population is difficult, especially in large cities. Thus, one might need to identify areawide variations for all hospitals in a small area. The task is much easier when dealing with well-defined geographic areas served by only one hospital.

QUALITY ASSESSMENT IN HEALTH CARE

The following discussion shifts from health care for a population to the assessment of care at the level of the individual provider and patient. As noted in previous chapters, there are annually more than 1 billion visits to physicians in the United States. While some care might be for trivial reasons, most of it has potential for either enhancing or harming the health of patients. It is essential, therefore, to use knowledge of the assessment and assurance of the quality of care to help to achieve improved health. Most of the knowledge acquired thus far has been based on care given by physicians, but the general principles apply to care given by other health professionals, especially nurses (10–12).

Before discussing specific methods of assessing quality of care, it is important to note that certain general issues of sampling and measurement have major relevance for the conclusions that might be drawn from any assessment of the quality of care.

FOCUS OF ASSESSMENT

Before embarking on any assessment of the quality of care, it is important to state specifically why the assessment is being performed and what is its target, or focus. At the extreme, studies are undertaken either because of substantive concern about problems in quality that may exist or because of a requirement of a regulatory group to demonstrate ongoing analysis of the quality of care. This issue may seem trite, but numerous professional groups have found that studies undertaken because of a perceived problem in quality are far more likely to yield important results than are assessments that are done simply to satisfy the requirements of external agencies. Also, studies performed because of a substantive concern about quality will more likely have a clear focal point, which is important in considering what sample of care will be reviewed. In general, the focal point of studies will be either specific providers, care for specific conditions, or care received by selected groups of patients.

Provider-based studies (e.g., physicians or hospitals) involve sampling of either selected aspects of care given by all providers rendering that care or all the care given for a large number of conditions by only a few providers. The specific sample chosen will depend on whether one assumes that deficiencies in care are likely to be randomly distributed across all providers, or whether poor care is more likely to be associated with only a few providers. If the latter is assumed to be true, one might attempt to identify providers whose practice pattern with respect to the use of such items as laboratory tests, drugs, or number of visits characterizes them as "outliers" in comparison to their peers.

An alternative assessment strategy is to select random persons, independent of the nature of their diagnosed medical problems or their usual provider, and determine whether they have received appropriate care. This approach is particularly helpful in evaluating case finding for an asymptomatic disease that may benefit from early treatment. It has been incorporated into a population-based quality assessment strategy known as the *tracer method* (13).

Finally, the focus of a study may be a specific medical topic (e.g., a particular disease, a specific treatment, or provision of preventive care). The sampling unit for such studies is either all patients receiving care or all patients at risk. The former is more appropriate for assessment of errors of commission; the latter two are appropriate for detecting errors of omission.

SOURCES OF DATA FOR QUALITY ASSESSMENT

Data sources that can be used to study the quality of care are numerous and include direct observation, video or audio recordings of patient–provider contacts, direct interviews and examinations of patients, review of medical records, review of insurance claims forms, and review of public documents such as birth or death certificates.

MEASUREMENT ISSUES

After specifying the subject or sample frame, topic, and data source, there are measurement problems that must be considered. Included are issues of validity, reliability, sensitivity, and specificity.

VALIDITY AND RELIABILITY

The validity of a measure is the extent to which it actually assesses what it purports to measure. For instance, if a measure is supposed to reflect the quality of care, one would expect improvements in quality to affect the measure positively. In this regard, it has already been noted that death rates may not be valid measures of care for a variety of disease processes. For instance, deaths due to cancer of the pancreas are, at the present time, not a good indicator of quality of care for that disease because it tends to be generally incurable. In general, the most valid measures of the quality of medical care will be defined quite narrowly (e.g., the proportion of patients in a given practice who have uncontrolled blood pressure).

Reliability reflects the extent to which the same result occurs from repeated application of a measure to the same subject. Reliability has been of considerable interest at two levels: the reliability of clinical observations by professionals and the reliability of the judgments of quality as assessed by certain methods. The reliability of a clinicial observation can be determined by having the same observer repeat the same examination of the same subject (e.g., a repeat physical examination or a rereading of x-ray films) to determine if the same results (e.g., normal versus abnormal, getting better versus getting worse, need for a treatment versus no need for treatment) are obtained. This phenomenon is termed *intraobserver reliability.*

A second method involves having different observers review the same subject and compare the results of the observations made. This phenomenon is termed *interobserver reliability* and is similar to what occurs in second-opinion surgery programs in which more than one surgeon determines whether surgery is indicated. The results of observer-reliability testing have generally demonstrated poor levels of reliability of clinician-based data and judgments (14). For example, substantial lack of reliability has been shown for such information as whether patients have a heart murmur, or a diagnosis of coronary artery disease, or whether they should have a certain elective surgical procedure. The order of magnitude of such disagreements varies from 5 to 40 percent using conventional reliability tests. When more sophisticated (kappa statistic) tests are performed, the results are even more disquieting. The advanced method adjusts for the expected distribution of agreement based on chance alone (14). The implications of these problems in the reliability of clinical observations have not been adequately explored, and most methods of assessing quality assume that clinical observations are correct.

RELIABILITY OF SECONDARY DATA SOURCES

Assuming that clinical observations are reliable, the next level of concern is the recording of data and its incorporation into data systems useful for quality assessment purposes. This process includes entering data into the medical record by providers, followed by abstracting or synthesis of that information by medical records personnel. Abstracts include discharge diagnoses listed on the cover or summary sheets of medical records, summary abstracts such as those prepared for the Commission on Professional and Hospital Activities, insurance claims forms, and hospital discharge summaries; these abstracted sources are termed *secondary* data. There have been very few studies of what bias occurs when the events occurring in a patient-provider encounter are recorded in the medical record. Studies have compared tape recordings of medical encounters to determine the extent to which the physician's notes of these encounters reflected the verbal content (15). Significant underrecording occurred and was most pronounced for information relating to patient education and number of pills prescribed. A study of patients undergoing tonsillectomy and/or adenoidectomy indicated that phrases in hospital records such as "frequent" and "numerous" episodes of tonsillitis were open to considerable variation in interpretation when compared to the actual disease experiences of the patients (16).

It is assumed that there is greater discordance between actual care provided and that recorded in office settings as compared to such discordance in inpatient settings. Indeed, one large study of office care provided for children documented numerous deficiencies in recording and found that more than half of the physicians felt that their records did not adequately reflect the care they provided (17).

Finally, with respect to data reliability, there is concern over information that is routinely abstracted from medical records and recorded on magnetic computer tapes. Studies conducted by the Institute of Medicine of the National Academy of Sciences assessed the reliability of hospital discharge diagnostic data and showed major disagreements on such critical information as principal diagnosis (18). As a result, concern has been raised regarding the utility of such data for many quality assessment programs. These studies do not negate the utility of such data systems for identifying possible areas for more intensive review at the individual case level. Reliable judgments of the quality of care at the individual level (either patient or physician) may require the use of the medical record, however, except for those few providers whose practice patterns are so deviant from the norm that problems such as those discussed above are inconsequential.

EVALUATING METHODS USED TO ASSESS QUALITY OF CARE

The sensitivity, specificity, and predictive value of methods of quality assessment have major implications for the efficiency of quality of review procedures. To illustrate these concepts, assume the presence of an omniscient quality assessor who knows whether or not people are sick, what happens to them, and what the relative contribution of medical care is to improving their illness. Such an assessor would provide a "gold standard" for true judgments against which other methods of assessing quality could be compared. If a new method of identifying cases of bad-quality care were proposed, a comparison of the new and true methods would result in a distribution of cases into four categories (Fig. 13-5). The sensitivity of the new method represents the extent to

Results by "New" Method	Results by "True" Method	
	Bad care	Good care
Bad care	a	b
Good care	c	d

Figure 13-5. Testing a new method of assessing the quality of care.

which it identifies all true cases of bad quality; in this case, sensitivity $= a/(a+c)$. Specificity reflects the extent to which cases that are classified as good by the test actually are good; specificity $= d/(b+d)$. At the operational level, methods that have high sensitivity and specificity are desirable. In general, increases in the sensitivity of a method achieved by loosening the criteria for bad versus good care, without changing the method itself, will tend to decrease the specificity of the method.

The concepts of positive or negative predictive value of a method are also of interest. In Figure 13-5 the new method attempts to identify bad care as indicated by a positive test result. The positive predictive value of the test is the probability that a positive result by the new method reflects a positive result by the true method; the positive predictive value $= a/(a+b)$. The accurate reflection of a negative result yields a negative predictive value $= d/(c+d)$.

Knowledge of these characteristics of a method for assessing quality of care helps one to use such methods. If the primary goal of an assessment of quality is to identify all episodes of bad care, then highest priority should be given to increasing the sensitivity of the method used. If a primary goal is to lower the cost of identifying a case of bad care, then the specificity or positive predictive value of the method is emphasized.

QUALITY ASSESSMENT METHODS

The preceding discussion sets the stage for presenting the categories of measures of quality that can be monitored. The selection and design criteria outlined above are generic and apply to all measures of the quality of care. Quality of care measures generally fall into one of three categories: (1) outcome measures that reflect the results or impact of care (e.g., changes in health status), (2) process measures that reflect what was done (e.g., number and types of laboratory tests performed), and (3) structural measures that reflect the setting in which care is provided (e.g., licensure of personnel or facilities).

OUTCOME MEASURES OF QUALITY

Outcomes of care reflect the net changes that occur in health status as a result of health care and are appealing because of their face validity; their use in assessing care has been extensively reviewed elsewhere (19,20). As discussed previously, many factors affect health. Therefore, if outcomes are to be used as an indicator of the quality of care, they must be sensitive to different levels in the quality of the process or content of care; that is, outcomes should change when the process changes.

The two major groups of outcome measures are general health status indicators and disease-specific indicators. A general health status measure is multidimensional and may include physical, emotional, and social aspects of health. The measures can be based on one's own perception of one's health or on independent assessments that do not rely on the patient's own perceptions (21–24). An example of a health status measure that relies on self-reported perceptions and covers several dimensions of health is the Sickness Impact Profile (25). This profile is an index based on patients' responses to a series of statements such as (1) I am going out less to visit people; (2) I do not walk at all; (3) I often act irritable toward my work associates, for example, snap at them, give sharp answers, criticize easily; (4) I am doing less of the regular daily work around the house than I usually do; and (5) I stop often when traveling because of health problems. Changes in these aspects of an individual's function can be produced by a variety of diseases.

General health status indicators have the advantage of reflecting changes in several dimensions of health that might not be detected by technically derived, disease-specific measures (e.g., changes in blood pressure level). They have the disadvantage of possibly being too sensitive to nonmedical factors. For instance, in assessing outcomes of care for an operation to fuse a spine because of back pain, a general health status instrument might detect deficiencies in work productivity and in the emotional state of the patient, but there are many factors other than the surgery that could affect a patient's productivity and propensity to depression.

Disease-specific outcome indicators include death rates due to a given disease, the presence of symptoms known to occur with a disease, or behavioral disabilities commonly associated with a specified disease. For example, in patients with coronary artery disease, assessments could be based on deaths from heart attacks, on the number of people with symptomatic chest pain on exertion, or on the avoidance of specific work or social activities by patients with heart disease due to fears of incurring a heart attack.

Data on many outcome measures must be obtained directly from patients because such data may not be recorded in the medical record. Obtaining reliable outcome information by either a self-administered or an interviewer-administered questionnaire may be expensive, and the cost may limit the usefulness of the outcome methods on a routine basis.

Outcome measures can be used in operational settings to assess quality of care. At the very least, adverse outcomes related to treatment can be monitored as indicators of suboptimal quality (e.g., infections after surgery). Similarly, while 5 years may have to elapse before one can determine if survivors of a surgical procedure have better or worse than expected death rates, immediate (within a short time period) surgical mortality can be used as an indicator of poor technical quality for such procedures as gastrectomies for patients with stomach cancer or replacement of heart valves in patients with rheumatic heart disease. Before passing judgment on such mortality data, however, the severity of illness in the patients treated must be considered, as was done in a study of the variation by hospitalization in surgical death rates (26). In this study, unadjusted death rates for various operations varied fivefold across study hospitals, but the differences were generally less than twofold after adjustments for case severity were made.

In addition to the use of treatment-related adverse outcome measures, quality of care can be reflected in intermediate outcomes that are known to relate to a final outcome that is a goal of care. For example, the treatment for high blood pressure seeks to avoid the future occurrence of stroke, heart attack, or heart failure by lowering blood pressure. Rather than waiting 10–14 years to determine if the incidence of stroke or heart failure has been altered by a treatment program, an intermediate outcome can be measured. In this case, one could assess the extent to which blood pressure has been reduced to levels that are known to be associated with a lower long-term probability of stroke or heart failure.

The use of intermediate outcomes is inherent in the staging approach to assessing quality of ambulatory care (27). This technique is very useful in the diagnosis of cancer, since death rates from certain cancers are related to how advanced the disease is at the time of detection. Many cancers should be detectable at an early stage if the quality of ambulatory care is high. The stage of a cancer is reflected in pathology, laboratory, and x-ray reports, and presumably a good-quality ambulatory care program will identify tumors at an early stage (i.e., the intermediate outcome) and improve long-term survival.

PROCESS MEASURES OF QUALITY

The process of care, as defined by Donabedian, refers to what is done to patients (28). DeGeyndt has elaborated this concept into the notion of the content of care (i.e., activities performed) and uses the word "process" to denote the sequence and coordination of these activities (29). A further refinement of the concept separates the technical aspects of care from the affective and interpersonal skills (how the patient was treated) implied in the art of care (30).

The use of process measures has considerable attraction because they are operationally much easier to collect than outcome measures. Specifically, they are less time dependent and less dependent on expensive patient follow-up studies because the medical record, despite its imperfections, does reflect certain processes of care reasonably well. Most of the process approaches to assessing care depend on the establishment of agreed-on criteria for good care and the application of these criteria to individual cases.

The most common process method used is based on the development of a list of elements of good care and on whether or not these elements are documented in the medical record. Physicians frequently argue that they do not think in checklist fashion or, more perjoratively, in a "laundry list" format. Instead, they argue correctly that in making decisions they use a contingency-based format that considers case severity, test results, and the presence or absence of certain signs and symptoms. Accordingly, simple checklists may not be the optimal or most relevant means of assessing the process of care.

An approach to assessing the process of care that more closely mirrors clinical decision making is the criteria-mapping approach (31). In this approach, criteria for good care can be met in a variety of ways depending on the presence or absence of certain signs, symptoms, laboratory test results, or more general reflections of case severity. The criteria-mapping approach should be as sensitive in detecting poor care as the list, but should also be more specific. Additionally, it may afford the possibility of identifying excess use of certain tests or procedures that should be done only in very selected circumstances. A comparison of criteria that might be used by these two approaches is shown in Table 13-1.

While assessment of the process of care is inherently attractive, several criticisms have been voiced about the use of process measures. The most common criticism is that outcomes should be of most concern, and few studies have demonstrated a strong relationship between the process and the outcome of care. While this contention is often correct, there are several biologic and methodologic reasons for this failure. The biologic explanation is that not all health care is necessarily efficacious. Accordingly, variations in the process of care will not alter outcomes. For example, in past years, many surgeons might have listed radical mastectomy as an element of good process for treating breast cancer. But this procedure is not clearly superior to a simple mastectomy, and no difference in outcomes may be measured for patients who had either a good or suboptimal process. Examples of process criteria for good care that have not been validated are numerous, including time-honored exhortations such as requiring all patients with sore throats to have a throat culture before antibiotic therapy is started (32).

There are also conceptual and methodologic deficiencies in those studies that demonstrate low (or even negative) correlations between process and outcome. The choice of the strategy used to assess the quality of care is critical; a strategy that emphasizes diagnosis rather than treatment ignores those aspects of process that are most proximate to determining a good outcome. For example, hypertension is a treatable condition, and therapy for it is efficacious. In more than 90 percent of treated cases, hypertension is *not* due to a readily identifiable etiology, yet it will respond to therapy. Process-oriented studies of the quality of care given to hypertensive patients frequently focus on the degree to which physicians establish the level of end-organ

TABLE 13-1. Comparison of Lists and Mapping Approaches for Assessing the Process of Care: Hypothetical Criteria for Diagnostic Tests in Patients with Newly Discovered Hypertension

Checklist Approach	Illustrative Criteria-Mapping Approach
Abdominal examination for bruits	Abdominal examination for bruits
Serum potassium level	Serum potassium level
Serum bicarbonate level	Serum bicarbonate level
Fasting glucose level	Fasting glucose level
Test of catecholamine or vanillylmandelic acid excretion for pheochromocytoma	Test for pheochromocytoma only if there is a history of palpitations, weight loss, elevated fasting glucose level, orthostatic drop in blood pressure without treatment, or a family history of this tumor
Plasma renin or intravenous pyelogram to rule out renal artery stenosis	Test for renal artery stenosis only if there is one of the following: abdominal or flank bruit, serum potassium less than 3.6 mEq/L or bicarbonate level greater than 28 mEq/L

damage when a hypertensive patient is identified, and the extent to which a differential diagnositc strategy is pursued to identify those few patients with a specific etiology for their hypertension. A more critical factor in changing outcomes, however, is whether an anithypertensive drug is prescribed. For the vast majority of patients, an antihypertensive drug is more important in determining whether blood pressure is lowered than a laboratory test to detect rare causes of hypertension. Accordingly, unless much greater weight is attached to initiation of therapy than to ruling out a rare diagnosis, there will be very little positive correlation between process and outcome assessments of the quality of care.

The use of criteria for good care that are process oriented but not of proven efficacy in operational quality assurance programs may result in the increased use of unnecessary tests and drugs without any improvement in outcome. Much of the concern about using a process-oriented approach can be alleviated if it is employed primarily to identify a lack of optimal process in cases with known poor outcomes, (e.g., use of antihypertensive drugs in patients with uncontrolled hypertension) or to discourage the use of practices that are known to be harmful (e.g., most applications of chloramphenicol in ambulatory care).

The lack of definitive studies on efficacy of some clinical strategies does not require that they be excluded from a quality of care study. Practicing physicians should not be expected to conduct basic research to demonstrate conclusively the efficacy of a procedure that overwhelming professional opinion already believes is appropriate to use; that should be the role of academic research centers. This reiterates the fundamentals of good care developed 50 years ago by Lee and Jones (33):

Good medical care is the kind of medicine practiced and taught by recognized leaders of the medical profession at a given time and period of social, cultural, and professional development in a community or population group . . . The concept of good medical care . . . is based upon certain "articles of faith" which can be briefly stated:

1. Good medical care is limited to the practice of rational medicine based on the medical sciences . . .

2. Good medical care emphasizes prevention . . .

3. Good medical care requires intelligent cooperation between the lay public and the practitioners of scientific medicine . . .

4. Good medical care treats the individual as a whole . . . . Good practice requires that the patient be considered as a person, a member of a family living in a certain environment. All factors which concern his [her] health—mental and emotional, as well as physiological—must be weighed in diagnosis, prevention, and treatment. It is the sick or injured person and not merely the pathologic condition which must be treated . . .

5. Good medical care maintains a close and continuing personal relationship between physician and patient . . .

6. Good medical is coordinated with social welfare, work . . . love of [people] must be clarified by an understanding of [people] and must take note of his [her] social environment and economic needs . . .

7. Good medical care coordinates all types of medical services . . .

8. Good medical care implies application of all the necessary services of modern scientific medicine to the needs of all the people. Judged from the viewpoints of society as a whole, the qualitative aspects of medical care cannot be dissociated from the quantitative. No matter what the perfection of technique of one individual case, medicine does not fulfill its functions adequately until the same perfection is within reach of all individuals.

STRUCTURAL MEASURES OF QUALITY

Measures of the structure of care relate to the personnel and facilities used to provide services and the manner in which they are organized. Examples of structural measures of care are presented in Table 13-2.

From an administrative viewpoint, structural assessments are attractive because much of the information they require can be readily obtained from existing documents or a simple inspection of a facility. Assessments based solely on the structure of care assume that if the structure is optimal, then the appropriate processes will necessarily follow and outcomes will be maximized. The assumptions underlying many structural criteria, however, have not been validated. For example, consider the criterion of whether or not the physicians in a hospital are board certified. Presumably physicians with longer training programs who become board certified in their specialty will treat diseases related to that specialty better than noncertified physicians. Much medical training, however, is oriented toward teaching the process of care as best known at the time of training. Because the presumed best process of care 10 years ago may not now result in the best outcome, board-certified status may not be a powerful prediction of quality of care.

There is also some evidence that better-qualified physicians do not necessarily perform at a substantially higher level, that is, have higher process scores, than similarly trained physicians who are not board certified. A large study in Hawaii showed that self-declared specialists tended to treat diseases related to their specialty better than nonspecialists, but it also found little difference in the quality of care provided by physicians with formal board certification in a specialty versus those who were self-identified specialists, but not board certified (34). This example is especially pertinent in view of recent trends stressing board certification as an indicator of quality in consumer's guides to choosing a physician, and as a mechanism to control the number of unnecessary surgical procedures. The objective of making all physicians board certified could increase the total costs of care for society substantially, with only a marginal effect on the quality of care, and perhaps no positive effect on outcomes. Similar concerns can be raised in regard to many other structural criteria for good care,

TABLE 13-2. Examples of Structural Measures of Quality

Resource	Illustrative Criteria
Facility	Does it meet fire and safety codes? Is it clean?
Personnel	Are the physicians licensed? Are the physicians board certified? Is the ratio of registered nurses to practical nurses over 0.3? Is the ratio of nurses to patients over 0.2?
Organization	Is there an organizational structure with clearly defined responsibility? Is there a mechanism for peer review?

including an increased interest in having only nurses with baccalaureate training be eligible for licensure as registered nurses.

Do limitations of structural measures mean that they should not be included as an element of a quality assessment or assurance program? While reliance on structural criteria does not guarantee that good processes and outcomes will follow, some level of structure must be obtained in areas such as professional responsibility, peer review, and life safety if good processes are to occur. Good structure is a necessary but not sufficient correlate of good care.

EFFICIENCY AND QUALITY

Efficiency of care reflects how much care of a given quality is provided for a specified cost, and can be expressed as net outcomes achieved per unit of cost. With concern over the rising costs of health care in relation to the gross national product (Chapter 11), increasing attention has been directed toward inefficient use of resources as reflected by such terms as *inappropriate hospitalization, unnecessary surgery,* and *defensive medicine.* A hypothesized relationship between costs and outcomes is presented in Figure 13-6. Initial investments in care produce rapid increases in positive outcomes (zone A). When only difficult and costly problems are left to be overcome, there is little and eventually no increase in positive outcomes from further investments (zone B). Finally, a negative slope could even occur in one of two ways (zone C). First, direct application of increased medical care at very intensive levels might produce more iatrogenic injury than benefit. Second, costs of care could become so high that resources that might be used to produce health through means other than medical care are diverted to medical care. Thus, auto safety devices may not be produced in favor of investments in medical care that product less impact on health. Note, however, that Figure 13-6 is very simplistic. A more complex figure would have a series of curves that takes account of the multidimensional nature of the outcome of care, (e.g., disability days, symptoms status, mortality) and relates each of these outcomes to costs of care.

Because outcomes are multidimensional, even a simple disease process produces a

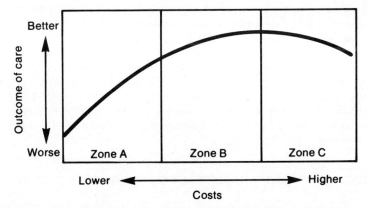

Figure 13-6. Hypothetical relationship between the outcomes and costs of care.

family of efficiency curves rather than a single curve; the trade-offs of favoring one efficiency curve over another must be understood. For example, two outcomes of interest in the management of high blood pressure might be work status and age-specific death rate. There is no question that investing more resources in the identification and adequate treatment of all hypertensives would reduce overall cardiovascular age-specific death rates. There may be, however, high rates of work loss in treated patients secondary to the psychologic effects of being labeled hypertensive, or because of complications of therapy such as depression. These latter effects occur when treated patients are in their third or fourth decade of life, while reduction in death rate might not occur until the fifth decade of life. The net effect might be substantially more disability days in a treated as compared to an untreated population in order to achieve a reduction in strokes and heart failure in later life. Many people who would never have had a stroke or heart failure are treated to prevent these events that will occur in some hypertensives. For those individuals who would never have developed a stroke or congestive heart failure, the treatment may have a negative effect on physical health. Unfortunately, trade-offs such as these are common in current medical practice and will need to be considered in efforts to improve the quality of care. Donabedian and colleagues have presented an integrated framework relating quality, costs, and health outcomes (35).

EFFICIENCY AND PROVIDER–PATIENT RELATIONSHIP

There has been considerable interest in increasing efficiency in recent years. When efficiency is stressed, providers must play a larger role of social police officer vis-à-vis their role of patient advocate. This shift in emphasis has substantial implications for patient–provider relationships, especially under prepayment arrangements.

For example, a physician may know that fewer than one out of 100 patients with adult-onset seizures have a treatable form of brain tumor. The physician may also know that certain associated signs and symptoms make that possibility more or less likely. The physician cannot determine with absolute certainty, however, whether a given patient is, or is not, that one in 100. It is unethical for the physician to tell the patient that there is a 100 percent likelihood that there is no serious and treatable problem. How many tests and what expense should be incurred to determine if the patient is the rare one with a treatable disease? What should be the provider's response to a patient who says, "Look, Doc, I'm fully covered by insurance, and I'd like you to order a computerized axial tomography scan for me because I just want to be sure?" These and similar questions have no simple answer, and they pose major ethical dilemmas for professionals entrusted with the dual functions of advocate and police officer. These dilemmas may prove to be too uncomfortable to place major emphasis on cost cutting in the individual patient–physician encounter. Rather, the emphasis might be placed at the institutional or payer level (e.g., restriction of benefits), so that patients and physicians do not develop a somewhat adversarial relationship concerning provision of certain services.

PATIENT SATISFACTION AND THE QUALITY OF CARE

Patient satisfaction is a measure that can reflect the outcome, process, and structure of care. Satisfaction has been viewed as a multidimensional concept involving the cost, convenience, technical and interpersonal aspects of care, and outcome of care (36,37). Satisfaction with care can be assessed for a specific illness episode, for a patient's personal care, or for medical care in general. From a technical medical perspective, satisfaction is important because it is positively correlated with patient adherence to prescribed therapeutic regimens. It may positively affect subsequent care-seeking behavior, and probably has some impact on the propensity to file a malpractice claim.

At any point in time, using existing measures, the overwhelming majority (usually more than 85 percent) of people are satisfied with their own health care. The level of satisfaction may appear to be high because most patients finally find a provider who meets their needs after a long odyssey, or because existing measures are not sensitive to all components of satisfaction. However, despite the generally high rate of satisfaction with most aspects of personal medical care, there is room for improvement, especially in the areas of interpersonal aspects of care and costs of care.

ACCESS TO CARE

Access to care, which has been discussed in earlier chapters, is an important element of quality assessment at the programmatic and social levels. Access to care as a dimension of quality at the individual provider level is more difficult to conceptualize and measure. A provider who agrees to be a regular source of primary care for a panel (those patients who identify that provider as their regular source of care) should be responsible for assuring access to services for those patients. Poor access may be reflected in delayed care seeking, absence of preventive care, and low patient satisfaction. Whether equity of access for all members of society is a measure of quality at the individual provider level is an unresolved issue. This issue includes questions about the extent to which individual providers should be accountable for assuring access to care by working longer hours, treating more patients, working more efficiently, or encouraging or actively seeking out potential patients with limited access to care, as reflected in the types of measures presented in Chapter 3.

A provider's patterns of practice can markedly affect access to care, and studies of physicians in group practices show large variations in the number of patients per physician and number of visits per patient despite relatively similar populations of patients (38). In the absence of optimal visit schedules for acute and chronic illnesses by which such data could be judged, it is difficult to determine which physicians are practicing better medicine or are requiring too many or too few follow-up visits. If providers who treat widely varying numbers of patients have similar outcomes, there should be considerable concern about the relationships among efficiency, quality, and access to care.

ILLUSTRATIVE STUDIES OF THE QUALITY OF CARE

The quality of care assessment literature has expanded rapidly in the past three decades. Selected major studies performed since 1950 are highlighted here for illustration purposes.

OUTCOME-ORIENTED STUDIES

Outcome-oriented studies have been based on death certificates, face-to-face and telephone interviews with patients, medical records, and secondarily abstracted medical records. Shapiro and associates studied the quality of care under two different organizational systems in New York by analyzing the perinatal mortality of infants born to low-income women (39). Their findings indicated a lower death rate for those infants whose mothers were enrolled in a prepaid practice plan. The study highlights the importance of defining a denominator population and raises several issues concerning epidemiologic and statistical adjusting procedures when dealing with problems of selection bias in quality of care studies based on outcome measures.

Forrest and associates studied the outcome of surgical care in 17 hospitals by making direct assessments of the status of patients during a 40-day postoperative period (26). They found significant variations across hospitals, with death rates that were nearly twice as high in the worst as compared to the best hospital in the sample. This study is important because it illustrates the need to adjust for case severity. Forrest and associates also found that the use of data from a medical abstracting service as opposed to a direct assessment produced results with similar trends but not similar magnitudes. This means that with proper adjustments for such factors as case mix, hospitals with unusually adverse outcome rates can potentially be identified for further investigation by means of analysis of data collected by a medical abstracting service. Additionally, the study identified some organizational features of hospitals that might be associated with better care (40). For example, both stringent control over membership on the surgical staff and the ratio of registered nurses to other nurses were positively related to better outcomes of care. Interestingly, teaching status, size of medical staff, and board certification of surgeons were not significantly correlated with quality of care. Because of the nature of the study, a causal relationship between these structural features and outcomes of care could not be inferred, but prospective studies using this information are clearly in order.

An analysis of death rates for selected surgical procedures was carried out by Luft using Medicare data. He demonstrated a significant association between better outcomes with higher volumes of procedures for some operations, but not for others (41,42). While the analyses were hindered by limited measures of case severity, and inadequate sample size for procedures with very low expectations of death, the data for several major surgical procedures do support the notion of better outcomes in institutions that have greater experience with selected procedures.

Kessner and associates conducted a population-based study of the quality of ambulatory care for children using the outcome-oriented tracer method (43). They assessed outcomes for iron deficiency, ear infection, and vision correction. The study sample consisted of 1436 families with 2780 children aged 6 months to 11 years in Washington, D.C. More than 25 percent of the children aged 6 months to 3 years had anemia, 20 percent had ear disease, and nearly 25 percent of those aged 4–11 failed a vision screening test. After controlling for the social class of the patients, no significant correlation between outcome and type of provider organization was found. Inappropriate or ineffective treatment was provided to a large proportion of children in the sample. Subsequent analyses of the same data did suggest different outcomes among different providers using a finer categorization of providers (44). In particular, it was suggested that outcomes were poorest among patients of solo practitioners.

Schroeder and Donaldson applied the outcome-oriented method known as *health accounting* to a Health Maintenance Organization (45). This method was developed by Williamson and requires a consensus estimate of what outcomes are achievable with specific interventions. The extent to which the outcomes achieved deviate from expected outcomes is then determined. The outcome assessment can usually be performed by telephone survey or mailed questionnaire. Applied to the diagnoses of depression, high blood pressure, and contraception, the method revealed major problems of underdiagnosis for all the conditions (44–74 percent) and unacceptable therapeutic outcomes for depression and high blood pressure. The operational difficulties for using this outcome-based method in ambulatory facilities delivering care to large numbers of disadvantaged people were also emphasized.

Intermediate outcomes have been assessed from medical records in several studies. Gonnella and colleagues applied the staging approach to hospitalized patients as an outcome measure of the quality of their ambulatory medical care (27). They studied 5000 patients admitted to hospitals in two cities in California. For six of the 18 conditions studied, they showed significant differences in the stages of disease present at the time of hospitalization in patients from various population groups. Disease was generally more severe in patients with government sponsorship other than Medicare.

PROCESS-ORIENTED STUDIES

Process-oriented studies can be conducted by direct observation of medical encounters, review of medical records, and review of insurance claims. Observational studies provide a wealth of information not otherwise obtainable, but suffer from high cost and potential alteration of behavior resulting from the presence of an observer. These problems notwithstanding, a few observational studies of process have been completed, the most noteworthy of which in the United States was a study of 88 general practitioners in North Carolina by Peterson and associates in 1953 (46). They developed a semistructured review protocol that included observable elements of history taking, physical diagnosis, use of laboratory services, preventive care, and clinical record keeping. In addition to an index score based on these observations, the authors developed a 5-point qualitative ranking system. With the ranking system, 8 percent of the physicians were in rank 5 (essentially outstanding) and 18 percent in rank 1. The physicians in rank 1 had a very superficial, disorganized approach to clinical medicine. Overall, 39 of the 88 physicians were in rank 1 or 2. This study was of considerable importance because it showed the feasibility of carrying out direct observations of practicing physicians in their offices and demonstrated major deficiencies in the level of care in office settings. The study also highlighted the need to assess the quality of care in an organized manner.

There have been numerous large-scale process-oriented studies of hospital and ambulatory care using medical records. In his pioneering work in Monroe County, New York, Lembcke identified numerous deficiencies in care given to patients undergoing hysterectomies (47). Similar findings were noted by Doyle in a study of more than 6000 hysterectomies in the Los Angeles area (48). More recently, major problems in surgery judged to be unnecessary by process criteria were noted in a population-based study of hysterectomies in Saskatchewan (49). McCarthy and Widmer have identified potentially unnecessary surgery in nearly one-third of patients recommended for a variety of elective procedures in a second surgical opinion program (50). They and others have found reductions in surgery after starting such programs, but the significance of the results is not yet clear.

In one of the largest studies of the process of care, Payne and Lyons found numerous deficiencies in care provided to patients admitted to hospitals in Hawaii. This study was based on a random sample of all hospital patients in the state who had selected discharge diagnoses in 1968 (34). A group of practicing physicians established criteria for good care that were then applied to the hospital records. For each disease, a physician's performance index (PPI) was developed that represented the percentage of process criteria (e.g., performance of certain laboratory tests) for which evidence of compliance could be found in the medical records. Overall, they found a PPI of 0.71 for hospitalized patients. In a companion study of office-based care in 1970, they found an average PPI of only 0.40 (34). These studies are important demonstrations of the feasibility of carrying out large-scale quality assessments. They have identified several organizational and structural features that tend to be associated with good care, even though the correlations were relatively low.

In addition to studies using direct observation or medical record review, the process of care has been studied through the use of claims forms. In Tennessee, Ray and associates established criteria for the appropriate use of certain drugs and applied them to claims data (51). Their first analysis was concerned with cholarmphenicol, a broad-spectrum antibiotic that can cause death due to agranulocytosis (absence of white cells necessary to fight infection). The use of this drug has been recommended only for serious, well-defined infections for which there are no reasonable therapeutic alternatives. The analysis indicated that nearly 6 percent of all antibiotic prescriptions filled by pharmacies were for this drug, and it was prescribed by 6 percent of the physicians participating in the Tennessee Medicaid program. About half of the prescriptions were for upper-respiratory-tract infections, for which the drug is never indicated. Most of the remaining prescriptions were also inappropriate. This study is important because it documented the ability to identify inappropriate practice patterns by analysis of claims data. In a similar study, Brook and colleagues analyzed the use of injectable antibiotics in Medicaid patients in New Mexico and showed that claims data could identify physicians whose practice patterns were both atypical and inappropriate (52). They further showed that practice patterns could be altered by the use of an ongoing monitoring system with feedback to physicians whose practice patterns were at variance with established and accepted standards.

QUALITY ASSURANCE IN MEDICAL CARE

The application of quality assessment methods in assuring acceptable care to patients is of considerable concern to providers. *Quality assurance* refers to those activities that are designed to guarantee, in part, that the care received meets reasonable professional standards. In general, there are two major mechanisms that serve this purpose: structure-oriented systems, or systems that actively monitor the events and outcomes of the care actually provided. The notion of assurance implies that when deficiencies occur, they will be corrected in some way, ultimately by changing physician behavior. As will be discussed below, our understanding of how to alter physician behavior is fragmentary, but there is accumulating evidence that some strategies are effective.

STRUCTURE-ORIENTED APPROACHES TO
QUALITY ASSURANCE: LICENSURE

The most pervasive, oldest, and most fundamental assurance mechanism is licensure. With rare but highly publicized exceptions, licensure assures a patient that a physician or nurse has a specified level of educational achievement relevant to the profession. For physician licensure, states require graduation in good standing from a recognized medical school, passing of a state-required examination or its equivalent (e.g., examinations offered by the National Board of Medical Examiners), no record of conviction for any major crime (such as a felony), and letters of recommendation from other licensed physicians. In addition, virtually all states require the applicant to have completed an accredited internship program. Persons not meeting these requirements are denied the right to practice their profession legally in a defined geographic area. In essence, the licensing mechanism sets a floor on the quality of the personnel available to provide care.

It is interesting to note that in professional licensure, the licensing body represents public interests, but the determination of whether certain schools are acceptable often lies (to a great extent) in the hands of nonpublic groups. In this instance, the accreditation of a given medical school is determined by a mixture of academic and professional organizations. This arrangement has raised the question of whether an organization representing professional interests, such as the American Medical Association, should have any direct or indirect influence in determining whether certain training programs are accredited because potential conflicts of interest might exist.

Licensure mechanisms are very general in relation to actual professional practice. For example, most physicians' licenses state only that they are physicians and surgeons; in theory, they are allowed to perform any act within the scope of medical practice. Accordingly, they could attempt procedures that they had not been specifically trained to do. For instance, there is great concern about the use of potentially toxic chemotherapeutic drugs in cancer patients by physicians not trained in this area. In view of such concern, the general nature of licensing laws may represent a substantial weakness. Because of this weakness, one could argue for the passage of limited licensure laws that would restrict surgery to those with surgical training in accredited programs, or the use of cancer drugs to oncologists. Obviously, such laws would be complex to administer and might reduce some of the highly beneficial flexibility given to practicing physicians. They presumably would, however, also prevent uncommon but egregious abuse of the medical license. Whether they would produce more good than harm is an open question.

A further weakness of licensure has been its static nature, although this situation appears to be changing in many states. Once licensed, individuals need only send in a fee on a regular basis, indicate that they had not been convicted of a felony in the past year, and provide other minimal information about themselves to be relicensed. Given the rapid changes in medical knolwedge and practice, it has been proposed that professionals should demonstrate evidence of up-to-date knowledge to be licensed. This concern has led to the development of relicensure requirements by which the individual must show proof of a certain amount of continuing medical education (CME). For instance, in several states, physicians must be able to document 150 hours of CME every 3 years to be relicensed. These CME credits can be obtained through attendance at special courses, teaching, independent study, and similar activities.

While mandatory CME resolves some of the problems inherent in what amounts to lifetime licensure, it does not resolve those related to the general nature of the license itself and, more seriously, does not address the failure of structural mechanisms to guarantee the appropriateness of care.

A few states (e.g., Washington) have strengthened their licensure systems through the establishment of medical disciplinary boards that have the power to revoke or severely restrict the licenses of physicians who are found to be impaired due to alcoholism or drug abuse, or who are involved in several malpractice cases or in professional misconduct.

Licensure has also been applied to hospitals and long-term care institutions. In general, such licenses heavily emphasize physical structure with a modicum of required organization structure. To the extent that medical care is provided in organized settings, institutional licensure represents a pervasive mechanism that can contribute to assuring the quality of care; however, given the present form of most licensing mechanisms, this potential might not be realized.

CERTIFICATION AND ACCREDITATION

The second most pervasive structural assurance mechanism has been voluntary professional certification and accreditation. For physicians, this procedure consists of certification by specialty boards that require completion of at least 3 years of postgraduate training and the passage of a special examination. Several specialty boards also require 1 or more years of practice and after completion of residency training and/or submission of a series of records of actual cases for review by members of the board.

Specialty certification goes one step beyond licensure in setting minimal standards of quality for the provider's training and knowledge; however, it has limitations similar to those of licensure. As in the case of relicensure, there has been a trend toward mandatory periodic recertification of many specialty boards to assure updating of knowledge. While recertification tends to be structure oriented and based on tests of knowledge, at least one board, the Academy of Family Practice, requires that records of selected cases be submitted for review.

Accreditation through the Joint Commission on Accreditation of Hospitals (JCAH) is the most pervasive and influential accreditation mechanism (see also Chapter 6). The JCAH functions as an independent accrediting body, with representation from the American Hospital Association, the American Medical Association, the American College of Surgery, the American College of Physicians and the American Dental Association.

For many years, the JCAH emphasized a structural approach to quality assurance, with formal requirements for such matters as the organizational framework of hospitals, adequacy of medical records, safety standards, a requirement for periodic review of tissue removed at surgery, hospital infections, and mortality reviews. In more recent years, the actual accreditation process has required demonstration of ongoing performance-based assessments of quality, including documentation that any deficiencies found were specifically corrected.

At the present time, the JCAH reviews the extent to which hospitals meet its quality assurance standard, which states: "There shall be evidence of a well-defined, organized program designed to enhance patient care thorugh the ongoing objective assessment of important aspects of patient care and the correction of identified problems" (53). Given the interpretation of this standard and other required activities of the JCAH, there are several dimensions of quality assurance that are expected of an accredited institution. These include an organized system for the granting of clinical privileges, with requirements for periodic review based on demonstrated performance; a system of evaluation studies of perceived problems in patient care; and a series of monitoring activities that may indicate when problems arise in selected areas such as tissue review, blood use, antibiotic use, or deviation in performance from other hospitals as reported by local peer review organizations.

As part of its standard, the JCAH requires coordination of quality assurance efforts throughout the hospital, and involves administrative, nursing, and other professional groups in addition to the medical staff.

Overall, the JCAH reviews about 75 percent of all hospitals for accreditation. Accreditation can be given for 3 years on an unconditional basis, or contingencies can be established for interim hospital reports and/or additional on-site review. About one-half of hospitals receive the full 3-year unconditional approval, and only about 1 percent are not approved for accreditation.

The historical impact of the JCAH and its current standards on quality of care are difficult to evaluate because this organization has had major direct and indirect effects on virtually all hospitals, even those it does not review. However, the emphasis on the coordination, delineation of accountability, and visibility of quality assurance efforts is consistent with existing research on organizational features that are positively associated with better quality of care using performance-based measures (54).

PERFORMANCE-BASED ASSURANCE APPROACHES

Structural mechanisms focus on the providers of care rather than care for selected patients or groups of patients, and generally do not rely on assessments of how the system is actually performing. In view of this deficiency, there is considerable interest in performance-based assurance programs that include use review and review of both processes and outcomes of care.

Use Review

Use review represents one of the earliest forms of process assurance to be instituted on a large scale. In essence, it assures that care is actually required and that the facility is not inappropriately costly for the level of care provided. Not surprisingly, use review developed out of a desire to control the costs of hospital care, and was developed through cooperation between insurers and professional groups. It grew slowly in the private sector in the late 1950s and 1960s and gained considerable attention in the public sector with the establishment of Medicare and Medicaid.

There are three forms of use review: review of the necessity of care before the provision of a service, review during the care process, and review after the care has been provided. These are known as *prospective, concurrent,* and *retrospective* review, respectively. In general, use review has been directed at costly institutionally based care, but it can also be applied in ambulatory care, dental care, and elsewhere.

How does use review relate to the quality of care? While it is true that efforts aimed at controlling inappropriate hospital admissions or lengths of stay in hospitals were begun because of interests in cost containment, they definitely represent a form of quality assurance. Patients spared admission to a hospital for surgical removal of a gallbladder because they do not require surgery as determined by a peer review group forego the pain, distress, and potential life-threatening hazards of major surgery; this is certainly a quality assurance function. Similarly, patients who might otherwise be kept in a hospital despite the availability of equally appropriate care at home, or in other less intense settings, are spared exposure to a host of nosocomial infections and other risks that can produce injury in the hospital. Because of their orientation toward cost control, use review programs are generally designed to avoid unnecessary care and do not specifically promote increased use where underprovision of services could occur (i.e., increased access).

The mechanism of review used by use review groups include establishment of explicit criteria for both appropriate indications for hospitalization and length of stay. Cases not meeting these criteria might not be reimbursed by the insurance program. In practice, the review body usually sets explicit criteria that can be applied by review coordinators, who most commonly are specially trained nurses or medical records personnel. Cases are reviewed shortly after admission (concurrent review) and periodically during the hospital stay. Cases that do not appear to meet the indications for hospitalization are then formally reviewed by a physician or panel of physicians. Most systems also include an appeal mechanism. Cases that are not found to meet indications for continued stay are then denied payment (after a small grace period) by the insurer for any further durations of stay.

Some use review programs have a mechanism for prehospital admission review that is applied to elective hospitalization. Second-surgical opinion programs represent such a review mechanism and require approval by an independent physician of the need for the planned surgery.

The extent to which use review programs have reduced inappropriate use or saved money spent for hospital care is unclear at present, and various studies suggest mixed results (55–59). It may be that there is a sentinel effect such that simple awareness of being watched has altered provider behavior substantially from what might have occurred had use review programs not been implemented. However, even if hospital costs are reduced, it does not necessarily follow that total medical care costs to individual persons or society are reduced because some substitution may occur.

Peer Review Assurance Programs

While the most use review programs represent forms of peer review, they are not designed to monitor patient-specific aspects of care once it has been decided that a certain procedure or level of care is appropriate. For example, once a decision has been made that a diseased gallbladder can be removed, use review systems are not designed to assess the technical adequacy of the procedure performed, or whether there were preventable operative complications. This latter question can be addressed only by peer review systems that focus on specific aspects of quality of care. Examples of peer review programs are provided elsewhere; this discussion will focus primarily on an approach originally known as *medical audits*, but now also termed *patient care evaluation studies* (59).

The medical audit concept has been embellished in recent years, but essentially consists of the following six steps: (1) selection of a topic for study, such as care for a specific disease or use of a certain procedure or drug; (2) selection of explicit criteria for good care using both process and outcome criteria, which might include whether specific diagnostic tests and treatments were performed, whether the status at discharge compared favorably with the expected status, and whether there were avoidable complications or unnecessary lengths of stay; (3) review of medical records to determine if the criteria for good care are met, usually by a medical records analyst; (4) review by professional peers of all cases that do not meet the criteria for good care; (5) development of specific recommendations for assuring that any deficiencies found will be avoided in the future (e.g., education programs, changes in administrative procedures, requirements for consultations); and (6) restudy of the topic at a future date to ascertain if deficiencies have actually been reduced or eliminated.

MALPRACTICE LITIGATION AND QUALITY ASSURANCE

The legal system plays a role in quality assurance because of patients' ability to sue for malpractice, which is to some extent a quality assurance mechanism (60). Despite possible abuses by a minority of patients and lawyers, most malpractice awards do relate to less than optimal care, and all physicians are aware that they are in jeopardy of suit for egregious deficiencies in the quality of care. Interestingly, until recently there was almost no linkage between the malpractice system and licensure. Thus, a physician could have been involved in several cases of malpractice, settled them out of court, and continued to maintain the license to practice without having it reviewed with extra scrutiny. However, some states now require insurance companies to report a physician to a state discipline board if a few malpractice cases involving the physician occur in a limited time period. The board may then make an independent judgment about this person's future suitability for practice.

Another trend in malpractice insurance that may have an effect on quality assurance is self-insurance by state medical societies and hospitals. As the size of the self-insurance unit becomes smaller than it was under usual insurance programs, it is highly likely that these units will be forced to exercise increasing self or peer vigilance. The net impact on quality of care of these newer aspects of the malpractice litigation and insurance systems cannot yet be ascertained. However, at this point, a positive impact is quite likely.

CURRENT DEVELOPMENTS AND FUTURE ISSUES
IN QUALITY OF CARE

What is happening currently with regard to the assessment and assurance of the quality of patient care in the United States? What are the issues that will be important in the future? At the present time, as the result of the institution of new payment mechanisms that encourage shorter length of hospital stay and earlier discharges [i.e., diagnosis-related groups (DRGs)], there is considerable concern that the quality of patient care may become compromised by the need to more rapidly and efficiently process patients through hospitals. With the pressures building to contain hospital costs by reducing utilization of services (and, indeed, by providing incentives that reward the use of *fewer* services), there has been worry that hospitals may be discharging patients "quicker and sicker." Public hearings held by the Special Committee on Aging of the United States Senate called attention to a number of seemingly flagrant examples of premature discharge and poor care (61), but detailed documentation of a significant trend has not been presented. As eloquently pointed out by Avedis Donabedian in the 1986 Michael Davis Lecture at the University of Chicago (62), this tension between cost constraints on one hand and quality enhancement on the other hand will be a major feature of the years ahead. It will only heighten the need for more accurate and exact quality of patient care measurements, since it would be difficult to document that quality has declined if there are not sufficiently sophisticated benchmark measures of quality to begin with.

A second major trend has been and will continue to be the movement of quality of care issues into the very center of hospital organization and policy. It might fairly be said that interest in the measurement of the quality of patient care was a somewhat peripheral issue in hospitals in the past, a set of activities that were carried out because they had to be and not necessarily because the vast majority of hospital personnel felt that quality assurance was important. In recent years, quality assessment and assurance has moved more directly into the center of hospital life and activities, as shown by the recent major emphasis by the JCAH to make hospital boards of trustees *directly* responsible for ensuring that quality of care measurements are actively carried out and quality assurance methods actively put into place (63); in the past, these responsibilities were delegated to the medical staff, and the trustees rarely had to be concerned about quality of patient care measurements. The new JCAH standards place the responsibility much more directly with the trustees.

This increased awareness and importance of better quality assessment and assurance methods is also shown by the JCAH's major thrust toward the use of "outcome" measures of quality, as opposed to its prior acceptance of "structure" and "process" indicators of quality (64). Outcome measures, although more difficult to implement (65), do provide a much more accurate indicator of the quality of care provided to patients and signal a much more meaningful commitment to quality assessment and assurance.

One of the most significant trends in quality assessment and assurance is the continued movement of quality measurement efforts into new parts of the American health care structure that have not previously been actively involved in such efforts. Within the last few years, the JCAH has expanded its efforts into areas of hospice care for the dying, mental health and psychiatric services, ambulatory patient care services, and long-term care, each with rather detailed guidelines for carrying out quality assessment and reassurance (66) and some with new standards for accreditation of these services. Therefore, in light of these developments, it seems clear that *all* aspects of health care will soon be actively involved in much more vigorous processes of quality evaluation.

Finally, the big unknown for the future is whether or not quality of patient care will become an important factor in the purchase and payment of patient care services. Will some purchasers intentionally opt for programs of care with demonstrably higher or demonstrably lower standards of quality, exercising a more discerning purchasing skill in selecting between programs of care that range from "Cadillac" to "jeep" in measured quality? If these economic purchasing choices do become more important, will this encourage the development of more accurate and sophisticated means of measuring patient care quality *solely* for its value in economic decision making? Will the overall quality of patient care actually fall when purchasers realize that there may be clearly discernible levels of quality ranging from "acceptable" to "outstanding" and with great pressure to financially support only an "acceptable" level through governmental or private insurance programs?

ASSESSMENT OF QUALITY OF CARE

This chapter has reviewed salient issues with regard to quality assessment strategies and described basic quality assurance mechanisms. The uncertainty concerning the impact of various medical strategies on the health of persons limits our ability to assess and assure the quality of medical care. However, there is sufficient medical knowledge to provide a solid foundation for systems of quality assessment and assurance that, as a minimum, could help us to avoid harmful strategies, promote known helpful strategies, and allow identification of practice patterns that deviate significantly from reasonable professional practice. While the chapter has dealt primarily with examples of physician and hospital behavior, the concepts presented are analogous for assessing care by other professionals or institutions.

A final note concerns the importance of personal motivation in improving the quality of health care. No matter how systems are structured, the final common pathway of assessment will rely on the best professional judgment of a variety of persons. The development, quality, and acceptance of those judgments will be a function of the professional's personal commitment to promoting good care in the context of a supportive organizational framework. Without strong positive commitments by practicing professionals, all of the structure will prove to be of no avail. Conversely, without appropriate structural support, the best professional commitments and energy expenditure will be as efficacious as Cervantes' sorrowful figure of the lone would-be knight tilting at windmills.

REFERENCES

1. Donabedian A: *Exploration in Quality Assessment and Monitoring,* Vol 1: *The Definition of Quality and Approaches to Its Assessment.* Ann Arbor, Mich, Health Administration Press, 1980.

2. Donabedian A: *Exploration in Quality Assessment and Monitoring,* Vol 2: *The Criteria and Standards of Quality.* Ann Arbor, Mich, Health Administration Press, 1981.

3. Williamson JW: *Improving Medical Practice and Health Care: A Bibliographic Guide to Information Management in Quality Assurance and Continuing Education.* Cambridge, MA, Ballinger, 1977.

4. Barro AR: Survey and evaluation of approaches to physician performance measurement. *J Med Ed* 1973; 48(Suppl):1047–1093.

5. Williams KN, Brook RH: Quality measurement and assurance, *Health Med Care Serv Rev* 1978; 1:3–15.

6. Bergman AB, Staemm SJ: The morbidity of cardiac non-disease in school children. *New Engl J Med* 1967; 276:1008–1013.

7. Sackett DL, Taylor DW, Haynes RB, et al: The short term disadvantage of being labeled hypertensive. *Clin Res* 1977; 25:266.

8. Neutra R: Indications for the surgical treatment of suspected acute appendicitis: A cost-effectiveness approach, in Bunker JP, Barnes BA, Mosteller F (eds): *Costs, Risks and Benefits of Surgery.* New York, Oxford University Press, 1977, pp 277–307.

9. Watkins RN, Howell L: A population based quality assessment of the treatment of appendicitis. Presented at the 105th Annual Meeting of the American Public Health Association, Washington, DC, November 1977.

10. Bloch D: Evaluation of nursing care in terms of process and outcome: Issues in research and quality assurance. *Nurs Res* 1975; 24:256–263.

11. Lang N: *Quality Assurance in Nursing. A Selected Bibliography,* Publ. No. 12, HHR-80-30. U.S. Department of Health, Education and Welfare, 1980.

12. Lang N (ed): *Nursing Quality Assurance Management/Leasing System.* Northridge, CA, American Nurses Association and Sutherland Leasing Association Inc, 1982.

13. Kessner DN, Kalk CE: *Contrasts in Health Status,* Vol 2: *A Strategy for Evaluation Health Services.* Washington, DC, National Academy of Science, 1973.

14. Koran LM: The reliability of clinical methods, data and judgments (parts 1 and 2). *New Engl J Med* 1975; 293:642–646, 695–701.

15. Zuckerman AE, Starfield B, Hochreiter C, et al: Validating the content of pediatric outpatient medical records by means of tape-recording doctor–patient encounters. *Pediatrics* 1975; 56:407–411.

16. LoGerfo JP, Dynes IN, Frost F, et al: Tonsillectomies, adenoidectomies, audits: Have surgical indications been met? *Med Care* 1978; 16:950–955.

17. Osborne CE, Thompson NH: Criteria for evaluation of ambulatory child health care by chart audit—development and testing of a methodology. *Pediatrics* 1975; 56(Suppl Part 2):625–692.

18. Demlo LK, Campbell PN, Spaght S: Reliability of information abstracted from patients' medical records. *Med Care* 1978; 16:995–1004.

19. Shapiro S: End-result measurements of quality of medical care. *Milbank Mem Fund Quart* 1967; 45:7–30.

20. Brook RH, Davis-Avery A, Greenfield S, et al: *Quality of Medical Care Assessment Using Outcome Measures: An Overview of the Method.* Santa Monica, CA, Rand Corp, 1976.

21. Stewart AL, Ware JE, Brook RH: *Conceptualization and Measurement of Health for Adults in the Health Insurance Study,* Vol 2: *Physical Health in Terms of Functioning.* Santa Monica, CA, Rand Corp, 1978.

22. Ware JE, Johnston SA, Davies-Avery A, et al: *Conceptualization and Measurement of Health for Adults in the Health Insurance Study,* Vol 3: *Mental Health.* Santa Monica, CA, Rand Corp, 1978.

23. Donald CA, Ware JE, Brook RH, et al: *Conceptualization and Measurement of Health for Adults in the Health Insurance Study,* Vol 4: *Social Health.* Santa Monica, CA, Rand Corp, 1978.

24. Ware JE, Davies-Avery A, Donald CA: *Conceptualization and Measurement of Health for Adults in the Health Insurance Study,* Vol 5: *General Health Perception.* Santa Monica, CA, Rand Corp, 1978.

25. Bergner M, Bobbitt RA, Krenel A, et al: The Sickness Impact Profile: Conceptual formulation and methodological development of a health status index. *Internatl J Health Serv* 1976; 6:393–415.

26. Forrest WH, Scott WR, Brown BW: *Study of the Institutional Differences in Postoperative Mortality,* Project report (PB 250-940). National Center for Health Services Research, Hyattsville, MD, 1974.

27. Gonnella J, Louis DZ, McCord JJ: The staging concept—an approach to the assessment of outcome of ambulatory care. *Med Care* 1976; 14:13–21.

28. Donabedian A: Promoting quality through evaluating the process of patient care. *Med Care* 1968; 6:181–202.

29. DeGeyndt W: Five approaches for assessing the quality of care. *Hosp Admin* 1970; 15:21–42.

30. Brook RH, Williams KN, Davis-Avery A: Quality assurance today and tomorrow: Forecast for the future. *Ann Intern Med* 1976; 85:809–817.

31. Greenfield S, Lewis CE, Kaplan SH, et al: Peer review by criteria mapping: Criteria for diabetes mellitus. The use of decision-making in chart audit. *Ann Intern Med* 1975; 83:761–770.

32. Tompkins RK, Burnes DC, Cable WE: An analysis of the cost-effectiveness of pharyngitis management and acute rheumatic fever prevention. *Ann Intern Med* 1977; 86:481–492.

33. Lee RI, Jones LW: *The Fundamental sof Good Medical Care.* Chicago, University of Chicago Press, 1933.

34. Payne BC, Lyons TF, Dwarshius L, et al: *The Quality of Medical Care: Evaluation and Improvement.* Chicago, Hospital Research and Educational Trust, 1976, pp 7–19.

35. Donabedian A, Wheeler JR, Wyszewianski L: Quality, cost, and health: An integrative model. *Med Care* 1982; 20:975–992.

36. Zyzanski SJ, Hulka BS, Cassel JC: Scale for the measurement of "satisfaction" with medical care: Modifications in content, format, and scoring. *Med Care* 1974; 12:611–620.

37. Ware JE, Davies-Avery A, Stewart PE: The measurement and meaning of patient satisfaction. *Health Med Care Serv Rev* 1978; 1:1–15.

38. Lyle CB, Applegate WB, Citron DF, et al: Practice habits in a group of eight internists. *Ann Intern Med* 1976; l84:594–601.

39. Shapiro S, Jacobziner H, Densen PM, et al: Further observation on prematurity and perinatal mortality in a general population and in the population of a prepaid group practice medical plan. *Am J Public Health* 1960; 50:1304–1317.

40. Scott WR, Forrest WH Jr, Brown BW Jr: Hospital structure and postoperative mortality and morbidity, in Shortell S (ed): *Organizational Research in Hospitals—An Inquiry Book,* Chicago, Blue Cross Association, 1976.

41. Luft HS, Bunker JP, Enthoven AC: Should operations be regionalized? An empirical study of the relation between surgical volume and mortlaity. *New Engl J Med* 1979; 301:1364.

42. Luft HS: The relation between surgical volume and mortality: An exploration of causal factors and alternatives models. *Med Care* 1980; 18:940—959.

43. Kessner DM, Snow CK, Singer J: *Contrasts in Health Status,* Vol 3: *Assessment of Medical Care for Children.* Washington, DC, National Academy of Sciences, 1974.

44. Dutton DB, Silber R: Children's health outcomes in six different ambulatory care delivery systems. *Med Care* 1980; 18:693–714.

45. Schroeder SA, Donaldson MS: The feasibility of an outcome approach of an outcome to quality assurance—a report from one HMO. *Med Care* 1976; 14:49–56.

46. Peterson OL, Andrews LP, Spain RS, et al: An analytic study of North Carolina general practice 1953–1954. *J Med Ed* 1956:31(12, Part 2):1–165.

47. Lembcke PA: Medical auditing by scientific methods: Illustrated by major female pelvic surgery. *JAMA* 1956; 162:646–655.

48. Doyle JC: Unnecessary hysterectomies—study of 6,248 operations in 75 hospitals during 1948. *JAMA* 1953; 151:360–365.

49. Dyck FJ, Murphy FA, Murphy JK, et al: Effect of surveillance on the number of hysterectomies in the province of Saskatchewan. *New Engl J Med* 1977; 296:1326–1328.

50. McCarthy E, Widmer G: Effects of screening by consultants on recommended elective surgical procedures. *New Engl J Med* 1974; 291:1331–1335.

51. Ray W, Federspiel CP, Schaffner W: Prescribing of chloramphenicol in ambulatory practice. An epidemiologic study among Tenessee Medicaid recipients. *Ann Intern Med* 1976; 84:266–270.

52. Brook RH, Williams KN, Rolph JE: Controlling the use and cost of medical services. The New Mexico experimental medical care review organization—a four year case study. *Med Care* 1978; 16(Suppl 9):1–76.

53. *Accreditation Manual for Hospitals,* 1983 ed. Chicago, Illinois, Joint Commission on Accreditation of Hospitals, 1982, p 151.

54. Shortell SM, LoGerfo JP: Hospital medical staff organization and quality of care: Results from myocardial infarction and appendectomy. *Med Care* 1981; 19:1041–1056.

55. Chassin M: The containment of hospital costs: A strategic assessment. *Med Care* 1978; 16(Suppl 10):1–55.

56. Ruchlin HS, Finkel ML, McCarthy EG: The efficacy of second-opinion consultation programs: A cost-benefit perspective. *Med Care* 1982; 20:3–20.

57. Martin SG, Shwartz M, Whalen BJ, et al: Impact of a mandatory second-opinion program on Medicaid surgery rates. *Med Care* 1982; 20:21–45.

58. Brook RH, Lohr KN: Second-opinion programs: Beyond cost-benefit analysis. *Med Care* 1982; 20:1–2.

59. Ertel PY, Aldredge MG (eds): *Medical Peer Review: Theory and Practice.* St. Louis, Mosby, 1977.

60. Brook RH, Brutoco RL, Williams KN: The relationship between edical malpractice and quality of care. *Duke Law J* 1976; 75:1197–1231.

61. *Quality of Care Under Medicare's Prospective Payment System: Hearings Before the Special Committee on Aging of the United States Senate, 1985.* (Senate Hearing No. 99-195), U.S. Government Printing Office, Washington, DC, 1986.

62. Donabedian A: The price of quality and the complexities of care. The 1986 Michael Davis Lecture, University of Chicago, May 9, 1986.

63. The governing body evaluates its own performance, Section 4.1.19. *Accreditation Manual for Hospitals,* Chicago, Joint Commission on Accreditation of Hospitals, 1986.

64. Quality gets a closer look. *Modern Healthcare,* February 27, 1987.

65. Schroeder S: Outcome assessment 70 years later: Are we ready? *New Engl J Med* 1987; 316:160–162.

66. *1987 Publications Catalog.* Chicago, Joint Commission of Accreditation of Hospitals.

CHAPTER 14

Evaluating Health Care Programs and Services

Arnold D. Kaluzny
James E. Veney

While the structuring of the health services system, including the regulation of its performance and the assessment of the quality of services provided, was discussed in Chapters 12 and 13, this chapter focuses on the *evaluation* of those services and the programs under which they are provided. Evaluation represents an important component of the overall process of assessing and regulating the performance of the health services system. While a great deal has been written about the techniques and methods appropriate to evaluation in various program and research activities, this chapter presents an overview of evaluation in the health services field. Specifically, it defines evaluation, illustrates various types of evaluation, and discusses the practical implications of evaluation to individuals in managerial positions. The chapter concludes with a historical perspective on evaluation—where it has been and where it is going.

WHAT IS EVALUATION?

Evaluation—or as it is often called, *evaluation research*—is defined as: "The collection and analysis of information by various methodological strategies to determine the relevance, progress, efficiency, effectiveness, and impact of health service program activities" (1).

Several points should be noted about this definition. First, it is *not* specific about the particular methodology that is used to gather and analyze information. Evaluation may employ a variety of methodologies, including monitoring, case studies, survey research, trend analysis, and/or experimental design. The critical element is that the evaluation is conducted in a systematic manner and focuses on achievement of program objectives as well as program process.

Second, information is used to make judgments and plan actions and thus is an integral part of the managerial process. Health service managers are forced daily to

438

make judgments and plan actions on the basis of program evaluations. Evaluations may deal with such apparently mundane affairs as determining whether program resources and personnel are in the right places at the right time (progress) or with more glamorous issues, such as whether a program has made any difference (impact). However, any activity aimed at making decisions about whether a program should be implemented, how the program should be carried out, whether program activities are being pursued in a timely manner, if the program is producing expected outcomes, or whether the outcomes are as desirable as anticipated is essentially evaluation.

Two views of evaluation and the role of each in the managerial process need to be considered: linear and nonlinear.

LINEAR PROCESS

One approach to evaluation and its role in the management process is consideration of a sequence of events in which program planning comes first, followed by implementation and finally by evaluation (2). This logical sequence of steps is often perceived as including feedback from evaluation to both planning and implementation, so that program modification occurs, allowing the program to proceed at a new level of effectiveness. Figure 14-1 presents this sequence of activities.

There is nothing basically wrong with this formulation; still, it is somewhat limited as far as the role of evaluation in program planning and implementation is concerned. The difficulty with the linear model is its assumption that evaluation takes place after program planning and implementation.

NONLINEAR PROCESS

An alternative view of evaluation, and the view taken here, is to consider evaluation as an integral part of the management cycle. Figure 14-2 shows a nonlinear model of planning, implementation, and control as three interconnected activities. From this perspective, program evaluation may accompany the planning and design stage of a program, focusing on such issues as the current state of the system to be affected by the program, the specific nature of problems to be addressed, and alternative approaches to solving those problems.

Once a program is in operation, a number of evaluation issues arise. A general question concerns whether the process works as intended. Do resources, funds, doses of vaccine, students to be trained, medical supplies, or other types of inputs arrive at

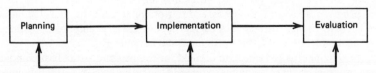

Figure 14-1. Linear model of program planning, management, and evaluation cycle. (SOURCE: Veney JE, Kaluzny, AD: *Evaluation and Decision Making in Health Service Programs.* Reprinted by permission of Prentice-Hall, Inc., Appleton-Lange, Englewood Cliffs, NJ, copyright 1983.)

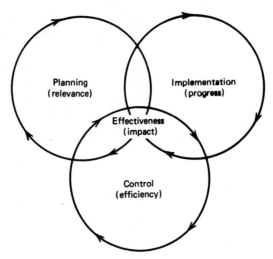

Figure 14-2. Nonlinear model of program planning, implementation, and evaluation. (SOURCE: Veney JE, Kaluzny, AD: *Evaluation and Decision Making in Health Service Programs.* Reprinted by permission of Prentice-Hall, Inc., Appleton-Lange, Englewood Cliffs, NJ, copyright 1983.)

the proper place, on time, and in sufficient quantity? Are activities undertaken in a timely manner and in proper order? Are various components of the program coordinated? These and many other questions are addressed as aspects of program progress.

Once the program has been implemented, is it effective and efficient? Are the costs of the program reasonable? Do the results expected from the program appear in the projected time frame? Are there other less expensive or more timely ways of producing the same results? Are the results of the program meeting predetermined objectives?

Finally, have the desired results been achieved? Has the problem the program was designed to solve been solved, or is being solved on a continuing bases? Would the problem have been solved in the absence of the program? Could any other program have solved the problem?

TYPES OF EVALUATION

As indicated in our definition, evaluations perform a variety of functions in order to determine the relevance, progress, efficiency, effectiveness, and impact of health service program activities. Below is a description of each of these functions, an illustration of the issues addressed by each function, and an example of specific types of evaluations involving health care programs and services (3).

Relevance concerns the question of need for the program—the basic rationale for having a program or set of activities to meet the health needs or service demands of a community. The development of relevance as a legitimate evaluation topic in health services is a recent phenomenon. Historically, health services have been considered relevant a priori, and the critical questions have focused on the delivery of services. In more recent years, the concern for delivery and extent of use have been supplemented by concern regarding the underlying rationale for the program. The very basis of a program in terms of objectives, scope, depth, and coverage becomes the primary issue. Questions central to this type of evaluation include the following:

What problem does the program address?
Does that problem need attention?
How accurate is the information about the problem?
How adequate is the definition of the problem?
How adequate is the definition of the program?
Is the program appropriate to the defined problem?

Consider the following example, entitled "King–Drew Needs Assessment" (4):

The evaluation was the effort by the King–Drew Medical Center in Los Angeles to meet the health needs of the inner-city community of Watts. The first step taken by the Center in attempting to assess needs of the community was to compile from literature, medical experts, and consumer advocates a list of 50 statements of objectives that a community health center should meet. The list included such statements as the following:

To teach individuals and families to identify the dangers of common health problems (e.g., lead poisoning, high blood pressure, obesity).

To reduce the time a patient has to wait to see a doctor.

To identify and assist with family problems that can threaten health, such as child abuse and alcoholism.

To care for normal pregnancies and deliveries.

After devising the list, three community groups, consumers (724), providers (224), and administrators (74), were approached to provide various types of input in regard to the final decision of which objectives should take priority for the Center. Each of the three groups were asked to rate each of the 50 objectives on a scale of five choices from "most important" to "least important." The respondents were asked to place at least two of the objectives in each of the importance categories to assure that all objectives were not rated equally important. They were also asked to rate each service on a 3-point scale of availability that included: "easily available," "available but difficult to get," and "not available as far as I know."

Physicians and administrators were asked to rate the feasibility of providing the services on a 3-point scale that included "easy to provide," "possible to provide but difficult," and "cannot be provided at this time."

The final decision was to concentrate on those objectives that had received a score greater than 4.0 on importance, less than 2.0 on availability, and greater than 2.0 on feasibility. The following 4 objectives out of 50 met these criteria:

To set up health services that are close to the people in the community.

To identify and assist with family problems that are threats to health.

To adequately treat common or frequent health problems in the same clinic.

To make better use of community resources.

Progress evaluation refers to the tracking of program activities. Here attention is focused on the degree to which program implementation complies with the predetermined plan. Traditionally, progress evaluation has been considered an integral part of the management process. Illustrative questions concerning progress include the following:

Are appropriate personnel, equipment, and financial resources available in the right quantity, in the right place, and at the right time to meet program needs?
Are expected products of the program actually being produced? Are these products of expected quality and quantity? Are these outputs produced at the expected time?

Consider the following example, entitled "Short Course Self-Learning Module Development" (5):

> This example of progress evaluation depends on the use of the Gantt Chart, a tool for assisting in the evaluation of progress. The actual chart is shown in Figure 14-3. The project was funded by the U.S. Public Health Service Program in Health Manpower Development to provide ways to make graduate-level training more accessible, flexible, economic, and learner-paced. The objective was to develop and produce nine health management method modules, each approximately equivalent to a 1-week workshop experience.
>
> The figure indicates each of the activities deemed necessary to carry out the development of the modules and the time at which these activities were expected to occur. It also indicates the precedence relationship of the activities, showing by arrows those activities that must be completed before others can begin. While in actual module development it was not possible to follow the exact sequence indicated in the figure at all times, this idealized sequence did serve as a model against which the progress of the project could be evaluated.

Efficiency evaluation concerns the relationship between the results obtained from a specific program and the resources expended for its operation. This form of evaluation is gaining increasing attention as programs compete for limited resources. It plays an important role in determining whether new programs are funded, continued or terminated, and expanded or contracted. Questions addressed by evaluations of efficiency include the following:

Are program benefits sufficient for the cost incurred?
Are program benefits more or less expensive per unit of outcome than benefits derived from other programs designed to achieve the same goal?

Consider the following example, entitled "Efficiency of Alternative Delivery Plans" (6):

> The research project evaluated health care services received by comparable populations with comparable benefits from a prepaid group practice and a fee-for-service system in the Seattle, Washington area. The study team examined use of physician and hospital services by four groups: participants covered for all services at virtually no cost to the beneficiaries, those sharing in costs of services received, subscribers to Group Health Cooperative of Puget Sound (GHC) receiving free GHC services, and a GHC control group randomly chosen from plan subscribers covered under a variety of arrangements from free services to some cost sharing.
>
> Hospital admission rates for both GHC groups were about 40 percent less than those for the two fee-for-service groups. Analysis of use of inpatient, outpatient, and preventive

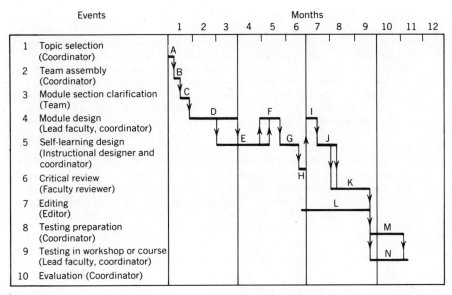

Figure 14-3. Sequence of events for one module through a single testing and evaluation. (SOURCE: Loddengaard, RA: Short Course Self-Learning Module Development. Public Health Special Projects Grant, Section 792. Department of Health Policy and Administration, School of Public Health, University of North Carolina at Chapel Hill, 1979. Reprinted by permission of R. A. Loddengaard.)

visits showed less striking differences, although clearly expenditures for GHC services were less than those for fee-for-service practice.

The study shows the prepaid plan delivers a less expensive type of care, mainly because of differences in hospitalization costs and questions the desirability of the group style of practice for future health status, patient satisfaction, and other dimensions of health care.

Effectiveness evaluation emphasizes program outputs and the immediate results of program efforts and considers their success in meeting predetermined objectives. Evaluations of effectiveness are aimed at improving program formulation and thus have a relatively short term perspective. The questions central to this type of evaluation include the following:

Did the program meet its stated objectives?
Were program providers satisfied with the effects of program activities?
Were program beneficiaries satisfied with the effects of program activities?
Are things better as a result of the program's existence?

Consider the following example, entitled "Effectiveness of Hospital Sponsored Primary Care" (7,8):

The Shortell and Aday studies evaluate the effects of the Community Hospital Program (CHP) funded by the Robert Wood Johnson Foundation to help hospitals to improve access to primary care in their communities. The Foundation allocated approximately $27 million in grants to 54 hospitals for a period of up to 4 years and amounts up to $500,000 to develop staff and facilities for programs to improve primary care services by providing more generalist care through partnerships of hospitals and physicians.

Shortell reports on achievement of organizational and financial program objectives. The analysis centers on three models—hospital service model, teaching model, and private practice model—and found that one-half to two-thirds of the hospitals improved primary care services, and "spin-off" services continued after expiration of the grant period. The study noted improvement in primary care services through organization of physicians into groups to provide more comprehensive and accessible services. Beneficiaries include many middle-class as well as poor patients who profited from linkage to a primary care physician. The program made a significant contribution in demonstrating the role of the hospital in acting as a catalyst for improving broad-based primary care services.

The Aday study found that the CHPs attracted patients who lacked a source of care as well as many patients of established primary care physicians. The study found that the CHPs did not increase use of inpatient and emergency room services and did improve patient access to appropriate primary care services.

Impact evaluation concerns the long-term implications of the program—the changes observed over time in characteristics that the program is designed to influence. While evaluation of effectiveness focuses on program outputs, impact evaluation considers whether program outputs have the desired effects on the fundamental problems the program is designed to solve. It is possible that a program may prove to be both efficient and effective in producing short-run outputs, yet have minimal long-term impact. Illustrative questions for this type of evaluation include the following:

Did a particular program produce the observed effects?
Could the observed effects occur in the absence of the program or in the presence of some alternative program?

Consider the following example, entitled "The Impact of Hospice Care" (9):

The study reports on a quasiexperimental study of the effects of hospice care in which terminally ill cancer patients at the Veterans Administration hospital were randomly assigned to receive hospice or conventional care. The 137 hospice patients received care in an inpatient unit and at home. The hospice patients and the 110 control patients in conventional care and their familial care givers (FCGs) were followed until the patient's death.

Hospice patients and their FCGs showed more satisfaction with care provided and also expressed less anxiety than the control group and FCGs. Otherwise, no significant differences were noted in measures of pain, symptoms, activities of daily living, number of therapeutic procedures per inpatient days, and so on. Costs of hospice care were at least as expensive as costs of conventional care.

The study suggests hospice services should be made available as a matter of choice for patients and FCGs who prefer the hospice style of care. The randomized control design ensured comparability of the different groups. However, studies based on data collected after the date of patient's death make up the bulk of studies of hospice services. More research of both types is needed to improve our understanding of the effects of different types of care for terminally ill cancer patients.

WHO DOES EVALUATION?

All health service managers need evaluation for various purposes. Many social scientists and persons involved in health services research have the skills necessary to conduct evaluation studies. The involvement of both groups depends on the degree to which formal evaluation research techniques are used and the extent to which the manager collaborates with persons skilled in their use.

Collaboration may be seen as a continuum having the various levels of involvement by managers and evaluation research personnel. At one end of the continuum, the manager has the most influence. Here, emphasis is on evaluation focusing on relevance and program progress. At the other end of the continuum, where researchers have the most influence, emphasis is on assessing impact and effectiveness. These evaluations involve more sophisticated methodologic approaches and techniques.

This continuum also illustrates an often made distinction between formative and summative evaluation (10). *Formative evaluation* concerns the activities associated with the ongoing operations of a program. Emphasis is placed on improving the management of the program through data gathering and analysis. *Summative evaluation*, on the other hand, refers to activities associated with more long-term effects of a program—whether the program has, in fact, had an impact on critical indicators or performance and/or meets specific previously determined program objectives.

In reality, evaluation requires collaboration between program administrators and persons trained in research and evaluation methodologies. The interface between program evaluation and management is much like the relationship between theory and practice (11:4):

> Theory and practice are not competing mistresses. Indeed, research that is useless to either the theoretician or the practitioner is suspect. If it is useful to the practitioner but not the theoretician, then one must wonder whether it is a valid finding and whether it has addressed the correct issue. If it is useful to the theoretician but not to the practitioner, then one must wonder whether the research is capturing a critical issue. Indeed, it can be argued that we should always ask two questions about research: is it useful for practice, and does it contribute to the body of scientific knowledge that is relevant to theory? If it fails either of these tests, then serious questions should be raised. It is a rare research study that can inform practice but not theory, or vice versa.

Collaboration requires considerable change in the way managers and evaluators function. For managers, collaboration requires recognition that they do not really know whether program X will be effective or is even relevant to the many problems faced by their organization. Instead of advocating a particular solution, the manager needs to present solutions as a series of options and develop ways to address them, at the same time considering affects on the community and organization. In essence, this approach requires (12:410):

> [a] shift from the advocacy of a specific reform to the advocacy of the seriousness of the problem, and hence to the advocacy of persistence in alternative reform efforts should the first one fail. The political stance would become: "This is a serious problem. We propose to initiate policy A on an experimental basis. If after 5 years there has been no significant improvement, we would shift to policy B." By making explicit that a given problem solution

was only one of several that the administrator or party could in good conscience advocate, and by having ready a plausible alternative, the administrator could afford honest evaluation of outcomes. Negative results, a failure of the first program, would not jeopardize his job, for his job would be to keep after the problem until something was found that worked.

For individuals involved in research and formal evaluation, an equally important shift must occur. Currently, many staff members view the research–evaluation community as the center of knowledge and its primary function as disseminator of information about program operations to the manager or community. A more realistic view for achieving collaboration is to recognize that much of the knowledge generated by social science represents only one approach to resolving important social problems (13). This perspective focuses on management as the center, with the various social sciences, including program evaluation, contributing to the main activity. To use evaluation studies for effective decision making, managers must be trained to understand research and evaluation skills as part of their overall arsenal in program management. In essence, given this approach, managers must be as knowledgeable about various evaluation methodologies as they are in other managerial skills, such as cost accounting and personnel management.

IMPLICATIONS OF EVALUATION

Health service managers are under increasing pressure to assure high performance. Utilization of information derived from the evaluation effort can be used to affect decisions at all stages of the managerial process: planning, implementation, and control. As described by Wholey et al. (14:12):

> Evalua[tion] can help managers establish and communicate clear, outcome-oriented objectives and performance indicators for organizations and programs. [It] can help managers assess performance in terms of those objectives and indicators. [It] can help managers stimulate improvements in performance. [It] can help managers communicate the value of organizational and program activities to people who work outside the organization as well as those who control needed resources . . .

Yet, any realistic assessment of the utilization of evaluation in the management process suggests that expectations far exceed reality. Several factors contribute to this discrepancy.

TIMELINESS

Timeliness, or rather lack of it, is often cited as an important factor in the nonutilization of evaluation studies. Evaluations of large health service programs may require years of study, but policymakers and project managers want to know study results within a few weeks or, at most, months. Since managers and policymakers have a propensity for action (15), evaluations, in order to be useful, must fit within management's limited time frame.

A good example of the lag between the need for information and completion of a program to satisfy that need is the Rand Corporation's experiment assessing the effect of various types of health insurance coverage on the use of services (16,17). The project began in 1972 and only recently produced final results. Although the project was well designed, the results have limited relevance to contemporary health care issues. The issue of national health insurance, important in the 1970s, has become more or less irrelevant to federal decision making in the mid 1980s. Perhaps new concerns with health insurance may emerge in the next decade; however, a study conducted in the 1970s may be considered too dated to be of value.

RELEVANCE

A second factor contributing to the failure of program evaluation to affect decision making is that evaluation has developed a dynamic of its own. In other words, evaluation activities have become increasingly professional, based on an expanding esoteric body of knowledge almost independent of basic service delivery activities. In essence, evaluation activities tend to be self-limiting and self-controlling, organized around their own technical requirements and processes. Administrators do not see the work of evaluators as relevant to their decision-making needs.

Resolution of this problem does *not* require that program evaluation redefine its task as purely a technical function or abandon methodologic rigor. Instead, evaluation must focus on questions of interest to program managers involved in decision-making processes necessary to direct a program. Often these questions have counterparts in theory: issues derived from theory can be translated into practical policy and administrative issues (18,19).

ALTERNATIVE DECISION MAKING

A third factor contributing to the apparent discrepancy between expectations and actual use is that information and analysis derived from program evaluation represent only one approach to the resolution of problems confronting decision makers. As described by Lindblom and Cohen (13:10):

> Information and analysis provides only one route because . . . a great deal of the world's problem solving is accomplished through the various forms of social interaction that substitute action for thought, understanding or analysis. Information and analysis are not a universal or categorical prescription for problem solving.

Lindblom and Cohen's challenging analysis indicates that a significant portion of decision making depends on ordinary knowledge, social learning, and interaction. *Ordinary knowledge* does not owe its origin, testing of degree of verification, truth status, or currency to distinctive evaluation or research methodologies and techniques. Instead, ordinary knowledge requires common sense, causal empiricism, and thoughtful speculation and analysis. Decision making regarding health programs will always depend heavily on ordinary knowledge.

Social learning results from actual participation and ongoing social phenomena through which persons learn new behavior. Information generated from evaluation is likely to be of little use until social learning occurs. In a sense, social learning must occur before researchers can raise the significant questions appropriate for evaluation.

Finally, decision making based on *interactive problem solving* is considered to be an important alternative to program evaluation and occurs through resolution of problems with actions substituting for thought. This method introduces solutions to resolve a problem or improve a situation without any understanding of the dilemma or systematic assessment of remedies or preferred outcomes. This approach to problems in health services is particularly pervasive because of the dominant role of physicians with their propensity for action (20).

LONG AND SHORT HISTORY OF PROGRAM EVALUATION

It is important to put evaluation into context. While evaluation may be considered a well established activity in health services, it has taken different forms over time. On one hand, it is part of a well established tradition of research and development characteristic of the medical field. As described by Freeman and Rossi (21:342):

> The R & D perspective is part of the vast medical research enterprise, dedicated to the detection, diagnosis, prevention, treatment, and management of disease. The evaluation of R & D efforts takes place at various levels within the medical enterprise. At one extreme, individuals and households are the targets of programs that seek to find efficacious ways to control or lessen harmful individual or household practices. Examples of such programs are those that seek to lower the incidence and prevalence of substance abuses—alcoholism, drug addiction, or smoking—or to instill health practice such as weight control or the use of dental floss, or to maximize participation in mass preventive efforts such as vaccinations, chest x-rays, or routine examinations for breast cancer.
>
> At the other extreme, the R & D efforts are directed at larger aggregates that include communities and the nation as a whole. Such programs are directed at improving public sanitation, abating noise, or controlling polluting substances.

On the other hand, it is also part of the emergent field of health services research. While the term "health services research" commonly refers to broad, heterogeneous activities, a fairly extensive review of the field defines it as inquiry to produce knowledge about the structure, processes, or effects of health services (22). The definition incorporates a number of program evaluation activities such as technology assessment, quality assessment, comparative use studies, and overall evaluation of the effects and impact of various types of health service programs.

Within this latter context, evaluation activities have taken on different forms and foci over the past 15 years. For example, during the early and mid 1970s, evaluation was focused primarily on fairly large scale and relatively long term activities (23). Many of these activities had an ideological fervor such as national health insurance studies (17) or integrated maternal–child health–family planning (24).

More recently, the focus shifted away from large-scale, long-term interventions to evaluation dealing with relatively small programs or incremental changes in existing programs focused on particular programmatic aspects and/or segments of the population. Table 14-1 presents a partial list of recent and/or ongoing evaluation projects illustrating the focus of evaluation efforts for one segment of the provider population.

TABLE 14-1. Selected Evaluation Studies

Project	Evaluation Focus	Period of Study	Sample Size	Results
NIH Consensus Development Program (Kanouse et al. 1986)	Impact on knowlewledge, attitudes, and behavior of selected NIH consensus development conferences	1984–1986	1453 physicians	Low levels of awareness about specific conferences— physician specialty differences
Community Hospital Oncology Program (Ford et al. 1986)	Effect of locally determined guideliness on patterns of care	1982–1984	23 CHOPs	Guideline development and dissemination have minimal effect on changing established practice patterns
Community Clinical Oncology Programs (NCII 1986)	Effects of protocols on accrual and patterns of care	1983–1986	62 CCOPs	CCOPs able to meet accrual standard— minimal diffusion effect
Strategies to Reduce Inappropriate Use of Blood Products (Avorn, 1986)	Education programs to influence physician decision making	1985–1989	7–9 hospitals	Pending
Communication Network and Physician Use of a Hospital Information System (Anderson, 1985)	Design, implement, and evaluate program to increase physician use of information systems	1985–1986	Physicians on 12 services in 1 hospital	Pending

SOURCES: Kanouse D, Winkler J, Berry S, Brook R: Physician awareness of the NIH Consensus Development Program. Rand Working Paper, April 1986; Anderson J: Communication networks and physician use of a HIS. Proposal funded, National Center for Health Services Research and Technology Assessment, 1985; Avorn J: Strategies to reduce inappropriate use of blood products. Proposal funded by National Center for Health Services Research and Technology Assessment, 1985; Ford L et al: Diffusion of information using patient management guidelines: The community hospital oncology program experience. National Cancer Institute, Bethesda, MD, 1985. National Cancer Institute: *Community Cancer Care Evaluation: Preliminary Findings.* Bethesda, MD.

Although it is difficult to speculate on the future, there is some indication that a new phase of evaluation activity is under way. Here evaluation efforts become an integral part of the managerial process, and as a result, attention is given to the link of evaluation to assuring high performance within organizations. The assessment of incremental changes in existing programs and evaluation of new program activities are emphasized. In short, evaluation becomes part of the strategic decision-making process of the organization. In this new role, several issues that will guide the role of evaluation in the foreseeable future need to be addressed:

It must be explicitly recognized that evaluation is only one method of resolving health services problems. Evaluation must not be considered a substitute for other types of problem solving. It merely supplements or complements other methods. Failure to recognize this fact reduces the overall effect of evaluation. As described by Lindblom and Cohen (13:54):

> [Evaluators] will indiscriminantly attempt too many tasks rather than selectively choosing critical supplements or complementarities to the other inputs; will spend their energies on tasks that they cannot do well, as well as those they need not do; and will fail to focus on tasks they can do.

To the extent that expectations can be reduced, and that evaluation can adapt to the realities of the problem-solving process, it will play an important role. Health services managers, for example, require information in order to improve decision making. Managers face problems of expanding or contracting services and recruiting, retaining, and allocating personnel, as well as deciding what types of service and personnel are required. To solve these problems, information generated by various evaluation methodologies is critical. Industrial managers spend a great deal of time and money to make these decisions more effectively. A similar investment is likely to be worthwhile for health services managers.

It must be recognized that evaluation resources, like program resources, are limited and should be allocated to activities likely to benefit from the process. Thus, while all programs can be evaluated, there is often merit in delaying any substantive evaluation until preliminary assessment of the program's basic design is made. Increased emphasis will be given to what Wholey (25) defines as *evaluability assessment*; that is, the process of determining whether objectives are well defined, whether program assumptions are plausible, and whether intended uses of evaluation information are clearly stated.

More selective identification of evaluation issues provides an opportunity to match types of evaluation with basic characteristics of the program within its political context. This approach is illustrated nicely by Shortell and Richardson's formulation of program evaluation using Thompson's (26) typology of organizational decision-making strategies. Table 14-2 presents the basic decision-making factors affecting the choice of future program evaluation activities, as well as the types of evaluation appropriate for these basic conditions.

As presented in Table 14-2, the type of evaluation that is appropriate is a function of whether there is (1) certainty or uncertainty about the desirability of program outcomes and (2) certainty about cause-and-effect relationships. Where there is certainty regarding both of these factors, a *progress* type of evaluation is considered the most appropriate. The purpose is simply to ensure that the program is following the expected plan.

Where there is certainty about cause-and-effect relationships but uncertainty about the desirability of possible outcomes, a far more elaborate evaluation effort is required. Here attention needs to be given to *effectiveness* and *efficiency* to determine whether the program is meeting stated objectives in the most efficient manner. Evaluation

TABLE 14-2. Decision-Making Factors Affecting the Choice of Future Program Evaluations

Beliefs about Cause–Effect Relationships	Preferences Regarding Desirability of Possible Outcomes	
	Certain	Uncertain
Certain	*Progress evaluation:* no need for formal program evaluation efforts, although ongoing monitoring is important	*Effectiveness–efficiency evaluation:* rigorous program evaluation efforts useful in selling and defending the program in political battles, particularly if program effects are small
Uncertain	*Impact evaluation:* impact, summative program evaluation most appropriate	*Relevance evaluation:* process-oriented formative evaluation most appropriate

SOURCE: Adapted from Shortell SM, Richardson WC: Health Program Evaluation. St. Louis, Mosby, 1978.

information becomes critical in providing a justification and/or defense for continuation of the program.

Where there is uncertainty about the cause-and-effect relationship but certainty about the desirability of possible outcomes, an *impact* type of evaluation is most appropriate. This approach determines whether observed effects occurred in the absence of the program or in the presence of some alternative activity.

Where there is uncertainty about both the cause-and-effect relationship and the desirability of possible outcomes, the basic issues is *relevance*, that is, whether the program is actually needed. The collection and analysis of information to define the problem and/or the nature of the services needed will reduce the level of uncertainty.

Failure to diagnose the basic problems accurately and to initiate the appropriate type of evaluation activity undermines the ability to respond to critical health service needs and demands. Unfortunately, there is often a preoccupation with issues of relevance when, in fact, there is certainty about cause and effect as well as about the desirability of outcomes. Similarly, there is often concern with progress when, in fact, there is uncertainty about cause and effect, as well as about the desirability of outcomes.

Finally, the role of evaluator needs to shift from critic to program advocate. Evaluation is an integral part of the managerial process and thus must be extremely sensitive to the organizational environment within which the critic or program advocate functions. Premium needs to be given to negotiating and communicating skills as well as the need to participate as part of a larger interdisciplinary team process. As described by Wholey et al. (14:289):

> The new evaluator is a program advocate—not an advocate in the sense of an ideal log willing to manipulate data and to alter findings to secure next year's funding. The new evaluator is some one who believes in and is interested in helping programs and organizations to succeed. At times the program advocate evaluator will play the traditional critic role: challenging basic program assumptions, reporting lackluster performance, or identifying inefficiencies. The difference, however, is that criticism is not the end of performance oriented evaluations; rather it is part of a larger process of program and organizational improvement, a process that receives as much of the evaluators attention and talents as the criticism function.

REFERENCES

1. Veney JE, Kaluzny AD: *Evaluation and Decision Making in Health Service Programs.* Englewood Cliffs, NJ, Prentice-Hall, 1983.
2. Borus ME, Buntz CG, Tash WR: *Evaluating the Impact of Health Programs: A Primer.* Cambridge, MA, MIT Press, 1982.
3. *Health Program Evaluation: Guiding Principles, Health for All,* Series No. 6. Geneva, World Health Organization, 1981.
4. Kosecoff J, Fink A: *Evaluation Basics, A Practitioner's Manual.* Beverly Hills, CA, Sage Publications, 1985.
5. Loddengaard, RA: Short Course, Self-Learning Module Development. Public Health Special Projects Grant-Section 792. Department of Health Policy and Administration, School of Public Health, University of North Carolina at Chapel Hill, 1979.
6. Manning WG, Leibowitz A, Goldberg GA, et al: A controlled trial of the effect of a prepaid group practice on use of services. *New Engl J Med* 1984; 310:1505–1510.
7. Shortell SM, Wickizer TM, Wheeler JRC: Hospital-sponsored primary care: Organizational and financial effects. *Am J Public Health* 1984; 74:784–791.
8. Aday LA, Andersen R, Loevy SS, et al: Hospital-sponsored primary care: Impact on patient access. *Am J Public Health* 1984; 74:792–798.
9. Kane RL, Wales J, Bernstein L, et al: A randomized controlled trial of hospice care. *The Lancet* 1984; 890–894.
10. Scriven M: The methodology of evaluation, in Tyler RW, Gagne RM, Scriven M (eds): *Perspective of Curriculum Evaluation.* Chicago, Rand McNally, 1967.
11. Lawler EE, Mohrman AM, Mohrman SA, et al: *Doing Research That Is Useful for Theory and Practice.* San Francisco, Jossey-Bass Publishers, 1985.
12. Campbell DT: Reforms as experiments. *Am Psychol* 1969; 24:409–429.
13. Lindblom CE, Cohen DK: *Usable Knowledge: Social Science and Social Problem Solving.* New Haven, CT, Yale University Press, 1979.
14. Wholey JS, Abramson MA, Bellavita C (eds): *Performance and Credibility.* Lexington, MA, Lexington Books, 1986.
15. Mintzberg H: *The Nature of Managerial Work.* New York, Harper & Row, 1973.
16. Newhouse JP: A design for a health insurance experiment. *Inquiry* 1974; 11:5–27.
17. Newhouse JP, Manning WG, Morris CN, et al: Some interim results from a controlled trial of cost sharing in health insurance. *New Engl J Med* 1981; 305:1501–1507.
18. Shortell SM: Organizational theory and health service delivery, Shortell SM, Brown M (eds): *Organizational Research in Hospitals,* Chicago, Blue Cross Association, 1976.
19. Kaluzny AD, Veney JE: *Health Service Organizations: A Guide to Research and Assessment.* Berkeley, McCutchan Publishing Co, 1980.
20. Friedson, E: *Profession of Medicine: A Study of the Sociology of Applied Medicine.* New York, Dodd, Mead & Co, 1970.
21. Freeman H, Rossi P: Social experiments. *Health Society: Milbank Mem Fund Quart* 1981; 59:340–373.

22. National Academy of Sciences: *Report of a Study, Health Services Research.* Washington, DC, National Academy of Sciences, 1979.

23. Greenberg D, Robins P: The changing role of social experiments in policy analysis, in Aiken L, Kehrer (eds): *Evaluation Studies: Annual Review,* Vol 10. Beverly Hills, CA, Sage Publications, 1985.

24. Ofosu-Amaah, Newmann AK: *The Danfa Comprehensive Rural Health and Family Planning Project, Ghana: Final Report.* Los Angeles, University of California at Los Angeles, Division of Population, Family and International Health, September 30, 1979.

25. Wholey JS: *Evaluation: Promise and Performance.* Washington, DC, Urban Institute, 1979.

26. Thompson J: *Organizations in Action.* New York, McGraw-Hill, 1967.

PART SIX

Health Care Policies and Politics

CHAPTER 15

Health Policy and the Politics of Health Care

Philip R. Lee
A. E. Benjamin

Political considerations have significantly affected nearly all the developments discussed in this book. However, the importance and central role of health care policy analysis and politics can best be highlighted by directly discussing these issues. That is the purpose of this chapter. While many of the topics mentioned here have been discussed from a variety of perspectives in other chapters, the policy and politics of changes in health care in the nation are the focus here, and examples of developments in health care serve as illustrations of the central role of political forces in shaping our health care system. The philosophies and processes discussed in other chapters, especially in Chapters 4 and 12, are further analyzed here.

Government plays a major role in planning, directing, and financing health services in the United States. The significance of the public sector is apparent as one considers the following: Public programs account for approximately 40 percent of the nation's personal health care expenditures, most physicians and other health care personnel are trained at public expense, almost 65 percent of all health research and development funds are provided by the government, and most nonprofit community and university hospitals have been built or modernized with government subsidies. The bulk of governmental expenditures are federal, with state and local government contributing significant, but much smaller, amounts.

Health policies and programs of the U.S. government have evolved piecemeal, usually in response to needs that were not being met by the private sector or by states and local governments. The result has been a proliferation of federal categorical programs administered by more than a dozen government departments. Over the years, new programs have been added, old ones redirected, and numerous efforts made to integrate and coordinate services. In recent years a major effort has been made by the Reagan Administration to significantly diminish the federal role in domestic social policy through the transfer of some programs to the states, reduced federal funding, or elimination of federal support entirely. The effort has been only partially successful and has not changed the basic configuration of publicly supported health programs. Functions of the public and private sectors have become increasingly interrelated, and roles are often poorly delineated. There can be little argument that the primary function of most government programs in health has been to support or strengthen the private sector (e.g., hospital construction, subsidy of medical student training, Medicare) rather than to develop a strong system of publicly provided health care.

Although U.S. government policies have evolved over a 200-year period, most of those affecting health services have developed since the enacement of the Social Security Act of 1935. Many federal health programs evolved because of failures in the private sector to provide necessary support—for example, biomedical research; others arose because results of the free market were grossly inequitable—for example, hospital construction; and some programs, such as Medicare and Medicaid, developed because health care was so costly that many could not afford to pay for necessary health services. Some federal health programs, such as biomedical research, potentially benefit everyone, while others, such as the Indian Health Service, reach only a small but needy segment of the population. Some programs, such as poliomyelitis immunization and health personnel development, have been effective in achieving their goals; others, such as health planning, have probably not realized even limited objectives; still others, such as Medicare, have reached some goals, although at a much higher cost than originally anticipated.

The process by which health policy is made in this country can be best understood by considering a fundamental paradox in American health care: government spends more and more money to support a wide range of health programs, services, and agencies, yet the role of government in the reform of our health care system remains limited and halting. Government is faced with a crisis in health care, defined primarily in terms of rising costs to public treasuries, while proposed solutions are framed in terms that do not address in a comphrensive fashion the sources of demand on the public purse. Indeed, solutions to the cost crisis have combined withdrawing benefits from those very recipient populations whose health care needs justify government intervention with attempts to reduce costs by either stimulating competition or regulating (reducing) payment to hospitals, nursing homes, and physicians. While federal policies may move in one direction, state policies may move in another. To understand this paradox, it is necessary to consider several characteristics of public policymaking and thus to explore the sources of the paradox and the nature of policy processes in health.

DIMENSIONS OF POLICYMAKING IN HEALTH

Policymaking in health care cross several levels of government and hundreds of programs, is complex, and no single analytical scheme can do it sufficient justice. Still, public policy students have identified five dimensions of the policy process: (1) the relationship of government to the private sector, (2) the distribution of authority within a federal system of government, (3) pluralistic ideology as the basis of politics, (4) the relationship between policy formulation and administrative implementation, and (5) incrementalism as a strategy of reform. Each will be considered in detail.

PUBLIC AND PRIVATE SECTOR POLITICS

Although the role of government in health care has grown considerably in recent years, that role remains relatively limited. The U.S. government is less involved in health care than are those of many other industrialized countries (1). This circumstance derives primarily from a persistent ideology that identifies the market system as the most appropriate setting for the exchange of health services and from a related belief that private sector support for public sector initiatives can be acquired only through accommodation to the interests of health care providers. The significance of the market ideology has been elaborated in analyses of the passage of Medicare and Medicaid in 1965 (2,3). The persistence of doubts about the appropriate role of government is certainly apparent in the renewed vitality of neoconservatism, in which it is argued that the market can better respond to the economic and social problems of our time if it is unfettered by government intervention (4).

Uncertainty about the role of government in health care has numerous consequences. The primary concern is the absence of any design or blueprint for governmental reform (5). Instead, the public sector (with its relatively immense capacity to raise revenues) is called on periodically to open and close its funding spigots to stimulate the health care market. Hospital construction and physician education are prominent examples of public activity. Not only is there no blueprint for public sector action, but governments in America harbor grave doubts about the appropriateness of regulation as a public sector activity. Dependence at the federal level on "voluntary approaches," such as the reduction of hospital costs in the late 1970s, delayed serious consideration of more stringent measures even as the costs to government of hospital care continued to rise dramatically (6).

A FEDERAL SYSTEM

The concept of federalism has evolved dramatically in meaning and practice since the founding of the republic more than 200 years ago. Originally, federalism was a legal concept that defined the consitutional division of authority between the federal government and the states. Federalism initially stressed the independence of each level of government from the other, while incorporating the idea that some functions, such as foreign policy, were the exclusive province of the central government, while other functions, such as education, police protection, and health care, were the resonsibility of regional units—state and local government. Federalism represents a form of governance that differs both from a unitary state, where regional and local authority derive legally from the central government, and from a confederation, in which the national government has limited authority and does not reach individual citizens directly (7,8).

Shifts in responsibilities assigned to various levels of government do not pose a serious problem for health policy if at least two conditions are met: (1) administrative or regulatory responsibilities and financial accountability are consonant, and (2) the various levels of government possess the appropriate capacities to assume those responsibilities assigned to them. Important questions can be raised regarding whether either of these conditions has been met in the development of health policy during the last two decades.

Analysis of federal–state relationships in programs as divergent as Medicaid, provider licensure, and family planning under Title X of the Public Health Service Act have suggested that the structure of these relationships produces outcomes widely held to be dysfunctional (e.g., Medicaid cutbacks) because one level of government (e.g., the states) can do nothing else under the conditions established by another (e.g., the federal government). The disjunction between administrative responsibilities and financial accountability (i.e., the terms of federalistic arrangements) in these cases has yielded results for which governments and the recipients of health care ultimately have paid a price. What seems to matter most in the structure of relationships within federalism is not so much the distribution of activities but the relationships among levels of government (9).

For allocations of authority among levels of government to work, it is important that governments possess those capacities appropriate to the responsibilities they confront. Governments must possess the capacity to generate revenue, the capability to plan and manage policies and programs, and the political will to plan and implement needed reform. State and local governments have been found wanting in each of these respects. Because state governments do not tax as heavily as the federal government (10), their capacity for generating new revenues is limited. Many states, moreover, are viewed as having inadequate administrative infrastructures, lacking sufficient sophisticated management techniques, and having limited capabilities in the conduct of policy analysis and planning.

Finally, there is evidence that state and local governments may have less political will to make decisions in the public interest than the federal government. Wide variations among states in program outputs (e.g., Medicaid) suggest significant inequities. The argument is not that every state, if freed from federal constraints, would establish standards for health programs that are certain to fall below former federal standards. Rather, it is that some states will surely exceed some federal standards and others will fall far below what is generally considered adequate. At the heart of this problem, many argue, is the reputedly greater susceptibility of state governments to interest group pressures and narrow conceptions of the public good.

Perhaps the most significant instance of the failure of the states to provide their citizens equal rights and equal protection has been in the area of civil rights. In education, housing, health care, and virtually every area of domestic social policy, it has been necessary for the federal government, particularly the federal courts, to require compliance with federal laws and regulations.

There is some countervailing evidence that the capacity and will to govern is becoming more widely diffused within the federal system. States (taken as a group) have spent a higher percentage of their budgets on health care than the federal government has, even though absolute federal expenditures for health have grown to more than double state and local health expenditures combined (11). A considerable increase at the state level in the conduct of policy analysis and its use in policy deliberations is one indication that state capacity to plan and manage is improving (12). Regarding inequities and political will, on the other hand, little counterevidence has emerged to challenge the argument that the states are more vulnerable to interest groups (e.g., provider groups in health) and that the result is a wide program variation among states in response to provider—not consumer—interests. The structure of federalism enables provider groups to maximize their power at the expense of consumer interests (9,13).

In a recent monograph on federalism and the national purpose, Brizius (14) groups the arguments favoring centralization into eight major clusters of related principles: (1) national purpose, (2) national security, (3) equity, (4) guaranteeing rights, (5) efficiency, (6) competence, (7) uniformity, and (8) unity. In contrast to the principles tending toward centralization are those that support greater decentralization and the maintenance of a truly federal system. Brizius groups 12 arguments for decentralization into seven principles: (1) diversity, (2) political sovereignty, (3) guaranteeing rights, (4) limits on power, (5) accountability, (6) efficiency and competence, and (7) competition.

The argument regarding centralization and decentralization has not been settled, despite a vigorous debate in the early years of the Reagan Administration. No agreement has been reached on the vital question of the distribution of authority and responsibility among various levels of government. The federal government finances hospital and medical services for the elderly through Medicare; it contributes at least 50 percent of health care costs for Medicaid beneficiaries, is the major supporter of biomedical research, provides a limited amount of support for a variety of health services (e.g., mental health, family planning, crippled children's services), is the sole regulator of the entry of new drugs into the market, and plays a critical role in the regulation of environmental and occupational health.

States spend a large portion of their general fund budgets on health care for the poor (Medicaid), on mental health services, on the support of a range of public health programs, and on the education and training of health professionals.

Local governments remain an important provider of health care, particularly hospital, outpatient and emergency care for the poor, mental health and substance abuse services, and a variety of public health services. Both state and local governments are mandated by higher levels of government (by either regulation or court order) to provide services or implement various environmental health or occupational health and safety regulations.

PLURALISTIC POLITICS

"Pluralism" is a term used by political theorists to describe a set of values about the effective functioning of democratic governments. Pluralists argue that democratic societies are organized into many diverse interest groups, which pervade all socioeconomic strata, and that this network of pressure groups prevents any one elite group from overreaching its legitimate bounds. As a theoretical framework for explaining the political context of policymaking, this perspective has been criticized relentlessly and appropriately (15,16). As an ideology that continues to influence the way elites and masses view government, pluralism becomes a basis for considering some essential elements of the process of public decision making in this country.

Interest groups play a powerful role in the health policy process. Most federal and state laws designed to address the health care needs of the population are shaped by the interaction between interest groups, key legislators, and agency representatives. Ginzberg (17) has identified four power centers in the health care industry that influence the nature of health care and the role of government: (1) physicians, (2) large insurance organizations, (3) hospitals, and (4) a highly diversified group of participants in profit-making activities within the health care arena.

The influence of these power centers is evident in policies at all levels of government. The development of Medicare and Medicaid policies reflects the powerful influence of physicians, hospitals, and nursing homes as well as their allies in the health insurance industry. For example, in enacting Medicare, Congress ensured that the law did not affect the physician–patient relationship, including the physician's

method of billing the patient. The system of physician reimbursement adopted by
Medicare is highly inflationary because it provides incentives to physicians to raise
prices and provide ancillary services, such as laboratory tests, electrocardiograms, and
x-ray films. Hospital reimbursement historically has been based on costs incurred in
providing care, creating strong incentives to provide more and more services. Despite
the impact of steadily rising Medicare costs on the Social Security trust fund, on Social
Security taxes (paid by employers and employees), and on the elderly, until recently,
Congress has steadfastly refused to alter Medicare's methods of payment to physicians
and hospitals. Also, many features of the program, patterned on principles developed;
by the medical industry, have had remarkable staying power.

The passage of a hospital prospective payment system (PPS) for Medicare by
Congress in 1983 signaled a potential shift in the power of key interest groups in health.
Recent history has made it clear that an apparent legislative defeat (e.g., the passage of
Medicare) can subsequently become an important source of benefits and power for
ostensibly losing interests (e.g., the medical lobby). The implementation of PPS has not
been a fiscal disaster for hospitals, as some predicted, and it remains to be seen whether
federal payment reforms will effect any fundamental alteration in the role of major
power centers in health care.

As the case of Medicare suggests, health policy in the United States has been a
product largely of medical politics (18). Marmor et al. (19) describe the political
"market" in health (i.e., institutional arrangements among actors in the political
system) as imbalanced. In an imbalanced market, participants have unequal power,
and those with concentrated rather than diffuse interests have the greater stake in the
effects of policy. At least until recently, provider interest groups have had a far greater
stake in shaping health policy than have consumer interests. Recently, large employers
have become increasingly important in the health policy debates at the federal and
state levels, particularly on issues related to health care cost containment.

Some observers argue that the rising costs of health care may be changing the
configuration of interest groups seeking to influence health policy. In recent years,
steadily escalating costs have stimulated other interests, especially labor, business, and
governments themselves, into giving greater attention to health policy and its
implications. In other words, their interests may be shifting from diffuse to concentrated.
The result may be that increased competition in the political marketplace from a more
diverse set of participants will lessen the dominance of medical provider groups (20).
The pluralist dream of effective interest groups that prevent any one group from
overreaching its legitimate bounds continues to influence our thinking about health
care.

POLICY IMPLEMENTATION

The nature of the health policy process is determined not only by the balance between
provider and consumer interests but also by the relationships of these interests to
government actors. Public policy students have observed that policymaking moves
through at least three stages: (1) agenda setting, the continuous process by which
issues come to public attention and are placed on the agenda for government action;
(2) policy adoption, the legislative process through which elected officials decide the
broad outlines of policy; and (3) policy implementation, the process by which
administrators develop policy by addressing the numerous issues unaddressed by

legislation (13,21). An important element of the health policy process involves the relative roles of elected officials and professional administrators. As one moves from agenda setting to policy adoption and implementation, it can be argued that the role of elected officials becomes more remote and that of administrators more crucial.

No policy theorist has pressed this argument with more conviction than Lowi (22). A central theme in what he calls interest-group liberalism is the growing role of administrators in politics. According to Lowi, in a period of resource richness and government expansion, such as the 1960s, government responded to a range of major organized interests, underwrote programs sought by those interests, and assigned program responsibility to administrative agencies. Through this process the programs became captives of the interest groups because the administrative agencies themselves were captured. Interest groups dominate the policy process, he argues, not only through their influence on the legislative process (policy adoption) but also through control of administration. In effect, governments in the United States make policies without laws, and they leave the lawmaking to administrators.

The study of policy implementation in health has received increased attention in recent years (23). Not surprisingly, the landmark legislation creating Medicare and Medicaid in 1965 has been the subject of much of this analysis. A study of Medicare by Feder is especially enlightening (24). She describes a number of crucial decisions related to the nature of the federal role that were not addressed by the legislation and discusses the process by which the Social Security Administration subsequently addressed these decisions. Feder argues that the agency could have pursued two fundamentally different strategies. Using a cost-effectiveness strategy, the agency could have assessed the impact of alternative approaches to a problem (e.g., hospital payment) on cost and quality and selected a course that would achieve maximum health care value per dollar spent. Alternatively, with a balancing strategy, the agency could have sought to identify relevant political actors (e.g., the American Hospital Association), weighed their capacity to aid or threaten program survival, and selected those policies that minimize political conflict (24).

Feder makes a persuasive argument that the Social Security Administration selected a balancing strategy. She traces the various consequences for the public interest of an approach that administratively transfers policy discretion to those provider groups with the greatest stake in the content of that policy. For those directly involved in the implementation of the Medicare program, the primary motivation was not to minimize political conflict, but to assure access for elderly Social Security beneficiaries to hospital and physician services. At one point these were jeopardized because of the vigorous enforcement of the Civil Rights Act by the U.S. Public Health Service and the Social Security Administration on instructions of the Secretary of Health, Education, and Welfare. When compliance with the Civil Rights Act was assured in hospitals, particularly in the South and Southwest, access barriers disappeared. Reimbursement policies followed the intentions of Congress and achieved the initial objective of assuring high levels of hospital and physician participation in Medicare.

INCREMENTAL REFORM

The powerful role of administrators in the implementation of policy is derived in part from the broad and ambiguous nature of much federal and state health legislation.

Despite dramatic improvements in the capacity of congressional staff to conduct policy analysis, the constraints of politics are such that ambiguity frequently is employed to assure the passage of legislation.

The public policy process in American government can best be described in terms of an incremental model of decision making (25,26). Simply stated, this model posits that policy is made in small steps (increments) and that policy is rarely modified in dramatic ways. Major actors in the political bargaining process, whether legislators, interest groups, or administrators, operate on the basis of certain rules, and these rules are founded in adherence to prior policy patterns. Because the consequences of policy change are difficult to predict and because unpredictability is risky in the political market, policymakers prefer reform in small steps to more radical change.

The incremental model was elaborated by decision theorists concerned with ways that policymakers managed a large information load and the uncertainty of their political environment. Quite a different view, but one that is compatible with this perspective, has been developed by Alford (27). Alford addresses the nature of reform in health care and its ideological basis. He identifies three approaches to reform, including market reformers, who call for an end to government interference in health care delivery and the restoration of market competition in health care institutions, and bureaucratic reformers, who blame market competition for defects in the system and call for increased administrative regulation of health care. What these perspectives share, notes Alford, is that each leads to incremental reform as well as the extent to which they challenge fundamental patterns of policy is limited. A third approach, the structural interest perspective, begins with an analysis of the ways in which the other two accept and benefit from current arrangements in health care. This perspective is formulated to challenge the effective, institutional control exercised by dominant structural interests that benefit from continuance of the system in its present form. As Alford makes clear, the market and bureaucratic approaches are descriptive of the limits of health care reform, and they underlie resistance to change in the health system.

Relatively little research in the United States has examined the institutional and class basis of public policy, including health policy (28). Those who hold that defects in health care are rooted deeply in the structure of a class society would radically alter the present health care system, creating a national health service, with decentralization of administration and community control over health care institutions and health professionals. Those who view defects in health care as having a class basis believe that tinkering with the health care system itself cannot achieve the desired outcomes but that these will follow major structural changes in society.

Policy developments of the coming decades will depend on which of these views of health care politics—pluralist, bureaucratic, or class—predominates. To date, the pluralists have played the most influential role in health care politics and policies.

A HISTORICAL FRAMEWORK:
THE DEVELOPMENT OF HEALTH POLICY
FROM 1798 TO 1988

Although the federal system in the United States has evolved continuously, at certain periods in our history the relationship between the federal, state, and local governments has undergone dramatic change. The major shifts in intergovernmental relations were often the result of a crisis (the Civil War, the Great Depression, civil rights issues) rather than the result of a critical examination of the issues.

Public health and health care did not loom large in the policy debate about federalism until the late 1940s, when President Truman advocated a program of national health insurance, and again in the 1960s, when the implementation of Medicare transformed the role of the federal government in health care. Over the years, however, health policy issues (e.g., federal regulation of food and drugs, federal support for biomedical research, hospital construction, and health professions education) have raised critical issues about the role of government in health care, intergovernmental relations, and the role of the private sector.

The private sector in the United States has always maintained a larger role in health care than it has in most other industrial nations. This has been true in both the financing and the delivery of services. While it is not possible to do full justice to the rich history of health care policy here, an effort is made to present highlights in the development of health policy that reflect the manner in which much has changed and much has stayed the same.

The slow emergence of public policies and programs related to health and health care in the United States has generally followed the pattern of other industrial countries, particularly those in western Europe (29). At least three stages in the process have been identified:

1. Private charity, including contracts between users and providers, and public apathy or indifference
2. Public provision of necessary health services that are not provided by voluntary effort and private contract
3. Substitution of public services and financing for private, voluntary, and charitable efforts

Although these three stages have been identified within many nations, different patterns have been observed among industrial countries. Political parties in the United States have been more reluctant than those in European countries or Canada to challenge the medical profession, hospitals, and the health insurance industry to promote health care reform.

The role of government at the federal, state, and local levels in public health and health care evolved in response to changes occurring in the health care system (30). With the major changes in health care that have occurred over the past 200 years, particularly those changes in the past 50 years, has come a transformation in the role of government.

THE EARLY YEARS OF THE REPUBLIC: A LIMITED ROLE FOR THE FEDERAL GOVERNMENT (1798–1862)

During the early years of the republic, the federal government played a limited role in both public health and health care, which were largely within the jurisdiction of the states and the private sector. Private charity shouldered the responsibility of care for the poor. The federal role in providing health care began in 1798, when Congress passed the Act for the Relief of Sick and Disabled Seamen, which imposed a 20-cent per month tax on seamen's wages for their medical care. The federal government later provided direct medical care for merchant seamen through clinics and hospitals in port cities, a policy that continues to this day. The federal government also played a limited role in imposing quarantines on ships entering U.S. ports in order to prevent epidemics (29). It did little or nothing, however, about the spread of communicable diseases within the nation, a problem that was thought to lie within the jurisdiction of the individual states.

Through the eighteenth, nineteenth, and early twentieth centuries, the major diseases in the United States, as in Europe, were infectious diseases, as discussed in Chapter 1. Tuberculosis, pneumonia, bronchitis, and gastrointestinal infections were the major killers. As the sanitary revolution progressed in the nineteenth century, social and economic conditions advanced, nutrition improved, and reproductive behavior was modified, and the burden of acute infection declined. National health policies during the nineteenth century were limited to the imposition of quarantines to prevent epidemics and the provision of medical care to merchant seamen and members of the armed forces. In laws beginning with the Port Quarantine Act, Congress preempted state and local authority and put an end to long-standing federal–state disagreements regarding the authority to prevent and control epidemics of yellow fever and cholera, as well as recurring outbreaks of plague and smallpox (31).

States first exercised their public health authority through special committees or commission. Most active concern with health matters was at the local level. Local boards of health or health departments were organized to tackle problems of sanitation, poor housing, and quarantine. Later, local health departments were set up in rural areas, particularly in the South, to counteract hookworm, malaria, and other infectious diseases that were widespread in the nineteenth and early twentieth centuries.

THE EVOLUTION OF HEALTH POLICY: THE EMERGENCE OF DUAL FEDERALISM AND THE TRANSFORMATION OF AMERICAN MEDICINE (1862–1935)

The Civil War brought about a dramatic change in the role of the federal government. The federal government not only engaged in a war to preserve the union but also began to expand its role in other ways that significantly altered the nature of federalism in the United States. This changing federal role was reflected in congressional passage of the first program of federal aid to the states, the Morrill Act of 1862, which granted federal lands to each state. Profits from the sale of these lands supported public institutions of higher education, known as *land-grant colleges* (32). Toward the end of the nineteenth century, the federal government began to provide cash grants to states for the establishment of agricultural experiment stations. While the federal role generally was expanding, the change had little impact on health care. An important exception occurred in the late 1870s when the Surgeon General of the Marine Hospital Service was given congressional authorization to impose quarantines within the United States. This marked the first time that the federal government assumed public health responsibility in an area where the states previously held jurisdiction.

While the first state health department was established in Louisiana in 1855, it was not until after the Civil War that the states began to assume a more significant role in public health. Massachusetts established the first permanent board of health in 1869. By 1909, public health agencies were established in all the states. During this period there also was a rapid development of local health departments. State and local governments based their policy changes and management practices on the rapid advances in the biological sciences. Drawing on these advances, state and local health departments moved beyond sanitation and quarantine to the scientific control of communicable diseases (33) (see Chapter 4).

The basic policies that created both state and local health departments derived from the police power of state governments (34). Thus the states, and not the federal government, were the key to translating the scientific advances of the late nineteenth century into public health policy and the dramatic improvements in public health that followed.

The most significant role played by state governments in personal health care was in the establishment of state mental hospitals. These first developed as a result of a reform movement in the midnineteenth century led by Dorothea Dix. Over the next century, state mental institutions evolved into isolated facilities for custodial care of the chronically mentally ill. The development of these asylums reinforced the stigma attached to mental illness and placed the care of the severely mentally ill outside the mainstream of medicine for more than a century (35).

Hospitals began to evolve in the nineteenth century from almshouses that provided shelter for the poor. Hospital sponsorship at the local level was either public (local government) or through a variety of religious, fraternal, or other community groups. Thus the nonprofit community hospital was born; this institution, rather than the local public hospital, gradually became the primary locus of medical care. Physicians provided voluntary services to the sick poor in order to earn the privilege of caring for their paying patients in the hospital (36). Hospital appointments became important for physicians in order to conduct their practices. Hospitals increased in the late nineteenth century and began to incorporate new medical technologies, such as anesthesia, aseptic surgery, and later, radiology. Although charity was the major source of care for the poor, public services also began to grow in the nineteenth century. Gradually, the public sector assumed responsibility for indigent care. The development of the hospital is discussed further in Chapter 6.

After the Morrill Act the next major change in the role of the federal government was in the regulation of food and drugs. After 20 years of debate and much public pressure, Congress enacted the Federal Food and Drug Act in 1906 to regulate the adulteration and misbranding of food and drugs, a responsibility previously exercised exclusively by the states. The law was designed primarily to protect the pocketbook of the consumer, not the consumer's health. While it provided some measure of control over impure foods, it had little impact on impure or unsafe drugs (37). The legislation not only represented a major change in the role of the federal government but also provided the constitutional basis for present-day regulation of testing, marketing, and promotion of prescription and over-the-counter drugs.

A number of other important developments in the early decades of the twentieth century had a strong impact on health care and health policy. Among the most significant were reforms in medical education that transformed not only education but also professional licensing and, eventually, health care itself. The American Medical Association and the large private foundations (e.g., Carnegie and Rockefeller) played a major role in this process. Voluntary hospitals also grew in number, size, and importance. Medical research produced new treatments. Infant mortality declined as nutrition, sanitation, living conditions, and maternal and infant care improved. Health care changed in significant ways, but it was little affected by public policy.

THE EVOLUTION OF HEALTH POLICY:
FROM DUAL FEDERALISM TO
COOPERATIVE FEDERALISM (1935–1961)

The Great Depression brought action by the federal government to save banks, support small business, provide direct public employment, stimulate public works, regulate financial institutions and business, restore consumer confidence, and provide Social Security in old age. The role of the federal government was transformed in the period of a few years. Federalism evolved from a dual pattern, with a limited role in domestic affairs for the federal government, to a cooperative one, with a strong federal role.

The Social Security Act of 1935 was certainly the most significant domestic social legislation ever enacted by Congress. This marked the real beginning of what has been termed "cooperative federalism." The act established the principle of federal aid to the states for public health and welfare assistance. It provided federal grants to states for maternal and child health and crippled children's services (Title V) and for public health (Title VI). It also provided for cash assistance grants to the aged, the blind, and destitute families with dependent children. This cash assistance program provided the basis for the current federal–state program of medical care for the poor, initially as Medical Assistance for the Aged in 1960 and then as Medicaid (Title XIX of the Social Security Act) in 1965. Both later programs linked eligibility for medical care to eligibility for cash assistance. More important, however, the Social Security Act of 1935 established the Old Age, Survivors' and Disability Insurance (OASDI) programs that were to provide the philosophical and fiscal basis for Medicare, a program of federal health insurance for the aged, also enacted in 1965 (Title XVIII of the Social Security Act). Passage of the Social Security Act was significant, for it provided the basis for direct federal income assistance to retired persons have established the basis for federal aid to the states in health and welfare; however, this legislation did not include a program of national health insurance. This was due principally to the opposition of the medical profession to any form of health insurance, particularly publicly funded insurance.

In 1938, after the death of a number of children due to the use of Elixir of Sulfonamide, consumer protection became a real issue. This disaster resulted in the enactment of the Food, Drug and Cosmetic Act of 1938, which required manufacturers to demonstrate the safety of drugs before marketing. This law was a further extension of the federal role and was consistent with other major changes in that role that occurred during the 1930s. After the passage of this act, little change was made in drug regulation law until the thalidomide disaster in the early 1960s.

Growing attention to maternal and child health, particularly for the poor, was reflected in grants to the states and in a temporary program instituted during World War II to pay for maternity care of wives of Army and Navy enlisted men. This means-tested program successfully demonstrated the capacity of the federal government to administer a national health insurance program. With rapid demobilization after the war and opposition by organized medicine, the program was terminated; but it was often cited by advocates of national health insurance, particularly those who accorded first priority to mothers and infants.

Introduction of the scientific method into medical research at the turn of the century and its gradual acceptance had a profound effect on national health policy and health care. The first clear organizational impact of the growing importance of research was the transformation of the U.S. Public Health Service Hygienic Laboratory, established in 1901 to conduct bacteriologic research and public health studies, into the National Institutes of Health (NIH) in 1930, with broad authority to conduct basic research. This was followed by enactment of the National Cancer Act of 1937 and the establishment of the National Cancer Institute within the framework of NIH. There followed multiple legislative enactments during and after World War II that created the present institutes, focused primarily on broad classes of disease, such as heart disease, cancer, arthritis, neurologic diseases, and blindness. In the 15 years immediately after World War II, NIH grew from a small government laboratory to the most significant biomedical research institute in the world. NIH became the principal supporter of biomedical research, quickly surpassing industry and private foundations. Indeed, in the period after World War II until the 1960s, federal support for biomedical research represented one of the few areas of health policy in which the federal government was active. The influence of organized medicine was a critical factor in limiting the federal role in other areas during this period.

In addition to federal support for biomedical research, largely through medical schools and universities, and a limited program of grants to states for public health and maternal and child health programs, federal policy related to hospital planning and construction became of primary importance, as discussed in Chapter 12. After World War II, it was evident that many of America's hospitals were woefully inadequate, and the Hill-Burton federal–state program of hospital planning and construction was launched in response. Its initial purpose was to provide funds to states to survey hospital bed supply and develop plans to overcome the hospital shortage, particularly in rural areas. The Hill-Burton Act was amended numerous times as its initial goals were met. This legislation provided the stimulus for a massive hospital construction program, with federal and state subsidies primarily for community, nonprofit, and voluntary hospitals. Public hospitals, supported largely by local tax funds to provide care for the poor, received little or no federal support until the needs of private institutions were met. The program became a model of federal–state–private sector cooperation in the distribution of substantial federal resources. It was a prime example of cooperative federalism and the major force—until enactment of Medicare and Medicaid—behind modernization of the voluntary community hospital system.

After World War II, President Truman urged Congress to enact a program of national health insurance, funded through federal taxes. President Truman's efforts and those of his supporters in Congress and organized labor were thwarted, again largely as a result of opposition by the American Medical Association. No progress was made in extending the federal role in financing of medical care because the medical profession argued that voluntary health insurance, such as Blue Cross, and commercial insurance could do the job.

By 1953, when the Department of Health, Education, and Welfare (now the Department of Health and Human Services) was created, the federal government's role in the nation's health care system, although limited, was firmly established. This role was designed primarily to support programs and services in the private sector. Biomedical research, research training, and hospital construction were the major pathways for federal support. Traditional public health programs, such as those for venereal disease control, tuberculosis control, and maternal and child health, were supported at minimal levels through categorical grants to the states. Federal support for medical care was restricted to military personnel, veterans, merchant seamen, and native Americans until 1960, when enactment of the Kerr-Mills law authorized limited federal grants to states for medical assistance for the aged. This program proved short-lived, but it highlighted the need for a far broader federal effort in medical care for the poor and the aged.

THE TRANSFORMATION OF HEALTH POLICIES:
THE NEW FRONTIER, THE GREAT SOCIETY,
AND CREATIVE FEDERALISM (1961–1969)

A number of major federal health policy developments took place between 1961 and 1969, during the presidencies of John F. Kennedy and Lyndon B. Johnson. Although federal suport was extended directly to universities, hospitals, and nonprofit institutes conducting research, most federal aid in health was channeled through the states. The term "creative federalism" was applied to policies developed during the Johnson Administration that extended the traditional federal–state relationship to include direct federal support for local governments (cities and counties), nonprofit organizations, and private businesses and corporations to carry out health, education, training, social services, and community development programs (7). The primary means used to forward the goals of creative federalism were grants-in-aid. More than 200 grant programs were enacted during the 5 years of the Johnson Administration.

The first major health policy changes after the election of President Kennedy again was the result of a crisis. The thalidomide disaster in Europe had little direct impact in the United States because the Food and Drug Administration had not approved the drug for marketing here. The disaster nonetheless focused renewed attention on the problems of drug safety, efficacy and promotion, and led to the most sweeping reforms of federal drug laws in 24 years. The 1962 amendments to the Food, Drug and Cosmetic Act specified that a drug must be demonstrated to be effective, as well as safe, before it could be marketed. Advertising also was strictly regulated, and more effective provisions for removal of unsafe drugs from the market were included (37).

The categorical programs that developed during the period of creative federalism were numerous and varied. Some programs were based on disease (heart disease, cancer, stroke, and mental illness); some, on public assistance eligibility (Medicaid); some, on age (Medicare, crippled children); some, on institutions (hospitals, nursing homes, neighborhood health centers); some, on political jurisdiction (state or local departments of public health); some, on geographic areas that did not follow traditional political boundaries (community mental health centers, catchment areas, the Appalachian Regional Commission); and some, on activity (research, facility construction, health professionals training, and health care financing) (31).

Among the more important new laws enacted during the Johnson Administration were the Health Professions Educational Assistance Act of 1963, which authorized direct federal aid to medical, dental, pharmacy, and other professional schools, as well as to students in these schools; the Maternal and Child Health and Mental Retardation Planning Amendments of 1963, which initiated comprehensive maternal and infant care projects and centers serving the mentally retarded; the Civil Rights Act of 1964, which prohibited racial discrimination, including segregated schools and hospitals; the Economic Opportunity Act of 1964, which provided authority and funds to establish neighborhood health centers serving low-income populations; the Social Security Amendments of 1965, particularly Medicare and Medicaid, which financed medical care for the aged and the poor receiving cash assistance; the Heart Disease, Cancer and Stroke Act of 1965, which launched a national attack on these major killers through regional medical programs; and the Comprehensive Health Planning and Public Health Service Amendments of 1966 and the Partnership for Health Act of 1967, which reestablished the principle of block grants for state public health services (reversing a 30-year trend of categorical federal grants in health). This legislation also created the first nationwide health planning system, which was dramatically changed in the 1970s to focus on regulation of health care as well as health planning (38) (Chapter 12). It should be noted that not until the Nixon and Reagan Administrations was the block grant concept widely applied to federal grants-in-aid to the states. Of the many new health programs initiated during the Johnson presidency, only Medicare was administered directly by the federal government.

The programs of the Johnson presidency had a profound effect on intergovernmental relationships, the concept of federalism, and federal expenditures for domestic social programs. Grant-in-aid programs alone (excluding Social Security and Medicare) grew from $7 billion at the beginning of the Kennedy and Johnson Administrations era in 1961 to $24 billion in 1970, at the end of that era. In the next decade the impact was to be even more dramatic as federal grant-in-aid expenditures for these programs grew to $82.9 billion in 1980. "Grants-in-aid," note Reagan and Sanzone (7), "constitute a major social invention of our time and are the prototypical, although not statistically dominant [they now constitute over 20 percent of domestic federal outlays], form of federal domestic involvement."

The programs of the Johnson Administration not only had a significant effect on the nature and scope of the federal role in domestic social programs but also had important consequences for health care. Federal funds for biomedical research and training, health personnel development, hospital construction, health care financing, and a variety of categorical programs were designed primarily to improve access to health care and secondarily to improve its quality. Increased attention during this period was given to the notion of health care as a right, a concept similar to the principle of the "earned right" that underlies the Social Security system (39,40).

Although there was a profound change in the role of the federal government, many policies adopted during this time reflected the interests of the medical profession, the hospitals, and the health insurance industry. Medicare and Medicaid hospital reimbursement policies were designed to assure hospital participation. Adoption of the cost-based method of reimbursement proved a boon for hospitals but was very costly for the taxpayer. Policies designed to meet the physician shortage of the 1960s eventually developed full support from organized medicine. Designed to strengthen the capacity of the nation's medical schools to respond to a nationally perceived need, these policies also provided direct benefit to an interest group of growing power—medical schools.

HEALTH POLICY IN AN ERA OF LIMITED RESOURCES: FROM CREATIVE FEDERALISM TO NEW FEDERALISM AND A RETURN TO DEPENDENCE ON COMPETITION AND THE PRIVATE SECTOR (1969–19??)

During the 1970s, President Nixon coined the term "New Federalism" to describe his efforts to move away from the categorical programs of the Johnson years toward general revenue sharing, through which federal revenues are transferred to state and local governments with as few federal strings as possible, and toward block grants, through which grants are allocated to state and local governments for broad general purposes. During the Nixon and Ford Administrations (1969–1977), considerable conflict developed between the executive branch and the Congress with respect to domestic social policy, including the New Federalism strategy originally advocated by President Nixon. Congress strongly favored categorical grants, with their detailed provisions, and was opposed to both revenue sharing and block grants. This period also witnessed an erosion of trust between federal middle management and congressional committees and subcommittees (41).

President Nixon also differed sharply from President Johnson in his explicit support for private rather than public efforts to solve the nation's health problems. On this fundamental issue the Nixon administration made its position clear: "Preference for action in the private sector is based on the fundamentals of our political economy—capitalistic, pluralistic and competitive—as well as upon the desire to strengthen the capability of our private institutions in their effort to provide health services, to finance such services, and to produce the resources that will be needed in the years ahead" (42).

Although the Nixon Administration attempted to implement its New Federalism policies across a broad front, progress was made primarily in the fields of community development, personnel training, and social services. Categorical grant programs in health continued to expand despite attempts by both the Nixon and Ford administrations to transfer program authority and responsibility to the states and to reduce the federal role in domestic social programs. During the period 1965–1975, more than 75 major pieces of health legislation were enacted by Congress, indicating continued support for the categorical approach by the federal government (38).

Although categorical health programs proliferated in the 1960s and 1970s, the expansion of two programs—Medicare and Medicaid—dwarfed the others. While these programs contributed to medical inflation, their growth was due largely to the rising costs of medical care in the 1970s. The federal and state governments became third parties that underwrote the costs of a system that had few cost-constraining elements, and the staggering expenditures had profound effects on health policy.

The federal government's response to skyrocketing health care costs (and thus governmental expenditures) assumed a variety of forms. Federal subsidies of hospitals and other health facility construction were ended and replaced by planning and regulatory mechanisms designed to limit their growth. In the mid-1970s health personnel policies focused on specialty and geographic maldistribution of physicians rather than physician shortage, and by the late 1970s, concern was expressed about an oversupply of physicians and other health professionals (43). Direct subsidies to expand enrollment in health professions schools were cut back and then eliminated. Funding for biomedical research began to decline in real dollar terms when an abortive "war on cancer" launched by President Nixon appeared to produce few concrete results and when Medicare and Medicaid preempted most federal health dollars.

More important than the constraints placed on resources allocated for health care were regulations instituted to slow the growth of health care costs (Chapter 12). Two direct actions were taken by the federal government: (1) a limit on federal and state payments to hospitals and physicians under Medicare and Medicaid (included in the 1972 Social Security Amendments) and (2) a period of wage and price control applied to the general economy when the Economic Stabilization Program was introduced to dampen increasing inflation. Wage and price controls on hospitals and physicians were continued after the general restrictions were removed. When controls were lifted in 1974, health care costs again began to climb.

Another regulatory initiative was designed to control costs through limiting the utilization of hospital care by Medicare and Medicaid beneficiaries. Although the original Medicare and Medicaid legislation required hospital utilization review committees, these appeared to have little effect on hospital utilization or costs. In 1972 amendments to the Social Security Act (PL 92-103) required the establishment of Professional Standards Review Organizations (PSROs) to review the quality and appropriateness of hospital services provided to beneficiaries of Medicare, Medicaid, maternal and child health, and crippled children programs (paid for under authority of Title V of the Social Security Act). PSROs were composed of physicians who reviewed hospital records in order to determine whether length of stay and services provided were appropriate. Results of these efforts have been mixed. In only a few are_s where PSROs have been in operation is there evidence that cost increases have been restrained, and in these areas it is not clear that the PSRO has been a critical factor.

An attempt also was made to control costs through major changes in the organization of medical care, as discussed throughout this book. Efforts were made to stimulate the growth of group practice prepayment plans, which provide comprehensive services for a fixed annual fee. These capitation-based prepayment organizations were defined in federal legislation enacted in 1973 as Health Maintenance Organizations (HMOs). Studies have demonstrated that HMOs provide comprehensive care at significantly less cost than fee-for-service providers, primarily because of lower rates of hospitalization (see Chapters 5 and 11) (44). Predictably, the federal stimulus for development of HMOs encountered strong resistance from organized medicine. Nevertheless, the program successfully enhanced professional and public awareness of HMOs and assisted in the development of a number of small prepaid group practices. The impact on costs at the national level, however, remained minimal.

An additional regulatory initiative enacted during President Nixon's second term was the National Health Planning and Resource Development Act of 1974 (PL 93-641). This law incorporated some of the planning principles from the Partnership for Health Act of 1967 and the Heart Disease, Cancer and Stroke Act of 1965, both of which were terminated with the enactment of PL 93-641. In addition to the health planning responsibility assigned to State Health Planning and Development Agencies (SHPDAs) and to local health systems agencies (HSAs), the law required that health care facilities obtain prior approval from the state for any expansion, in the form of a "certificate of need" (CON).

The National Health Planning and Development Act was enacted when decentralization of government authority and new federalism were primary strategies for achieving national objectives and when the role of special interests, such as organized medicine, was expanding at both federal and state levels. State and local health planning agencies created by the law resisted efforts to impose what they considered to be too much federal direction and regulation. With few exceptions, HSAs were not part of local government, but rather nonprofit private agencies strongly influenced by health care providers, particularly physicians and hospitals represented on their boards of directors. Although health planning agencies were concentrating their efforts on health care costs, particularly those generated by additional hospital beds and technology, these efforts appeared to have little effect in the face of inflationary pressures from the hospital reimbursement policies of Blue Cross, Medicare, Medicaid, and commercial health insurance carriers. The regulatory role that they were required to play, particularly the approval (or disapproval) of the certificate of need required for new hospital and nursing home construction, created growing resistance among providers. Although this regulatory role apparently has had little impact on total investments by hospitals (45), provider opposition to it has led to efforts to limit the authority of health planning agencies.

Although the New Federalism advocated by President Reagan was a dramatic departure from previous policies and trends because of the scope of his proposals, the roots of these policies were first evident in the comprehensive Health Planning and Public Health Service amendments enacted in 1966 during the presidency of Lyndon Johnson. They were increasingly evident in both the policy initiatives and the budgetary decisions of Presidents Nixon and Ford. The Nixon and Ford New Federalism policies were not only similar to those later advocated by President Reagan but their fiscal and monetary policies also were designed to reduce the growth of federal spending and program responsibility.

During the presidency of Jimmy Carter (1977–1981), there were few new health policy initiatives. The Carter Administration tried without success to get Congress to enact hospital cost-containment legislation. Special interests, particularly hospitals and physicians, again prevailed. They were able to convince Congress that a voluntary effort would be more effective. Escalating health care costs did moderate during the debate in Congress, but when mandatory controls were discontinued, costs rose at a record rate. The picture in the late 1970s was one of frustration with efforts to control costs. Concern about access to care became a secondary consideration.

In 1979, when legislative authority for health planning was renewed, two conflicting congressional attitudes emerged: (1) an antiregulatory, procompetitive sentiment that was to grow in the 1980s (46) and (2) a continuing movement toward decentralization of existing planning and regulatory programs, providing state and local authorities with increasing responsibility. Congress was not anxious to spend more money on medical care, and the procompetitive approach was promoted as a more effective means of cost containment than continued expansion of regulatory cost controls.

Since it is inherently difficult to make specific changes in health planning and regulatory processes that increase beneficial competition, these new provisions simply added impossible goals to the already lofty purposes identified for health planning— improving access and assuring quality of care while controlling costs. These procompetitive, antiregulatory, and prodecentralization forces found full expression 2 years later with the enactment of the Omnibus Budget Reconciliation Act of 1981 and in efforts in 1982 to eliminate federal support for local health planning efforts.

The Reagan Administration accelerated the degree of pace of change in policy that had been developing since the early years of the Nixon Administration. The most prominent shifts in federal policy advanced by the Reagan Administration that have directly affected health care are (1) a significant reduction in federal expenditures for domestic social programs; (2) decentralization of program authority and responsibility to the states, particularly through block grants; (3) deregulation and greater emphasis on market forces and competition to stimulate health care reform and more effective control of health care costs; (4) tax reductions, despite significant increases in the national debt, with a resulting decline in the fiscal capacity of the federal government to fund domestic social programs; and (5) Medicare cost containment through the implementation of a prospective payment system for hospitals based on costs per case, using diagnosis-related groups (DRGs) as the basis for payment.

An important consequence of the block grants enacted by Congress at the urging of the Reagan Administration is that the wide discretion that they provide to the individual states fosters inequities in programs among the states. This, in turn, makes it impossible to assure uniform benefits for target populations, such as the poor and the aged, across jurisdictions or to maintain accountability with so many varying state approaches (13). Because the most disadvantaged persons are heavily dependent on state-determined benefits, they are especially vulnerable in this period of economic flux. These policies also have increased pressure on state and local governments to underwrite program costs at the same time that many states, cities, and counties are under great pressure to curb expenditures.

Although the Reagan Administration strongly favors deregulation and stimulation of procompetitive market forces, this has had little impact on federal health care policies except in the health planning area. Indeed, in the Medicare program, the use of regulations to limit hospital reimbursement and physician fees has increased. At the state level, however, major changes are under way that respond to the growing influence of the free market ideology. In California, major reforms were enacted in 1982 in an attempt to increase competition among hospitals and reduce the costs of Medicaid in that state. Private insurance companies were also authorized to contract directly with hospitals through preferred provider contracts in an attempt to stimulate price competition among hospitals.

Congress has considered a number of procompetition proposals related to Medicare, Medicaid, and private health insurance. Although the proposals differ in detail, several elements characterize the procompetitive approach: (1) changes in tax treatment for employers, employees, or both, regarding employer contributions to health insurance plans (not supported by Congress and unlikely to become policy); (2) establishment of incentives or requirements for employers to offer employees multiple choices of health insurance plans, subject to certain limitations with respect to coverage of services and cost sharing, including catastrophic illness benefits and preventive care; and (3) establishment of Medicare voucher systems under which elderly and disabled persons would receive a fixed value voucher that could be used toward the purchase of a qualified health insurance plan (unlikely to be enacted).

Although President Reagan's New Federalism and procompetition–deregulation policies have attracted the greatest attention, it is the dramatic reduction in federal fiscal capacity due to tax cuts and high interest rates that have had the most immediate effect on health services. While the federal government is debating cost-containment strategies, a number of states have moved to restrict expenditures for Medicaid beneficiaries because of the continued impact of high costs on Medicaid expenditures at the state and federal levels. Several states, including California, have enacted dramatic policy changes, restricting patients' freedom to choose providers, reducing levels of hospital and physician reimbursement, and shifting the burden of large numbers of poor patients back to local government.

The politics of limited resources began to dominate the U.S. political scene in the 1970s, and this continues into the 1980s, with little prospect of change. Controlling the costs of health care has become a critical need at the federal and state levels. In the 1970s, policy efforts focused more on limiting federal and state expenditures in Medicare and Medicaid than they did on dealing with the root causes of the problem— reimbursement incentives in Medicare, Medicaid, and private insurance mediated through the fee-for-service health care system that have led to enormous inflation in health care costs. With the advent of the prospective payment system (PPS) for Medicare, enacted by Congress in 1983, federal policymakers have begun to attack these perverse reimbursement incentives. Similarly, the introduction of competitive contracting at the state level addresses problems created by traditional retrospective reimbursement.

Whether these approaches to restraining hospital expenditures are effective remains to be seen. Given a policy process characterized by limited government roles, federalism, pluralism, administrative bargaining, and incrementalism, prospects remain relatively dim for controlling expenditures in ways that protect vulnerable groups such as the poor and the elderly. It is increasingly evident that those groups whose needs originally inspired special programs are relinquishing the gains achieved in access to care.

The cost-containment strategies of the past decade, particularly those since 1981, combined with the effects of the recession of 1981-1982 on unemployment and access to private health insurance; the growth of the undocumented alien, immigrant, and refugee populations; and the diminishing commitment to provide for the near poor and the working poor has led to a significant increase in the number of uninsured and underinsured. Census Bureau data for 1984 revealed that 17 percent of the population under age 65 years (35 million people) lacked any health insurance, an increase of more than 20 percent since 1979 (47).

Federal policies related to Medicare and Medicaid, taxes, and refugees and undocumented aliens; state policies related to health care cost containment and Medicaid, ranging from California's procompetitive approach to New York's regulatory strategy; and the policies of private insurance companies and employers related to private health insurance, competition, and cost containment have all contributed to the rising number of uninsured and underinsured. Because the working poor, the disabled, refugees, new immigrants, undocumented aliens, and workers in small businesses do not have the influence of the large employers, the insurance industry, physicians, hospitals, and other influential participants in health policy, it is unlikely that their voices will be heard, unless the costs of their care impose such a burden on state and local governments and community hospitals (i.e., bad debt and charity care) that these groups will gain allies willing to advocate on their behalf. Because the interests of these groups remain diffuse in terms of potential for political action, it is unlikely that they can compete effectively in the policy process with the interest groups that have long influenced the shape of public policy in health.

The changes in public policy, health care financing, and health care organization have been viewed as both evolutionary and revolutionary. Like Canada, Australia, New Zealand, and the countries of western Europe, the United States has moved from a phase of rapid expansion with an emphasis on access to care to a phase of containment with an emphasis on cost containment (48). This latter phase began in the early 1970s and has yet to reach its peak.

While two fundamentally different approaches to cost containment have been advocated and applied in the past 15 years—regulation and competition—it appears that a mixed system will emerge in the United States because of the strong role of the private sector, a federalist system of government, the dominance of pluralistic politics, and a penchant for incremental reform.

In his critical analysis of health planning in the United States, France, England, and Quebec Province in Canada, Rodwin calls for "regulated competition" (48). Enthoven (49), in his most recent contribution to the policy debate about the role of competition, calls for both "managed competition" and universal health insurance. Whether health policymakers decide on competition, regulation, "regulated competition," or "managed competition," there is no way to escape the need to link health planning and health care financing. It is critical that reimbursement systems— whether capitation or fee-for-service—encourage hospitals, physicians, nursing homes, pharmacists, and other providers to pursue society's interests as well as their own.

There are signs of an emerging consensus amid all the conflicts and tensions engendered by the need to constrain the growth in the health care sector. Various forces will affect future policies: some, such as the aging of the population, are beyond the control of policymakers; others, such as the rapid increase in physician supply and the use of an increasing number of new technologies in health care, are amenable to more direct policy interventions. One of the keys will be to reach agreement on the nature and scope of universal health insurance. Another will be to modify reimbursement policies to achieve appropriate policy goals. Another will be to deal realistically with the failure of the "free market" and unregulated competition to assure equity. These tasks can be accomplished, and the current experimentation at the state level will provide the models for national health policy.

REFERENCES

1. Jonas S, Banta D: Government in the health care delivery system, in Jonas S (ed): *Health Care Delivery in the United States.* New York, Springer, 1981.
2. Marmor TR: *The Politics of Medicare.* Chicago, Aldine, 1973.
3. Vladeck BC: *Unloving Care: The Nursing Home Tragedy.* New York, Basic Books, 1980.
4. Wade RC: The suburban roots of new federalism. *The New York Times Magazine,* August 1, 1982:20, 21, 39, 46.
5. Ginzberg D: Health reform: The outlook for the 1980s. *Inquiry* 1978; 15:311–326.
6. Pechman JA (ed): *Setting National Priorities: The 1980 Budget.* Washington, DC, The Brookings Institution, 1979.
7. Reagan MD, Sanzone JG: *The New Federalism,* 2nd ed. New York, Oxford University Press, 1981, p 7.
8. Hale GE, Palley ML: *The Politics of Federal Grants.* Washington, DC, Congressional Quarterly Press, 1981.
9. Vladeck BC: The design of failure: Health policy and the structure of federalism. *J Health, Politics, Policy, Law* 1979; 4:522–535.
10. Reagan MD: *The New Federalism.* New York, Oxford University Press, 1972.
11. Clarke GJ: The role of the states in the delivery of health services, in Jain SC (ed): *Role of State and Local Governments in Relation to Personal Health Services,* 1981. Reprinted from *American J Publ Health* 1981; Vol. 71.
12. Lee RD, Staffeldt RJ: Executive and legislative use of policy analysis in the state budgetary process. *Policy Analysis* 1977; 3:395–405.
13. Estes CL: *The Aging Enterprise.* San Francisco, Jossey-Bass, 1980.
14. Brizius JA: *Federalism and National Purpose* (Working Paper 2, Project on the Federal Social Role). Washington, DC, National Conference on Social Welfare, 1984, pp 72–98.
15. Schattschneider EE: *The Semisovereign People.* New York, Holt, Rinehart & Winston, 1960.
16. Bachrach P: *The Theory of Democratic Elitism: A Critique.* Boston, Little, Brown, 1967.

17. Ginzberg E (ed): *Regionalization and Health Policy.* Washington, DC, U.S. Government Printing Office, 1977.

18. Silver GA: Medical politics, health policy, party health platforms, promise and performance. *Internatl J Health Serv* 1976; 6:331–343.

19. Marmor TR, Wittman DA, Heagy TC: The politics of medical inflation. *J Health, Politics, Policy, Law* 1976; 1:69–84.

20. Feldstein PJ: The politics of health, in Lee PR, Brown N, Red IVSW (eds): *The Nation's Health: Article Booklet.* San Francisco, Boyd & Fraser, 1981, pp 40–42.

21. Sabatier B, Mazamania D: Conditions of effective implementation. *Policy Analysis* 1979; 5:481–504.

22. Lowi TJ: *The End of Liberalism: The Second Republic of the United States.* New York, Norton, 1979.

23. Silver GA: *Preface: Uncertainties of Federal Child Health Policies.* Hyattsville, MD, National Center for Health Services Research, 1978.

24. Feder JM: *Medicare: The Politics of Federal Hospital Insurance.* Lexington, MA, Lexington Books, 1977.

25. Lindblom CE: The science of "muddling through." *Public Admin Rev* 1959; 10:79–88.

26. Wildavky A: *The Politics of the Budgetary Process.* Boston, Little, Brown, 1964.

27. Alford RR: *Health Care Politics: Ideological and Interest Group Barriers to Reform.* Chicago, University of Chicago Press, 1975.

28. Estes CL: Austerity and aging in the United States: 1980 and beyond. *Internatl J Health Serv* 1982; 12:573.

29. Lee PR, Silver GA: Health planning—a view from the top with specific reference to the USA, in Fry J, Farndale WAJ (eds): *International Medical Care.* Oxford, Medical and Technical Publishing Co, Ltd, 1972.

30. Torrens PR: Overview of the health services system, in Williams SJ, Torrens PR (eds): *Introduction to Health Services.* New York, Wiley, 1980.

31. Lewis I, Sheps C: *The Sick Citadel: The American Academic Medical Center and the public Interest.* Cambridge, Oelgeschlager, Gunn and Hain, 1983.

32. Hale GE, Palley ML: *The Politics of Federal Grants.* Washington, DC, Congressional Quarterly Press, 1981.

33. Miller CA, Moos MK, Kotch JB, et al: Role of local health departments in the delivery of ambulatory care, in Jain SC (ed): *Role of State and Local Governments in Relation to Personal Health Services.* Chapel Hill, University of North Carolina, 1981.

34. Miller CA, Gilbert B, Warren DG, et al: Statutory authorizations for the work of local health departments. *Am J Public Health* 1977; 67:940–946.

35. Foley HA: *Community Mental Health Legislation.* Lexington, MA, Lexington Books, 1975.

36. Silver GA: *A Spy in the House of Medicine.* Germantown, MD, Aspen Systems Corp, 1976.

37. Silverman M, Lee P: *Pills, Profits, and Politics.* Berkeley, University of California Press, 1974.

38. U.S. Department of Health, Education, and Welfare: *Health in America 1776–1976*. DHEW Publication No. (HRA) 76-616. Government Printing Office, 1976.

39. Lee PR, Jonsen AR: The right to health care. *Am Rev Resp Dis* 1974; 109:591–593.

40. Callahan D: Health and society: Some ethical imperatives. *Daedalus* 1977; 106:1.

41. Walker D: *Toward a Functioning Federalism.* Cambridge, MA, Winthrop, 1981.

42. Richardson EL: *Towards a Comprehensive Health Policy in the 1970s.* Washington, DC, Department of Health, Education, and Welfare, 1971.

43. Lee PR, LeRoy L, Stalcup J: *Primary Care in a Specialized World.*

44. Luft HS: *Health Maintenance Organizations: Dimensions of Performance.* New York, Wiley-Interscience, 1980.

45. Salkever DS, Bice TW: The impact of certificate-of-need controls on hospital investment. *Milbank Mem Fund Quart* 54:185–214, 1976.

46. Budetti P: Congressional perspectives on health planning and cost containment: Lessons from the 1979 debate and amendments. *J Health Human Resources Admin* 1981; 4:10–19.

47. Blendon RJ, Aiken LH, Freeman HE, et al: Uncompensated care by hospitals or public insurance for the poor. *New Engl J Med* 1986; 314:1160–1163.

48. Rodwin VG: The Health Planning Predicament. Berkeley, University of California Press, 1984, 303.

49. Enthoven AC: Managed competition and health care and the unfinished agenda. *Health Care Fin Rev* 1986(Annl Suppl); 150–120.

EPILOGUE

Issues for the Future

In this book we have looked at what has happened in the past and is happening in the present in health care in the United States. Before concluding the book, it is imperative that we also look toward the future. What is the future of the American health care system? What are the issues and pressures that will shape and mold the American health care system in the future?

A number of key issues and forces will be increasingly important in determining what kind of health care system we have in the future. It is absolutely essential that health care workers in the future be aware of these issues and trends, not just so that they can function more effectively as managers and planners, but also so that they can take an active part in developing the future of health care in the United States. This epilogue briefly identifies some of these key issues and discuss why they will probably be important to our future.

THE REAL PURPOSE OF HEALTH CARE

At the present time, the United States really has a "sickness care" system, not a "health" system. Tremendous amounts of money, energy, and personal resources are presently being spent on the treatment of illnesses after they have started, sometimes *long* after they have started. While this country probably has the most sophisticated and elaborate technology establishment in the world for the treatment of illness, it must be admitted that this is probably the wrong part of the disease spectrum in which to excel. If excellence in health is what we want, we should be trying to attack disease earlier, when it may be amenable to simpler treatment or even when it may still be preventable.

The challenge for the future will be one of remaking and reshaping a health care system so that it emphasizes methods of preventing illness from happening rather than treating an illness after it is already present. This process will involve a change in values and attitudes, a change in reimbursement patterns, a change in the provider system, and most important of all, a change in the power structure of health care. None of these changes will occur easily, and perhaps none of them will occur at all, but one thing is certain: the next health care "revolution" in this country, the next major advance, will certainly have to be the establishment of a system that actively promotes healthier

480

lifestyles and works to prevent or limit the occurrence of accidents, many acute illnesses, and most chronic diseases in all its aspects.

THE ESTABLISHMENT OF PRIORITIES FOR HEALTH CARE AND THEIR IMPLEMENTATION

In 1985 U.S. citizens spent $425 billion, or 10.7 percent of the gross national product (GNP), on health care. This amounted to $1721 for every person in our country (see Chapter 11).

While the amount is staggering and the percentage of GNP spent on health care is immense, these two factors by themselves are not the major reasons for concern. What should really worry all interested people is that we have no idea if these funds were intentionally channeled toward those problems that have the most direct relationship to the *real* health status of our people. There is absolutely no indication that these funds were spent according to any sort of priority ranking, by either disease condition or population group.

In the United States today, while we have the means of identifying the major health problems and their impact on the real health status of our people, we have absolutely no means of establishing any set of priorities for organized or concerted action to alleviate those problems. Further, even if we *did* have a system for identifying the most important problems and establishing priorities, there is virtually no means of focusing the efforts of our health care system in a coordinated and directed fashion toward those particular problems. Our health care system is a collection of absolutely independent entities, each of which choose their own priorities and determine their own course of action, regardless of the real needs and priorities in health care for our society as a whole. We do not operate in health care as a whole society, but rather as a loose collection of individual and independent programs and institutions.

For the future, one of the greatest challenges facing our health care system, particularly as it experiences the economic realities of budget limitations and reductions, is to establish a means whereby our nation can focus its combined resources and energies on those health problems that are most critical to solve. Although it will certainly take a Herculean effort and test the goodwill and good spirits of everyone involved, we can no longer afford the scattered and random approach of spreading our national resources over as wide an array of situations and conditions as possible with the hope that by using enough money and resources, we will somehow impact everything important. There simply will not be enough money available. We must establish a more rational and organized system of identifying real needs, establishing definite priorities, and intentionally channeling resources toward the conditions and populations of highest priority.

THE CONFLICT BETWEEN COST AND QUALITY OF CARE

For the future, there will continue to be a great need to control the rising costs of health care. In the last few years, mechanisms have been developed [such as the use of diagnosis-related groups (DRG) prospective payment systems for hospitals and the enrollment of Medicare recipients in Health Maintenance Organizations (HMOs)] that show promise of slowing the rate of increase in health care costs.

Unfortunately, however, there is a growing suspicion in some parts of the American health care system that the control of health care costs is being carried out now and may be carried out in the future at the expense of decrease in quality of patient care. Regardless of whether these suspicions are valid, the concern is a very real one: the scarcity of financial resources available to provide health care may lead to a decrease in the quality of patient care provided.

For the future, it will be important to be able to document accurately (indeed, much more accurately than now) the actual quality of patient care being delivered. Without accurate measurements of *real* quality as a baseline, it will be absolutely impossible to detect anything but the grossest decline in the quality of patient care. Without accurate measurements of *all* aspects of care provided by the American health care system in the future, the quality of patient care provided by that system may be quietly and gradually eroded, and many years of progress and improvement may slip away unnoticed.

The pessimistic observers say that there is no way that the present level of the quality of patient care can be maintained if the total level of financial support is not maintained as well. The more optimistic observers, however, point out that much of our present health care financial resources are really wasted on nonessential or unnecessary procedures, tests, and materials. A more optimistic viewpoint suggests that a *shift* in resources away from unnecessary and nonproductive use of health care services and *toward* those items and elements that *really* do contribute to quality of patient care, can actually lead to an era of increased quality and stabilized (or declining) health care costs. Whichever camp one tends to agree with, the relationship of health care costs and quality must be continuously borne in mind in the future.

DECREASING SIZE OF CERTAIN PORTIONS OF THE AMERICAN HEALTH CARE SYSTEM

Since the earliest days of the American health care system, one of its strongest characteristics has been growth and expansion in size. Almost since its inception, there has been an uninterrupted increase in the amount of money provided to the American health care system, the size and scope of our hospitals, and the numbers of physicians, nurses, and other health care personnel.

It has become apparent in the last few years that the American health care system reached maximum size, at least in many parts of the system, and most probably now will see a decrease in size and numbers. Certainly with regard to the supply of physicians, it seems clear that the United States has overproduced physicians in the last few years and that there will be attempts to cut back on the total numbers of physicians as well as on the number of certain specialist physicians. It seems clear that hospitals are currently decreasing the total volume of their beds and that a small number of hospitals are actually closing in various parts of the United States. Whether this will be a long-term and continuous trend is not clear at this time; however, certainly there seems to be a general sense of contraction with regard to the numbers of hospital beds and actual operations throughout the United States. With regard to the financial support made available to the health care system, 1984 was the first time in more than 40 years that the country spent a slightly smaller proportion of its GNP on health care than it did in the preceding year (10.6 percent for 1984 as compared to 10.7 percent for 1983; the figure for 1985 returned to 10.7 percent) (see Chapter 11).

The move away from the "growth ethic," away from the era of "bigger is better," will provide certain significant challenges to the thinking of everyone in the health care system who has been used to thinking of success as doing more, getting bigger, having greater numbers. In the era ahead, health care workers will have to measure their organizations' success or failure with new criteria that has nothing to do with size or numerical increases. Rather, the entire question of what is a successful health care program or institution in the future will have to be based on more pertinent and direct measures of success, such as improvement in the quality of care, improvement in patient satisfaction, or improvement in ultimate outcomes. For generations of health care workers who have been accustomed to measuring success in terms of sheer volume, the shift to new measures of success, both for the entire health care system and for the individual institutions and programs within it, will call for careful thinking through what are and what will be the *real* measures of success in the future.

NEW ORGANIZATIONAL FORMS IN HEALTH CARE

In the past few years we have witnessed the development of a wide variety of new organizational forms in health care in the United States, and we can be assured that this change in organizational structure throughout the American health care system will continue in the future. With regard to the individual hospital, we have seen very extensive corporate reorganization, with multiple, linked corporate units replacing the previous single-corporate structure. In the individual hospital, we have seen the development of numerous new products, many of which have little to do with traditional inpatient services, but that are now focused on outpatient care and the provision of services used widely in the community. We have seen the idea of "joint venture" become increasingly prominent, with hospitals joining in partnerships with physicians on their medical staffs, with nursing home organizations, with home health care agencies, and even with other hospitals with whom they would ordinarily be in direct competition. Also with regard to hospitals, we have seen the development of the multihospital organizations, first in the proprietary, for-profit sector and more recently in the nonprofit, voluntary hospital sector. Indeed, we have seen the growth of the "mega-hospital" organizations, such as Voluntary Hospitals of America and American Health Care Systems, each with hundreds of hospitals participating in a new form of joint affiliation.

With regard to the provision of physician services, we have seen the rapid growth and expansion of HMOs, particularly of the nationwide, proprietary type, whose stock is traded actively on various stock exchanges across the country. Individual hospitals and physicians' organizations have formed more locally based HMOs as well, some of which have been purchased or otherwise absorbed by larger HMOs. Indeed, one of the major characteristics of HMOs (and of many other types of health care organization as well) has been the tendency toward purchase and absorption of smaller, local or regional organizations into larger, statewide or nationwide organizations, often of a proprietary, for-profit nature.

In the area of financing, we have seen the development of a number of new organizational forms, including (among others) the development of nationwide insurance company–hospital affiliations. This has been paralleled by the development of nationwide HMO insurance vehicles, as mentioned in the previous paragraph. Local and regional employer health cost coalitions have begun to play an active part on the health care scene, influencing (and even, occasionally, controlling) the management of various employer-sponsored health insurance plans. In many areas, the Preferred Provider Organization (PPO) has appeared on the scene, to act as broker for employers, insurance carriers, physician groups, and hospital groups, either seeking or offering a discount from the usual price for health care services.

The development of these new organizational forms will certainly continue rapidly, and probably *should* continue since they lend vigor and creative energy to our health care system. There are, however, several aspects of these developments that health care workers must keep actively in mind as they watch and participate in the growth of these new organizational entities.

First, health care workers should be encouraging the exploration into and the development of new organizational forms in health care for the future, since the development of new organizations and systems can possibly help us solve many of our present problems and avoid future problems. Moving away from our traditional organizational forms that developed to serve us under the conditions of the past may very well allow us to better deal with the new conditions of the future.

Countering that positive aspect of new organizational development in health care is the fear that new organizational forms may develop for the *wrong* reasons and may merely compound or confuse the normal, productive functioning of health care organizations in the future. It may very well be that economic considerations of profit, monopoly, and control of market share may be the overriding factors in the development of new organizational forms, and these may ultimately have a more negative than positive effect on our health care system. There is nothing that is automatically and necessarily positive and productive about a new organizational unit or entity. Therefore, the development of new forms in the future will have to be watched very closely in order to ensure that they are really more productive and beneficial to the society and the people being served than to the units they replaced.

Finally, the growth of new organizational forms in health care in the past (and most probably in the future) has tended to lead to larger and larger organizations, with more and more control and decision making geographically and organizationally removed from the site of delivery of health services. This tendency can lead to a comparative isolation as far as decision making is concerned, with the decision makers being far removed from the daily pulse and throb of the health care organizations and the patients for whom they are making decisions. This may lead to vastly inferior and more impersonal decisions and may eventually cause a deterioration in the personal quality of our health care services.

Furthermore, the development of the large multi-unit or mega-unit organization may create much further distance between those actually doing the work to provide the health care services and those in controlling and decision-making positions. This may lead to a sense of alienation, frustration, and deterioration of commitment to an organization for the people who are actually providing the care, if they are not also able to feel that they are playing an active part in shaping their particular unit. In many ways, the American health care system has prospered marvelously because of the personal commitment of the individual workers in that system, and the development of larger and larger corporate entities may inadvertently damage or destroy that sense of personal involvement.

It is clear that the American health care system is entering a period in which new organizational forms and models will be developed and tried on all sides. This could be one of the most exciting times in health care in this country for many years to come, if the development of these new models is done carefully and thoughtfully by all concerned.

SPECIAL AREAS OF INTEREST OR NEED

In the future, there will be a number of disease states, life situations, or population subgroups that will require special emphasis and attention, since their problems present important challenges that have not been met adequately in the past and will be increasingly important in the future. What are some of these high-priority areas, and what are the disease states or population groups that will need special attention in the future?

Certain disease states or conditions such as alcoholism and substance abuse, depression, and mental illness of all kinds have never received the attention and the financial support that they deserve; they certainly must be high on our list of priorities for special attention in the future, as it is clear that many of the most disabling health conditions now are related to mental and emotional disabilities. As people live longer and longer, new forms of care for the elderly—primarily at home and then in first-stage care facilities—will have to be developed, and the skilled nursing facilities and nursing homes that already exist will have to be improved; the population most at risk for physical and mental disability in the future will be the elderly (particularly the *old* elderly), and the health care system will have to devote special attention to their particular needs and concerns.

In recent years, it has become evident that many of our present disease and disability states are the products of our life-styles. What we eat and drink, how much stress we take upon ourselves, what overindulgence in alcohol and other drugs we impose on our systems . . . all these factors are now understood as being major causes of many of the chronic disease and disability states with which the system must deal. In the future, programs of life-style change and health promotion that aim at influencing these precursors to chronic disease will have to be much more greatly supported, in both personal and financial ways. Problems related to the environment and to hazards that are breathed in, ingested, or otherwise absorbed without our knowledge must be handled more directly and adequately in the future. Programs to promote safety at the worksite and programs that use the work environment for general health education and promotion must be explored and expanded.

Indeed, one major feature of the health care system that needs to be developed in the future is the ability to identify special areas of interest and need and to focus resources primarily on those areas of high priority. In the future, we must resist the temptation of pouring more and more resources into the old, well-established channels simply because they exist and because it is easier to do that than to develop new channels, new targets, and new priorities.

TECHNOLOGY AND HEALTH CARE

The whole issue of technology—its development, distribution, and use—will have to be carefully reviewed in the future. The explosion of health care technology that has taken place since World War II shows no signs of abating; indeed, it gives every indication of expanding. Expansion by itself is neither bad nor good, but if it is not controlled by thoughtful people, technology will continue to absorb vastly inappropriate amounts of financial resources, diverting funds away from potentially more important patient care services of a non-technological nature.

An even more important challenge of technology is the potential threat that it poses to patient care values. As technology becomes more sophisticated and elaborate, it tends to assume an importance in its own right, not just because of what it can possibly accomplish for the patients being served. The technology becomes an end in itself, sometime clothed in the aura of scientific investigation and progress, and workers in the health care system unconsciously become distracted from the personal and compassionate aspects of health care by the sometimes more impersonal and scientifically exciting aspects of technology. The place of technology in health care value systems must be very carefully watched so that it continues to be the servant of patient care rather than the master.

At the same time, it must be pointed out that the actual distribution of the benefits of our present technology is spotty and frequently inequitable. There are significant subgroups in our population who do not have adequate access to the technology that is available today, because they have neither the health insurance coverage nor the personal financial resources to purchase it. For these subgroups, the fact that American health care is the most technologically advanced in the world may be irrelevant, since their easy access to it may be considerably hampered. For the future, it will be very important to develop systems that ensure an appropriate access to the benefits of modern technology to all parts of our population.

THE CONTROL AND DIRECTION OF THE AMERICAN HEALTH CARE SYSTEM

In an earlier section of this epilogue, reference was made to the need for a means of establishing and implementing social priorities for health care. Parallel to the issue of better social priorities is the question of control and direction of the American health care system, when (and if) those priorities are ever established. At the present time, as a society we do not have the ability to insist that appropriate social priorities for health are actually carried out, if and when they are established.

The American health care system is a far-flung, eclectic, and internally unrelated collection of separate institutions, programs, and personnel . . . a genuine nonsystem, to use a much overused term. There is no central organizing or controlling force, either nationally or locally, that can ensure that any portion of the health care system will respond to the highest social priorities, if those priorities are ever set. Instead, by default, power in the health care system has been exercised by indirection and almost by accident. For a while, power rested solely in the hands of physicians and the medical profession. Later, it was jointly held by physicians and hospitals acting in concert. Then power began to move into governmental regulatory and planning agencies. Most recently it has moved to the major health insurance plans, such as Medicare and Medicaid, Blue Cross, and the employer purchasers of health insurance. Indeed, it would have to be said today that the most powerful directing forces in health care are the third-party payers and, to a certain degree, the employer purchasers of health insurance. Frequently, almost by default, the health insurance mechanisms become a means for *establishing social priorities*, rather than a means for paying bills. As a people, we have not developed a means whereby all the parties involved can cooperatively and voluntarily come together to create a set of priorities and a set of directions under which all parts of the health care system can move forward in a coordinated and cooperative manner.

This is not to say that there is a need for a rigid, single, governmentally operated national health care system. Rather, the point needs to be made that unless there is developed a more acceptable means for establishing social control and direction of our health care system and its parts, we will waste our resources needlessly and never achieve the maximum effect on our most important health care priorities.

RATIONING OF HEALTH CARE

It has been suggested very recently that perhaps there will be a need for rationing of certain health care services in the future, as we begin to reach the limits of our economic resources. Examples have been drawn from other countries' health care systems where specific examples of rationing of services have been put into effect, with the implication that similar steps may be unavoidable here in the future. The idea of rationing and its implementation is almost certainly unacceptable to virtually everyone concerned with health care in the United States, but the issue deserves considerable thought and attention if it is to be avoided in the future.

It should be pointed out that a form of rationing exists at the present time, and that certain parts of our population are restricted in their use of health services either because they do not have appropriate health insurance coverage or because they do not have personal financial resources to purchase health care at the prices presently in effect. People in these population subgroups are then forced to use local government health care systems, where the crowding, waiting time, and lack of access can often be considerably more severe than in the private sector. In effect, these population subgroups have had a type of rationing applied to them, a rationing by price and by ease of access to health care.

In many ways, it is unthinkable that a country such as ours should even have to consider the specter of rationing, when we as a people devote more of our GNP to health care than almost any other country in the world, a GNP that is itself the largest in the world. Rationing is a phenomenon and a process that is usually associated with scarcity rather than abundance such as we have in health care in the United States. Indeed, it would seem that if we used our abundant resources more carefully, more appropriately, and less wastefully, there would be adequate resources available for all the important things that need to be done for a long time in the future, and rationing would be an unnecessary specter to consider. Unfortunately, our capacity to consume resources in a luxuriant and profligate manner may almost insist that we develop rationing procedures, ironically enough, in the midst of great abundance.

If the idea of rationing of health care services to the people of this country is to be avoided in the future, appropriate steps must be taken in the present to ensure that our resources are used as wisely and as productively as possible.

MAINTENANCE OF PRIDE, CONFIDENCE, AND HOPE

Perhaps the most difficult challenge for the future will be for health care workers to maintain their sense of equilibrium in the midst of the vigorous challenges they will face, and their sense of pride in the face of serious criticism and occasional bad publicity. One of the saddest commentaries on the state of health care in our country at the present time is the frequent expression of frustration and occasional hopelessness that one hears from health care workers throughout the country.

There is, in fact, no need for sadness, frustration, or hopelessness about health care in the United States, either now or in the future. Indeed, although the challenges are stronger and more immediate than they have ever been in the past, the status of health care in the United States has never been better. The health care system is better supported, both financially and emotionally, by the people of this country than it has ever been before. What health care workers are able to offer their patients and what can be accomplished by health care services is now more impressive than ever before. Results are obtainable now for patients in this country that were formerly unheard of and that still cannot be obtained in most other countries of the world. The challenges will certainly remain and perhaps even grow, but it is important for health care professionals to maintain a sense of pride in what they have been able to achieve and confidence that good health care will continue to be available to the people of this great country.

Index